3rd edition
pathology

National Medical Series

In the basic sciences

anatomy, 2nd edition
behavioral science, 2nd edition
biochemistry, 3rd edition
clinical epidemiology and
    biostatistics
genetics
hematology
histology and cell biology,
    2nd edition

human developmental anatomy
immunology, 2nd edition
introduction to clinical medicine
microbiology, 2nd edition
neuroanatomy
pathology, 3rd edition
pharmacology, 3rd edition
physiology, 2nd edition
radiographic anatomy

In the clinical sciences

medicine, 2nd edition
obstetrics and gynecology,
    3rd edition
pediatrics, 2nd edition
preventive medicine and
    public health, 2nd edition
psychiatry, 2nd edition
surgery, 2nd edition

In the exam series

review for USMLE Step 1,
    2nd edition
geriatrics

The National Medical Series for Independent Study

3rd edition
pathology

EDITORS

Virginia A. LiVolsi, M.D.

Professor of Pathology
Department of Pathology
  and Laboratory Medicine
University of Pennsylvania
  School of Medicine
Director, Surgical Pathology Section
Hospital of the University
  of Pennsylvania
Philadelphia, Pennsylvania

Maria J. Merino, M.D.

Chief, Surgical Pathology
Senior Investigator
National Cancer Institute
National Institutes of Health
Bethesda, Maryland

John S.J. Brooks, M.D., MRCPath

Chairman, Department of Pathology
Roswell Park Cancer Institute
Vice Chairman, Department
  of Pathology
State University of New York
  at Buffalo Medical School
Buffalo, New York

Scott H. Saul, M.D.

Adjunct Associate Professor
  of Pathology
Department of Pathology
  and Laboratory Medicine
University of Pennsylvania
  School of Medicine
Adjunct Associate Professor
  of Pathology
Department of Pathology
Jefferson Medical College
Philadelphia, Pennsylvania
Staff Pathologist
Chester County Hospital
West Chester, Pennsylvania

John E. Tomaszewski, M.D.

Associate Professor of Pathology
Department of Pathology
  and Laboratory Medicine
University of Pennsylvania
  School of Medicine
Staff, Surgical Pathology Section
Hospital of the University
  of Pennsylvania
Philadelphia, Pennsylvania

Harwal Publishing

Philadelphia • Baltimore • Hong Kong • London • Munich • Sydney • Tokyo

A Waverly Company

Harwal

Sponsoring Editor: Debra Dreger
Managing Editor: Jane Velker
Production: Laurie Forsyth, Joan Leary
Editorial Assistant: Anne Praino

Library of Congress Cataloging-in Publication Data

Pathology / editors, Virginia A. LiVolsi . . . [et al.] —3rd ed.
        p.   cm.—(The National medical series for independent study)
    Includes index.
    ISBN 0-683-06243-3 (pbk. : alk. paper)
    1. Anatomy, Pathological—Outlines, syllabi, etc.   I. Livolsi,
Virginia A.   II. Series.
    [DNLM: 1. Pathology—examination questions.   2. Pathology—
outlines.   QZ 18 P2965   1993]
RB32.P37   1993
616.07—dc20
DNLM/DLC
for Library of Congress   93-16371
                                                                                                      CIP

©1994 by Harwal Publishing

10 9 8 7 6 5 4 3 2 1

Contents

Preface

The third edition of NMS *Pathology,* like its predecessors, is not intended to be a reference book but, rather, a comprehensive outline of the scientific principles and phenomenology that underpin the field of basic and organ-system pathology. In each chapter, we have attempted to highlight what are considered the key concepts and pertinent facts. With the current explosion of medical knowledge, the factual content of most chapters has necessarily increased. As in the earlier editions, however, we have continued to extract and underscore the most critical concepts and data.

In this edition, a new chapter has been added on transplantation pathology, reflecting the increasingly important role of organ transplantation in modern medicine. All other chapters have been substantially updated and enhanced with the addition of charts and tables enumerating the most essential information.

The self-testing feature continues to be a principal element of the book, with study questions included within each chapter and in the Comprehensive Exam at the end of the book. Detailed answers are provided for each question. In this edition, many of the questions have been modified to include a case-based orientation. This will allow the student to practice applying pathology-related data to patient care.

Whether used as a comprehensive review tool or a primary study guide, we hope that the third edition of NMS *Pathology* is a substantial aid for guiding the medical student's study efforts.

Virginia A. LiVolsi
Maria J. Merino
John S.J. Brooks
Scott H. Saul
John E. Tomaszewski

To the Reader

Since 1984, the National Medical Series for Independent Study has been helping medical students meet the challenge of education and clinical training. In today's climate of burgeoning information and complex clinical issues, a medical career is more demanding than ever. Increasingly, medical training must prepare physicians to seek and synthesize necessary information and to apply that information successfully.

The National Medical Series is designed to provide a logical framework for organizing, learning, reviewing, and applying the conceptual and factual information covered in basic and clinical sciences. Each book includes a comprehensive outline of the essential content of a discipline, with up to 500 study questions. The combination of an outlined text and tools for self-evaluation allows easy retrieval of salient information.

All study questions are accompanied by the correct answer, a paragraph-length explanation, and specific reference to the text where the topic is discussed. Study questions that follow each chapter use the current National Board format to reinforce the chapter content. Study questions appearing at the end of the text in the Comprehensive Exam vary in format depending on the book. Wherever possible, Comprehensive Exam questions are presented as clinical cases or scenarios intended to simulate real-life application of medical knowledge. The goal of this exam is to challenge the student to draw from information presented throughout the book.

All of the books in the National Medical Series are constantly being updated and revised. The authors and editors devote considerable time and effort to ensure that the information required by all medical school curricula is included. Strict editorial attention is given to accuracy, organization, and consistency. Further shaping of the series occurs in response to biannual discussions held with a panel of medical student advisors drawn from schools throughout the United States. At these meetings, the editorial staff considers the needs of medical students to learn how the National Medical Series can serve them better. In this regard, the Harwal staff welcomes all comments and suggestions.

1
Inflammation
John S. J. Brooks

I. GENERAL FEATURES OF INFLAMMATION

A. Definition and etiology

1. Inflammation is the directed tissue response to noxious and injurious external and internal stimuli. Inflammation can occur in response to anything that damages the tissues, such as:
   a. Toxic chemical agents
   b. Physical factors (e.g., heat, cold, electricity, radiation, trauma)
   c. Microorganisms and their metabolic by-products
   d. Immune responses (hypersensitivity, immune complex, or autoimmune reactions)

2. Every organ and tissue type is susceptible to inflammation; the degree and nature of the inflammatory response are governed by a person's state of health, nutrition, and immunity as well as by the nature and severity of the noxious stimuli.

B. Advantages and disadvantages

1. **Advantages**
   a. Inflammation serves to **localize and isolate** the injured (or infected) tissue area, thereby protecting the surrounding healthy tissue.
   b. It tends to **neutralize and inactivate** the toxic substances that are produced by humoral factors and enzymes.
   c. It **destroys** or limits the growth of **infecting microorganisms** and counteracts their effects.
   d. It **prepares the area for** wound **healing and repair** by disposing of devitalized tissue and cell debris.

2. **Disadvantages** (see also section VI B)
   a. The pain and swelling associated with inflammation lead to varying degrees of **disability**.
   b. Inflammation may lead to **rupture of a viscus** (e.g., perforating appendicitis) or to serious hemorrhage (e.g., from an enlarging pulmonary tuberculous granuloma).
   c. It can lead to the formation of **excessive scar tissue,** with contractures, adhesions, and keloids.
   d. It may result in **fistula formation,** such as an abdominal perineal fistula or a bronchopleural fistula and pleural empyema, with accompanying normal tissue breakdown by neural proteases.
   e. Inflammation may propagate **further inflammation** by destruction of the surrounding healthy tissue.
   f. Damage caused by inflammation can lead to the **development of inflammatory diseases,** such as:
      (1) Glomerulonephritis
      (2) Arthritis
      (3) Allergic reactions (e.g., allergic bronchitis)
      (4) Myocarditis
      (5) Encephalitis

II. CELLS INVOLVED IN INFLAMMATION

A. Neutrophils [also known as polymorphonuclear neutrophils (PMNs), granulocytes, "polys," and pus cells] are the predominant cells in acute inflammation as well as in abscess formation, loculation, and empyema. They are the white blood cells (WBCs) most responsible for the leukocytosis that occurs in response to an inflammatory or infectious crisis.

1. **Morphology.** Neutrophils are granular leukocytes with a multilobate nucleus and fine cytoplasmic granules that stain readily with neutral dyes.

2. **Functions**
   a. In the inflammatory response, neutrophils are the first cells to arrive at the injured area. They leave the vascular system by **diapedesis** (see IV B 2) and are directed to the tissue site by **chemotaxis** (see IV B 3).
   b. The major activity of neutrophils is **phagocytosis** of invading bacterial cells, with subsequent destruction of the cells through the release of lysosomal enzymes.
      (1) Intracellular granules (**lysosomes**) within neutrophils contain several active enzymes.
         (a) **Myeloperoxidase (MPO)**, the major active component of granulocytes, is the main antibacterial enzyme. It operates by combining with hydrogen peroxide and a halide ion.
         (b) **Acid hydrolases** act on organic matter, including bacteria.
         (c) **Proteases** cause degradation of proteins, including elastin, collagen, and the proteins found in basement membranes.
         (d) **Lysozyme** (muramidase) acts on microorganisms through hydrolysis; it is found in monocytes (macrophages, histiocytes) as well as neutrophils.
         (e) **Cationic proteins** inhibit bacterial growth, cause monocyte chemotaxis, and increase vascular permeability.
      (2) The extracellular release of the highly irritating **lysosomal enzymes** into tissues contributes to the local inflammation.

B. Basophils

1. **Morphology.** Basophils (basophilic granulocytes) contain granules that stain blue with Wright's stain. The granules contain histamine, heparin, and slow-reacting substance of anaphylaxis (SRS-A).

2. **Functions**
   a. Basophils are involved in type I [i.e., immediate, or immunoglobulin E (IgE)-mediated] hypersensitivity reactions. When an IgE-specific antigen enters the body, basophils stimulate the formation of IgE, which binds to the surface of the antigen. The basophilic granules then release histamine and other vasoactive substances to produce anaphylactic reactions in susceptible persons.
   b. Basophils also play a role in type IV (i.e., delayed) hypersensitivity reactions, such as contact dermatitis.

C. Eosinophils

1. **Morphology.** Eosinophils (eosinophilic granulocytes) have a characteristic bilobate nucleus and cytoplasmic granules that stain orange with Romanovsky's stain and red-orange with eosin. The granules contain hydrolytic enzymes (e.g., histaminase, which inactivates histamine; arylsulfatase B, which inactivates SRS-A). The granules also contain a poorly understood major basic protein.

2. **Distribution.** Although they also can be found in peripheral blood, a number of the body's eosinophils exist in hypersensitivity sites within the tissues, where they can abort hypersensitivity reactions. Eosinophils are increased in the peripheral blood in the presence of allergy and parasitic infestation.

3. **Functions**
   a. Eosinophils are readily chemotactic upon the release of eosinophil chemotactic factor (ECF) from IgE-sensitized mast cells—an occurrence in anaphylaxis.
   b. Eosinophils also are phagocytic, although phagocytosis is a minor function.

D. Mast cells resemble basophils in both structure and function. Whereas basophils are present mainly in the peripheral blood and at sites of inflammation, mast cells are connective tissue cells found close to small blood vessels.

1. Mast cells contain numerous granules that stain metachromatically with basic dyes. Like basophilic granules, mast cell granules release histamine, heparin, and SRS-A during type I reactions. In addition, mast cell granules release ECF.

2. Agents that cause inflammation (e.g., physical factors, drugs, immunoglobulins, complement components C3a and C5a, cationic proteins) may cause histamine release from mast cells.

E. Macrophages. The mononuclear phagocyte system (also known as the monocyte–macrophage system and reticuloendothelial system) is an extensive network of macrophages that exists throughout the body.

1. **Cellular components**
   a. Components of the system include:
      (1) Pulmonary alveolar macrophages
      (2) Pleural and peritoneal macrophages
      (3) Kupffer cells of the liver
      (4) Histiocytes of mesenchymal and connective tissue
      (5) Mesangial cells of the kidney
      (6) Both fixed and mobile macrophages in the lymph nodes, spleen, and bone marrow
   b. Macrophages in the body tissues develop from monocytes that have left the peripheral blood. The monocytes originally derive from bone marrow precursors.
   c. Monocytes in the bone marrow and the peripheral blood can be converted rapidly into additional macrophages when needed.

2. **Phagocyte functions.** Macrophages dispose of noxious matter within tissues, for example, microorganisms and necrotic tissue or other debris. Macrophages also appear to serve in tumor cell killing.
   a. **Endocytosis** is the first step in the process.
      (1) In **phagocytosis,** the cytoplasmic membrane extends around particles and engulfs them, forming an intracellular vacuole.
      (2) In **pinocytosis,** the cell membrane engulfs extracellular fluid along with the particles.
   b. **Digestion** of the engulfed matter within the vacuole is the next step.
      (1) The lysosomes of macrophages contain degradative substances similar to those in neutrophils (e.g., proteinases, acid hydrolase, lysozyme, and MPO).
      (2) In their microbicidal function, macrophages are most effective against intracellular or encapsulated organisms, such as *Mycoplasma, Salmonella, Listeria,* and *Cryptococcus.*
   c. **Opsonization.** Macrophages have surface receptors for the Fc segment of the immunoglobulin G (IgG) molecule and for complement component C3b. These aid the macrophage in phagocytosis of opsonized microorganisms (i.e., organisms coated with IgG or C3b).

3. **Immune functions.** Macrophages are important components of the immune system. Their involvement begins with the initiation of the immune response, and they interact closely with T lymphocytes (T cells).
   a. **T-cell activation**
      (1) During phagocytosis, the macrophage "processes" the antigenic component of foreign matter within its vacuole. The macrophage then "presents" the processed antigen to T cells in conjunction with **major histocompatibility complex (MHC)** molecules on the macrophage surface. This combined presentation of processed antigen and MHC molecules is required in the sensitization and activation of T cells.
      (2) Macrophages release **interleukin-1 (IL-1),** a substance that stimulates sensitized T cells to release **interleukin-2 (IL-2)** [see III F 4]. IL-2 allows full T-cell activation to proceed and causes the various T-cell subsets to proliferate.
   b. **Macrophage activation**
      (1) T cells, once activated, cause the mobilization and metabolic activation of macrophages by releasing various **lymphokines.*** (See III F 1–3 for more information about lymphokines that act on macrophages.)
      (2) The activation of macrophages is immunologically specific. However, once activated, the macrophages attack and devour organisms without regard to their antigenic makeup.

---

*Nonimmune mediators also can activate macrophages. These mediators include components of the clotting and complement cascades.

(3) Activated macrophages prolong the inflammatory process and cause tissue destruction by releasing their highly irritative enzymes. This process also has a protective function, thereby amplifying the immune response.

c. B-cell activation. Macrophages also serve in this phase of the immune response, although their role is not essential.

(1) B-cell activation requires IL-1, which is secreted by macrophages (and some other cells).

(2) B-cell activation also requires that antibody on the B-cell surface match its specific antigen. Antigen on the macrophage surface can serve this purpose.

(3) B-cell activation is aided by the presence of **helper–inducer T cells**. These cells proliferate in response to IL-2, which in turn is induced by IL-1.

4. Other functions

a. Secretory function. Macrophages release substances other than IL-1, such as:

(1) Colony-stimulating factor (CSF) and **tumor necrosis factor (TNF),** which serve in the immune response

(2) Alpha interferon (IFN-α), which aids in blocking viral replication

(3) Precursors of prostaglandins, which, in conjunction with IL-1 (a pyrogen), induce acute-phase signs of inflammation, such as **fever** and **peripheral blood leukocytosis** (i.e., a shift to the left with an increase in immature neutrophils)

b. Healing and repair. Macrophages aid in healing after inflammation subsides by:

(1) Cellular debridement through phagocytosis

(2) Release of fibroblast proliferating factor

F. Lymphocytes (see also Chapter 6 II A)

1. General considerations. Lymphocytes and their derivatives are found in the tissues in all types of inflammation, especially after the acute ingress of neutrophils.

a. Source and distribution. All lymphocytes are derived from bone marrow stem cells.

(1) Stem cells differentiate into lymphocytes in the primary lymphoid organs (i.e., the thymus and bone marrow).

(2) From these locations, some lymphocytes migrate—via the circulation—to secondary lymphoid organs, namely, the spleen, lymph nodes, and lymphoid germinal centers throughout the body (e.g., tonsils, Peyer's patches of the gastrointestinal tract, appendix).

b. Types

(1) Lymphocytes are divided into two major types—**T cells and B cells**—which serve different functions. The two types are given initials that signify their site of processing: "B" cells are named after the **bursa of Fabricius** in chickens and other birds (the human counterpart of the bursa is unknown), and "T" cells are named after the **thymus**.

(2) A third population of lymphocytes—referred to as **null cells**—have none of the characteristics of T cells or B cells.

2. T cells are found in the **paracortical areas** of lymph nodes, between the follicles. They comprise about 70% of the peripheral blood lymphocytes.

a. Types. T cells differentiate into several subsets that can be distinguished because their **cell surface markers** are detected by monoclonal antibodies. The **cellular differentiation or cluster designation** (CD) series of markers formerly were called **T** or **OKT** (e.g., CD4$^+$ refers to OKT4 or T4).*

(1) All T cells are CD2$^+$, CD3$^+$. The CD3 marker is closely associated with the T cell's antigen receptor, a heterodimer composed of α and β polypeptide chains.

(2) T cells differ from all other cells in that they contain a gene rearrangement in surface receptor genes ($\alpha \beta \gamma$). These genes produce proteins that become cell–surface receptor molecules and have a conformation similar to the surface immunoglobulin on the B cell. Only T cells possess these cell–surface proteins, and only T cells show the corresponding gene rearrangements.

b. Function in inflammation

(1) Lymphokines produced and released by T cells attract cells (e.g., macrophages, basophils) that serve as nonspecific mediators of inflammation.

---

*A plus sign ($+$) indicates the presence of a marker; a minus sign ($-$) indicates its absence.

       (2) Cytotoxic T cells lyse target cells—an important function in viral infections and in graft rejection.

       (3) Sensitized T cells are responsible for initiating delayed hypersensitivity reactions (e.g., contact hypersensitivity, tuberculin-type hypersensitivity). The sensitized T cells interact with macrophages by releasing lymphokines, which, in turn, activate and attract macrophages to the site of inflammation, thus enhancing the local response.

          (a) The lymphokine-induced local inflammation causes killing of "innocent bystander" cells.

          (b) In contrast, lysis by cytoxic T cells affects target cells only, with no destruction of neighboring cells.

   3. B cells are found in the **peripheral cortical areas** of lymph nodes and in the germinal centers of secondary follicles. They comprise about 15% of circulating lymphocytes.

     a. Definition and description

       (1) B cells differ from all other cell types in that they have rearrangement of the genes that code for the light and heavy immunoglobulin chains.

       (2) Antigen receptors are found in the immunoglobulin molecules that are part of the B-cell membrane and are the products of the gene rearrangement process. B cells also have surface receptors for the Fc portion of IgG and for C3b and C3d.

       (3) B cells may differentiate into immunoglobulin-producing **plasma cells**. Each plasma cell produces one type of immunoglobulin: IgG, IgM, IgA, IgD, or IgE.

     b. Function in inflammation. The various immunoglobulins have several functions in inflammatory processes.

       (1) Antibodies neutralize toxins produced by bacteria.

       (2) IgG functions in opsonization: It agglutinates certain bacteria, stopping organisms in their tracks and making it easier for macrophages to engulf them.

       (3) Antibodies specific to the surface antigens of gram-negative bacilli cause bacteriolysis in the presence of complement.

   4. Null cells are cytotoxic lymphocytes that are not definable by T-cell and B-cell criteria (i.e., they lack the surface antigens that identify T cells and B cells).

     a. Natural killer (NK) cells comprise the majority of the null cells.

       (1) Morphology

          (a) NK cells are large granular lymphocytes. They may be related to T cells, since they share some molecular features. For example, NK cells are $CD2^+$, and some have T-cell–like surface receptors.

          (b) NK cells have surface receptors; but, in contrast to K cells (see II F 4 b), they are cytotoxic in a nonspecific manner.

       (2) Function

          (a) NK cells are important in the rejection of bone marrow transplants and are a form of first-line defense against viral infection and tumor development.

          (b) Without prior sensitization, NK cells are capable of lysing leukemia–lymphoma cells experimentally.

     b. Killer (K) cells have IgG Fc receptors in their cell membrane and are able to lyse target cells coated with specific antibody. Because T-cell activation also is involved, this property is known as **antibody-dependent cell-mediated cytotoxicity**.

     c. Lymphocyte-activated killer (LAK) cells are morphologically and functionally similar to NK cells but have a greater range of target cells. LAK cells become cytotoxic under the stimulation of IL-2, the lymphokine that autoactivates T cells.

III. CHEMICAL MEDIATORS OF INFLAMMATION. A variety of chemical substances are synthesized and emitted during the inflammatory process. These substances are responsible for controlling the response. The actions of these chemicals also produce the observable signs (edema, erythema) and the symptoms (pain, fever) of inflammation.

   A. Vasoactive amines (e.g., histamine and serotonin) are responsible for hemodynamic and vascular changes.

     1. Histamine

       a. Source. Most of the body's histamine is stored in the granules of mast cells. It is also found in basophils and platelets.

    b. Release. Histamine is released by **degranulation** in response to various stimuli, such as physical factors (heat, cold, trauma, radiation), type I hypersensitivity reactions, C3a and C5a (referred to as **anaphylatoxins**), and cationic lysosomal proteins.

    c. Actions

       (1) Once released, histamine causes direct vascular effects. Some degree of vasoconstriction (which varies according to animal species) almost always occurs, followed by vasodilation (which is the stage of observable hyperemia). Histamine also causes an increase in the vascular permeability of small veins and venules.

       (2) Histamine has also been shown to be chemotactic for eosinophils.

2. Serotonin

    a. Source. Most of the body's serotonin is stored in the gastrointestinal tract and central nervous system (CNS); a much smaller proportion exists in the dense granules of platelets.

    b. Actions. Although serotonin is known to have the same vascular effects as histamine in rodents, its role in inflammation in humans is not well understood.

B. Plasma factors

1. The **kinin system,** when activated, leads to the formation of **bradykinin.**

    a. Generation of bradykinin. When plasma comes in contact with collagen, endotoxin, or basement membrane proteins, **clotting factor XII** (Hagemen factor) is activated. This step is followed sequentially by **kallikrein** formation, which then converts **high-molecular-weight kininogen (HMWK)** to bradykinin.

    b. Actions. Although bradykinin is not chemotactic, its actions are much like those of histamine. It causes increased vascular permeability, vasoconstriction, smooth muscle contraction, and pain.

2. The **complement system,** an important mediator of the inflammatory process, contains nine major plasma proteins, termed **complement components** (see Chapter 6 II D).

    a. Activation of complement. Critical to the biologic actions of the complement system is the activation, or cleavage, of complement component C3, which forms **C3a.** This cleavage can occur in two ways.

       (1) In the **classic pathway,** circulating antigen–antibody complexes activate the system and, by successive steps of cleavage and combination, generate complement components C3a and C5a.

       (2) In the **alternative pathway,** nonimmunologic stimuli (e.g., bacterial endotoxin) activate the system and lead to the cleavage of C3.

    b. Actions

       (1) Both C3a and C5a are chemotactic for neutrophils and play an important role in the increased vascular permeability caused by histamine release from mast cells.

       (2) Following complement cascade activation (by either pathway), C5, C6, and C7 in combination also become chemotactic.

       (3) C5b and C9 (termed the **membrane attack sequence**) appear to be involved in injury to parenchymal cells.

C. Arachidonic acid metabolites

1. Prostaglandins are a group of compounds derived from arachidonic acid via the **cyclooxygenase pathway.**

    a. Prostaglandin production. Most mammalian cells, including endothelial and inflammatory cells, have the potential to produce prostaglandins. Nonsteroidal anti-inflammatory agents (e.g., aspirin, indomethacin) inhibit cyclooxygenase and, therefore, interrupt the synthesis of prostaglandins.

    b. Actions. Prostaglandins are involved in a variety of biologic and physiologic activities.

       (1) Prostaglandin E_2 (PDE_2) and PGI_2 (also called **prostacyclin**) are potent vasodilators and, although they do not directly affect vascular permeability, are involved in edema formation by potentiating the effects of histamine.

          (a) In addition, PGE_2 produces pain as well as potentiating this effect of bradykinin, and it acts on the hypothalamic mechanism of fever production.

          (b) PGI_2 also inhibits platelet aggregation.

       (2) Other prostaglandins are vasodilators (e.g., PGD, $PGF_{2\alpha}$) as well as vasoconstrictors and agents of platelet aggregation (e.g., PGG, PGH, thromboxane A_2).

2. Leukotrienes, like prostaglandins, are derived from arachidonic acid, but by the **lipoxygenase pathway**. They have the following actions.

a. Chemotaxis. Leukotriene B$_4$ (LTB$_4$) is a potent chemotactic agent for neutrophils and monocytes–macrophages. The 5-hydroperoxy derivative of arachidonic acid, referred to as **5-HPETE,** has similar, although less powerful, chemotactic activity.

b. Vascular effects. LTC$_4$, LTD$_4$, and LTE$_4$ are powerful stimulators of vascular permeability, with 1000 times the potency of histamine. They also cause vasoconstriction and broncho-constriction.

D. Leukocyte substances, such as proteases, hydrolytic enzymes, and cationic proteins, are activators of inflammation and are discussed in II A 2 b.

E. SRS-A is a low-molecular-weight lipid found in mast cells and is now known to be composed by LTC$_4$, LTD$_4$, and LTE$_4$. It also may be produced by neutrophils and macrophages.

1. SRS-A accounts for many of the clinically dramatic (and potentially lethal) reactions that occur during anaphylaxis because of vasoconstrictive and bronchoconstrictive effects.

2. SRS-A also causes edema because of its powerful effect on vascular permeability.

F. Lymphokines are biologically active substances produced and released by T cells during immune reactions, particularly cell-mediated immune reactions and antibody responses. Several lymphokines have been identified, a few of which are described here (see also Chapter 6 II A 1 c).

1. Chemotactic factors. Sensitized lymphocytes produce factors that attract specific leukocytes to inflamed tissues. There are lymphokines that are selective for monocytes–macrophages [macrophage chemotactic factor (MCF)], neutrophils (NCF), eosinophils (ECF), and basophils (BCF).

2. Migration-inhibiting factor (MIF) arrests the intrinsic mobility of macrophages, serving to keep them in the area of inflammation where they are needed.

3. Macrophage-activating factor (MAF) promotes the bactericidal and tumoricidal activities of macrophages by stimulating macrophage growth; an increase in mitochondria, lysosomes, and hydrolytic enzymes accompanies the increase in cell size.

4. Interleukin-2 (IL-2), formerly referred to as T-cell growth factor, is produced by T cells that have been stimulated by antigen in the presence of IL-1, which is a product of macrophages. IL-2 causes nonspecific amplification of activated T-cell production (i.e., both helper T cells and cytotoxic T cells proliferate).

5. Interferons are glycoproteins that have widely varied antiviral and antitumor cell activities.

IV. INFLAMMATORY RESPONSE. The inflammatory response involves vascular and cellular events that are mediated by the various chemical substances described in III.

A. Vascular phase of the inflammatory response. Alterations in the blood vessels and capillary beds of the injured site begin almost immediately within the site of primary injury and variably within the peripheral tissue adjacent to the site.

1. Vasoconstriction. The initial reaction to injury is a momentary vasoconstriction of the small blood vessels in the area; this reaction lasts seconds to minutes and may be neurogenic in origin.

2. Vasodilation. The initial vasoconstriction phase is followed by massive vasodilation in the arterioles and capillaries in the injured area.

a. This vasodilation leads to postcapillary venule dilation and allows increased blood flow to the site (**hyperemia**), which is reflected clinically by heat and erythema—the **flare phenomenon**.

b. If intracapillary hydrostatic pressure exceeds capillary bed tissue pressure, the resulting movement of fluid (i.e., **transudate**) into the tissue causes **edema,** which results in a **wheal**.

3. **Increased vascular permeability.** A release of chemical substances causes an increase in vascular permeability, with passage of plasma (i.e., colloid and water), resulting in further edema and vascular stasis. The increase in vascular permeability is due, in part, to widened junctions between vascular endothelial cells.

   a. **Effects of increased vascular permeability**

   (1) The extravasated fluid that forms is an **exudate** (see V A 3), which has a higher specific gravity than the transudate, which forms earlier in the inflammatory process. This is due to its high plasma protein and leukocyte content. Exudation of fluid from the capillaries into the injured area helps to dilute the toxic or irritating agent and brings antibodies, complement, leukocytes, and chemotactic substances to the area.

   (2) The loss of plasma due to increased vascular permeability leads to vascular stasis and sluggish movement of red cells through the microcirculation. Eventually, blood clots form in the small capillaries that supply the inflamed area, helping to localize the effects of the injury.

   b. **Types of increased vascular permeability**

   (1) The **immediate transient response** involves small and medium-sized venules. Heat and histamine cause contraction of endothelial cells, resulting in widened intercellular gaps. This type is characteristic of type I hypersensitivity reactions.

   (2) An **immediate sustained response** is seen with severe vascular injury (e.g., in severe burns). The vascular permeability continues beyond one day and affects venules, arterioles, and capillaries alike.

   (3) A **delayed prolonged response** begins after a delay of several hours. It is seen in type IV (delayed) hypersensitivity reactions, overexposure to ultraviolet light radiation injury, and moderate thermal burns.

B. **Cellular phase of the inflammatory response.** Leukocytes have four specific actions in inflammation.

1. **Margination and pavementing**

   a. During the vascular stasis stage of hyperemia, leukocytes (principally neutrophils and monocytes) begin to line the endothelial surfaces of the affected vessels (**margination**). Leukocytes adhere to the vascular endothelium (**pavementing**) in preparation for migration into the extravascular space.

   b. Chemotactic factors probably influence the attraction of leukocytes to the vessel periphery, and microcirculatory stasis aids in the margination of leukocytes along the endothelial surface. Cell membrane electronegativity and divalent calcium probably play a role in leukocyte adherence to the endothelial surfaces.

2. **Diapedesis** (also called **emigration**) refers to the process by which leukocytes migrate from blood vessels.

   a. Leukocytes develop pseudopods and emigrate, without accompanying loss of fluid, through gaps between the endothelial cells. The emigration is purposeful, directed, and ameboid, and it occurs without endothelial cell contraction.

   (1) Neutrophils are the first to emigrate outside the vascular compartments. They are short-lived, with a life span of 24 to 48 hours, and they contain a chemotactic factor for monocytes (MCF).

   (2) Monocytes follow neutrophils into the site of inflammation, apparently on cue from the chemotactic factor elaborated by neutrophils (NCF). Monocytes are referred to as macrophages or **histiocytes** after emigrating.

   b. All leukocytes—neutrophils, basophils, eosinophils, lymphocytes, and monocytes—emigrate in the same manner. Occasionally, passive emigration of red cells may accompany leukocyte diapedesis.

3. **Chemotaxis** is the process by which leukocytes are directed to the site of injury. Leukocytes appear to have cell–surface binding receptors for peptides of chemotactic factors. Following exposure to a chemotactic agent, random motion of the leukocyte begins. The microtubular system and contractile proteins are involved in cell locomotion.

   a. **Chemotactic factors for neutrophils** primarily include:

   (1) Bacterial proteases, which are soluble, low-molecular-weight factors that are elaborated from both gram-positive and gram-negative organisms

   (2) Complement component C5a, which is activated by the complement cascade

   (3) LTB_4 and other products of the lipoxygenase pathway of arachidonic acid metabolism

    b. Chemotactic factors for monocytes–macrophages include:
  - **(1)** Complement components C5a and C3a
  - **(2)** LTB$_4$
  - **(3)** Bacteria-related substances
  - **(4)** Neutrophil components
  - **(5)** Lymphokines generated in response to exposure of sensitized lymphocytes to antigens
  - **(6)** Fibronectin fragments

    c. Chemotactic factors for eosinophils. Eosinophils are attracted to sites of immediate hypersensitivity reactions (anaphylaxis), some immune complex reactions, and parasitic infestation. The chemotactic factor, ECF, is emitted by mast cells, basophils, and sensitized lymphokines.

4. Phagocytosis is the process by which **phagocytic cells**—mainly neutrophils and monocytes–macrophages—recognize and then engulf and dispose of foreign particles (e.g., bacteria) [Figure 1-1].

    a. Recognition of a particle to be phagocytosed involves cell–surface receptors that attach to **opsonins** coating the particle. Neutrophils and macrophages have surface receptors for the Fc portion of IgG and for C3b, which act as opsonins in phagocytosis.

    b. Engulfment. A **phagolysosome** is formed when the cytoplasmic membrane of the phagocyte extends around the attached particle, forming a vacuole that connects with a lysosome.

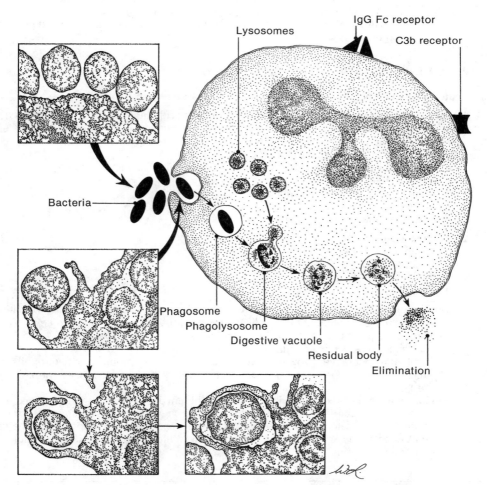

Figure 1-1. Composite schematic and corresponding electron microscopic representation of the phagocytosis of a bacterium by a neutrophil. (Reprinted with permission from Hyde RM, Patnode RA: *Immunology.* Malvern, PA, Harwal Publishing, 1992, p. 4.)

(1) Phagolysosome formation is accompanied by the release of peroxides and hydrolytic enzymes into the extracellular space, which may result in some injury to surrounding tissue.

(2) Acid hydrolases, then, are released into the phagolysosomes.

(3) Both divalent calcium and divalent magnesium are required for engulfment of particles.

c. Degradation

(1) Oxygen-dependent mechanism

(a) Oxidase-mediated bactericidal activity, which is initiated by cell membrane oxidase, converts oxygen to hydrogen peroxide.

(b) Hydrogen peroxide then combines with MPO (present in neutrophil granules) and chloride ion in the phagolysosome. This chemical combination is the most important and powerful bactericidal agent of leukocytes.

(c) Superoxide free radicals are formed in other reactions, being stimulated during oxidative metabolism following phagocytosis. They are independent of MPO and have bactericidal activity.

(2) Oxygen-independent mechanism

(a) Leukocyte bactericidal activity that is independent of oxygen involves certain proteins, including:

(i) Lysozyme, which hydrolyzes bacterial wall gycopeptides in a powerful bactericidal activity

(ii) Cationic proteins, which also have a deleterious effect on bacterial cell walls

(iii) Lactoferrin, an iron-binding protein with bactericidal activity

(b) Hydrogen ions are released into the phagolysosome, creating an acid pH to suppress bacterial growth.

V. TYPES OF INFLAMMATION include acute and chronic.

A. Acute inflammation is the hallmark of mammalian tissue response to injury.

1. The acute inflammatory process involves vascular and cellular events that occur with the help of a variety of chemical mediators (see III and IV). In order of occurrence, the processes involved in acute inflammation are:

a. Vasodilation, which causes local heat and redness

b. Increased vascular permeability, which causes local edema and swelling

c. Influx of neutrophils

d. Influx of monocytes–macrophages

e. Phagocytosis

f. Release of intracellular enzymes from phagocytes

2. Cardinal signs of acute inflammation are:

a. Local heat (calor)

b. Redness (rubor)

c. Swelling (tumor)

d. Pain (dolor)

3. Morphologic patterns. The acute inflammatory response is characterized by the formation of an exudate (i.e., a mixture of fluid, cells, and proteins exuded from damaged cells). The exudate contains protein in excess of 3 g/dl and has a specific gravity exceeding 1.015.* There are four major types of acute inflammatory exudate.

a. Purulent (suppurative, pyogenic) **exudate** consists of large amounts of neutrophils, often accumulated in response to bacterial infection, which may lead to abscess formation (Figure 1-2).

b. Fibrinous exudate is characterized by a large amount of protein (albumin, fibrinogen) from plasma, with visible deposits of fibrin coagulum; it often is bloody (sanguineous). Examples of fibrinous exudate include tuberculous pleuritis and rheumatic pericarditis. The coagulum exudate may become organized by neovascularity and fibroblast formation, with consequent scarring.

---

*A **transudate,** in contrast to an exudate, is a noninflammatory fluid characterized by few cells, a protein content less than 3.0 g/dl, and a specific gravity less than 1.015. A transudate does not imply altered vascular permeability and results from increased hydrostatic pressure within capillaries.

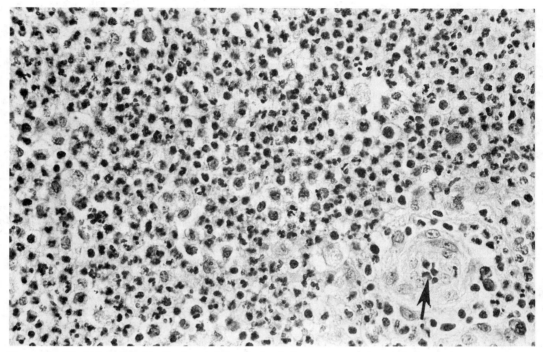

Figure 1-2. The histologic hallmark of acute inflammation is the presence of numerous acute inflammatory cells in the form of neutrophils with multilobate nuclei. Monocytes and macrophages also are scattered throughout and are readily visible by their single oval or round nuclei. A reactive capillary is seen in the *lower right*.

    c. Serous exudate occurs with mild inflammation. Characteristically, it involves fewer cells and less protein than the other types of exudates contain. Serous exudates generally form in body cavities (pleural, pericardial, peritoneal) and in the spinal fluid. Examples are the fluids in second-degree thermal burns, viral meningitis, and joint and pleural effusions.

    d. Catarrhal exudate refers to the type of exudate that forms on mucous membranes and is characterized by a high mucus content. An example is the exudate that occurs in allergic rhinitis (coryza) and bronchitis.

B. Chronic inflammation occurs when healing of acute inflammation is incomplete, when noxious stimuli are ongoing or recurrent, or when responses to immunologic reactions are present. Chronic inflammation, in contrast to acute inflammation, is not a natural defense mechanism. It always is pathologic.

  1. The chronic inflammatory process

    a. Cells involved in chronic inflammation are monocytes–macrophages, lymphocytes, and plasma cells. Monocytes that are derived from the peripheral blood become tissue macrophages.

    b. Granulation tissue forms from budding capillaries, with fibroblast proliferation and variable degrees of collagen deposition. Granulation tissue response may be slight and inapparent. However, in long-standing chronic inflammation, fibrous tissue proliferates and tends to replace functional tissue.

    c. Tissue healing and scarring may be concurrent.

    d. Chronic inflammation may coexist with acute inflammation, as in repeated episodes of acute cholecystitis (with gallstones), osteomyelitis, and pilonidal sinus.

  2. Morphologic patterns

    a. Nonspecific chronic inflammation causes diffuse accumulation of macrophages and lymphocytes at the affected site. Rather than walling off the site, the accumulated macrophages stimulate fibroblast proliferation, resulting in scar formation that typically replaces normal supporting or functional tissues. An example is **chronic glomerulonephritis,** an inflammatory process that results in the loss of functional nephrons. A wide variety of diseases cause chronic inflammation, and its morphologic features vary with the particular site of inflammation.

    b. Granulomatous inflammation is an important subtype of chronic inflammation, and its presence implies some degree of immune capability. It is characterized by **granulomas** (i.e., discrete aggregates of epithelioid macrophages, lymphocytes, and multinucleate giant cells). The granuloma is a type IV immune reaction or cell-mediated hypersensitivity (see Chapter 6 III D). The main cell of the granuloma is the epithelioid macrophage, which may have a secretory function. The giant cells are formed by fusion of multiple macrophages. Blood monocytes transform into epithelioid cells at the tissue site. The granuloma forms in response to a persistent antigen.

        (1) Infectious granulomas form in response to the following conditions.

            (a) Mycobacterial infection is caused by acid-fast bacilli and may result in granuloma formation. Examples include tuberculosis, leprosy, and intracellular infections caused by *M. avium–intracellulare, M. kansasii,* and *M. marinum.* Tuberculous granulomas are characterized by central caseating **necrosis**.

            (b) Brucellosis (i.e., infection by species of *Brucella*) is a granulomatous condition, as is **glanders** (a disease caused by *Pseudomonas mallei*) and **tularemia**.

            (c) Lymphogranuloma venereum is an infectious disease caused by *Chlamydia trachomatis*.

            (d) Cat-scratch disease is caused by a newly discovered bacteria that stains with silver; granulomas with central necrosis are seen.

            (e) Fungal infection by species of *Coccidioides, Cryptococcus,* and *Histoplasma* can produce infectious granulomas.

            (f) *Treponema,* a type of spirochete, causes syphilis, pinta, and yaws; the syphilitic granuloma is called a **gumma**.

            (g) Parasitic infestation, such as schistosomiasis, also produces granuloma formation.

        (2) Foreign-body granulomas typically are **nonnecrotic** and form in the presence of the following:

            (a) Particulate matter (e.g., glass, soil, gravel, metal) [Figure 1-3]

            (b) Synthetic material (e.g., surgical sutures)

            (c) Vegetable matter (e.g., cellulose, which may occur due to fecal contamination of tissues in the presence of a fistula or perforated bowel)

            (d) Beryllium poisoning

        (3) Unknown causes. Sarcoidosis is caused by epithelioid granulomas and may involve the lungs, liver, spleen, lymph nodes, and skin. The granulomas are **nonnecrotic,** uniformly sized, and multiple.

VI. CONSEQUENCES OF INFLAMMATION

    A. Wound healing and repair. Eventual healing is the goal of all inflammatory processes.

        1. Mechanisms of repair. Tissue restoration begins almost at the onset of inflammation itself. Complete restoration of injured tissue requires the removal or destruction of the injurious agent.

        a. Repair by regeneration of cells can occur only in injured tissues that have retained their cell division capability. Restoration occurs by regeneration of cells and tissue specific for the damaged site. The regenerative ability of cells is described in three ways.

            (1) Labile cells possess a constant capacity for regeneration, multiplying continuously to replace old cells that are lost in normal physiologic activities. Lymphoid and hematopoietic cells as well as epithelial cells in the gastrointestinal tract, respiratory tract, urinary bladder, male and female genital tracts, and skin are all labile cells.

            (2) Stable cells have a limited regrowth capacity; they can undergo cell division in order to replace dead cells but normally are not actively multiplying. The liver, pancreas, kidney, endocrine glands, and blood vessels are composed of stable cells. For normal structural restoration to occur in these organs, basement membrane zones must be in contact with the supporting stroma of the organs.

            (3) Permanent cells do not have the ability to reproduce and, once destroyed, cannot be replaced. Neurons and cardiac muscle cells are examples of permanent cells.

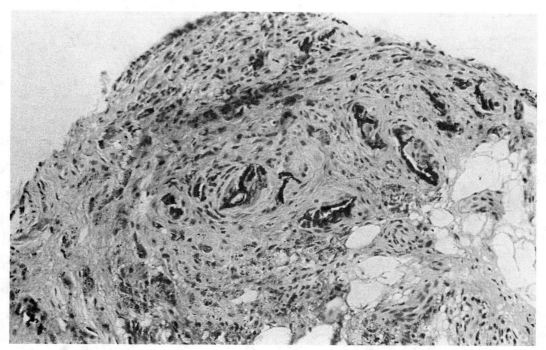

Figure 1-3. Chronic granulomatous inflammation. Multinucleate giant cells are seen engulfing dark-staining particulate foreign material. The granuloma also is rimmed by fibrous connective tissue and chronic inflammation.

   b. Repair by granulation tissue formation, with eventual scarring, is the typical outcome of tissue injury. The process may be quick, as in the healing of surgical wounds that have been cleanly and neatly sutured (a process referred to as **primary,** or **first-intention, healing**). Areas of extensive tissue damage take longer to heal, as the necrotic debris and abscesses must be diminished before granulation tissue formation can occur (a process referred to as **secondary,** or **second-intention, healing**).
   (1) Neocapillary growth (i.e., buds of proliferating endothelial cells) and fibroblastic proliferation begin during the macrophage activity stage, about 36 hours after injury.
   (2) By 100 hours after injury, inflammation is accompanied by well-developed granulation tissue formation, unless abscess formation causes delay (Figure 1-4).
   (3) Fibroblasts synthesize collagen and glucose aminoglycan ground substance.
   (4) Eventually, fibrosis (scar tissue) occupies the defect left by inflammation.

   2. Factors inhibiting repair. Many factors inhibit the desired tissue restoration after inflammation.
   a. Old age. The ability to mount an adequate inflammatory response decreases with advancing age.
   b. Nutrition. Cell metabolism and activation for defense are affected adversely by malnutrition.
   c. Immune depression. Decreased cell-mediated immunity because of familial or acquired disease (e.g., AIDS) may allow inflammation to become chronic–active or to disseminate (e.g., as in disseminated tuberculosis).
   d. Certain diseases. For example, diabetic patients usually are slow to heal properly because of impaired vascularity.
   e. Malignancy. Malignant neoplasms, including leukemias and lymphomas, adversely affect mobilization and activation of leukocytes.
   f. Drugs. Antiinflammatory drugs and antineoplastic agents cause bone marrow suppression, with subsequent leukopenia and reduced response to noxious stimuli.
   g. Superimposed infection. Opportunistic invasion of injured tissue by bacteria (e.g., *M. avium–intracellulare*), yeasts (e.g., *Candida albicans*), or fungi can occur.
   h. Inflammatory tissue damage. Inflammation progressing to formation of fistulous tracts, perforations, or abscesses inhibits healing.

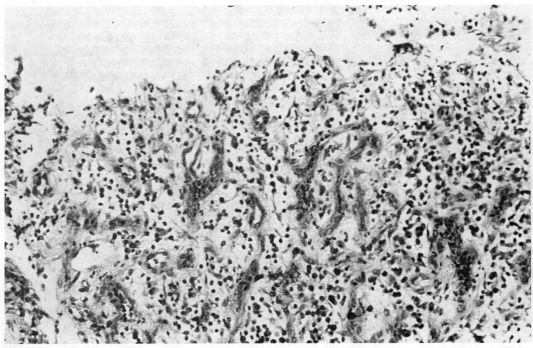

Figure 1-4. Repair by granulation tissue formation. The developing granulation tissue shows characteristic budding capillaries (neovascularization), stromal edema, and red cells. Accompanying the granulation tissue are persistent, chronic inflammatory cells. This type of repair mechanism is effective for healing large tissue defects.

B. Untoward effects of inflammation and repair

1. **Perforation.** Expanding masses of inflamed tissue in the acute inflammatory phase may lead to viscus wall weakening and potential rupture.
    a. A ruptured appendix with spillage of the contents into the abdominal cavity results in purulent peritonitis.
    b. Exudative perihepatitis can occur secondary to tuboovarian pyogenic infections [e.g., pelvic inflammatory disease (PID)] due to gonorrhea.
    c. Chemical peritonitis can occur as a complication of perforated gastric ulcer.

2. **Advancing planes of inflammatory tissue** (fistulous tracts) also may result.
    a. A bronchopleural fistula can form from a pulmonary staphylococcal abscess, with consequent purulent pleuritis (empyema).
    b. Acute mediastinitis can result from an eroding inflammatory tracheoesophageal fistula.
    c. Perirectal and ischiorectal fossa fistulas can form from expanding perineal abscesses.

3. **Extensive fibrosis.** The following are problems related to fibrosis and scar formation after healing.
    a. **Keloids** are excessive accumulations of collagen, which can form in susceptible persons during the healing process. This excess collagen results in a protuberant scar that extends beyond the region of the original injury.
    b. **Bowel obstruction** can occur if adhesive fibrous bands form after repair of abdominal trauma (e.g., surgery, knife wounds).
    c. **Sterility** can result from fibrous obliteration of the fallopian tubes after healing of salpingitis.

4. **Complications** may result from sequelae to an inflammatory process.
    a. Ascending pyelophlebitis of the portal vein system and cholangitis can be caused by a ruptured appendix.
    b. A large abscess may form in the liver, brain, or body cavities, with a thickened fibrous capsule on the exterior that prevents resolution and healing.
    c. Infection may occur and spread through the draining lymphatics, with regional lymphadenitis. The lymphangitis appears as reddish streaking, which is visible through the skin.

STUDY QUESTIONS

Directions: Each of the numbered items or incomplete statements in this section is followed by answers or by completions of the statement. Select the **one** lettered answer or completion that is **best** in each case.

1. Fluid that collects during acute inflammation and that has a protein content exceeding 3 g/dl and a specific gravity exceeding 1.015 is referred to as

(A) edema
(B) an effusion
(C) a transudate
(D) serum
(E) an exudate

2. Which cell type differentiates into morphologically distinct cells capable of immunoglobulin production?

(A) Neutrophils
(B) Basophils
(C) B cells
(D) T cells
(E) Plasma cells

3. The adherence of neutrophils and monocytes to the vascular endothelium prior to movement into the extravascular space is called

(A) margination
(B) diapedesis
(C) pavementing
(D) emigration
(E) clotting

4. An exuberant, hypertrophic, collagenous reaction that can occur following an injury is referred to as

(A) a callus
(B) a cicatrix
(C) a contracture
(D) a keloid
(E) an adhesion

5. Cells that are capable of phagocytosis of particulate matter include

(A) neutrophils, macrophages, eosinophils
(B) lymphocytes, mast cells
(C) T cells, null cells
(D) basophils, stem cells
(E) endothelial cells, plasma cells

6. The unidirectional migration of leukocytes toward a target is referred to as

(A) diapedesis
(B) chemotaxis
(C) opsonization
(D) endocytosis
(E) margination

7. If eosinophils and mast cells are identified in a tissue biopsy from an inflammatory process, which type of immune reaction is most likely occurring?

(A) Type I
(B) Type II
(C) Type III
(D) Type IV
(E) Type V

8. Black carbon particles, cleared from the blood by the reticuloendothelial system of a laboratory animal, can be seen in cells in all of the following organ components EXCEPT

(A) lymph node sinuses
(B) glomeruli
(C) intestinal epithelium
(D) liver sinuses
(E) splenic cords

9. All of the following statements describing leukocyte emigration from vessels in areas of inflammation are true EXCEPT

(A) leukocytes pass through gaps between the vascular endothelial cells
(B) neutrophils are the first cells to emigrate
(C) leukocytes develop pseudopods to aid in emigration
(D) a small loss of fluid accompanies leukocyte emigration
(E) accompanying loss of red cells is passive

1-E	4-D	7-A
2-C	5-A	8-C
3-C	6-B	9-D

10. Once damaged, a tissue or organ usually attempts to regenerate itself. All of the following cell types are capable of regenerating tissue EXCEPT

(A) hepatocytes
(B) colonic mucosal cells
(C) vascular endothelial cells
(D) myocardial cells
(E) bone marrow myeloblasts

11. The inflammatory response serves all of the following EXCEPT

(A) isolation of infected tissues
(B) inactivation of causative agents
(C) neutralization of toxins
(D) removal of devitalized tissue debris
(E) fistula formation

Directions: The group of items in this section consists of lettered options followed by a set of numbered items. For each item, select the **one** lettered option that is most closely associated with it. Each lettered option may be selected once, more than once, or not at all.

Questions 12–16

Match each description of an inflammatory cell to the most appropriate cell type.

(A) Macrophage
(B) Mast cell
(C) Neutrophil
(D) Eosinophil
(E) Basophil

12. These cells are the first to arrive at a site of injury

13. These cells can abort hypersensitivity reactions

14. These cells have metachromatic granules and are found mainly in the tissues

15. These cells are involved in both type I and type IV hypersensitivity reactions

16. These cells are particularly effective against intracellular or encapsulated microbes

---

10-D	13-D	16-A
11-E	14-B	
12-C	15-E	

ANSWERS AND EXPLANATIONS

1. The answer is E *[V A 3]*.
An exudate is the fluid and cells that collect during acute inflammation; the fluid contains protein in excess of 3 g/dl and has a specific gravity exceeding 1.015. Exudates often have abundant neutrophils as their cellular element. In contrast, a transudate is a noninflammatory fluid that is characterized by few cellular elements, a protein content less than 3 g/dl, and a specific gravity less than 1.015. Edema is fluid collected in tissue as a result of various processes [e.g., congestive heart failure (CHF), liver failure, hypoalbuminemia, a blocked lymphatic vessel]; the fluid accumulates because of osmotic pressure, not as a result of acute inflammation; and it does not have a high protein content. An effusion is the accumulation of any type of fluid (exudate or transudate) into a body space, such as the pleural cavity. Serum is the cell-free portion of the blood that remains after the blood has clotted—and has nothing to do with inflammation.

2. The answer is C *[II F 3 a (3)]*.
B cells differentiate into plasma cells, which produce immunoglobulins. Each plasma cell apparently manufactures only one class of immunoglobulin. Plasma cells are the mature and already differentiated form of cells; they are called "end cells" because they no longer divide. B cells are stimulated to differentiate into plasma cells under the influence of antigens, T-cell interaction, and macrophage interaction.

3. The answer is C *[IV B 1]*.
As the vascular phase of the inflammatory response progresses, neutrophils and monocytes move toward the periphery of the microcirculatory vessels (a process referred to as margination) and then adhere to, or pavement, the vascular endothelium in preparation for migration into the extravascular space. To migrate, leukocytes develop pseudopods and move, without accompanying loss of fluid, through gaps between the endothelial cells—a process termed diapedesis. In the latter part of the vascular phase, increased vascular permeability causes loss of plasma with resultant venous stasis and, eventually, clotting in the small capillaries local to the inflamed area.

4. The answer is D *[VI B 3 a]*.
A keloid is an excessive accumulation of collagen that can form during the healing process, resulting in a protuberant scar that extends beyond the region of the original injury. Keloid formation can be a problem in both primary and secondary forms of healing in genetically predisposed persons. Keloids that form in exposed areas of the skin can cause considerable cosmetic problems, as repeated excision of the scar tissue may result in a cycle of subsequent keloid formation. Contractures (i.e., fixed high resistance to passive stretch muscles, as in a fixed elbow) and adhesions (i.e., fibrous bands that cause abnormal adherence of structures, such as bowel loops) are other adverse effects of healing caused by extensive fibrosis and scar formation. A callus forms by hyperplasia of the stratum corneum in areas of the skin that are exposed to excessive or repeated friction or pressure. A cicatrix simply refers to the new tissue (i.e., scar) that forms in the healing of an injury; it is not hypertrophic.

5. The answer is A *[II A, C, E]*.
Neutrophils and macrophages are the inflammatory cells that participate most actively in the acute phases of inflammation through phagocytosis of particulate matter (e.g., microorganisms, cell fragments). Cell surface receptors on these phagocytic cells are responsible for identifying opsonized material [i.e., material coated with immunoglobulin G (IgG) or complement component C3b], which is to be ingested and destroyed enzymatically. Eosinophils can also phagocytose. Lymphocytes and plasma cells participate very little, if at all, in the phagocytic process but contribute in chronic inflammation and in immunologic reactions. Basophils are concerned with the release of vasoactive amines (e.g., histamine) after complexing with IgE to promote type I (IgE-mediated) hypersensitivity reactions.

6. The answer is B *[IV B 3]*.
During the vascular stasis stage of the inflammatory response, neutrophils and monocytes move toward and then adhere to the vascular endothelium of microcirculatory vessels prior to migration into the extravascular space; this two-step process is known as margination and pavementing. Leukocytes, then, emigrate through gaps between the endothelial cells in a process known as diapedesis. Once outside the vessels, leukocytes undergo unidirectional migration toward the agent causing the inflammatory response. Several chemotactic factors have an apparently specific influence on the rate of movement of selected cell types. Endocytosis is the process by which leukocytes engulf the injurious agent once they

have reached it. Opsonization refers to the coating of injurious agents with substances (e.g., immuno-globulins, complement) that enhance the phagocytic process.

7. The answer is A *[II C, D]*.
Eosinophils, basophils, and mast cells are the hallmarks of an immediate hypersensitivity (type I) reaction. These cells would be seen in sputum samples from a patient with asthmatic bronchitis. Cytotoxic (type II) reactions attract neutrophils, lymphocytes, and complement and ultimately lead to lysis or inactivation of target cells; necrotizing transplant vasculitis is an example of a type II reaction. Immune complex (type III) reactions mainly involve lymphocytes and complement, although neutrophils also are present; rheumatoid arthritis, systemic lupus erythematosus, and many types of glomerulonephritis are immune complex–mediated diseases. The hallmark of delayed hypersensitivity (type IV) reactions is the accumulation of macrophages and histiocytes, as in the granulomatous reaction to tuberculosis. There is no type V reaction.

8. The answer is C *[II E 1]*.
One of the major functions of the reticuloendothelial system (i.e., the body's storehouse of monocytes, histiocytes, and macrophages) is to clear the blood quickly of noxious matter such as bacteria, foreign particles, and cellular debris. For example, if particulate carbon were injected into the bloodstream, within minutes the carbon would be extracted from the blood by the reticuloendothelial system. The system consists of cells found in many organs, including the histiocytes in lymph node sinuses and splenic cords, the histiocytes lining hepatic sinuses (called Kupffer cells), and the histiocytes in glomeruli (called mesangial cells). Intestinal epithelial cells are not monocytes and are not directly related to the bloodstream; they can only absorb or engulf carbon from the gut lumen.

9. The answer is D *[IV B 2]*.
Emigration (also called diapedesis) of motile leukocytes from blood vessels into tissues surrounding an area of inflammation is a vital component of the inflammatory response. To emigrate, leukocytes insert pseudopodia into endothelial cell junctions and show active, purposeful movement through the endothelial gaps, without evidence of phagocytic movement by the endothelial cells. No loss of fluid accompanies leukocyte emigration; however, passive emigration of red cells may occur. The first, or immediate, wave of migration is predominantly that of neutrophils, closely followed by monocytes.

10. The answer is D *[VI A 1 a]*.
Many cells and tissues have the capacity to regenerate to some extent. This is particularly true for the so-called "labile" cells (e.g., colonic mucosal cells, bone marrow myeloblasts), which multiply continuously, even in the absence of injury. To a slightly lesser extent, the so-called "stable" cells have this capacity; examples of stable cells include hepatocytes (which may nearly completely regenerate even after removal of up to half of the liver) and vascular endothelial cells (which grow to form vessels into an avascularized tissue or wound). Some cells, once damaged, are permanently lost. These permanent cells include the myocardial cells and the neuron and its process in the peripheral nerve.

11. The answer is E *[I B 1]*.
The inflammatory response is a direct reaction against injurious agents or organisms that threaten the homeostasis of the host. Inflammation serves many useful purposes ultimately aimed at restoring host homeostasis, including isolation of infected tissues, inactivation of noxious agents and organisms, neutralization of toxins, and cleanup of devitalized tissues in preparation for tissue repair. Not all effects of inflammation are favorable, however. Beyond the simple discomfort and disability that may be associated with inflammation are a variety of more serious complications of the inflammatory process, such as rupture of a viscus, excessive scar tissue formation, fistula formation, and the development of certain inflammatory diseases (e.g., glomerulonephritis, arthritis, myocarditis).

12–16. The answers are 12-C *[II A 2]*, **13-D** *[II C 2]*, **14-B** *[II D 1]*, **15-E** *[II B 2]*, **16-A** *[II E 2 b (2)]*.
A variety of cells are involved in the inflammatory response, including granulocytes (i.e., neutrophils, eosinophils, basophils, and mast cells) and macrophages. Neutrophils (i.e., neutrophilic granulocytes) are the white blood cells (WBCs) that are most responsible for the leukocytosis that occurs in response to an inflammatory or infectious crisis. They are the first cells to arrive at the site of injury after emigrating from neighboring vessels. Neutrophils are directed toward the injurious agent by chemotactic substances and, upon reaching their target, are involved in phagocytosis of the agent.

Eosinophils (i.e., eosinophilic granulocytes) have cytoplasmic granules containing enzymes that inactivate histamine, which is a chemical mediator of immediate (type I) hypersensitivity reactions. Most of the body's eosinophils exist in the tissues at sites of immune reactions, where they can abort hypersensitivity reactions.

Mast cells contain granules that stain metachromatically with basic dyes. The granules release histamine upon degranulation during type I hypersensitivity reactions. Mast cells are connective tissue cells found close to blood vessels.

Like mast cells, basophils (i.e., basophilic granulocytes) have cytoplasmic granules that contain histamine. When an immunoglobulin E (IgE)-specific antigen enters the body, basophils stimulate the formation of IgE, which binds to the surface of the antigen. The basophilic granules then release histamine, producing an anaphylactic (type I) reaction. In addition to this role, basophils also are involved in type IV (delayed) hypersensitivity reactions, such as contact dermatitis.

Macrophages, like neutrophils, play a major role in the disposal of noxious matter within tissues, such as microorganisms and necrotic tissue. They also have important functions in the immune response. In their microbicidal function, macrophages are most effective against intracellular or encapsulated organisms, such as *Mycoplasma, Salmonella,* and *Cryptococcus.*

Special Diagnostic Techniques

John S. J. Brooks

I. OVERVIEW. In hospitals, diagnostic pathology involving human tissue is called **anatomic** pathology and consists of **surgical** pathology (which receives all material removed at surgery) and **cytology** (e.g., pap smears, fine needle aspirations (FNAs), sputum cytology). Diagnoses must be accurate because patient therapy is intimately connected to and dependent on the tissue diagnosis. While many diagnoses are straightforward and require only the microscope, others are more difficult and require additional information. All future clinicians should recognize that modern pathologists cannot operate in a vacuum, but must coordinate their impressions with the clinical situation.

A. Clinical information. All pertinent clinical details should accompany any pathology or cytology request form. Many times such information is absent, resulting in delays in diagnosis.

1. Basic data. Patient age, sex, location of biopsy, and problem or question to be addressed

2. Additional data. Pertinent laboratory values, x-ray findings, and infectious precautions

B. Special techniques. These procedures include electron microscopy (EM), immunohistochemistry (IHC), cytology, flow cytometry for DNA analysis, in situ hybridization (ISH), and DNA gene rearrangement studies.

C. Diagnostic process. When a biopsy is received, the problem or disease to be identified is assessed, and tissue is preserved for possible use as follows.

1. IHC occasionally uses frozen tissue, but most antibody markers work in routinely processed tissue (paraffin-embedded tissue).

2. EM uses fresh tissue, special fixative, and small (1-mm) tissue fragments.

3. Flow cytometry uses 5 mm of fresh tissue for either DNA analysis or immunophenotyping for lymphomas or leukemias.

4. Molecular biology analysis uses fresh or fixed tissue as follows.
a. DNA gene rearrangements for lymphomas. Analysis uses fresh tissue, the same material used for flow cytometry for immunophenotyping.
b. ISH. Analysis can utilize routinely processed fixed tissue—no special processing is necessary.
c. Other. Analysis for other genes may require additional fragments preserved as fresh or fixed tissue.

D. Specimen handling. Modern pathology analysis is a complex process which may require fresh tissue to address certain problems. Whenever possible, the clinician should put a biopsy **fresh tissue in saline** for analysis by the pathologist.

II. CYTOLOGY. This study of disease processes involves cell smears from various orifices (e.g., vagina, mouth, bronchus) or the fine-needle aspiration (FNA) of any mass or lymph node. The needle is so thin that no adverse tissue damage results, even if deep within internal organs; it is often guided by computerized tomography (CT) x-rays.

A. Benign disease

1. Cytologic smears of skin vesicles and the cervix can identify viral diseases such as herpes. These procedures can take place in the office or emergency room.

2. In AIDS patients, **sputum cytology** is a quick and accurate way to diagnose pneumocystis pneumonia and saves the patient a more costly and risky biopsy.

B. Cancer studies

1. The value of diagnostic cytology in modern cancer detection cannot be overemphasized. The **microscopic examination of scrapings and brushings** from minimally invasive lesions allows the early diagnosis of cancers of the bronchus, esophagus, stomach, colon, breast, and many other sites.

2. **Neoplastic cells** can be identified in several ways from the interpretation of cytologic smears, since malignancy is associated with changes in chromosomal and membrane composition. Visually, these changes are reflected in the nucleus and nucleolus of the cells and in cellular and nuclear shapes, sizes, and configurations.
   a. Nuclei of benign cells usually are small and oval; nuclei of malignant cells often are large, irregular, and even bizarre. Nuclear changes are the most specific morphologic change for malignancy.
   b. The appearance of the cytoplasm distinguishes the type of malignancy and also reflects genetic abnormalities.

3. Recent research has attempted to elucidate **cell membrane changes** as cell-to-cell communication and contact inhibition as well as the development of metastases.
   a. In vitro, normal cells cease dividing when they become crowded (**contact inhibition**). Malignant cells do not stop dividing, despite cell-to-cell contact; instead, they pile up.
   b. The uncontrolled, often rapid growth presents a problem to the neoplasm—how to obtain and maintain adequate nutrients. Therefore, **necrosis** often is observed in malignant tumors.
   c. Also, neoplastic cells, because of loss of contact inhibition, tend to be **less sticky** and are exfoliated and scraped off more easily than their normal counterparts.

C. Smears. The examination of isolated cells in smears is the basis for modern diagnostic cytology. Specimens may be obtained in several ways.

1. Cells may be collected from areas where they normally exfoliate (e.g., from the vagina and cervix uteri). The squamous cells may show inflammatory reactive changes, varying degrees of dysplasia, or carcinoma.

2. Cells may be obtained from sites where they normally desquamate but remain for periods of time (e.g., from sputum and urine). Urine specimens contain cells from the entire collecting system (i.e., from the renal pelvis to the bladder); in contrast, prostatic cells rarely are found.

3. Cells may be coaxed to exfoliate through various washing methods (e.g., from bronchial or bladder washings).

4. Cells may be brushed or scraped from lesions, either directly (e.g., from oral lesions) or by means of endoscopy (e.g., from pulmonary or gastrointestinal lesions).

5. Cells may be aspirated from proliferative lesions, such as breast masses, thyroid nodules, salivary gland tumors, and enlarged lymph nodes.

6. Cells may be aspirated from effusions (e.g., from pleural effusions, which may form due to pneumonia, mesothelioma, or adenocarcinoma).
   a. In women, a breast adenocarcinoma is the most likely source.
   b. In men with effusions due to a malignancy, lung cancer is very likely.

D. FNA biopsy is a method of taking a cytology sample by means of a fine needle with negative pressure supplied by an attached syringe. When performed during exploratory surgery, the procedure can provide a rapid diagnosis that helps to determine the extent of surgery needed. However, this method cannot fully evaluate lesions or diseases that require attention to tissue architecture as opposed to cellular cytology (e.g., follicular lymphomas).

1. **Uses** for the technique are as follows.
   a. Aspiration of **superficial breast masses,** whether found by palpation or roentgenography, has proved particularly advantageous.
   b. During a laparotomy, the **pancreas** can be examined safely, or suspicious **hepatic nodules** can be aspirated.

    c. The **lung** can be aspirated during fluoroscopy.

    d. Deep organs can be penetrated by cutaneous biopsy with the aid of ultrasonography or CT.

  2. Advantages of the technique are myriad.

    a. The equipment and technique are simple, and the procedure is safe. For a superficial lesion, the procedure can take place in the office the first time a patient is seen; the biopsy takes 1 minute, and the specimen can be processed and interpreted within 15 minutes.

    b. The procedure has an accuracy of 80% to greater than 95%.

    c. For some patients, aspiration biopsy may eliminate hospitalization or surgery, and for others it may shorten the hospital stay.

  3. Complications have been reported.

    a. Thousands of biopsies reported from Scandinavia have shown no significant seeding of malignant cells through the needle tract.

    b. Pulmonary hemorrhage is a very rare complication of fine-needle lung biopsy; spontaneously resolving pneumothorax occurs in 10% to 30% of the cases.

E. Cytology special analysis. Many of the special techniques described can be applied to cytology specimens, thus increasing diagnostic accuracy.

III. IMMUNOHISTOCHEMISTRY (IHC)

A. Definition and uses. IHC is defined as the use of antibodies (both polyclonal and monoclonal) to tissue markers for diagnostic or research purposes. A diluted antibody solution is applied to a tissue section where the antibody sticks to its specific antigen; it is then detected by either a fluorescent probe or an enzymatic system such as peroxidase. The presence or absence of the antigen impacts on the diagnosis.

B. Immunofluorescence. This method is now used only on biopsies from certain sites—skin, kidney, and lung—to detect microscopic deposits in medical diseases.

  1. Technique. Antiserum can be combined chemically with small quantities of a **fluorescent dye** [usually fluorescein isothiocyanate (FITC)] without loss of its specific antibody properties. The fluorescein-conjugated antiserum can then be examined by fluorescence microscopy for histologic localization of the corresponding antigens.

  2. Uses

    a. The **detection of autoantibodies** by immunofluorescence has wide applications.

      (1) In clinical practice, the specificity of these reactions is deduced from the histologic localization of the patient's antibody on the substrate tissue.

      (2) In the **indirect technique** that is generally used, the tissue is treated first with the patient's serum; after removal of uncombined serum proteins by washing, the attached human antibody is demonstrated by a fluorescent anti–human immunoglobulin serum.

    b. The technique can also be used to **localize tissue antigens** (serum proteins and certain hormones) and to **identify microorganisms** in tissues. Specifically, it is most useful in identifying **immune complex deposits** containing immunoglobulins IgG, IgA, or IgM or in identifying **complement proteins** in certain skin and kidney diseases. In this one area, it still is preferred over the immunoperoxidase (IP) method.

  3. Disadvantages include the following.

    a. Samples fade, requiring photography to document results.

    b. Reading slides may be difficult because of autofluorescence.

    c. Fresh-frozen tissue is required for reliable results.

C. Immunoperoxidase staining. This enzymatic detection system is the one most commonly used; other enzymes, such as alkaline phosphatase, can replace IP. Its advantage is its high sensitivity, the production of a permanent slide, and the ability to use fixed paraffin-embedded tissues.

  1. Techniques. IP staining procedures take advantage of the ability of an enzyme to catalyze a substrate exponentially, resulting in a vast amount of visible, insoluble product at the site of a tissue antigen. In today's parlance, the technique has a high signal-to-noise (antigen-to-nonantigen) ratio.

   a. The four basic **variations of the IP method** follow.
   (1) The **indirect method** employs a primary antibody (usually from the rabbit or mouse) to the required antigen and a secondary antibody to the species immunoglobulin; the secondary antibody is conjugated to peroxidase. With this method, one enzyme molecule is present per antigen molecule detected.
   (2) The **enzyme-bridge method**—also called the **peroxidase–antiperoxidase (PAP) method**—employs three antibodies, a primary and a secondary antibody as described, and a third, or antiperoxidase, antibody from the same species as the primary; the third antibody is the one coupled to peroxidase. In this way, three enzyme molecules are present per antigen molecule detected, so this method is more sensitive than the indirect method. The **steps in the PAP method** are as follows.
   (a) Dilute rabbit anti–human chorionic gonadotropin (anti–hCG)—the "primary"—is applied to a tissue section.
   (b) Dilute sheep anti–rabbit IgG—the "secondary"—is then applied. (This antibody is bivalent: One end links to the primary antibody, the other end to the third antibody. Thus, it is also called the "link" antiserum.)
   (c) Dilute rabbit anti–peroxidase complex is then added. (This **PAP complex** includes two antibodies and three enzymes bound together, that is, three enzyme molecules per antigen molecule.)
   (d) The section is then developed with a substrate for peroxidase, often diaminobenzidine (DAB), which gives a brown color.
   (3) The **avidin–biotin complex (ABC) method** follows the same steps as the PAP method, except that the three-enzyme PAP method is replaced by the **ABC method,** with five to seven enzymes per antigen molecule; the ABC method is the most sensitive of the three.
   (4) The **strep–avidin (STA) method** is a further refinement of the ABC method, with added gain in sensitivity. Primary antibodies can now be used at very high dilution (1:10,000 to 1:20,000), and background problems are almost nonexistent.
   b. Antibodies. Two types of antibodies are used for IHC purposes—-polyclonal and monoclonal.
   (1) Polyclonal antibodies usually are raised in rabbits and, thus, are used as antiserum (i.e., rabbit serum containing the wanted specificities). However, unwanted antibodies may be present in the immunized rabbits, and these antibodies may cause problems. On the other hand, polyclonal antibodies are inexpensive and often valuable because they are reactive against a variety of epitopes on a given antigen.
   (2) Monoclonal antibodies (MoAbs) usually are raised in tissue culture or as ascites fluid in animals injected with clones of mouse myeloma cells selected to produce antibodies to a substance. The clones are first produced by cell fusion of the myeloma cells with splenic lymphoid cells from mice immunized with the substance wanted.
   (a) MoAbs usually are considered superior to polyclonal antibodies and are used more often for several reasons.
   (i) MoAbs are absolutely specific for a given epitope of an antigen.
   (ii) They cause no problems of background cross-reactivity, as they have no other unwanted specificities.
   (iii) They can be constantly produced from the clone.
   (b) However, MoAbs have occasional disadvantages.
   (i) Sometimes they are reactive to an epitope that does not survive fixation and, thus, will not detect the tissue antigen.
   (ii) Sometimes the small epitope they are raised against is repeated in another antigen, causing a different type of cross-reactivity.
   (iii) Also, they may not have high-affinity binding to the antigen.
   c. The IP techniques have a number of **advantages** over immunofluorescence.
   (1) They are far **more sensitive.** If immunofluorescence is assigned a sensitivity value of 1, then indirect IP has a value of about 10 to 100; PAP, about 1000; and ABC, about 10,000.
   (2) They result in a **permanent preparation** that can be reexamined or sent to other hospitals.
   (3) Conjugation is not required, and any commercially available primary antibody can be used (without modification).
   (4) IP can be used on frozen tissues (e.g., for fragile lymphocyte surface markers), but it is most often employed on **paraffin-embedded tissues**. This use is ideal because:
   (a) The pathologist can judge from the histology which antigens might be the most useful aids in defining the process or type of tumor.

    (b) The cell detail is better preserved.

    (c) The method is sensitive enough to detect most tissue antigens or substances, even those partially lost during processing.

  d. The **disadvantages** to IP methods no longer exist. In the past, the indirect and PAP methods gave a light background staining, but that problem has been eliminated with the ABC method. Further, antibodies last longer, as they are used at great dilution (1:1000 to 1:10,000).

2. Uses

  a. Immunocytochemistry, especially the ABC IP method, has made it possible to demonstrate the presence of antigens in a tissue section, thus allowing pathologists to investigate the functional aspects and histogenesis of many diseases. Immunocytochemical methods provide a bridge between the morphologic and functional or biochemical aspects of a lesion since they permit examination in situ.

  b. Some **major applications** of immunocytochemistry methods are as follows.

    (1) **Identifying the cell of origin of neoplasms** (e.g., lymphoma versus carcinoma versus sarcoma). Carcinomas express the intermediate filament cytokeratin (CK), lymphomas express leukocyte common antigen (LCA), and sarcomas have neither.

    (2) **Identifying oncofetal antigens in neoplasms** [e.g., alpha-fetoprotein (AFP) and carcinoembryonic antigen (CEA)]. These substances, which are synthesized during fetal life, also appear in adults with certain types of tumors (e.g., germ-cell tumors). A variety of neoplasms are associated with elevated levels of these antigens.

    (3) **Identifying tumor-specific** and **tissue-specific markers in neoplasms**

      (a) Tissue-specific markers (Table 2-1) are antigens that are present in only a few tissues; thus, they are extremely useful in diagnostic pathology since they can be used to determine the histogenesis of a neoplasm. For example, myoglobin is produced only by skeletal muscle cells and tumors thereof (rhabdomyosarcomas).

      (b) Identification of tumor-specific markers has helped pathologists in resolving difficult differential diagnosis of malignancies. Knowledge of the exact nature of a neoplasm is often vital to oncologists when determining the appropriate chemotherapy to apply. For example, prostatic-specific antigen is valuable in identifying prostatic cancer, and CEA aids in distinguishing metastatic adenocarcinoma (CEA-positive) from mesothelioma (CEA-negative).

    (4) **Detecting the loss of a normal antigen in a neoplasm.** Blood group antigens in bladder and breast neoplasms are examples.

Table 2-1. Selected Examples of Tumor Markers

Marker	Type of Tissue or Cancer
Intermediate filaments	
Cytokeratin	All epithelial lesions (carcinomas)
Vimentin	Mesenchymal lesions (sarcomas; also epithelial tumors)
Neurofilament	All neuronal and many neuroendocrine cells
Glial fibrillary acidic protein (GFAP)	Nonneuronal brain tissue
Desmin	Muscle cells
Other general markers	
Leukocyte common antigen (LCA)	Lymphomas (not carcinomas or sarcomas)
S100 protein	Melanomas; various other cell types (Schwann cells; chondrocytes; some carcinomas)
Carcinoembryonic antigen (CEA)	Carcinomas (not mesotheliomas)
Alpha-fetoprotein (AFP)	Germ cell tumors (embryonal carcinoma of testis)
Tissue-specific markers	
Prostate-specific antigen (PSA)	Prostate cancer
Thyroglobulin	Thyroid cancer
Calcitonin	Medullary carcinoma of thyroid
Various polypeptides	Neuroendocrine tumors (carcinoid; islet cell tumors)
Coagulation factor VIII–related antigen	Angiosarcoma
Myoglobin; muscle-specific actins and myosins; desmin	Rhabdomyosarcoma

(5) **Detecting hormones and hormone receptors.** Immunocytochemical techniques have contributed to the identification of neoplastic and hyperplastic lesions of endocrine organs.

    (a) Detection of hormones in neoplasms gives information about neoplastic histogenesis. The immunocytochemical procedure is so sensitive that an extremely small amount of hormone can be detected, as in cases of clinically nonfunctioning neoplasms. Immunocytochemical techniques have produced evidence that many neoplasms of endocrine organs contain multiple hormones.

    (b) Estrogen receptor can now be detected in paraffin-embedded tissue specimens in breast cancer. This information is clinically useful in identifying patients who may benefit from tamoxifen therapy. Small tumors can today be tested as never before.

(6) **Localizing enzymes.** Many enzymes have been localized in tissue sections by immunocytochemistry. Some enzymes, such as prostatic acid phosphatase or lysozyme, are used as tissue-specific markers to ascertain the histogenesis of neoplasms. (Certain enzymes can be detected by standard enzyme histochemical methods, but these methods require fresh or specially handled tissues.)

(7) **Studying lymphomas.** IP techniques can be used to distinguish:

    (a) A B-cell lymphoma from a reactive proliferation by detecting a single class of an immunoglobulin light chain in the lymphoma, thus establishing its monoclonal nature

    (b) A large-cell lymphoma from an undifferentiated carcinoma by detecting LCA

    (c) To distinguish the type of lymphoma (B cell, T cell, true histiocytic). This is currently done on frozen tissue due to the fragility of the surface markers (e.g., T-cell surface receptors CD2$^+$ or OKT11). However, antibodies that can be used in paraffin-embedded tissue are becoming available.

(8) **Detecting an abnormal distribution or number of cells** (e.g., hyperplasia or hypoplasia of endocrine cells)

(9) **Detecting autoantibodies,** using the patient's serum against some tissue, such as liver. (A positive stain in this case would indicate that the patient has autoantibodies to liver cells.)

(10) **Identifying viral antigens in tissues**

    (a) An important example is the localization of hepatitis B virus (HBV) surface antigen (HBsAg) and core antigen (HBcAg). HBsAg is present in the cytoplasm of affected hepatocytes; HBcAg is present in hepatocyte nuclei. Immunocytochemical methods of HBsAg staining correlate well with histochemical methods (orcein staining); moreover, positive cells are demonstrated more intensely by immunocytochemical staining.

    (b) Identifying cytomegalovirus (CMV) in the lung is another example of this use.

(11) **Identifying microorganisms.** If antibodies against microorganisms are available, a specific method to identify these microorganisms can be developed, such as staining for *Legionella* in a lung biopsy.

c. Prognostic immunohistochemistry. Testing tumors for markers of possible prognostic significance has become increasingly important and places further emphasis on the entire pathology analysis of a patient's neoplasm. These markers include the following.

    (1) **Oncogene proteins.** Also known as oncoproteins, these proteins may be applicable to a specific tumor (e.g., **c-erbB2** in breast cancer) or to a large group of cancers (e.g., **p53** oncoprotein in lung, breast, prostate cancers and sarcomas).

    (2) **Enzyme activity.** Certain enzymes like **clathepsin** may be prognostically significant in breast and colon cancer.

    (3) **Tumor-immune response markers.** Whether tumor cells express or lose histocompatibility antigens **HLA-ABC** or **HLA-DR** has prognostic significance in melanoma, certain sarcomas, and breast and colon cancer.

IV. TECHNIQUES FROM MOLECULAR BIOLOGY.
These research tools are beginning to show their clinical utility, most notably in the pathologic diagnosis of various malignancies.

A. Flow cytometry for DNA analysis

1. **Purpose.** Flow cytometry is commonly used in academic centers to determine the DNA ploidy values of neoplastic tissues. For some tumors, this information has prognostic clinical significance, since aneuploidy may indicate a tumor that is clinically aggressive and difficult to treat. However, a large number of aggressive neoplasms are diploid.

    a. Diploid lesions may be reactive or neoplastic, benign or malignant. Reactive and benign lesions almost always are diploid.

    b. Aneuploid lesions usually are neoplastic and malignant, but exceptions do occur. **Aneuploidy is not equivalent to malignancy.**

2. Procedure

    a. A tissue sample is treated to liberate and isolate the cell nuclei, so that their DNA will not mix and give false-high values. Although fresh tissue is often used, formalin-fixed tissue can be tested as well.

    b. The isolated nuclei are extracted, stained, and analyzed in a flow cytometer. The amount of DNA per cell is determined from the amount of emitted light of a specified wavelength (corresponding to the type of stain used).

    c. The information is used to generate a DNA histogram, from which the number of resting diploid cells, dividing cells, and tetraploid or aneuploid cells can be determined.

3. Tumor prognosis. Whether malignancies are diploid or aneuploid or have a high proliferative component has prognostic value. Examples are as follows.

    a. Breast cancer. A high proliferative component (S-phase) correlates with the absence of estrogen receptor; as a rule, aneuploid tumors are more aggressive.

    b. Neuroblastoma. In some childhood tumors like this one, aneuploidy aparadoxically connotes a favorable prognosis.

    c. Sarcomas. Aneuploid adult tumors connote a prior prognosis.

    d. Other cancers. For practically every adult cancer type (e.g., lung, colon, stomach, bladder), aneuploid (or nondiploid) tumors behave more aggressively.

B. Hybridization procedures

1. Purpose. Hybridization techniques allow researchers to isolate and identify DNA fragments, which are sometimes as minute as four to six base pairs, from the genome of virtually any organism. These techniques are beginning to be clinically useful in three areas.

    a. Identification of microbes in body fluids or tissues of patients with infectious disease

        (1) Relatively simple hybridization methods using radiolabeled DNA fragments (**"DNA probes"**) from known pathogens allow the detection of a suspected pathogen in a tissue or fluid sample by in vitro autoradiography.

        (2) ISH techniques allow viral identification within a tissue section.

    b. Gene studies in inherited conditions

        (1) The hemoglobin S gene of sickle cell anemia can be detected in amniotic fluid cells or in a person with sickle cell trait.

        (2) Histocompatibility gene alleles can be identified, and this capability should prove valuable in pretransplant tissue typing.

    c. Diagnosis of malignancies

        (1) Hybridization techniques are now being used clinically in the differential diagnosis of **lymphoproliferative disorders**.

            (a) DNA probes have been developed to identify **gene rearrangements** in immunoglobulin genes and in T-cell receptor genes. These gene rearrangements are a normal part of B-cell and T-cell maturation and serve as a unique marker for each B or T cell and for any clone that arises from it. The same unique gene rearrangements occur during monoclonal (i.e., malignant) lymphocytic proliferation.

            (b) Therefore, hybridization methods employing the DNA probes can identify **monoclonal lymphoproliferation** and determine whether it is of B-cell or T-cell origin.

        (2) Hybridization techniques underlie the explosion of knowledge about viral **oncogenes** and their association with malignant tumors. However, the clinical utility of this information lies in the future.

2. Procedures

    a. Various **"blot" techniques** (southern, northern, and dot blot) are available. The widely used **southern blot procedure** is described.

        (1) DNA fragments from tissue extracts are separated by electrophoresis, blotted onto nitrocellulose paper, then hybridized to a molecular probe.

        (2) This probe consists of a known DNA or RNA sequence that has been labeled with a radioisotope. The nucleic acid sequences of the probe combine with the complementary sequences in the blot, forming hybrid helices.

(3) The original, unknown nucleic acid fragments in the hybrid can then be identified by autoradiographic techniques.

b. DNA gene rearrangement assays in lymphomas

(1) DNA probes are hybridized to fresh tissue by a method much like that of ISH. Only 1% of the lymphocytes in a biopsy specimen need be the malignant clone for positive detection.

(2) Nonmalignant lymphoid disorders and carcinomas show a nonrearranged, or germ-line, configuration of the immunoglobulin and T-cell receptor genes.

(3) Lymphomas and lymphoid leukemias will show gene rearrangements.

(a) These will be in heavy-chain or light-chain immunoglobulin genes if the malignant neoplasm is of B-cell origin.

(b) The rearrangements will be in T-cell α, β, or γ-receptor genes if the malignancy is of T-cell origin.

(4) Analysis of gene rearrangements is used primarily when standard immunologic and IHC techniques cannot define a clonal B-cell or T-cell population. In these instances, DNA gene rearrangement studies are quite helpful; in fact, they have become the best way to determine the presence of T-cell clonal proliferation.

(5) Gene rearrangement studies also corroborate the genetic markers that can be identified by karyotypic analysis in the leukemias and lymphomas, such as the reciprocal 9;22 chromosomal translocation that occurs in chronic myelogenous leukemia.

(6) In the future, similar technology employing gel electrophoresis may be used to detect specific genetic defects, either in tissue samples or in buffy-coat preparations.

c. ISH is derived from the various blot techniques. It allows analysis of a tissue section, rather than an extract, as in blot techniques; the pathologist can see where the probe is in the tissue.

(1) The tissue section is incubated with a probe (labeled with either a radioisotope or biotin), at about 80°C. The incubation denatures the tissue nucleic acids and allows the hybridizing to occur.

(2) The hybrid sequences are then identified by autoradiography or by the use of avidin-linked enzymes or antibiotin antibodies.

(3) With DNA ISH, mainly **viral information** is being detected clinically. Viral infections (e.g., due to CMV) produce multiple copies of DNA per cell, enabling easy detection. However, detection of oncogenes is more difficult in tissue sections of tumors, because multiple copies often are not present.

(4) With mRNA ISH, messenger RNA can be detected readily in fixed tissues. Since many copies are present, no amplification is required. Tests being developed include assays for growth factors (EGF, TGF-B) and specific cell products (actin).

d. ISH-polymerase chain reaction (ISH–PCR). Using a DNA or RNA polymerase, the nuclei acid of a specific sequence can be amplified using highly specific probes, enabling detection of genes present in small copy numbers (1–3). This emerging technology allows assessment of integrated viral DNA as a cause of neoplasia (e.g., human papillomavirus (HPV) in cervical and oral cancer) and detects the presence of mutated oncogenes (e.g., p53).

e. Future procedures. All these trabecular techniques utilize biopsy tissue and will pave the way toward integration of molecular biology in diagnostic surgical and cytopathology laboratories.

V. ELECTRON MICROSCOPY. Studying tissues at the ultrastructural level by means of both **transmission and scanning EM** allows a better understanding of many disease processes. EM used to be the sole special technique in diagnostic pathology. Its role now is limited to evaluation of rare infections, immune complex disease, and tumor samples when other methods have yielded equivocal results.

A. Infectious agents. Screening to detect microorganisms always should use light microscopy, not EM. Examples of uses for EM are the following:

1. Confirmation of the initial light microscopy impression, especially when cultures are not available (i.e., organisms that cannot be cultured routinely)

2. Confirmation of the diagnosis of Whipple's disease from a gastrointestinal or lymph node biopsy (i.e., large accumulations of histiocytes containing bacterial organisms on ultrastructural examination)

3. Search for viral particles in skin biopsy specimens (see V D 5)

4. Examination of neural tissues for infectious agents or their cytopathic effects (see V D 4)

B. Immune complex diseases

1. Immune complex–mediated reactions are type III hypersensitivity reactions, which involve the following processes.
   a. Antigen–antibody complexes are deposited on the basement membrane of blood vessels or other tissues.
   b. The immune complexes lead to complement activation, neutrophil chemotaxis, and an acute inflammatory reaction accompanied by the release of lysosomal enzymes that destroy the basement membrane.

2. The immune complexes frequently are visible by EM as electron-dense deposits along the basement membrane in the skin (e.g., in pemphigus), in blood vessels (e.g., in vasculitis), in the renal glomerulus (e.g., in immune complex glomerulonephritis), or in the lung (e.g., Goodpasture's syndrome).

C. Neoplasms

1. **Ultrastructural analysis** is helpful in identifying the nature of a neoplasm and the cells of its origin, but neoplastic cells may be difficult to distinguish from normal regenerating cells at the ultrastructural level. When EM is used to help in establishing the diagnosis of a neoplastic disease, it must be combined with clinical findings and light microscopy, and the biologic characteristics of the cells must be considered.

2. **Diagnostic structures.** Certain subcellular organelles and structures are characteristic of various bodily cell types. These include:
   a. **Junctional complexes between cells.** These complexes are often defective in neoplasms. **Desmosomes** abound in well-differentiated carcinomas, but usually are sparse in poorly differentiated ones. Nonetheless, finding them can distinguish a carcinoma from a lymphoma (which lacks desmosomes).
   b. **Surface villi.** The length of the microvilli can be helpful in identifying tumor type (Table 2-2).
   c. **Mitochondria.** The shape and number can be helpful.
   d. **Dense core granules.** Characteristic **granules** often are present and can aid in the diagnosis of certain tumors.
      (1) The dense core of granulated vesicles that are typical of endocrine cells often can permit recognition of carcinoids when the light microscopic morphology is deceptive.
      (2) Diagnosis of melanomas can be a problem when they are undifferentiated (inconspicuous pigment). Melanosomes and premelanosomes, however, often can be recognized by their characteristic elongated granules on EM, which can be of great help in the diagnosis (see V D 5 c).

Table 2-2. Selected Examples of Diagnostic EM Findings in Tumors

Tumor	Structure	Comment
Thymoma	Desmosome	Epithelial differentiation eliminates mediastinal lymphoma
Histiocytosis X	Birbeck granule	This granule is present only in this disease of Langerhans' histiocytes
Melanoma	Premelanosome	This type of dense core granule is not present in carcinomas
Rhabdomyosarcoma	Z-bands	Skeletal muscle differentiation eliminates other round cell tumors
Liposarcoma	Lipid droplet	The droplet is not present in other sarcomas
Carcinoid	Dense core granules	These granules are absent from nonneuroendocrine tumors
Islet cell tumors	Dense core granules	Each type of granule has a specific shape (e.g., insulin, glucagon)
Mesothelioma	Long microvilli	Pleural tumor is confirmed
Adenocarcinoma	Short microvilli	Metastatic tumor to pleura is confirmed

3. Diagnosis by EM
   a. Although EM is not a substitute for the light microscope, **ultrastructural features** of the cell can help in establishing the diagnosis of various types of tumors. Thus, EM studies may be of value when the surgical pathologist (who reads all biopsies and resections from surgery) is confronted with any of the following situations:
   (1) Differential diagnosis of carcinomas, sarcomas, and lymphomas
   (2) Confirmation of the diagnosis of thymoma
   (3) Unequivocal diagnosis of histiocytosis X, melanoma, rhabdomyosarcoma, leiomyosarcoma, angiosarcoma, and neurogenic sarcomas
   (4) Differentiation between fibrous histiocytoma and liposarcoma
   (5) Identification of cell type in islet cell, carcinoid, and other related tumors in order to distinguish them from poorly differentiated ductal carcinomas
   (6) Differential diagnosis of undifferentiated small round cell tumors
   b. Examples (see also Table 2-2)
   (1) The ultrastructural diagnosis of **squamous cell carcinomas** (SCC), regardless of origin, is based on the presence of desmosomal attachments and cytoplasmic tonofibrils, the morphologic ultrastructural counterparts of keratinization. Desmosomes, although not usually prominent in poorly differentiated neoplasms, do persist in even the poorly differentiated SCCs, as exemplified in the lymphoepithelial carcinoma of the nasopharynx, a neoplasm often difficult to differentiate from lymphoreticular lesions.
   (2) The presence of desmosomes almost always excludes the possibility of **sarcoma or lymphoma**. It must be appreciated, however, that simple cell junctions (as opposed to the fully developed desmosome) do occur in sarcomas as well as in carcinomas, and focal thickening of opposed cell membranes is not uncommon in sarcoma.
   (3) With **adenocarcinomas,** desmosomes are present, as well as tight junctions between neighboring cells and true acini. Microvilli usually are present (though **short**), recapitulating the glandular formations of the parent tissue. However, all adenocarcinomas appear similar.
   (4) In diffuse pleural **mesotheliomas,** mesothelial cells are joined by desmosomes, have abundant tonofilaments, and are studded with very **long** microvilli; adjacent cells delineate systems of communicating channels.

D. Examples of EM use for specific systems

1. Liver
   a. Many hepatic diseases are impossible to diagnose precisely by light microscopy, and new pathologic entities (e.g., new viruses) are being revealed through the use of EM. Hepatic parenchymal cell damage can be estimated with EM.
   b. In the future, morphometric techniques (which measure cell size and shape) should provide more accurate correlations with liver function tests.

2. Kidney. Often correlated with immunologic results, the ultrastructural analysis of renal diseases has important clinical and prognostic relevance.
   a. Modern nephrology relies on EM for diagnosis of the primary lesion, analysis of therapeutic effects, and analysis of types of rejection in transplant patients.
   b. Certain renal disorders (lipoid nephrosis, minimal lupus nephritis) show no light microscopic lesions but do exhibit ultrastructural abnormalities.

3. Hematopoietic system
   a. Ultrastructural studies of hematopoietic tissues, particularly blood buffy-coat and marrow samples, have helped pathologists reach more precise diagnoses in a variety of serious hematologic conditions, including the acute leukemias, hairy-cell leukemia, Sézary syndrome, granulocytic sarcoma, and "nonsecretory" myeloma.
   b. Ultrastructural studies of hematopoietic tissues meet two major objectives:
   (1) The solution of diagnostic problems that cannot be resolved by routine light microscopy, such as distinguishing a lymphoma from a chloroma (a local collection of leukemic cells)
   (2) A better understanding of both the cytogenesis and pathogenesis of blood diseases

4. Nervous system. EM has replaced the special stains of the past because of its ease of use and the reproducibility of results.
   a. EM permits the **characterization of abnormalities** that are poorly definable by light microscopy (e.g., inclusion bodies, storage substances).

    b. Even in autopsy material, EM allows the **identification of virions** and other infectious agents and portrays cytopathic effects that are currently attributed to "slow" viruses.

5. Skin. Ultrastructural investigations have shed new light on the pathogenesis of certain skin diseases, such as the bullous diseases, some of which have been shown to have immune deposits or complexes. EM of skin biopsy specimens may be classified by the type of structure identified.

    a. Intracellular virus particles (e.g., molluscum contagiosum virus, herpesvirus) can be identified readily in infected cells through EM, although not all viruses can be distinguished structurally from others of the same group.

    b. Cell types in insufficiently differentiated tumors frequently may be identified by EM demonstration of specific organelles or other ultrastructural features.

    c. Malignant melanoma may be identified by the presence of melanosomes or unpigmented premelanosomes.

        (1) EM provides results even when the amount of melanin formed is too small to be seen through light microscopy.

        (2) This use of EM is especially valuable in the differential diagnosis of metastatic melanoma when no primary tumor has been identified, because a **metastatic melanoma** is more frequently **unpigmented** compared to a primary malignant melanoma. Metastases may become clinically evident years after the removal of a presumed mole or in the absence of any known primary lesion in patients with metastatic melanoma.

6. Endocrine system

    a. An endocrine cell examined by light microscopy often is distinguished by the number of endosecretory (neurosecretory or dense core) granules in the cytoplasm. However, EM is necessary for adequate evaluation of the granules, especially when they are sparse. Correlation of EM findings with IHC findings allows even better definition of the cell type and product.

    b. EM has identified unrecognized tumors as probably derived from endocrine cells. For example, direct EM, used with silver stains and ultrastructural immune techniques, may permit early identification of endocrine cells in utero and help to determine the origin of such cells.

    c. EM is helpful in identifying tumors that occur in families with multiple endocrine neoplasia syndrome, but it does not differentiate between tumors that are associated with the syndrome and those that occur separately.

E. Disadvantages of EM

1. Instrumentation, technical assistance, and special processing are **expensive**.

2. Special preparation of tissues is a requirement.

    a. For optimal results, the freshly removed sample has to be placed in appropriate fixative immediately.

    b. If EM examination is performed on tissue routinely processed for conventional microscopy, the artifacts of inadequate tissue preservation make the examination suboptimal at best.

3. Although some rapid methods for EM are available, many laboratories require **several days for processing** and diagnostic interpretation.

4. In tumor diagnosis, **sampling error** is occasionally a major problem. It can occur if the minute EM specimen is taken from a nondiagnostic site in the tumor, which may show only reactive rather than neoplastic cells.

STUDY QUESTIONS

Directions: Each of the numbered items or incomplete statements in this section is followed by answers or by completions of the statement. Select the **one** lettered answer or completion that is **best** in each case.

1. A biopsy should be sent to pathology in which of the following modes?

(A) Fixed in formalin
(B) Fixed in alcohol
(C) Fresh in saline
(D) Frozen
(E) Fixed in a generic fixative

2. Cytologic examination of pleural effusions in a woman without a known primary cancer is most likely to reveal cells derived from which of the following malignant tumors?

(A) Lymphoma
(B) Mesothelioma
(C) Carcinoma of the breast
(D) Carcinoma of the lung
(E) Leiomyosarcoma

3. The cytologic abnormalities of malignant cells can be explained best by

(A) chromosomal anomalies
(B) excessive mucin content
(C) cell surface alterations
(D) a decrease in cellular glycogen content
(E) mitotic activity

4. The best method for detecting a clonal T-cell process is by

(A) in situ hybridization (ISH) for T-cell DNA
(B) immunohistochemistry (IHC) for T-cell markers
(C) cytologic examination for nuclear irregularity
(D) DNA gene rearrangement studies
(E) electron microscopic (EM) inspection of nuclear features

5. For immunohistochemical (IHC) analysis, employing either immunofluorescence or immunoperoxidase (IP) techniques, which characteristic is true?

(A) IHC can be used to define the origin of many tumor types
(B) Immunofluorescence methods provide a permanent slide
(C) The peroxidase method is less sensitive
(D) IP methods are preferred to identify immune complexes
(E) Polyclonal antibodies cannot be used

6. All of the following information should accompany a biopsy EXCEPT

(A) patient age and sex
(B) biopsy site
(C) pertinent laboratory values
(D) x-ray findings
(E) family history

7. Electron microscopy (EM) is useful for all of the following diagnostic purposes EXCEPT

(A) identifying viruses in tissues
(B) classifying a lymphoma as a B-cell or T-cell type
(C) making a diagnosis of Whipple's disease
(D) classifying a bullous skin disease as pemphigus
(E) identifying immune complexes in renal glomerulonephritis

8. Urinary cytology can detect all of the following disorders with great accuracy EXCEPT

(A) prostatic carcinoma
(B) lead poisoning
(C) papillary transitional carcinoma of the bladder
(D) cytomegalovirus (CMV)
(E) in situ carcinoma of the bladder

1-C	4-D	7-B
2-C	5-A	8-A
3-A	6-E	

9. The fine-needle aspiration (FNA) biopsy method of obtaining a cytology sample is useful for all of the following reasons EXCEPT

(A) safety factor
(B) extreme accuracy
(C) cellular morphology preserved
(D) architectural details
(E) open biopsy elimination sometimes

10. Flow cytometry for DNA ploidy analysis can determine all of the following features of blood cells EXCEPT

(A) the number of dividing cells
(B) the number of resting cells
(C) the presence or absence of aneuploidy
(D) diploidy in malignant lesions
(E) presence of pathogens

11. Hybidization procedures, either by blot techniques or in situ methods, are useful for all of the following purposes EXCEPT

(A) identifying viral DNA in a specimen
(B) classifying a lymphoma to be of T-cell origin
(C) diagnosing certain types of anemia
(D) distinguishing breast cancer from ovarian cancer
(E) determining whether a lymph node is benign or malignant

Directions: The group of items in this section consists of lettered options followed by a set of numbered items. For each item, select the **one** lettered option that is most closely associated with it. Each lettered option may be selected once, more than once, or not at all.

Questions 12–15

Match each use for cancer diagnostic techniques with the appropriate response.

(A) Electron microscopy (EM)
(B) Immunohistochemistry (IHC)
(C) Both
(D) Neither

12. Differentiation between prostate cancer and gastric cancer

13. Differentiation between lymphoma and carcinoma

14. Differentiation between adenocarcinoma and mesothelioma

15. Localization of the primary site of a squamous cell carcinoma (SCC)

9-D	12-B	15-D
10-E	13-C	
11-D	14-C	

ANSWERS AND EXPLANATIONS

1. The answer is C *[I D]*.
When in doubt, a clinician should send a fresh specimen to pathology. This practice allows the pathologist or a clinical colleague acting as a consultant to deal best with the tissue and aliquot portions in various ways for the tests, which may be required for a proper diagnosis.

2. The answer is C *[II C 6]*.
Numerous studies have shown that when malignant disease causes pleural effusions in patients without known cancer, most of the effusions contain adenocarcinoma cells. Statistically, the usual primary sites for such tumors are the breast in women and the lung in men. Lymphoma, mesothelioma, and leiomyosarcoma are rarely diagnosed by cytologic studies, although cells from such tumors may appear in pleural effusions.

3. The answer is A *[II B 2]*.
Only alterations in the nucleus that reflect chromosomal changes (e.g., increased size, abnormal shape) are diagnostic of malignancy. Cell surface alterations give rise to cytologic abnormalities but these are not diagnostic. Mitotic figures are not specific for cancer, since such changes also are seen in granulation, tissue repair, and other processes. The presence or absence of glycogen or mucin may aid the pathologist in defining tumor type, but not in determining whether a tumor is malignant.

4. The answer is D *[IV B 1 c, 2 b]*.
A clonal T-cell lesion can be identified by the fact that one of the T-cell receptor genes is rearranged. Cytologically and ultrastructurally, T cells do have more nuclear irregularity than B cells, but this will not differentiate a clonal process from a reactive one. Currently, no T-cell–specific DNA is available for in situ hybridization (ISH). Immunohistochemical (IHC) markers may determine a large percentage of T helper cells in a lesion (e.g., in mycosis fungoides or cutaneous T-cell lymphoma), but no marker detects T-cell clonality, unlike the case in B-cell neoplasms, which show either kappa (κ) or lambda (λ) expression.

5. The answer is A *[III B 2 b, C 1]*.
Immunohistochemical (IHC) analysis for tumor markers has revolutionized pathology because many antigens remain preserved in paraffin-embedded tissues—the routine way tissues are processed. The immunoperoxidase (IP) staining method provides a permanent slide (a major advantage of this method over immunofluorescence, which provides only temporary slides that may be difficult to read). Moreover, the IP method allows later review of the slide without loss of immunoreactivity. This method has greatly aided in tumor diagnosis by defining antigens in many tumor types. When comparing IP methods, the more enzyme molecules localized to the antigen site, the more substrate will be deposited there, making the method more sensitive. Because immune complexes are so small, they are better seen with the higher contrast of immunofluorescence—the one preferred use of this technique over IP methods. Polyclonal antibodies can be used although they have some disadvantages.

6. The answer is E *[I A]*.
Pathologists do not diagnose lesions in a vacuum, although a common misconception is that they do. Many decisions require the entire clinical picture. Information on the request form enables the pathologist to determine whether preliminary thoughts fit the usual clinical picture of a disease state.

7. The answer is B *[V A 2, 3, B 2]*.
Electron microscopic (EM) study of tissues allows identification of a variety of disease processes. Ultrastructurally, it is easy to identify viruses, bacteria (e.g., as seen in Whipple's disease histiocytes), and immune deposits (e.g., as seen in the skin in pemphigus and in the renal glomeruli in glomerulonephritis). However, only immunohistochemistry (IHC) or DNA gene rearrangements can distinguish one type of lymphoma from another.

8. The answer is A *[II C 2]*.
Normally, very few prostatic cells, whether benign or malignant, are exfoliated into the urine. Bladder lesions, in situ cancer, invasive papillary or nonpapillary cancer, and lead poisoning can be detected readily by appropriate examination of urine specimens prepared and screened adequately. Cytomegalovirus (CMV) inclusions in bladder epithelium also have a characteristic cytologic appearance, which can be readily diagnosed.

9. The answer is D *[II D].*
Only individual cells or small groups are seen and, therefore, tissue architecture cannot be evaluated by this method (as it can be in an ordinary biopsy). This drawback of fine-needle aspiration (FNA) biopsy makes it inappropriate for the diagnosis of certain lesions (e.g., follicular or nodular lymphoma) that require attention to tissue patterns or architecture. The FNA biopsy method of obtaining cytology specimens is a safe, simple, quick, and very accurate procedure; it can be used to diagnose tumors in some situations and may eliminate the need for surgery. Cellular morphology (i.e., cell size and shape) is well preserved by this method.

10. The answer is E *[IV A 2, 3].*
Flow cytometry can determine the number of dividing cells (those in cell cycle phases S and G_2) and the number of resting cells (those in phases G_0 and G_1). This quantitation is clinically useful information. Most carcinomas and many sarcomas are aneuploid; however, a high frequency of diploidy is found in leukemias and lymphomas and in some carcinomas and sarcomas. Therefore, diploidy in a lesion is not equivalent to benignancy. Detection of pathogens is accomplished with hybridization techniques.

11. The answer is D *[IV B].*
Currently, there is no way to distinguish various types of carcinomas by hybridization techniques. These techniques do allow the isolation and identification of minute DNA fragments. DNA probes to various substances enable hybridization techniques to be quite valuable in the diagnosis of infectious diseases, inherited disorders, and malignancies. Viral DNA and abnormal hemoglobins, such as hemoglobin S in sickle cell anemia, can be identified. Likewise, probes for rearranged immunoglobulin or T-cell receptor proteins characterize malignant lymphomas; they will not be found in a reactive (benign) lymph node.

12–15. The answers are: 12-B, 13-C, 14-C, 15-D *[III C 2 b (1), (3) (b); V C 2 a, b, 3 b].*
Both prostate cancer and gastric cancer are adenocarcinomas; and, structurally, they appear similar under the electron microscope (EM). However, the two cancers can be distinguished by immunohistochemical (IHC) testing for prostatic-specific antigen, a tissue marker that is valuable in identifying prostatic cancer.

Carcinomas reveal cell-to-cell junctions (called desmosomes) when viewed with an EM; lymphomas do not demonstrate these ultrastructural components. The IHC profile of a carcinoma is cytokeratin (CK) positive and leukocyte common antigen (LCA) negative, whereas a lymphoma is CK negative and LCA positive.

EM examination reveals long microvilli in a mesothelioma and short microvilli in an adenocarcinoma. IHC analysis usually reveals the presence of carcinoembryonic antigen (CEA) in adenocarcinomas, whereas most mesotheliomas do not express CEA.

All squamous cell carcinomas (SCC), regardless of origin, look alike ultrastructurally. Unfortunately, no markers currently used in IHC can help to identify the primary site of an SCC.

3
Neoplasia
Virginia A. LiVolsi

I. INTRODUCTION

A. Definitions and nomenclature. In a number of instances, exceptions to the following definitions have been established by long use; the most common ones are mentioned.

1. **Neoplasia** is the autonomous proliferation of cells without response to the normal control mechanisms governing their growth. As used by investigators, clinicians, and the laity alike, neoplasia is often the equivalent of cancer. However, neoplasia may be benign or malignant.
   a. **Benign neoplasms** extend but do not invade local tissues or spread to other sites. They are generally associated with a good prognosis.
   b. **Malignant neoplasms,** commonly called **cancers,** can invade local tissue and can disseminate (**metastasize**) to other tissues and organs. They are generally associated with a poor prognosis. Malignant neoplasms are named on the basis of their cellular origin.
      (1) **Carcinomas** are malignancies that derive from the ectoderm and endoderm.
      (2) **Sarcomas** are malignancies of mesodermal origin.
      (3) Carcinomas and sarcomas have further descriptive terms that indicate their histopathology; examples are **leiomyosarcoma** (smooth muscle), **squamous cell carcinoma** (SCC), and **adenocarcinoma** (glandular).
      (4) **Leukemias** are malignancies of the hematopoietic series; **lymphomas** are malignancies of the immune system.

2. **Hypertrophy** is an enlargement in **individual cell size,** causing a corresponding increase in tissue mass. Cellular proliferation is controlled.

3. **Hyperplasia** is an increase in the **number of cells,** causing a corresponding increase in tissue mass.

4. **Metaplasia** is the replacement of one adult tissue type by another; usually the replacement (i.e., the metaplastic tissue) is simpler in form.

5. **Dysplasia** literally means any abnormal growth. However, the term has come to have several more restricted meanings.
   a. It covers such congenital defects as dysplastic (malformed) kidneys.
   b. More commonly, dysplasia connotes cytologic abnormalities that most believe to be precursors of malignant neoplastic changes. These abnormalities include disorderly architectural changes and pleomorphism (a multiplicity of sizes and shapes); frequent mitoses, often in odd locations; and unusually large, hyperchromatic (deeply staining) nuclei.

6. **Anaplasia** is a loss of the cell's normal morphologic and functional characteristics. In practice, anaplasia equals malignancy (i.e., with cancer).
   a. Anaplastic cells resemble more primitive cells of similar tissue. The more primitive (embryonic) the cells appear, the more anaplastic they are.
   b. Anaplasia literally means "backward formation." However, the anaplastic process is a failure to develop into a differentiated cell, not a progressive loss, or dedifferentiation, of cellular specialization. Hence, the earlier concept that malignancy is due to dedifferentiation has disappeared.

7. A **tumor** is, literally, any swelling, including an inflammatory mass (e.g., an abscess), but the term has become a synonym for neoplasm, and thus is equivalent to the term cancer.

B. Epidemiology

1. **United States.** Cancer is the second leading cause of death, accounting for 20% of deaths compared to 38% from cardiac conditions, 10% from cerebrovascular disease, and 5% from accidents of various types.

2. **Worldwide.** By contrast, cancer is a less significant disease worldwide: In underdeveloped countries, malnutrition and parasitic infections (e.g., malaria) still account for more deaths than cancer does.

3. **Risk factors.** Four important factors said to increase the incidence of cancer are age, diet, environment, and genetic makeup.
   a. **Age**
      (1) With the population increasing in age, carcinogens have more time to exert their effects; additionally, the immunologic defenses of the elderly may be less effective than those of young people.
      (2) The crucial point is that cancer can occur at any age. Neoplasms may be congenital; and in the 1- to 14-year-old age-group, cancer accounts for 11% of deaths, second only to accidental death.
   b. **Diet**
      (1) Geographic differences in cancer rates partially reflect dietary differences.
         (a) The smoking of foods is known to produce chemical carcinogens. Icelandic people, who have an exceedingly high rate of esophageal cancer, eat large amounts of smoked fish.
         (b) A diet rich in fiber and low in animal fat and refined carbohydrates seems to discourage colorectal cancer. The African Bantus, on such a diet, have almost no incidence of colorectal cancer.
         (c) Japanese people who live in Japan have a high rate of cancer of the stomach, twice the rate of Japanese who have migrated to Hawaii and have adopted a Western diet. However, diet alone cannot be the total answer, since Japanese in Hawaii still have a higher rate of gastric cancer than do non-Japanese in the same environment.
      (2) Alcoholic beverages affect carcinogenesis when they are consumed frequently and excessively over long periods.
         (a) Although the alcohol per se appears not to be carcinogenic, it may potentiate effects of other substances in alcoholic beverages or may allow increased absorption of carcinogens.
         (b) The carcinogenic impact of alcohol is especially pronounced on hepatic cells and, when combined with tobacco use, even more pronounced on the mucosa of the esophagus, pharynx, and oral cavity. Coexisting (multiple primary) cancers occur twice as often among cirrhotic persons as among the noncirrhotic.
   c. **Environment.** The environmental agents associated with a high incidence of cancer include radiation and chemical pollution. Industrialization and development, along with the conquest of infection and malnutrition, bring an increase in cancer incidence.
      (1) An urban setting, with greater air and water pollution than a rural environment, leads to higher rates of cancer, especially lung cancer.
      (2) Smokers get lung cancer much more frequently than do nonsmokers. Smoking has also been linked to oral, pharyngeal, laryngeal, and bladder carcinoma.
      (3) Industrial workers exposed to agents such as asbestos and vinyl chloride develop cancer more often than do nonexposed groups.
      (4) Sexual activity may be related to cancer.
         (a) Possible carcinogens or cocarcinogens (e.g., certain viruses) may be venereally transmitted.
         (b) In the female reproductive tract, the uterine cervix has the highest association with malignant disease and its precursors.
            (i) The cervix shows an increased vulnerability to neoplasia after exposure to infection, particularly human papillomavirus (HPV) infection.
            (ii) Since squamous cervical neoplasia begins in the squamocolumnar junction, hyperplasia in this area that results from the irritation of infection may be one cause.
   d. **Genetic makeup.** In some families, predisposition to cancer appears to be hereditary. Nonhereditary chromosomal abnormalities also increase the risk of certain cancers.

(1) Clinical observations indicate that some forms of cancer have a mendelian basis of inheritance. For example, in families affected with xeroderma pigmentosum, familial polyposis of the colon, or multiple endocrine neoplasia syndromes, neoplasms are common and multiple; moreover, they often are found at an early age.

(2) Children with primary immunodeficiency disorders have an extremely high rate of lymphoid malignancies.

(3) The incidence of acute leukemia is 4 to 30 times higher in persons with Down syndrome than in the normal population.

(4) Translocation of chromosomes 8 and 14 is associated with Burkitt's lymphoma.

II. MECHANISMS OF CARCINOGENESIS.

A variable number of steps occur during the change from the normal to the fully malignant cell. The first step apparently occurs in a single cell (i.e., cancer is a monoclonal disease). The change (mutation) in the first neoplastic cell is a random process. Any given etiologic factor simply increases the probability that any particular cell will transform, but how this happens is still unknown.

A. Role of genetic instability

1. Initial transformation

a. Because of genetic instability (apparently greater in the neoplastic state), mutant cells are produced. Some are destroyed by metabolic disadvantage or immune mechanisms, but an occasional cell expresses a selective advantage over the original neoplastic cells and will give rise to the predominant subpopulation.

b. In time, this selection process leads to increasingly abnormal cells with the acquired properties of the fully developed cancer.

2. Subsequent role

a. The cancerous phenotype itself is unstable. With continued cell division and progression of the neoplastic process, a variety of subclones may appear as the progeny of a single cancer.

b. This clonal heterogeneity may manifest itself morphologically or biochemically. Each of the subclones can show differences in morphology, special product elaboration, and antigenicity.

c. Cancer cells display a type of clonal evolution that enables the insidious selection of the most aggressive, rapidly growing, and invasive clones. This selection process gives rise to subclones that are fiercely resistant to all known modes of therapy and eventually prove lethal.

3. Mutation hypothesis

a. Most neoplasms accompany a heritable alteration in the involved cells; that is, the transformation of a normal to a neoplastic cell involves changes within the genetic apparatus of the cell (**mutation**). Heredity, chemicals, physical agents, radiation, and viruses may be factors in this change.

b. Most investigators feel that neoplasia involves a multifactorial, multistage process of progressive mutation in the genetic makeup of cells. Several arguments favor this mutation hypothesis.

(1) All carcinogens (including chemicals, radiation, and viruses) are mutagenic.

(2) Defective DNA repair mechanisms, as occur in xeroderma pigmentosa, accompany an increased risk of neoplasia.

(3) Neoplasia is a clonal disease.

B. Role of carcinogens

1. A constant feature of carcinogens is their demonstrated **interaction with DNA**. This interaction is readily apparent for the three major classes of carcinogens, namely chemicals, viruses, and ionizing radiation. Each of these classes can intercalate with nuclear DNA and induce miscoding of genetic information.

2. Many carcinogens (often chemical by nature) must be metabolically **activated by cellular enzymes**. In the absence of the appropriate enzymes, transformation cannot occur.

3. Neoplasia has a minimum of two stages (at least in experimental settings): **initiation** (primary insult) and **promotion** (requiring other agents for full expression of the neoplasm).

a. An **initiator** causes alterations in DNA structure and is mutagenic.

b. A **promoter** stimulates replication of the mutant cells, apparently by acting on cell membranes. Alone, promoters are not carcinogens, and they must act after the initiator to produce cancer.

c. Two or more initiators, acting in combination, can induce transformation (**cocarcinogenesis**).

C. Role of viruses

1. General concepts

a. Functionally speaking, viruses are blocks of genetic material. Thus, once viruses are inside a cell, they can change the genetic information that the cell transmits to all its progeny.

b. Viruses of either the DNA or RNA type can cause the genetic transformation; and in some experimental systems, the viral genes seem necessary in maintaining the transformed state. The neoplastic change involves the integration of new genetic information from the virus—in the form of DNA nucleotide sequences—into the host's cellular genome.

2. Retroviruses and oncogenes

a. Retroviruses are RNA viruses. They replicate by forming a proviral DNA that integrates into host-cell DNA. The integrated provirus then acts just like host-cell genes, transmitting genetic information to the cell's progeny.

(1) Some retroviruses contain one or more nucleotide sequences capable of inducing malignant transformation. These sequences are called **viral oncogenes (v-*oncs*)**. Several v-*oncs* have been proven to induce cancers in experimental systems; none are definitely known to produce cancer in humans, although some viruses show strong evidence of doing so.

(2) Eukaryote cells contain genes with nucleotide sequences that are identical or closely similar (homologous) to v-*oncs*. These **proto-oncogenes,** or **cellular oncogenes (c-*oncs*),** are thought to be v-*oncs* precursors, picked up by retroviruses in the course of evolution.

b. Oncogenes probably confer a growth advantage on tumor cells.

(1) Different oncogenes appear to have different functions.

(a) Platelet-derived growth factor (PDGF) is encoded for by *sis*.

(b) An epidermal growth factor **receptor** is encoded for by c-*erb* B2.

(c) The genes that appear to be involved in transmitting signals from receptors are *ras* oncogenes.

(2) Certain oncogenes appear to interrelate. Stimulation of tumor cells with PDGF (the product of *sis* oncogene) leads to increased expression of other oncogenes, *myc* and *fos*.

(3) Some oncogenes have tyrosine kinase activity related to that of receptors for hormones and growth factors at the cell membrane.

c. Tumor suppressor genes. In some tumors, **loss** or **deletion** of certain genes **promotes** tumor growth.

(1) The **retinoblastoma (Rb) gene,** when added to cultured human osteosarcoma cells or retinoblastoma, depresses tumor growth. Studies of hereditary forms of retinoblastoma, in which bilateral tumors are found at a very young age or are a congenital condition, have given rise to the **Knudsen "two-hit" hypothesis** of tumor development. The first hit is a germinal mutation in all cells of the retina. The second hit involves an additional retinal cell mutation leading to tumor development. The gene involved—the Rb gene—has suppressor activity in the nonmutated form.

(2) The **p53 gene** and its encoded p53 protein product have unknown functions in normal cells. Addition of p53 gene into breast cancer cells in culture can suppress their growth. Mutations of p53 have been identified in many human tumors; these alterations in the gene theoretically remove suppressor activity and allow the tumor to grow.

(3) The rare **Li-Fraumeni** familial syndrome, in which multiple malignancies develop in family members at young ages, has been associated with germ-line mutation of the p53 gene.

d. Certain oncogenes have been found in patients with specific **human cancers,** although causation has not been proven.

(1) The oncogene c-*myc* is associated with a translocation between chromosomes 8 and 14 in Burkitt's lymphoma.

(2) The oncogene *ras* is associated with loss of the small arm of chromosome 11 in Wilms' tumor.

(3) The c-*erb* B2 oncogene is **overexpressed** in some breast cancers; this overexpression correlates with a poor prognosis.

(4) The n-*myc* oncogene **amplification** in childhood neuroblastoma correlates with a favorable prognosis.

(5) The *ras* oncogene **activation** in lung adenocarcinoma correlates with a poor prognosis.

3. DNA viruses

   a. Less is known about the role of DNA viruses in tumorigenesis.

   b. Carcinogenic DNA viruses code for certain proteins that are prerequisites for the transformation of cells, such as the SV40 virus **T antigens**. These substances, like the protein products of v-*oncs,* are membrane-associated and have protein kinase activity.

D. Role of endogenous factors

   1. The change from normalcy to malignancy is associated with increasing inflexibility of enzyme patterns. The reasons are unknown but may reflect the far greater number of free ribosomes in malignant cells than in normal cells.

   2. It is possible that all tumors pass through stages when they still depend on physiologic factors, but this concept has been documented only for endocrine-dependent tissues, such as the female breast. With time, due to tumor progression, a tumor loses its endocrine dependency, and hormonal manipulation ceases to influence its growth.

III. CHARACTERISTICS OF NEOPLASMS. Groups of abnormally proliferating cells can arise in any part of the body. These neoplasms share certain characteristics, both in vitro and in vivo. Besides the major components found in all neoplasms, important properties include clonality, autonomy, a blood supply, and, in malignant neoplasms, the capacity to metastasize.

A. Components. All neoplasms have a parenchyma and a stroma.

   1. The **parenchyma** comprises the neoplastic proliferating cells. Parenchymal morphology underlies the name assigned to a neoplasm, and parenchymal behavior determines whether a neoplasm is benign or malignant.

   2. The **stroma** comprises the supporting connective tissue and blood supply that allows the neoplasm to grow.

B. Clonality. In theory, a neoplasm represents the **progeny of one cell,** a clone, and in many neoplasms all cells show the same abnormal karyotype. Even when several chromosome patterns are present, marker chromosomes in each cell suggest that the different subpopulations derive from a common stemline, as in the following examples.

   1. Immunoglobulins from a myeloma (a plasma cell neoplasm) display a homogeneity that is characteristic of a single clone.

   2. Women have two types of cells: In one, the active X chromosome is maternally derived; in the other, it is paternally derived. If a woman who is heterozygous for an X-linked gene should develop cancer, all the cancer cells will be homozygous for that gene, strongly suggesting descent from a common precursor.

C. Autonomy. Neoplastic cells exhibit **uncontrolled proliferation;** that is, they are autonomous.

   1. Normally, inhibitory influences control cell growth and proliferation; for example, cell movement stops when two cells growing in tissue culture collide. Neoplastic cells, by contrast, tend to grow over one another.

   2. The property of autonomy is probably a factor when neoplastic cells show changes in morphology and membrane composition and, hence, in receptor sites.

D. Blood supply. Solid neoplastic growth requires the development of a blood supply to the neoplasm; that is, **neovascularization**. Without such a blood supply, solid neoplasms cannot grow beyond 2 to 3 mm in diameter.

   1. Various experiments have shown that neovascularization does not require direct cell-to-cell contact, either between neoplastic cells or between these cells and endothelial cells in blood vessels near the lesion.

2. The protein **tumor angiogenesis factor** stimulates endothelial cell mitosis and new vessel growth in tumors.

E. **Metastasis.** The major characteristic of cancer is its capacity to metastasize.

1. As the neoplastic clone undergoes mutation, the more aggressive subpopulations selected tend to be those with metastasizing potential.

2. Not only can such subpopulations travel, via the bloodstream or lymphatics, away from the initial focus of cancer, but they can also grow in organs other than those of their origin (e.g., liver or lung). Reasons for this ability remain unknown. However, such cell groups must be capable of both binding the body's defense mechanisms and penetrating lymphatic and vascular channels.

3. Each neoplasm tends to have **sites of predilection** for metastasis.
   a. Some of these patterns are determined by purely anatomic considerations; for example, the lung capillary bed is the first vascular sieve that "catches" intravenous tumor cells.
   b. Other patterns of tumor metastasis are explained only as more favorable sites for that particular neoplasm.

4. The **biochemical basis** of invasion and metastasis involves several factors.
   a. Cells of a malignant neoplasm are less tightly adherent than normal cells.
      (1) The calcium content in the malignant cell wall is lower than that in normal cells.
      (2) The negative surface charge of malignant cells tends to be high, and the cells tend to repel one another.
   b. Some neoplasms produce hyaluronidase and other enzymes, which may facilitate invasion through tissue ground substance.

F. **DNA ploidy.** The majority (more than 70%) of malignant neoplasms show abnormal DNA content by cytometric measurements; that is, they are **aneuploid**. Normal cells show **diploid** DNA patterns. This finding is of clinical use in that aneuploid tumors (in breast, colon, or ovarian cancer) confer a poor prognosis.

IV. **IMMUNE HOST RESPONSES TO MALIGNANT NEOPLASMS.** At least in animal studies, autoimmune reactions to cancer cells are common. However, the ability of cancer cells to stimulate the immune mechanism in humans is usually quite small and is probably inconsequential as a defense mechanism.

A. **Tumor antigens**

1. Some antigens on the surface of cancer cells are much the same as those on normal cells (e.g., organ-specific antigens and histocompatibility antigens).

2. Most cancer cells also appear to possess antigenic specificities that are nonexistent in normal cells. Some of these, such as carcinoembryonic antigen (CEA) and alpha-fetoprotein (AFP), may result from derepression of the parts of the genome that normally function only in embryonic life.

3. Animal studies have identified tumor antigens that are capable of stimulating resistance to a tumor implant in normal animals. They are called **tumor-specific** or **tumor-associated transplantation antigens** (**TSTA** or **TATA**), depending on whether they are found only on tumor cells or also on normal cells.

B. **Cellular and humoral defenses**

1. Because immunodeficient persons are prone to develop malignancies, a normal immunologic defense system against malignancy would seem likely. In vitro and animal studies have produced the following **data in support** of this assumption.
   a. **Cells that seem to destroy tumor cells** include:
      (1) Cytotoxic T cells that become sensitized by specific tumor antigens
      (2) Killer (K) cells that also recognize specific antigens
      (3) Natural killer (NK) cells that are not specifically sensitized
      (4) Macrophages, some activated by gamma-interferon, and some nonspecifically activated

    b. Immunoglobulins aroused by tumor antigens seem to aid in tumor destruction by:
       (1) Activating complement
       (2) Coating tumor cells, thereby enhancing their destruction by NK cells and macrophages.

  2. Several **findings oppose** the concept of **immunosurveillance against tumors**.
    a. The malignancies found in immunodeficient persons are mostly lymphomas, not the common epithelial cancers with high incidence rates.
    b. Immunologic mechanisms can also promote tumor growth, as well as fight it, through the actions of suppressor T cells and of unidentified humoral blocking factors, which appear to act via antigen–antibody complexes.

C. Immunotherapy potential

  1. Although immunologic surveillance may be weak to the point of nonexistence, immunotherapy for cancer may become possible, especially in tumors with strong in vitro evidence of an immune response to tumor cells.

  2. Since most, perhaps all, tumors have TSTAs, it may be possible to activate the important immune defense mechanism to greater levels of effectiveness. Clinical trials have been started with IFN and with interleukin 2 (IL-2)—both of which activate NK cells—and with NK cells themselves.

V. THE DIAGNOSIS OF CANCER. Many of the techniques being used in the diagnosis of malignant neoplasms are described in Chapter 2.

A. Identification of malignancy. Once a lesion has been identified as neoplastic, a prime duty of the pathologist is to determine whether the neoplasm is benign or malignant.

  1. The **gross appearance** of a lesion may suggest its degree of malignancy.
    a. Benign lesions tend to grow by expansion, compress surrounding structures, and often produce a well-defined capsule.
    b. Malignant lesions, by contrast, tend to infiltrate the surrounding tissues so that the borders of the lesions are not discrete, and no capsule is formed.

  2. The **histologic appearance** is of major diagnostic importance.
    a. The edges of malignant lesions are usually poorly demarcated, and individual neoplastic cells infiltrate the surrounding normal tissue.
    b. Lesions invade lymphatic channels and blood vessels.
    c. Anaplasia, or **lack of differentiation,** is a major indicator of malignancy.
       (1) In principle, the prime feature of neoplastic progression to malignancy is the stepwise loss of characteristics of the tissue of origin. Clinicopathologic studies have shown that in many types of cancer the better the differentiation, the better the prognosis.
       (2) In practice, malignant neoplasms range in histologic appearance from well differentiated to markedly anaplastic. Whereas a well-differentiated appearance may be seen in either a benign or a malignant neoplasm, anaplasia usually signifies malignancy.
       (3) The following are **features of anaplasia**.
         (a) Cells tend to be **pleomorphic,** that is, to vary in size and shape. **Giant cells** are common.
         (b) Cell **nuclei** also tend to be **large,** so that the nuclear:cytoplasmic ratio is higher than normal. Multiple and prominent **nucleoli** may be present, and **chromatin clumping** is seen.
         (c) **Mitotic figures** are numerous and often abnormal. Karyotypic analysis shows that many, although not all, malignant tumors are **aneuploid,** with an abnormal number of chromosomes.

B. Identification of precancerous lesions

  1. In many—if not all—systems (e.g., cervix, lung, colon), clinicopathologic studies have demonstrated that initial neoplastic change can be recognized in a preinvasive stage. Such changes can progress over a prolonged time span.
    a. Whether all malignant neoplasms arise as benign lesions, which then undergo progression, or whether some are highly malignant from the start is debatable.

    b. However, all neoplasms probably go through a benign preinvasive phase, even if this phase is often not recognized clinically.

  2. The morphologic alterations of cancer allow the trained pathologist to recognize not only the invasive malignant process, but also the preinvasive lesions (**carcinoma in situ**).

    a. In situ carcinomas are usually recognized in epithelial malignancies (not in sarcomas or lymphomas). They show the various morphologic changes of malignancy, but remain confined to the epithelial or mucosal surface.

    b. Developments in histopathology and cytopathology enable the screening of preinvasive (usually asymptomatic) cancer; once such a lesion is recognized, it can be effectively treated.

C. Grading and staging of malignancies. These prognostic measures attempt to express the degree of malignancy and aggressiveness of a tumor, as a guide to its clinical behavior and the probable outcome of therapy.

  1. The **grade** of a tumor describes its histologic degree of anaplasia and extent of invasion. Grade levels of I to IV are often used.

  2. The **stage** of a tumor describes its size, the extent of regional lymph node spread, and the presence or absence of metastases. Several **systems for staging** are in use.

    a. The **TNM system** assigns a **T** level of 1 to 4 for **t**umor size; an **N** level of 0 to 3 for **n**odal involvement; and an **M** level of 0 or 1 for **m**etastases.

    b. A simpler system incorporates this information into stages 0 to IV.

  3. Staging has proved more useful clinically than grading.

D. Tumor markers [see also Chapter 2 III C 2 b (3)]

  1. In some forms of cancer, a particular protein or other substance is found consistently enough in patients' serum that the substance can be used to screen for the cancer and to monitor cancer patients for recurrences. The substance may be an abnormal counterpart of a known body component, an excess of a normal component, or the reexpression of a fetal or embryonic substance. Two examples follow.

    a. From 40% to 90% of primary liver cancers show an associated elaboration of **AFP,** a substance regularly made by developing embryonic liver cells but not by normal adult tissue.

    b. The hormone **calcitonin,** normally produced by thyroid parafollicular cells, is elevated in the serum of patients with medullary thyroid cancer.

  2. Finding cancer-specific oncogenes or chromosomal abnormalities could provide invaluable new tumor markers. Besides serving a diagnostic or posttherapeutic use like the tumor markers previously described, these markers could be useful for identifying cancer-prone patients.

VI. CLINICAL MANIFESTATIONS OF CANCER

A. Both benign and malignant neoplasms can produce the following manifestations.

  1. They can be **asymptomatic**. Such a neoplasm might be noticed incidentally at physical examination, at unrelated surgery, or at autopsy.

  2. They can produce a **lump**.

  3. They can cause **obstruction**. A benign tumor, such as a leiomyoma of the small bowel, just like a malignant lymphoma of the small intestine, can occupy the lumen and obstruct it.

  4. They can cause **bleeding**. Benign neoplasms usually produce bleeding by expansive growth and erosion of the overlying surface. Cancers are more likely to invade the overlying surface tissues and ulcerate, as in adenocarcinoma of the stomach, or to infiltrate vessels and rupture them.

  5. They can produce **abnormal function**.

    a. In endocrine organs, for example, either a benign or malignant neoplasm can produce an excess of a specific hormone, since the neoplasm is not bound by normal feedback control mechanisms.

    b. Symptoms will be those of hormonal excess. Examples include hypercalcemia from a parathyroid adenoma and Cushing's syndrome from an adrenal adenoma.

6. They can **interfere with function**. A benign pituitary adenoma, for example, can replace the normal gland and lead to pituitary hormonal deficiencies. Similarly, a histologically benign glioma in the thalamic region of the brain can expand and lead to brain edema, herniation, and death.

B. **Problems more likely to occur with malignancies** include the following.

1. **Anemia**
   a. As a consequence of chronic low-grade blood loss (usually associated with gastrointestinal or genitourinary neoplasms), an iron deficiency anemia may be responsible for the initial symptoms (weakness and fatigue) of a cancer.
   b. Anemia also may result from poor nutrition, especially in oral and esophageal cancers, or from metastatic replacement of the red-cell–producing bone marrow.

2. **Malnutrition**
   a. This condition is most often noted in patients who have cancer of the head and neck or the upper gastrointestinal tract. However, many other cancer patients also exhibit poor nutrition.
   b. Sometimes malnutrition accompanies the gastric distress, nausea, and vomiting resulting from radiotherapy and chemotherapy.
   c. Carcinomas also may produce substances that interfere with intestinal absorption or produce anorexia. Although poorly characterized, such substances are strongly suspected to exist.

3. **Loss of function** can result from the mass effect of a cancer or from the replacement of normal tissue.

4. **Paraneoplastic syndromes.** These symptom complexes seen in cancer patients are not caused by the tumor, by its metastases, or by hormones secreted by the tumor's tissue of origin. The following are two of the most common.
   a. **Ectopic hormone production**
      (1) Peptide hormones such as adrenocorticotropic hormone (ACTH) and antidiuretic hormone (ADH) may be increased in some forms of lung cancer. The consequent symptoms of hormonal excess (e.g., Cushing's syndrome, hyponatremia) may become a life-threatening clinical problem.
      (2) These syndromes suggest that the regulation of cell differentiation tends to occur in bizarre and unexpected ways. These changes are not completely random, however, since particular types of tumors show particular patterns of aberrant differentiation.
   b. **Hypercoagulability.** This symptom can result in nonbacterial thrombotic endocarditis or venous thrombosis.

5. **Infections** are common in patients who have cancer and may occur for several reasons.
   a. An **obstructive** neoplasm (e.g., of a bronchus) can lead to postobstructive infection (e.g., pneumonia).
   b. **Altered host resistance** may permit relatively avirulent organisms (e.g., normal bacterial bowel flora) as well as common fungi, parasites, or viruses to cause infection and death.
      (1) **Serologic factors.** In lymphomas and leukemias, normal immunoglobulins are decreased, resulting in an increased susceptibility to and severity of infection.
      (2) **Cellular factors**
         (a) Decreased total mature granulocyte counts are found in patients with acute leukemia or with other neoplasms involving the bone marrow and also often follow intensive chemotherapy. Neutrophil function, as well as total count, is critical, since immature granulocytes phagocytize and kill bacteria less efficiently than mature leukocytes. Quantitative and qualitative abnormalities of neutrophil function include defects in chemotaxis, phagocytosis, and bactericidal capacity.
         (b) Patients with lymphoid malignancies (especially Hodgkin's disease) have alterations of cell-mediated immunity.
      (3) **Cytotoxic chemotherapy** has significant adverse effects on both B- and T-cell functions, resulting in diminished opsonization, inadequate lysis of bacteria, and defective neutralization of bacterial toxins.
      (4) Integumentary and mucosal **barriers can be disrupted** by a tumor or by its treatment (surgery, radiation), providing a nidus for microbial colonization and a portal for invasion. Breakdown of mucous membranes may lead to sepsis resulting from normal bowel flora.

    c. Malnutrition promotes infection by contributing to the loss of integrity of the skin and mucosal barriers, impairing phagocytosis, and depressing lymphocyte function.

    d. Microbial flora. Some 80% of infections that occur in cancer patients arise from endogenous flora. The flora can be altered by antibiotic and cancer chemotherapy agents; when such microbial changes occur in conjunction with other host defects, life-threatening infection can result.

6. Associated disorders may be of clinical or epidemiologic importance. For example, in medullary carcinoma of the thyroid, the finding of multiple nodules of tumor or hyperplastic parafollicular cells strongly suggests the presence of multiple endocrine neoplasia syndrome; since family members of an affected patient may be affected, they should also be evaluated.

STUDY QUESTIONS

Directions: Each of the numbered items or incomplete statements in this section is followed by answers or by completions of the statement. Select the **one** lettered answer or completion that is **best** in each case.

1. When histologically benign neoplasms prove fatal, they most likely do so because they

(A) cause extensive bleeding
(B) are multifocal
(C) fail to invoke an immune response
(D) interfere with organ function
(E) transform into carcinoma

2. Epidemiologic studies reveal a relationship between cancer incidence and all of the following factors EXCEPT

(A) advanced age
(B) nonhereditary chromosomal abnormalities
(C) air pollution
(D) bacterial infection
(E) diet

3. All of the following conditions can increase tissue mass EXCEPT

(A) hypertrophy
(B) inflammation
(C) neoplasia
(D) hyperplasia
(E) anaplasia

Directions: Each group of items in this section consists of lettered options followed by a set of numbered items. For each item, select the **one** lettered option that is most closely associated with it. Each lettered option may be selected once, more than once, or not at all.

Questions 4–7

Match each condition below with the related type of cancer.

(A) Malignant lymphoma
(B) Leukemia
(C) Uterine cervical cancer
(D) Hematoma

4. Down syndrome

5. Cirrhosis

6. Human papillomavirus (HPV) infection

7. Primary immunodeficiency

Questions 8–12

Certain oncogenes have prognostic implications in human tumors. Match the oncogene with the human tumor that is most commonly associated with it.

(A) Neuroblastoma
(B) Lung adenocarcinoma
(C) Breast carcinoma
(D) Burkitt's lymphoma
(E) Retinoblastoma

8. *ras*

9. n-*myc*

10. Rb

11. c-*myc*

12. c-*erb* B2

1-D	4-B	7-A	10-E
2-D	5-D	8-B	11-D
3-E	6-C	9-A	12-C

ANSWERS AND EXPLANATIONS

1. The answer is D *[VI A 6]*.
Although malignant transformation of a benign neoplasm may occur, it is rare. More often, fatality due to a benign neoplasm is the result of interference with the function of a vital organ. Bleeding due to the expansive growth of a benign tumor is less likely than bleeding due to the invasion and ulceration of tissues or to the infiltration and eventual rupture of vessels by a malignant tumor. Occasionally, multifocal benign neoplasms are found, but they are not a likely cause of death. Any neoplasm can invoke an immune response.

2. The answer is D *[I B 3]*.
The incidence of cancer tends to increase with age, possibly because of the cumulative effects of carcinogen exposure and the diminished immune defenses with advancing age. Certain cancers (e.g., multiple endocrine neoplasia syndromes) exhibit a mendelian basis of inheritance; other genetic factors (e.g., chromosome translocation, trisomy) also have been associated with an increased incidence of certain cancers. Environmental agents (e.g., air pollutants, industrial chemicals, cigarette smoke) are strongly associated with increased cancer rates, especially lung cancer. Certain dietary habits have been linked to decreased rates of cancer (e.g., a high-fiber, low–animal fat and protein diet with a reduced rate of colorectal cancer), whereas other habits have been associated with increased cancer rates (e.g., a diet high in smoked foods with an increased rate of esophageal cancer).

3. The answer is E *[I A 1–3, 6, 7]*.
Hypertrophy (i.e., an increase in the number of cells) and hyperplasia (i.e., an increase in the size of individual cells) are two processes that cause an increase in tissue mass. Edema and cells in inflammation cause the formation of a mass, and neoplasms produce mass lesions. Anaplasia is loss of a cell's morphologic and functional characteristics.

4–7. The answers are 4-B *[I B 3 d (3)]*, **5-D** *[I B 3 b (2) (b)]*, **6-C** *[I B 3 c (4) (b)]*, **7-A** *[I B 3 d (2)]*.
In some cancers, a substance (often a protein) is found in the serum of a significant number of patients and becomes regarded as a "marker" for that cancer. The substance, then, can be used to screen patients for the cancer and to monitor cancer patients for recurrences. Alpha-fetoprotein (AFP) is such a tumor marker, in that it is found in 40% to 90% of patients with hepatocellular carcinoma.

The incidence of many cancers appears to be affected by factors related to a patient's genetic makeup, age, dietary habits, environment, and general health. A few examples of such associations are given.

Genetic predisposition to cancer has been documented for a variety of malignancies. The incidence of acute leukemia is 4 to 30 times higher in persons with Down syndrome (a trisomy involving chromosome 21) than in the normal population. Also, children with primary immunodeficiency disorders have an extremely high incidence of malignant lymphoma.

Dietary habits that have been linked to the development of certain malignancies include heavy consumption of smoked foods, foods high in animal fat and protein, and alcohol. The carcinogenic impact of alcohol is particularly hard on the liver. In patients with alcoholic cirrhosis, the incidence of multiple primary tumors is twice as high as in noncirrhotic persons.

Environmental agents associated with cancer include irradiation, chemical pollution, and tobacco smoke as well as certain sexually transmitted viruses that act as cocarcinogens. Human papillomavirus (HPV) is one virus that appears to be able to reprogram the nuclei of growing cells and, perhaps, lead to certain cancers (most notably uterine cervical cancer).

8–12. The answers are: 8-B, 9-A, 10-E, 11-D, 12-C *[II C 2 e, f]*.
Amplification of n-*myc* oncogene is associated with improved prognosis in childhood neuroblastoma. Patients who have adenocarcinoma of the lung with amplification of *ras* oncogene fare less well than patients with a similar tumor stage but without *ras* amplification. Women who have breast cancers that overexpress c-*erb* B2 have poorer prognoses than women whose breast cancers do not. The oncogene c-*myc* is found in Burkitt's lymphoma, and the Rb suppressor gene was identified from retinoblastomas.

4

Environmental Pathology

John S. J. Brooks

I. SCOPE. Environmental pathology encompasses a group of disease states that result from any of a variety of environmental factors. Immediately apparent are physical agents (e.g., radiation, ultraviolet light, burns) and chemical factors (e.g., drugs, heavy metals, industrial organic compounds). However, humans are also affected by other types of environmental influences, which can be classified as cultural (e.g., alcohol, smoking), nutritional (e.g., diet, inadvertent toxic compounds in food), and occupational (e.g., pneumoconioses). Besides their environmental origin, a common denominator in all of these diseases is some degree of potential control by the individual or society. Even remote environmental issues, such as the "greenhouse" effect of increased atmospheric carbon dioxide or the depletion of the ozone layer, will ultimately affect human health.

II. PHYSICAL INJURY

A. Mechanical injury may result in a **contusion** (interstitial bleeding from blunt trauma), a **laceration** (a tear in tissues), or an **abrasion** (loss of superficial tissue layers).

B. Injury due to extremes of temperature

  1. Injury due to cold

  a. Frostbite results from prolonged exposure to freezing temperatures. Tissues appear white because of their inadequate blood supply, which results from vascular thromboses. Gangrenous necrosis may ensue.

  b. Hypothermia is a generalized condition in which the body temperature is lowered below normal. The skin is extremely pale because of marked vasoconstriction. While anyone may develop hypothermia when subjected to prolonged outdoor exposure to cold weather, the elderly are particularly susceptible and may develop hypothermia inside houses without adequate heating.

  2. Injury due to heat

  a. Heat stroke, the inability to dissipate body heat, may be seen in febrile patients or in those exposed to elevated ambient temperatures.

  (1) Physiologic cooling processes (e.g., sweating) are overwhelmed and become inactive; patients are, thus, dry and hot to the touch.

  (2) Persistent body hyperthermia results in and further causes generalized vasodilation, decreased effective blood volume, cellular hypoxia, and eventual life-threatening hyperkalemia.

  b. Thermal burns. The clinical significance of burn injury is related to its severity and extent. Severity, formerly categorized as first-, second-, or third-degree burns, is now classified as partial-thickness or full-thickness burns.

  (1) **Partial-thickness burns** are reddened areas that may show blisters but that are capable of self-repair.

  (2) **Full-thickness burns** are open wounds that result in the loss of large volumes of body fluids; they frequently require skin grafts. Systemic reactions, such as shock, result when the burns cover more than 20% of the body surface. Sepsis, often from *Pseudomonas aeruginosa,* is the most important cause of death. Modern management of burns has markedly reduced fatalities from thermal injury.

  (3) **Pulmonary injury** also occurs in patients **due to smoke inhalation**. Bronchial irritation may be severe, and noxious fumes may cause diffuse alveolar damage.

C. Electrical injury

1. The outcome of an electrical injury depends on the **type of current** (alternating or direct), the **amperage and voltage,** the **path** it takes through the body, and the **duration of contact**.

2. An **alternating current** is more dangerous than a direct current because it causes strong muscular contractions, often preventing the person from letting go of a high-tension wire.

3. **Flow of current** through the brain may disrupt critical cardiopulmonary functions and result in death.

D. Radiation injury

1. **Sources of radiation.** A person can be exposed to ionizing radiation from a number of sources.
   a. Daily **low-level radiation** from the sun is ever-present and (combined with ultraviolet rays) may be a factor in the development of skin cancers and melanoma in individuals with prolonged exposure.
   b. Direct **environmental exposure to large doses** (e.g., Hiroshima and Chernobyl) is associated with severe effects on multiple organ systems (see II D 4).
   c. **Diagnostic and therapeutic procedures** expose a person to additional irradiation.

2. **Mechanisms of injury**
   a. The following theories are proposed.
      (1) The **direct,** or **target, theory** states that radiant energy exerts its effect by direct hits on target molecules, such as DNA within cells. Single or multiple hits might be required for damage or cell killing.
      (2) The **indirect action theory** states that effects result from production of free radicals within cells, which, in turn, react with critical cellular components, such as membranes, nucleic acids, and enzymes.
   b. The biologic effect may not be apparent for some time—even decades; radiation damage, therefore, has a **latency period**. The indirect theory better explains the latent effects of radiation.

3. **Variables influencing degree of injury**
   a. **Quantity (dose) of radiation**
      (1) The **roentgen (R)** gives a **measure of radiation exposure** in air and applies only to x-rays and gamma rays.
      (2) More important is the **quantity absorbed** in the tissues.
         (a) The unit of measure is the **rad** (**r**adiation **a**bsorbed **d**ose), which applies to all forms of ionizing radiation. One rad equals the energy absorption of 100 ergs/g [in International System (SI) units, 0.01 joule/kg].
         (b) Recently introduced is the **gray (Gy),** the SI unit of absorbed dose; 1 Gy equals 1 joule of energy per kg of tissue. Thus, 1 Gy equals 100 rads, and 1 rad equals 0.01 Gy, or 1 cGy (centigray).
   b. **Time frame.** Not only the total dose of radiation absorbed, but also the **dose rate** influence the effects of radiation.
      (1) A large dose of radiation received all at once has a far greater effect, particularly on normal tissues, than the same total dose given as fractional doses over several incidents.
      (2) Therapeutic radiation is always split into fractions [commonly 200 rads (2 Gy) each] given over weeks to months until the selected total dose is reached.
   c. **Type of radiation**
      (1) **Electromagnetic waves,** in the form of x-rays, for example, are far less destructive than the same dose in the form of particles.
      (2) **Particles** of higher mass, such as alpha particles, are more damaging than beta particles.
   d. **Linear energy transfer (LET)** defines the amount of energy transferred to the tissues per unit length of path; it relates to such variables as mass and velocity.
      (1) For the equivalent amount of energy, **beta particles** are smaller, move faster, and penetrate deeper than alpha particles, but they deliver less energy per unit length (and, thus, have a lower LET value).
      (2) **Gamma rays** also have a lower LET value, because they have greater penetrability and dissipate energy over a longer distance.
   e. **Relative biologic effectiveness (RBE)** relates to the amount of actual cellular damage

caused by a specific radiation dose. The RBE relates the absorbed dose (equivalent in the following examples) to the actual biologic effect.

   (1) X-rays, when uniformly distributed in a tissue field, may affect all cells but none seriously (**lower RBE**).

   (2) Alpha particles, which are heavier, would hit the tissues randomly but would be lethal to the subpopulation of cells that were hit (**higher RBE**).

f. Tissue properties

   (1) Penetrance. Some tissues (e.g., subcutaneous adipose tissue and certain organs) offer far less resistance to radiation than does the outer cutaneous shell.

   (2) Oxygenation. Radiation affects hypoxic central regions of tumors less than it affects the more oxygenated tumor periphery and surrounding normal areas.

g. Cell type

   (1) Cells are affected in direct proportion to their normal rate of mitotic activity and reproduction and in inverse proportion to their level of specialization.

   (a) High radiosensitivity. Rapid cell turnover is characteristic of the hair follicles, gastrointestinal tract, bone marrow, lymphoid system, and germ cells. Acute radiation sickness, thus, results in hair loss, nausea, vomiting, diarrhea, and susceptibility to bleeding and infection.

   (b) Low radiosensitivity. The cells of certain organs (e.g., kidney, liver, pancreas) and tissues (e.g., mature cartilage, muscle) rarely divide and are, thus, relatively less affected by radiation. Gradual loss of function may result when such organs are within a therapeutic radiation field.

   (c) Intermediate radiosensitivity. Most other body tissues (e.g., connective tissue, vessels, urothelium) lie between the two extremes just described.

   (2) Tumor cell types generally reflect their normal counterparts in terms of radiosensitivity. Thus,

   (a) Lymphomas and germ cell tumors may be cured by radiation if localized. Leukemic cells are also radiosensitive.

   (b) Intraabdominal tumors are difficult to reach with an effective dose without causing significant gastrointestinal complications.

   (c) The postoperative site of an extremity sarcoma may be sterilized since a higher dose can be achieved without a significant effect on surrounding structures.

4. Tissue effects of radiation

a. General changes include cytoplasmic swelling; formation of bizarre pleomorphic nuclei in both tumor cells and surrounding fibroblasts; vascular damage, including thrombosis and perivascular and intimal fibrosis; and tissue necrosis.

   (1) Cells in the G_2 and M phases of the cell cycle are more vulnerable than those in the G_1 and S phases.

   (2) Tissues not killed by therapeutic radiation "remember" its effects, and reirradiation of an area is generally avoided because it results in substantial loss of normal tissues through necrosis.

b. Effects on specific tissues

   (1) Organs. Due to the effect of radiation on the vasculature, a common result is partial or complete organ atrophy with fibrosis.

   (2) Skin. Radiodermatitis appears as thin, atrophic, hyperpigmented or depigmented skin. Changes may persist for decades.

   (3) Blood. Whether peripheral blood cytopenias occur depends on the **field of exposure**.

   (a) With a large field, lymphopenia may appear in hours, granulocytopenia in a week, and thrombocytopenia thereafter. Anemia may not occur for several weeks [red blood cells (RBCs) are radioresistant] but may persist because of marrow damage. Marrow recovery takes several months.

   (b) A small field may produce no appreciable effects on blood cells.

   (4) Gonads. Sterility is a common result if gonads are included in the field of exposure. Ovarian follicles are relatively more radiosensitive than the testes. Menses may cease, temporarily or permanently.

   (5) Lungs. Pulmonary interstitial fibrosis may lead to shortness of breath and even to acute respiratory insufficiency within weeks or even months. The alveolar septae are widened, and fibrosis prevents air exchange in those affected.

   (6) Intestines. Mucosal atrophy and ischemia may lead to bowel necrosis or stricture formation.

(7) **Nervous tissue.** Adult nervous tissue is relatively resistant, but high cranial doses can cause brain necrosis. In children, the long-term effects of radiation may be severe because further development of the brain is impeded.

5. **Dosage levels and bodily effects of radiation**
   a. **Total-body radiation**
      (1) The **lethal range** for humans begins at about 300 rads. About 50% of people die in one month when exposed to 350 to 500 rads. Above that level nearly all die, and death within days is certain at 1000 rads.
      (2) An **acute radiation sickness** occurs in those exposed to 100 to 300 rads, but no deaths are expected. A whole-body dose of 10 to 50 rads generally produces no obvious effect.
   b. **Limited fields** (e.g., those treated in cancer therapy) are often given a high dose (exceeding 4000 rads) without significant systemic effect.
   c. **Diagnostic x-rays,** by contrast, use only minor dosages: A chest x-ray delivers about 0.02 rad; intravenous pyelography, or a barium enema, 0.1 to 0.2 rad; an abdominal computed tomography (CT) scan, about 1.5 to 2.5 rads. Such levels are associated with a very low, and hypothetical, risk of inducing future neoplasms.

6. **Long-term effects of radiation.** The late carcinogenic effect of radiation is clear. Some of the more common tumors that develop after therapeutic radiation are shown in Table 4-1. Many other tumors in almost any site or organ have been reported as late complications of radiation.

7. **Nuclear disasters.** Occasionally, dangerous levels of radiation are released into the atmosphere from a nuclear accident such as the one at Chernobyl. Thus, the following actions form the basis of a medical response.
   a. The **weather pattern** should be determined in order to chart the area of greatest damage.
   b. **Animals and food** derived from animals should be protected from the effects of radiation (e.g., cow's milk may show radioactivity in several forms and should not be marketed).
   c. **Iodine** should be given to all potential victims to prevent thyroid uptake of radioactive iodine.
   d. **Acute radiation sickness** can be expected in those closest to the disaster.
   e. The **water supply** should be tested and, if unsafe, an external source provided.
   f. An **evacuation of the area** should be undertaken as soon as possible.
   g. The **long-term effects** of radiation should be monitored. Subsequent development of leukemias, thyroid cancer, and other tumors is to be expected, therefore, periodic examinations should be conducted.

III. CHEMICAL INJURY. Adverse reactions to medicinal agents are discussed in V.

A. **Methyl alcohol (methanol, wood alcohol).** This type of alcohol is found in solvents, Sterno, paint removers, and antifreeze. The toxic dose is small (20 mg).

1. Metabolites, such as formic acid and formaldehyde, produce a **metabolic acidosis**.

Table 4-1. Tumors Developing as Late Complications of Radiation Therapy

Initial Site Irradiated	Later Tumor Development	
	Type of Tumor	Delay in Appearance (years)
Skin	Squamous cell carcinoma (SCC)	8–50
	Lymphomas, leukemias	5–20
Tumors of head, neck, mediastinum	Thyroid cancer	5–20
Soft tissue, bone	Sarcoma [most commonly malignant fibrous histiocytoma (MFH) and osteosarcoma]	5–20

2. These metabolites are toxic to the retina and cortical neurons; they may also cause central nervous system (CNS) depression. Although **visual changes** are reversible if the injury is mild, blindness may result.

B. Kerosene. Generally, intoxication comes from inhaling fumes in poorly ventilated homes. Fulminant bronchopneumonia results, together with drowsiness from its CNS depressant action. Patients are mainly children age 1 to 6.

C. Chloroform and carbon tetrachloride. These agents, found in cleaning fluids, induce centrilobular fatty changes or necrosis of the liver. Renal tubular necrosis may also occur and lead to oliguria. Toxicity may persist for long periods because these substances are slowly released from fatty stores.

D. Insecticides and polychlorinated biphenyls (PCBs)

    1. Insecticides produce acute or chronic toxicity.

        a. Acute toxicity is found in farmers or other occupational users who absorb these agents through the skin or the respiratory and gastrointestinal tracts. Since insecticides persist in soil and water for long periods, they contaminate the food chain and then travel to concentrate in adipose tissue where they are stored.

        b. Chronic toxicity may result from long-term exposure to small daily quantities, as in contaminated food.

    2. Common insecticides

        a. Chlorinated hydrocarbons [chlordane, aldrin, dichlorodiphenyltrichloroethane (DDT)] produce hyperexcitability followed by delirium and convulsions.

        b. Organophosphates (malathion, dimpylate, pyrophosphates) inhibit acetylcholinesterase (AChE), causing muscle twitching, flaccid paralysis, and cardiac arrhythmias.

    3. PCBs are related to DDT and were once used in adhesives. Their use is now restricted to closed industrial systems since they persist in the environment forever and have contaminated the food chain. Human exposure to PCBs produces chloracne, impotence, and—possibly—infertility.

E. Mushroom poisoning. Different mechanisms account for the toxicity of the following most dangerous types of mushrooms.

    1. *Amanita muscaria* produces a toxin with almost **immediate parasympathomimetic effects**— salivation, sweating, pupillary constriction, gastrointestinal symptoms, bradycardia, and hypotension. Recovery is the rule.

    2. *Amanita phalloides,* by contrast, is associated with a death rate of 30% to 50%. Its main toxin, amanitine, inhibits RNA polymerase, and its effects show **delayed onset** of 6 to 24 hours. Severe gastrointestinal and cardiac symptoms then develop with collapse, convulsions, and coma. Centrilobular hepatic necrosis and acute renal tubular necrosis also result.

F. Carbon monoxide (CO)

    1. This odorless, tasteless gas acts as a systemic asphyxiant by forming stable **carboxyhemoglobin,** which is incapable of binding oxygen. The affinity of CO for hemoglobin is 200 times the affinity of oxygen.

    2. The **cherry-red color of both blood and dependent skin is the hallmark** in acute poisoning; it results from the carboxyhemoglobin. Diffuse punctate hemorrhages, hypoxia, coma, and death ensue quickly.

    3. CO is released by **incomplete combustion**. Concentrations of 1% CO can be fatal in 10 to 20 minutes. The 7% CO of automobile exhaust can produce lethal blood levels (60% to 70% hemoglobin saturation) within 5 minutes in a closed garage.

    4. Chronic exposure to CO (e.g., from air pollution) can produce headaches.

G. Cyanide

    1. An inhibitor of oxidative respiration via the **cytochrome oxidase system,** cyanide is highly lethal. With cyanide gas, death ensues in minutes. With ingestion of inorganic salts, as little as 100 mg results in death within hours. Chronic poisoning, although rare, causes headaches and cyanosis.

2. The following information regarding cyanide is important.

   a. Cyanide is present in the **pits of peaches, apricots** (and, therefore, in the drug amygdalin), **bitter almonds,** and the **wild black cherry**.

   b. Blood and dependent tissues are **cherry-red** (as in CO poisoning) because of the fully oxygenated blood unused by poisoned tissues.

   c. A **bitter almond odor** on the patient's breath, detected clinically, is an aid in diagnosis.

   d. **Nitrite** is a life-saving **antidote** if given promptly. It produces methemoglobin, which complexes with and dissociates the enzyme-bound cyanide.

H. Heavy metals

1. Arsenic. Binding to sulfhydryl groups, arsenic interferes with many essential enzymatic processes.

   a. Acute arsenic poisoning (now rare) produces nausea, vomiting, and abdominal pain, followed by vascular collapse due to visceral hemorrhages.

   b. Chronic toxicity is now the rule. It is due to prolonged exposure to arsenicals in fruit sprays, weed killers, rat poisons, and industrial compounds.

     (1) Detectable amounts are found in hair, nails, and skin. Characteristic skin pigmentation forming dark brown to black areas aids in the diagnosis.

     (2) Chronic exposure results in weakness, malaise, gastrointestinal bleeding, and—occasionally—paralysis. The liver and kidney may develop fatty changes and necrosis.

     (3) Long-term toxicity (e.g., in vineyard workers) has been associated with an increased incidence of hepatic angiosarcoma and lung cancer.

2. Mercury. Also binding to sulfhydryl groups, mercury has its greatest effect on mitochondrial oxidative processes. Mercuric salts are more toxic than mercurous ones; organic mercurials are also toxic.

   a. Acute poisoning outbreaks usually occur from the accidental ingestion of contaminated fish or grain, but individuals may occasionally and unintentionally swallow a mercuric salt. Acute poisoning causes erosion of oral and gastric mucosa, acute tubular necrosis, and cerebral edema.

   b. Chronic poisoning from fungicides or dermatologic ointments produces metal deposits on the gingiva similar to the "lead line" of lead poisoning. CNS symptoms include headache and memory loss. Chronic gastritis and a nephrotic syndrome (from membranous or proliferative glomerulonephritis) also occur. Characteristic **eosinophilic globules** appear in renal tubules.

3. Lead. Absorption is through the lungs or gastrointestinal tract and causes chronic poisoning from the gradual bodily accumulation of toxic lead levels above the accepted blood level of 30 μg/dl. Lead is deposited in the bones and may be gradually released.

   a. Etiology. Disease caused by air pollution has been reduced by the use of lead-free gasoline.

     (1) In **adults,** the primary source is occupational exposure from battery production or burning, from paint spraying, or from highway work.

     (2) In **children,** despite restrictions, lead in paints is still the primary source of toxicity, particularly in older housing within slum areas.

   b. Effects

     (1) Neurotoxicity occurs. In children, this poisoning takes the form of encephalopathy from cerebral edema. In adults, peripheral neuritis causes footdrop and wristdrop.

     (2) Renal proximal tubular acidosis (Fanconi's syndrome) may result from altered function of tubular enzymes. Characteristic and diagnostic **acid-fast tubular intranuclear inclusions** are seen in the proximal tubules.

     (3) The **gastrointestinal tract** is affected, and children may present with **lead colic,** a poorly localized abdominal pain.

     (4) Anemia is typically present, with fragility and basophilic stippling of red cells. The red cells are mainly affected, because lead inhibits enzymes involved in red cell metabolism. Since one of these is aminolevulinic acid (ALA) dehydratase, urinary ALA is increased.

   c. Diagnosis

     (1) Lead poisoning is suspected in **adults** with anemia, basophilic stippling, and the appropriate blood lead level. Finger, wrist, or footdrop are also telltale signs.

     (2) In **children,** the diagnosis can be difficult because the development of lethargy and ataxias is insidious. Radiodensities along epiphyseal lines can be seen.

     (3) The dark **gingival "lead line"** and an increase in **urinary ALA** are helpful diagnostic features.

IV. TOBACCO, ALCOHOL, AND DRUG ABUSE. Although these substances are chemicals, they are discussed separately to emphasize the very common medical problems which arise from them and to outline concepts of addiction, withdrawal, and psychological dependence (see IV D).

A. Tobacco use and smoking. About 20% (or 55 million) Americans still smoke; however, nearly 90 million smoked in 1960. Currently, society has less tolerance for the smoker, and smoke-free areas are now common. This change has resulted from the now-known harmful effects of so-called "passive smoking"—that is, the inhalation of air contaminated by the smoking of others. The legal and social pressure on smokers is increasing, and more individuals are attempting to quit. However, the nicotine in cigarette smoke is very addictive, and many individuals fail to quit on the initial attempt. The major effects of tobacco use on a variety of organs are listed along with associated diseases and cancers.

1. Toxins and carcinogens. All forms of tobacco have toxins (e.g., CO) and carcinogens. It is estimated that about 40 carcinogens are present in cigarette smoke.

2. Effects of tobacco use. The deleterious effects of the use of any tobacco (i.e., chewing, cigars, cigarettes) are noted only after years of use.
   a. Chewing tobacco is associated with an increased risk of oral cancer, particularly squamous cancers of the gums and floor of the mouth.
   b. Cigars. The use of cigars has been strongly associated with an increased risk of developing cancers of the lip, oral cavity, and larynx.
   c. Cigarettes. Because cigarette smoke is inhaled, it has more widespread bodily effects.
      (1) In addition to being associated with oral and laryngeal cancer, cigarettes are known to increase the risk of the following cancers:
         (a) Bronchogenic carcinoma, particularly squamous and oat cell types
         (b) Gastric cancer
         (c) Esophageal cancer
         (d) Pancreatic cancer
         (e) Renal cell carcinoma
         (f) Bladder cancer, transitional cell carcinoma
         (g) Lymphoma
      (2) Aside from malignancies, cigarette smoke is strongly associated with the following medical diseases:
         (a) Myocardial infarction
         (b) Congestive heart failure (CHF)
         (c) Atherosclerosis (general)
         (d) Stroke and cerebrovascular accidents (CVA)
         (e) Chronic bronchitis and emphysema
         (f) Peripheral vascular disease

3. Effects of passive smoking. Those who live with smokers may have so-called "passive smoking" diseases, which can include the following.
   a. Asthma. The incidence of childhood asthma is higher when the parents of these children smoke.
   b. Irritations. The toxic smoke irritates the mucous membranes of the eyes and nasal passages.
   c. Cancer. The development of cancer is calculated to be proportional to overall exposure. This relationship explains the higher incidence of cancer in nonsmoking spouses of smokers.

4. Methods to quit tobacco use. The medical profession should encourage patients to quit smoking, but not merely by mentioning it. Physicians should encourage patients to enroll in low-cost programs or to use nicotine substitutes.
   a. Physicians should remember that a true addiction to nicotine is unlikely to be altered by a casual approach. Rather than preach, doctors should be sympathetic to those who are addicted.
   b. Nicotine substitutes are available in chewing gum or time-release patches. The physician should caution the patient about nicotine toxicity, which can occur if the patient uses nicotine substitutes while still smoking.
   c. The patient will usually require multiple attempts to be successful, and clinicians should recognize this aspect of addiction and be supportive.

B. Ethyl alcohol (ethanol). Heavy drinkers comprise 8% to 12% of the United States population, and the number of true alcoholics is much higher.

1. Acute intoxication. Alcohol is a **CNS depressant**.

   a. The **rate of alcohol metabolism** is relatively constant at 150 mg/kg of body weight per hour (about 1 oz of 90 proof whiskey or 10 oz of beer per hour).

   b. Consumption beyond this rate leads to increasing blood alcohol levels and consequent effects, as outlined in Table 4-2. Fatal blood levels (400 mg/dl or higher) are usually prevented by vomiting and stupor.

2. Chronic alcohol abuse

   a. Nutritional deficiencies, drug abuse, and infections often accompany alcohol abuse, making separation of specific toxic effects difficult. It is thought that the most toxic metabolite is **acetaldehyde**.

   b. Complications and sequelae are many; the following is a partial list:

   (1) Acute fatty liver, with fever and hepatomegaly

   (2) Alcoholic cirrhosis, with associated portal hypertension, life-threatening esophageal varices, gradual hepatic insufficiency, and late development of hepatocellular carcinoma

   (3) Acute and chronic gastritis (atrophic gastritis may lead to pernicious anemia)

   (4) Acute and chronic pancreatitis, leading to pancreatic insufficiency

   (5) Alcoholic cardiomyopathy

   (6) Peripheral neuritis due to degeneration of myelin sheaths

   (7) Cerebral atrophy and dementia

   (8) Korsakoff's syndrome and Wernicke's encephalopathy, both of which respond to thiamine

C. Drug abuse

1. Marijuana. Regardless of the social implications and complications related to this substance, clearly it can cause human disease.

   a. Chronic bronchitis can result from prolonged use.

   b. Neoplasia can develop in long-term users, since marijuana contains several known carcinogens.

2. Heroin

   a. Overdose of this potent narcotic may cause sudden death from depressed respiration. Fatal acute pulmonary edema or cardiac arrest may also occur; in some cases, these conditions may be due to such substances as quinine, which is used to "cut" heroin.

   b. Intravenous drug abuse leads to various consequences.

   (1) Nonsterile injections result in bacterial infections of the skin and various internal organs. Individuals are also susceptible to viral diseases transmitted by blood (e.g., hepatitis, AIDS).

   (2) Contaminated foreign debris may be deposited in the lungs and eventually cause pulmonary vascular disease or fibrosis.

3. Cocaine. After alcohol, cocaine is the major drug of abuse in the United States. Cocaine is a CNS **stimulant** which acts at dopaminergic synapses by blocking reuptake of neurotransmitters, resulting in enhanced synaptic activity.

   a. Systemic effects include increased heart rate and blood pressure, dilated pupils, peripheral vasoconstriction, rise in body temperature, and relaxation of bronchial muscles.

   b. Methods of abuse

   (1) "Snorting" cocaine may cause mucosal ulceration and perforation of the nasal septum if use of the drug is chronic.

   (2) Intravenous use achieves a more rapid onset but has a greater likelihood of seizures.

Table 4-2. Blood Alcohol Levels and Their Effects

Blood Level (mg/dl)	Effect
100*	Ataxia; decreased motor response times
200	Drowsiness
300	Stupor
400 or higher	Profound anesthesia (may be fatal)

*Legal intoxication level.

(3) The mass-produced solid form of free-base alkaloidal cocaine is called "crack." When heated and inhaled through a pipe, this form of cocaine gives the user an intense "high." Crack is the most addictive substance encountered clinically, with dependence appearing in days.

c. **Acute cocaine toxicity** is dose-related and consists of sympathomimetic effects (e.g., tachycardia, hypertension, hyperthermia, arrhythmias). These conditions may be followed by seizures, brain-stem depression, and cardiorespiratory collapse. Patients may experience stroke, coma, myocardial infarction, and sudden death following cocaine binges.

d. **Chronic cocaine abuse.** Chronic users neglect hygiene and are susceptible to infections. Schizophrenic disorders also occur. Cocaine abuse among pregnant women results in a high incidence of low-birthweight premature infants with neurological abnormalities.

D. **Addiction** is defined as the state of dependence on a given substance which may be psychological, physical, or both.

1. **Psychological dependence** is a self-perpetuating behavioral conditioning whereby the act of substance abuse is rewarded by the attendant pleasure and is reinforced by subsequent use. Subjective symptoms of craving result.

2. **Physical dependence** is the result of developing a tolerance to a substance through metabolic changes and physiologic resistance to a given quantity of the substance.
   a. Physical dependence becomes evident when a withdrawal syndrome occurs.
   b. Increased quantities of the substance are required to produce the same effect because the body adapts by increasing its tolerance level. For example, degradative enzymes can break down larger amounts of a substance in a shorter time.
   c. Physical dependence eventually results in excessive drug use, with gradual changes in both personality and ability to work (as occurs in the alcoholic or drug abuser).

3. Substances not generally considered in drug abuse, (e.g., caffeine) may also cause psychological and physical dependence (i.e., addiction). Recent evidence shows a withdrawal syndrome even among mild-to-moderate coffee drinkers: they experience headaches and lethargy when they stop drinking coffee.

V. **ADVERSE EFFECTS OF MEDICINAL AGENTS.** The known side effects of therapeutic or diagnostic agents are myriad.

A. **Causes** for adverse reactions to drugs also show considerable variety.

1. **Accidental poisonings,** involving many substances, occur at the rate of about 300,000 annually.

2. **Purposeful overdosage** may be tried as a lifesaving measure in a patient whose disease is refractory to therapy (e.g., **digitalis** in cardiac failure).

3. **Adverse drug interactions** are all too common in this day of multiple drug usage, especially in the elderly. Adverse interactions may **inhibit or potentiate** the desired effect. **Phenobarbital,** for example, induces the enzymatic machinery that metabolizes a number of substances, thereby reducing their effect.

4. **Idiosyncrasy,** which may cause an unpredictable response, can occur with almost any substance. The reaction can be severe and life-threatening.

5. **Hypersensitivity reactions** can be mild or severe. A life-threatening anaphylactic response may occur in a previously exposed individual; it occurs most commonly with **penicillin** and related compounds but may also occur with **methyldopa.**

B. **Manifestations** can be grouped by the affected body system.

1. **Skin.** Perhaps the most common type of drug reaction, skin eruption may take the form of macules, papules, and vesicles. Erythema multiforme may be caused by **sulfonamides** or **barbiturates**.

2. **Liver.** Hepatic reactions range from relatively innocuous (e.g., cholestasis from **chlorpromazine,** fatty change from **tetracycline**) to serious (e.g., hepatitis from a variety of drugs, massive necrosis from **halothane**).

3. **Kidney.** Interstitial nephritis may result from hypersensitivity (e.g., to **methicillin**) or direct toxicity (e.g., from **amphotericin**). Papillary necrosis of the medulla may follow **analgesic abuse**.

4. **Lung.** Pneumonitis and interstitial fibrosis may result from a variety of antineoplastic agents (e.g., **bleomycin, busulfan, methotrexate**). Some reactions are dose-related, and the restriction of pulmonary capacity may be severe. Atypical alveolar lining cells are seen histologically.

5. **Bone marrow.** Some reactions affecting the blood are immunologic in nature (e.g., hemolytic anemia from **penicillin** or **methyldopa**). Most others are due either to idiosyncrasy (e.g., agranulocytosis from **chloramphenicol**) or to direct toxicity (e.g., pancytopenia from **cytotoxic agents**).

C. **Specific examples** of reactions to commonly used drugs include the following.

1. **Aspirin**
   a. Fatalities in children result from ingestion of 2 to 4 g (6 to 12 adult tablets). In adults, the fatal dose is about 15 g. Respiratory stimulation causes respiratory alkalosis, followed by metabolic acidosis; severe vomiting, hypokalemia, bleeding, and coma ensue.
   b. Aspirin in usual doses may cause life-threatening **Reye's syndrome** in children with viral illness. Coma and microvesicular fatty change in the liver may ensue, or hypersensitivity reactions may develop, ranging from mild rash to severe anaphylaxis.

2. **Phenacetin.** Chronic analgesic abuse with this drug, taken alone or with aspirin, causes **analgesic nephropathy,** including **renal papillary necrosis**. Affected individuals have consumed a cumulative dose of more than 3 kg over a period of years.

3. **Barbiturates**
   a. Accidental or deliberate **overdosage** is common with these CNS depressants.
      (1) Potentially fatal doses of barbiturates are about 3 g for short-acting types and 5 g for long-acting types.
      (2) Systemic hypoxia results from a decreased respiratory rate and leads to shock and coma. The patient who survives the hypoxic episode may develop bronchopneumonia, renal tubular necrosis, and cutaneous "barbiturate blisters."
   b. Rarely, a hypersensitivity vasculitis similar to polyarteritis nodosa may be seen.

4. **Steroid hormones**
   a. These agents are associated with a number of **malignancies**.
      (1) **Clear cell adenocarcinoma of the vagina** in teenage daughters has been etiologically associated with **diethylstilbestrol (DES)** use by the mother during pregnancy.
      (2) **Endometrial cancer** has been linked to prolonged use of **exogenous estrogens**.
      (3) **Breast cancer** has **not** shown a clear-cut link with exogenous estrogens, but further study is necessary.
      (4) **Liver tumors** (hepatic adenomas and hepatocellular carcinomas) have been associated with long-term use of **anabolic steroids** and **oral contraceptives**.
   b. **Gallstones** in women have doubled in incidence since they began using **estrogens** or **oral contraceptives**.
   c. **Oral contraceptives** also have been linked to the following conditions (negative effects refer to past preparations; newer combinations may be safer).
      (1) **Circulatory disease,** with the potential for causing death from myocardial infarction or cerebral thrombosis and hemorrhage, shows a fivefold increased risk. Smoking increases the risk further. In **nonsmokers,** the overall risk of circulatory disease is lower than the risk of complications from pregnancy.
      (2) **Breast cancer** shows a questionable increased risk.
      (3) A **protective effect** against endometrial cancer and fibrocystic breast disease has been found.

VI. EFFECTS OF AIR POLLUTANTS

A. **Overview.** Breathing contaminated air is a daily part of life in urban America. Pollutants abound, including heavy metals, chemical vapors, and dusts.

1. Many of the important agents cause specific **pulmonary reactions,** the largest group of which are the **pneumoconioses** from inhaled mineral or organic dusts. In addition to those discussed here, the many other inhalation-related pulmonary diseases include **byssinosis** (chest tightness

from cotton and hemp fibers) and **interstitial pneumonitis** from hypersensitivity to any number of inhaled resins, pollens, molds, or other organic or chemical dusts.

2. **Chronic bronchitis** is seen with a variety of inhalants, including all dusts at certain exposure levels.

3. **Neoplasia** can be a consequence, particularly with asbestos exposure and cigarette smoking and, rarely, with radioactive dust exposure.

B. Acute pulmonary toxicity

1. **Acute pulmonary edema** may result from inhaling oxides of nitrogen (as in silo-filler's disease) or paraquat insecticide (as in marijuana smoking).

2. **Asthmalike reactions** occur in wood workers exposed to red cedar dust and in refinery workers exposed to platinum or aluminum dust.

C. Pneumoconioses. Types of pneumoconioses, their pathologic features and relationship to other diseases can be found in Table 4-3.

1. **General considerations.** This group of diseases is due to **chronic exposure** to various inhalants. The extent of disease is influenced by the nature of the substance, its concentration, its size and shape, and the duration of exposure.
   a. **Particle size** is especially important. Particles about 3 to 5 μ in size can pass into the alveoli and persist there, whereas most smaller particles exit with the expired air; larger particles are trapped in the major bronchi by the mucus barrier.
   b. When they reach the alveoli, most particles (90%) are still cleared from the lungs by mucociliary action. Those remaining may be injurious. **Pulmonary alveolar macrophages** then become the only remaining defense and, indeed, may clear the lungs of large quantities of relatively inert substances (e.g., carbon pigment), removing such particles via lymphatic channels to regional lymph nodes.

2. **Anthracosis.** The accumulation of carbon dust is seen in every urban dweller and is accentuated in the cigarette smoker. Black pigment within macrophages accumulates around terminal bronchioles but causes little harm. The exception is the **smoker,** where additional destructive mechanisms are at work, resulting in **centrilobular emphysema**.

3. **Silicosis.** Silica dust is a potent lung irritant. Particularly at risk are sand blasters, glass workers, miners, metal grinders and polishers, and cement workers.
   a. **Acute exposure** to large quantities of silica may result in an **exudative pneumonitis**. Histologically similar to alveolar proteinosis, it may cause death within 1 or 2 years from a gradually worsening respiratory failure.

Table 4-3. Summary of Pneumoconioses

Type	Pathologic Features	Comments
Silicosis	Upper lobe nodules, eggshell calcification	Increased tuberculosis, no increase in mesothelioma
CWP	Small upper lobe nodules, emphysema	No increase in lung cancer
PMF	2–10-cm nodules	Increased tuberculosis, no increase in lung cancer
Caplan's syndrome	Pulmonary nodules and rheumatoid arthritis	Can occur in silicosis, CWP, or PMF; must be distinguished from tuberculosis
Asbestosis	Finely nodular x-ray and pleural plaques	Need not be present for risk of mesothelioma
Asbestos exposure	Essentially normal lungs	Increased mesothelioma and lung cancer
Berylliosis	Hypersensitivity reaction, with granulomas in finely nodular x-ray	Bronchial biopsy helpful; increased lung cancer

CWP = coal workers' pneumoconiosis; PMF = progressive massive fibrosis.

b. Chronic silicosis develops over years to decades, with the formation of collagenous **silicotic nodules** and marked **fibrotic changes** in the lungs. Due to the persistence of silica within the lungs, the disease may progress or even present long after the period of exposure.

   (1) Pathogenesis. Silica is a stimulant to fibroblasts, and the membrane injury to macrophages probably initiates an inflammatory response.

   (a) The tetrahedral structure of silicon dioxide somehow is related to the fibrogenic response of the lung. The **three crystalline forms** are fibrogenic in the following order: **tridymite** (most), **crystobalite** (intermediate), and **quartz** (least). **Particle size** is also important, with 1 to 2 μ being the most dangerous size.

   (b) General agreement exists on the following **sequence for fibrogenesis:** Alveolar macrophages phagocytose the silica dust and die after rupture of silica-laden phagolysosomes. The released material is re-engulfed by other macrophages, and the cycle is repeated.

   (c) More controversial is the **mechanism of fibrogenesis;** it may be due to a fibroblast growth factor released by the macrophages. Also, partial dissolving may create hydroxyl groups on the silica, fostering damage to cell membranes.

   (2) Clinical features and complications

   (a) Chronic silicosis is insidious and relentless. The gradual reduction in lung capacity is asymptomatic at first but later causes **dyspnea** on exertion; it may progress to an incapacitating condition.

   (b) Patients with chronic silicosis have an increased risk of both **pulmonary tuberculosis** and the associated rheumatoid arthritis (**Caplan's syndrome**) but show no increased incidence of lung cancer or mesothelioma.

   (3) Pathology

   (a) Tiny collagenous nodules are initially present in the upper lobes and slowly enlarge into visible circular scars. Dense fibrosis is present in these nodules, which are relatively hypocellular; polarized light reveals minute flecks of the **polarizable silica particles** among the lamellated collagen bands, a fact of diagnostic importance.

   (b) With further nodular growth, coalescence may occur. **Central cavitation** may develop as a result of ischemia or superimposed tuberculosis.

   (c) Similar reactions to those found in the lung occur within the hilar lymph nodes (where nodules undergo peripheral calcification), giving rise to the classic "**eggshell**" radiologic appearance.

   (d) Any **cellular infiltrate** in the lungs or lymph nodes, such as true granulomas, should prompt suspicion of tuberculosis.

4. Coal worker's pneumoconiosis (CWP). This disease is present in some degree in every long-term coal worker and is a significant cause of morbidity and mortality in this occupational group. Two main categories exist: **simple CWP,** which is usually asymptomatic, and **progressive massive fibrosis (PMF),** which resembles chronic silicosis in its insidious nature and late symptomatology.

   a. Pathogenesis. The **mechanisms of CWP and PMF** are probably similar to those in pure silicosis, namely fibroblast stimulation and an inflammatory response to macrophage injury. The factors controlling the **transformation of CWP into PMF** are more difficult to outline clearly, but the following are possible factors:

   (1) Total quantity of dust, which appears to correlate with the severity of disease

   (2) Obliterative vasculitis, with ischemic extension of damage

   (3) Concomitant silicosis, since the level of quartz in coal dust may be related to progression of disease

   (4) Immunologic mechanisms (postulated but not well supported)

   (5) Presence of **intercurrent tuberculosis,** occurring in 40% of PMF cases (seems coincidental)

   b. Clinical features and complications

   (1) A chronic dry cough may accompany simple **CWP** but may relate to emphysematous changes.

   (2) In contrast, **PMF** is a severely disabling disease, with dyspnea on exertion progressing to dyspnea at rest.

   (a) Jet-black sputum is produced, and patients may have poorly localized chest pain. Fever should raise suspicion of tuberculosis, which occurs in 40% of patients.

(b) Complications include right ventricular hypertrophy, with pulmonary hypertension and cor pulmonale.

(c) Caplan's syndrome (rheumatoid arthritis with pulmonary nodules) is also seen.

(d) The increased incidence of gastric carcinoma in CWP and PMF is not true of lung cancer.

c. Pathology

(1) CWP. Early on, the distinction between CWP and anthracosis is blurred, but the eventual fibrosis of CWP is a later distinguishing feature.

(a) The **pleura** and cut surfaces of the lung are blue-black, but the pleura is not thickened.

(b) Minute (up to 1 cm) pigmented foci (**coal macules**) initially are seen concentrated in the upper lobes. These macules are composed of intact pigmented macrophages around bronchioles and adjacent alveoli.

(c) As the process continues, mild **fibrosis** develops in the form of fine reticulin fibers deposited together with increasing amounts of collagen. At this stage, **nodules** (up to 2 cm) become apparent but contain no visible macrophages; rather, the pigment is dispersed within the collagen.

(d) Expansion next to vessels produces an obliterative **vasculitis,** and **centrilobular emphysema** is also seen.

(2) PMF. In contrast to CWP, PMF is characterized by pleural thickening and by large, occasionally massive, regions of black scars that exceed 2 cm in size (some are as large as 5 to 10 cm). The upper regions of the upper and lower lobes are most affected, along with the lower region of the upper lobes.

(a) Often occurring on a background of CWP, PMF scars are quite irregular and eventually coalesce to produce **black lung disease**.

(b) Dense collagen peppered with black pigment is seen. Polarized light reveals the presence of **silica**. Trapped vessels develop thick walls and become obliterated. Hypoxia may cause central blackish liquefaction of the scars. Cellular infiltrates of lymphocytes and macrophages are scanty; finding **caseating granulomas** strongly suggests tuberculosis (as does cavitation on x-ray).

5. Asbestos-related disease. The morbidity and mortality associated with asbestos exposure is one of the medical disasters of the twentieth century. Numerous deaths have occurred, and many will yet result from either severe pneumoconiosis or malignancy.

a. Risk factors

(1) Importantly, **no known threshold of exposure** exists. Certainly, those exposed to high asbestos levels over long periods are at great risk, but even indirect exposure (as in those who live with asbestos workers) has resulted in neoplastic disease.

(2) Persons at risk occupationally include shipyard, roofing, brake lining, and insulation workers. At **unknown risk** are those exposed in older buildings (e.g., schoolchildren).

(3) Fiber type affects pathogenicity. Fibrous silicates (i.e., asbestos fibers) are either curled **serpentines** (chrysotile) or straight **amphiboles** (crocidolite and amosite). All types are thin but long (1 × 30 to 50 μ).

(a) Although **chrysotile** is the major air pollutant, it tends to fragment and be cleared by the respiratory tract.

(b) Cancer is more strongly associated with amphiboles, particularly **crocidolite**. The straight form offers less air resistance, and fibers are carried to the lung periphery.

(4) Cigarette smoking markedly increases the risk of lung cancer in asbestos-exposed workers; however, it does **not** increase the risk of mesothelioma.

b. Clinical diseases

(1) Asbestosis is the name for the **pneumoconiosis** which presents clinically as a diffuse, nonspecific, chronic interstitial pneumonitis. Complications include bronchiectasis, cor pulmonale, and cancer. Asbestosis need not be present for malignant neoplasia to develop—and often is not.

(2) Malignancies of several types occur, and a rough correlation does exist between bodily asbestos burden and the development of asbestos-related cancers.

(a) Mesothelioma shows a marked (100-fold) increase in incidence. Both pleural and peritoneal mesotheliomas occur, with the former the most common. Mesothelioma occurs in up to 10% of heavily exposed persons, presenting 20 to 40 years after exposure has ceased. All patients with this tumor die within an average of one year.

       (b) Bronchogenic carcinomas are 4 to 5 times more likely to occur in this exposed group than in nonexposed individuals. **Cigarette smoking** markedly increases the risk; the likelihood is 50 to 90 times that of the general population.

       (c) Other cancers that show an asbestos-related increased incidence include gastric, colonic, and renal adenocarcinomas, and gastrointestinal lymphomas.

    c. Pathogenesis

      (1) Concerning **fibrogenesis,** the mechanism may be similar to that of silicosis, with membrane damage and release of fibroblast-stimulating cell products. Some asbestos fibers directly stimulate reticulin and collagen production in tissue culture.

      (2) Asbestos may act as a tumor promoter for **carcinogenesis**.

      (3) Interestingly, **transport** of asbestos fibers may be through the lymphatics, a mechanism invoked in the explanation of pleural plaques and mesotheliomas.

    d. Pathology

      (1) Fibers, when phagocytosed, acquire a proteinaceous, iron-rich coating that gives rise to beaded **"asbestos bodies"** with clubbed ends, which constitute the hallmark of asbestos exposure. These bodies may be seen **in the absence of disease,** suggesting the importance of host factors in the development of disease. No correlation exists between the amount of visible pulmonary asbestos (much of which is uncoated) and later disease.

      (2) In **asbestosis,** a **diffuse interstitial fibrosis** of the lower lobes is seen, with asbestos bodies and calcified and noncalcified **pleural plaques**. The pleura becomes thickened with fibrous adhesions, which encase the lungs.

       (a) The **fibrosis** starts peripherally and extends centrally, ultimately producing the end-stage or "honeycombed" lung.

       (b) The **pleural plaques** are distinctive (but not pathognomonic of asbestosis) and asbestos bodies are typical (but not pathognomonic); similar **ferruginous bodies** form around other kinds of inhaled particles.

6. Berylliosis. Beryllium is used in the electronic, ceramic, aerospace, and nuclear industries because of its high tensile strength. Disease occurs in only 2% of those exposed, underscoring a striking individual susceptibility.

    a. Acute berylliosis, a toxic acute pneumonitis, is induced by finely powdered dust. Histologically, it resembles an acute bronchopneumonia with alveolar neutrophils. It is nongranulomatous. Healing may cause pulmonary septal fibrosis. Acute berylliosis resolves within weeks, but 5% to 10% of cases may progress to chronic granulomatous disease.

    b. Chronic berylliosis is characterized by sarcoidlike **noncaseating** peribronchial and perivascular granulomas. The granulomatous reaction is consistent with a **type IV hypersensitivity reaction;** in fact, affected patients show sensitivity through a positive skin test.

      (1) Clinical features

       (a) Patients present with dyspnea on exertion and give a history of beryllium exposure; nodular densities are seen on chest x-ray. Progression of the disease occurs over decades, resulting in some deaths from respiratory failure.

       (b) The incidence of bronchogenic carcinoma shows a twofold increase.

      (2) Pathology

       (a) The **pulmonary granulomas** of chronic berylliosis closely resemble those of sarcoidosis. Granulomas may also be found in other organs, including the liver, kidney, skin, and lymph nodes.

       (b) Inclusions seen within granulomas include Schaumann's bodies, calcium carbonate spicules, and asteroid bodies (stellate eosinophilic proteinaceous material); none of these is specific for berylliosis.

STUDY QUESTIONS

Directions: Each of the numbered items or incomplete statements in this section is followed by answers or by completions of the statement. Select the **one** lettered answer or completion that is **best** in each case.

1. An individual cell would be most harmed by which type of radiation?

(A) X-rays
(B) Alpha particles
(C) Beta particles
(D) Gamma rays
(E) Electrons

2. Which statement accurately describes therapeutic radiation?

(A) The kidney is especially radiosensitive
(B) The skin is rarely affected
(C) The internal part of a tumor is less affected due to hypoxia
(D) Germ cell tumors are radioresistant
(E) Radiosensitivity is unrelated to the rate of cell division

3. Patients presenting with sweating, narrow pupils, a slow heart rate, and low blood pressure are most likely to have been poisoned with

(A) *Amanita muscaria*
(B) methyl alcohol
(C) chloroform
(D) heroin
(E) cocaine

4. What is the term given to the group of lung diseases that result from the chronic inhalation of particulate or gaseous agents as a result of occupational exposure?

(A) Granulomatous disease
(B) Pneumoconiosis
(C) Mycobacteriosis
(D) Pseudolymphoma
(E) Bronchiectasis

5. Large irregular densities and apparent cavitation with air–fluid levels are noted on the chest x-ray of a coal miner. These findings are most suggestive of

(A) chronic silicosis with eggshell calcifications
(B) superimposed tuberculosis
(C) simple coal worker's pneumoconiosis (CWP)
(D) asbestosis
(E) Caplan's syndrome

6. Asbestos-related disease is best characterized by which statement?

(A) Asbestosis is often seen in patients with mesothelioma
(B) Mesothelioma may occur years after holding a job for 6 weeks as a ship worker
(C) Fiber type and shape are not significant
(D) Ferruginous bodies are nonspecific findings
(E) Asbestos exposure increases the risk of tuberculosis

7. Characteristics of thermal burns include all of the following EXCEPT

(A) partial-thickness burns may appear red and blistered
(B) shock may ensue with severe burns
(C) diffuse alveolar damage may result from smoke inhalation
(D) full-thickness burns usually are capable of self-repair
(E) wounds may become infected with *Pseudomonas*

8. Clinical and laboratory findings in alcoholic patients may include all of the following EXCEPT

(A) a macrocytic anemia
(B) decreased deep tendon reflexes
(C) a leukocytosis
(D) right lower quadrant pain
(E) vomiting of blood

1-B	4-B	7-D
2-C	5-B	8-D
3-A	6-B	

9. The tumor and causative agent are correctly matched in all of the pairs EXCEPT

(A) hepatic angiosarcoma—arsenicals
(B) endometrial carcinoma—exogenous estrogens
(C) vaginal carcinoma—diethylstilbestrol (DES)
(D) mesothelioma—beryllium

10. The causative agent and untoward effect are correctly matched in all of the pairs EXCEPT

(A) halothane—massive hepatic necrosis
(B) lead—renal tubular intranuclear inclusions
(C) oral contraceptives—liver tumors
(D) bleomycin—renal papillary necrosis

Directions: Each group of items in this section consists of lettered options followed by a set of numbered items. For each item, select the **one** lettered option that is most closely associated with it. Each lettered option may be selected once, more than once, or not at all.

Questions 11–15

For each pathologic response, select the disease with which it is most likely to be associated.

(A) Silicosis
(B) Asbestosis
(C) Tuberculosis
(D) Chronic berylliosis
(E) Coal worker's pneumoconiosis (CWP)

11. Caseating granulomas

12. Centrilobular emphysema

13. Noncaseating granulomas

14. Pleural calcifications

15. Polarizable flecks in nodules

Questions 16–19

For each clinicopathologic finding, select the agent with which it is most closely associated.

(A) Cyanide
(B) Carbon monoxide (CO)
(C) Both
(D) Neither

16. Cherry-red color of blood

17. Bitter almond odor on breath

18. Blindness

19. High affinity for hemoglobin

9-D   12-E   15-A   18-D
10-D   13-D   16-C   19-B
11-C   14-B   17-A

ANSWERS AND EXPLANATIONS

1. The answer is B *[II D 3 c, d, e].*
X-rays, gamma rays, and electrons are very penetrating, but the amount of energy per hit is small. Alpha particles are heavier and, thus, would have a higher relative biologic effectiveness (RBE) and would be most likely to be lethal to individual cells. Beta particles have a lower linear energy transfer (LET) value and a lower RBE than alpha particles.

2. The answer is C *[II D 3 f, g, 4 b].*
The effect of radiation is best seen at the highly oxygenated tumor periphery; the central regions of tumors are least affected by radiation because oxygen saturation is lowest there. When external radiation is given, the skin often shows changes: erythema, loss of hair, and reduced thickness. Deep organs (e.g., the kidneys) are radioresistant, but cells showing a high rate of cell division (e.g., bone marrow, gastrointestinal tract) are particularly radiosensitive. Germ cell tumors are also radiosensitive.

3. The answer is A *[III E 1].*
The mushroom *Amanita muscaria* causes muscarinic effects on the nervous system (i.e., sweating, narrow pupils, a slow heart rate, and low blood pressure); but, in contrast to poisoning with *Amanita phalloides,* patients usually recover without more severe problems. Methyl alcohol may cause blindness, and chloroform causes liver toxicity, which would not produce this patient's symptoms. Nasal bleeding secondary to perforation is a common presentation of cocaine sniffers. In heroin overdose, shortness of breath due to pulmonary edema is often seen.

4. The answer is B *[VI C 1].*
Pneumoconiosis is a pathologic lung condition produced by chronic inhalation of particulate or gaseous matter, which generally occurs in the course of certain occupations. Anthracosis is observed in miners and occasionally in people who live in congested urban environments. Silicosis is seen in miners, metal grinders, and others who are chronically exposed to silica particles. Asbestosis is a particularly widespread form of pneumoconiosis and can lead to the development of malignant mesotheliomas.

5. The answer is B *[VI C 3 b (2) (b), (3) (b)–(d)].*
Any cavitary lesions, whether in chronic silicosis, simple coal worker's pneumoconiosis (CWP), or progressive massive fibrosis (PMF), are highly suggestive of superimposed tuberculosis. The eggshell appearance of the hilar lymph nodes in chronic silicosis is due to outer calcification and does not imply infection. Simple CWP has only small irregular densities, as does asbestosis; no cavitation is seen. Although granulomas are noted in rheumatoid arthritis complicating CWP (Caplan's syndrome), they do not appear as cavitary lesions.

6. The answer is B *[VI C 5].*
Although there is a rough correlation between total asbestos burden and the development of malignancy, there is no dose-response curve and no real threshold of exposure to cause disease. It is well known that a 6-week exposure to asbestos has resulted in mesothelioma 20 years later, but many mesothelioma patients have had very high exposure. Oddly enough, mesothelioma patients do not frequently show the interstitial lung nodules of asbestosis. Fiber types are important; for example, cancer is most strongly associated wth amphiboles. Ferruginous bodies are quite typical and characteristic of asbestos exposure but are rarely seen in other inhaled substances; thus, finding them should alert the pathologist to the possibility of asbestos exposure. Tuberculosis is not increased in persons exposed to asbestos.

7. The answer is D *[II B 2 b].*
Full-thickness burns are wounds with such complete skin loss that they require skin grafts to heal. The red and blistered partial-thickness burn wounds often repair themselves. Open wounds may become infected with *Pseudomonas,* which, in turn, may cause septicemia. In a fire, smoke inhalation may cause pulmonary injury, including severe bronchial irritation and alveolar damage.

8. The answer is D *[IV B 2].*
Although alcoholics may present (rarely) with the right lower quadrant pain of appendicitis, this condition is not connected in any way to ethanol abuse and would not be expected. Alcoholics, through either atrophic gastritis or lack of dietary intake, may develop pernicious anemia with large or macrocytic red blood cells. They may have a peripheral neuritis, causing decreased deep tendon reflexes. A leukocytosis may be seen as a result of either alcoholic hepatitis or pancreatitis. Esophageal varices may bleed, causing vomiting of blood.

9. The answer is D *[III H 1; V C 4; VI C 6 b].*

Mesothelioma follows exposure to asbestos. Chronic berylliosis is associated with a twofold increase in the incidence of bronchogenic carcinoma, but it is not linked to mesothelioma. Chronic exposure to arsenical products has been associated with an increased incidence of hepatic angiosarcoma and lung cancer. Endometrial cancer has been linked to long-term estrogen therapy, and diethylstilbestrol (DES) therapy during pregnancy has been linked to the later development of clear cell adenocarcinoma of the vagina in the teenage daughters of these women.

10. The answer is D *[III H 3; V B 2–4, C 4].*

Bleomycin commonly produces pulmonary fibrosis, whereas renal papillary necrosis can be caused by analgesic abuse. Halothane has caused fatal hepatic necrosis. In lead poisoning, both the gingival lead line and the characteristic intranuclear inclusions of kidney tubules are helpful diagnostic markers. Contraceptives are well known to be associated with the hepatic adenoma.

11–15. The answers are: 11-C *[VI C 4 c (2) (b)]*, **12-E** *[VI C 4 b]*, **13-D** *[VI C 6 b]*, **14-B** *[VI C 5 d (2)]*, **15-A** *[VI C 3 b (3) (a)].*

Caseating granulomas are found in tuberculosis, whereas noncaseating granulomas are seen in berylliosis as well as many other diseases. Simple emphysema has a variety of causes, such as smoking, but the emphysematous changes seen in the pneumoconioses are not simple. Pleural calcifications are typical of asbestosis, and nodules with polarizable silica are seen in silicosis.

16–19. The answers are: 16-C, 17-A, 18-D, 19-B *[III F, G].*

Both cyanide and carbon monoxide (CO) produce a cherry-red appearance of blood and dependent tissues. However, cyanide acts by inhibiting the cytochrome oxidase system (thus blocking oxidative respiration) whereas CO binds avidly to hemoglobin (thus acting as a cellular asphyxiant). Only cyanide causes the diagnostic almond odor on a patient's breath, and neither cyanide nor CO poisoning is characterized by blindness, which is a characteristic of methanol poisoning.

5
Nutritional Pathology
Virginia A. LiVolsi

I. INTRODUCTION. In the United States, the pathology of nutrition and its aberrations is of concern currently because the American diet is high in calories, in fats, in salt, and in refined sugar—that is, Americans eat "fast foods." In addition, large quantities of food additives, some of which may have carcinogenic potential, are ingested.

II. OVERNUTRITION. Obesity is the excess storage of fat and a body weight more than 15% to 20% above "ideal" weight as defined by standard height–weight tables.

   A. General considerations. About 25% of all American adults are obese, and most of this obesity is idiopathic and related directly to overeating.

   1. The causes of obesity are complex and involve hereditary, environmental, and psychosocial factors.

   2. The overall death rate in obese persons is about 50% higher than in the general normal-weight population.

   B. Associated disorders

   1. Many diseases are more frequent or more severe in the obese. Obesity is a major contributing factor in atherosclerosis, hypertension, diabetes, gallbladder disease, and probably some forms of carcinoma, such as breast and colon cancer.

   2. Diabetes mellitus type II (non–insulin-dependent) is influenced by nutritional factors. Type II diabetes accounts for 90% of all cases of diabetes mellitus and affects about 10% of elderly Americans. In this disease, insulin is adequate, but there is resistance to insulin at the level of the insulin receptor.
      a. Type II diabetes shows a close correlation with obesity and, especially, with excessive fat consumption early in life.
      b. Good dietary control in type II diabetes can reduce the need for oral hypoglycemic agents; such control also can significantly reduce both morbidity and mortality.

III. UNDERNUTRITION. Starvation is a caloric intake inadequate to sustain normal metabolic processes.

   A. In affluent communities, starvation is unusual except in certain psychological disorders such as **anorexia nervosa**—a disease of self-induced severe weight loss observed primarily in young women.

   B. In underdeveloped countries and in conditions of poverty or deprivation, severe **protein–calorie malnutrition** may be found readily; particularly affected are infants and children.

   1. Severely malnourished individuals are at increased risk for infections, because starvation interferes with immune mechanisms. Humoral antibody production, cell-mediated immunity, and phagocytic activity all are impaired. In addition, collagen synthesis is inadequate.

   2. Severe protein–calorie malnutrition in young children takes two forms.
      a. Marasmus is severe emaciation that usually occurs in the first year of life. Characteristics are a loss of subcutaneous fat, marked muscle wasting, and atrophy of most organs.

b. **Kwashiorkor** is a disease of severe malnutrition usually seen in children.
  (1) Affected patients are edematous and have a protuberant abdomen due to ascites, which is caused by hypoalbuminemia. The skin is dry and thickened, and the hair is fine and brittle. Diarrhea and anorexia are common.
  (2) **Hepatosplenomegaly** is seen. The liver is fatty and may in time become cirrhotic. The gastrointestinal tract and endocrine organs often are markedly atrophic.

IV. **VITAMINS.** These essential organic substances normally are present in mammalian tissues in trace quantities. Usually they cannot be synthesized and must be obtained from exogenous sources (e.g., from dietary intake). Table 5-1 shows the results of many vitamin deficiencies.

A. **Fat-soluble vitamins**

  1. **General considerations**
    a. **Vitamins A, D, K, and E** are absorbed together with lipids. Thus, deficiencies can occur despite adequate intake (e.g., in gastrointestinal diseases characterized by malabsorption of fat, including Crohn's disease, chronic pancreatic insufficiency, and short-bowel syndrome).
    b. Hypervitaminosis involving vitamins A and D is caused by increased dietary intake.

  2. **Vitamin A,** important in vision, is required when light absorbed by the rod cells of the retina is converted to a nerve impulse.
    a. **Vitamin A deficiency** in children is reflected in retarded growth, hyperkeratosis of the skin, and a variety of ocular changes, including **xerophthalmia** (i.e., extreme dryness of the conjunctiva and cornea, which may lead to ulceration and eye infection). In adults, the major finding is impaired visual acuity in dim light (**night blindness**).
    b. **Hypervitaminosis A** is seen in individuals taking huge quantities (over 50,000 units) of vitamin A per day. In children, alopecia and radiologic evidence of periosteal new bone formation are seen. In adults, hepatic injury results in portal hypertension and ascites.
    c. Vitamin A deficiency or excess also affects bone, as discussed in Chapter 23 I E 3.

  3. **Vitamin D** is the collective name for a group of chemically related sterols that play a role in the intestinal absorption of calcium and the remodeling of bone.
    a. **Formation.** 7-Dehydrocholesterol, when subjected to ultraviolet radiation through exposure of the skin to sunlight, is converted to cholecalciferol (vitamin D_3). This vitamin is converted to 25-hydroxyvitamin D_3 [25-(OH)D_3] in the liver and then to 1,25-dihydroxyvitamin D_3 [1,25(OH)$_2D_3$; calcitrol] in the kidney. This final product is the **active form** of vitamin D.

Table 5-1. Vitamin Deficiencies

Vitamin	Deficiency
Fat soluble	
A	Night blindness; growth retardation; skin hyperkeratosis
D	Rickets in children; osteomalacia in adults
E	Unknown in humans
K	Bleeding
Water soluble	
B_1	Beriberi
B_2	Glossitis; stomatitis; dermatitis
B_6	Seizures; polyneuritis; anemia
B_{12}	Pernicious anemia; subacute combined degeneration of spinal cord
Niacin	Pellagra
Folate	Megaloblastic anemia
C	Scurvy

    b. Deficiency of vitamin D can result from prolonged lack of exposure to sunlight, from dietary deprivation or from fat malabsorption. Vitamin D deficiency also occurs in chronic renal failure, because the kidney is unable to convert 25-$(OH)D_3$ to the active 1,25-dihydroxyvitamin D_3.

        (1) Severe deficiency of vitamin D results in inadequate absorption of calcium and phosphorus and in impaired deposition of mineral in the bone.

        (2) In children, the resulting bone disease, known as **rickets,** is characterized by osteoid overgrowth and bone deformities. In adults, the bone disease is known as **osteomalacia,** which is characterized by demineralization of bone (see Chapter 23 I E 1).

    c. Hypervitaminosis D (vitamin D intoxication) is manifested by symptomatic hypercalcemia, simulating the symptoms of hyperparathyroidism, for example, renal stones and bone pain. Hypervitaminosis D results from excessive intake of dietary vitamin D.

  4. Vitamin K is essential for blood clotting. It is involved in the hepatic synthesis of prothrombin and coagulation factors VII, IX, and X.

    a. Deficiency of vitamin K is manifested by bleeding.

    b. Hypervitaminosis K is not known to occur.

  5. Vitamin E has been studied mostly in animals; their deficiencies are associated with muscular atrophy and sterility. In humans, it is difficult to document **vitamin E deficiency,** although some patients with severe fat malabsorption may show muscle weakness and atrophy.

B. Water-soluble vitamins

  1. General considerations

    a. In the body, most water-soluble vitamins (except vitamin C) undergo metabolic transformation, becoming parts of coenzymes. Vitamin C acts as a cofactor without undergoing such change.

    b. Hence, lack of these vitamins results in decreased activity of the specific enzyme systems in which they are involved, affecting whichever organ or organs require these enzymes.

    c. Water-soluble vitamins are not stored in the body and, therefore, do not cause hypervitaminoses.

  2. B complex vitamins

    a. Vitamin B_1 (thiamine) deficiency, or **beriberi,** is seen in developed countries chiefly among alcoholics with poor nutritional intake. The major organs affected by thiamine deficiency are the heart and the nervous system. Peripheral neuropathy, muscle weakness, and cardiac failure are the clinical manifestations.

    b. Vitamin B_2 (riboflavin) deficiency is observed in chronic alcoholics or, in underdeveloped countries, as a prominent aspect of a generalized nutrient-deficient state. Riboflavin deficiency causes changes in mucous membranes and skin, producing glossitis, stomatitis, and seborrheic dermatitis.

    c. Niacin (nicotinic acid, niacinamide) deficiency causes the disorder known as **pellagra**.

        (1) Niacin deficiency is seen in persons whose diet is low in both niacin and tryptophan (from which the body can synthesize niacin); for example, it occurs when corn is the main dietary staple.

        (2) Secondary niacin deficiency can occur in prolonged diarrhea, in alcoholism or cirrhosis, during therapy with isoniazid (a biochemical competitor), and in carcinoid syndrome (because tryptophan is preempted for serotonin synthesis).

        (3) Manifestations of **pellagra** include the **four Ds:** dermatitis, diarrhea, dementia, and death.

    d. Vitamin B_6 (pyridoxine) deficiency can be found in infants who are fed formulas deficient in the vitamin, in persons receiving drugs that inactivate it (isoniazid, penicillamine), and in chronic alcoholics. In infants, the clinical manifestations are generalized seizures; in adults, polyneuritis and anemia are seen.

    e. Vitamin B_{12} deficiency

        (1) Causes

            (a) Vitamin B_{12} deficiency is usually due to a lack of **gastric intrinsic factor,** which is required for B_{12} absorption in the intestine. Intrinsic factor is absent in patients with gastric atrophy or after extensive gastric surgery.

            (b) Inadequate dietary intake of vitamin B_{12} may be seen in strict vegetarians.

            (c) Impaired absorption and consequent vitamin B_{12} deficiency may occur in extensive small bowel disease, such as Crohn's disease, celiac disease, fistulas and diverticula, or blind loop syndrome after intestinal surgery.

        (d) The fish tapeworm, *Diphyllobothrium latum,* may compete for vitamin B_{12} in the small intestine.

    (2) Clinical syndromes

        (a) Pernicious anemia, a megaloblastic anemia, results from ineffective erythropoiesis. DNA synthesis is defective and cell maturation is impaired. This combination results in large red cells (macrocytes) and in white cells with hypersegmented nuclei. The incidence of gastric carcinoma is significantly higher in patients with pernicious anemia than in the general population.

        (b) Subacute combined degeneration of the spinal cord (i.e., degeneration of both the dorsal and lateral columns of the cord) is manifested by paresthesias, slowed reflexes, weakness, and ataxia (see Chapter 21 IV A).

  f. Folate (folic acid) deficiency causes a macrocytic anemia with megaloblastic changes similar to those seen in vitamin B_{12} deficiency, except that folate deficiency does not cause neurologic damage.

    (1) Causes include insufficient intake (alcoholism, poor diet), defective absorption (small bowel disorders), or increased utilization or demand (pregnancy). Certain drugs interfere with folate metabolism or absorption, notably the anticancer drug methotrexate and the anticonvulsant drug phenytoin.

    (2) When a patient has a **megaloblastic anemia,** it is critically important to rule out B_{12} deficiency, since folate therapy may reverse the hematologic changes but will not prevent the neurologic damage associated with B_{12} deficiency.

3. Vitamin C (ascorbic acid) deficiency results in **scurvy.** The principal manifestations are bleeding gums, perifollicular skin hemorrhage, petechiae, and conjunctival hemorrhages. These conditions result from functional and structural abnormality of the connective tissue due to defective hydroxylation of lysine and proline.

V. ESSENTIAL TRACE ELEMENTS

A. General considerations. Normal metabolism requires the presence of a number of inorganic elements. Though needed in only small amounts, these trace elements serve a variety of essential functions.

B. Specific essential elements

  1. Sodium, potassium, chloride, and **magnesium** are important in extracellular and intracellular fluid metabolism and in neuromuscular excitation.

  2. Calcium and **phosphorus** are important in bone metabolism.

  3. Zinc, present in the liver and muscle, acts as a cofactor for certain enzymes. **Zinc deficiency** occurs when the diet is devoid of animal protein and rich in bread and beans. The clinical manifestations are growth failure, hypogonadism, poor wound healing, anemia, and hepatosplenomegaly.

  4. Manganese is required for the action of enzymes involved in protein digestion and fatty acid biosynthesis. Specific deficiency syndromes have not been observed in humans; in rats, deficiency is associated with infertility and osteodystrophy.

  5. Copper is involved in electron transport and neurotransmitter metabolism.

    a. Copper deficiency is rare in humans, occurring either in malnourished infants or in adults maintained for long periods on intravenous hyperalimentation. Clinically, these patients have anemia and leukopenia. In animals, neurologic disturbances also have been reported.

    b. In the inherited abnormality of copper metabolism, **Wilson's disease,** copper is deposited in the tissues, especially the liver, brain, and cornea (see Chapter 15 IX C 3).

  6. Iron is involved in the production of normal red cells.

    a. Iron deficiency is quite common, especially in women of reproductive age. It may be caused by insufficient intake or excess loss due to bleeding, and it is associated with a microcytic, hypochromic anemia.

b. Iron excess occurs in several well-defined clinical situations (see also Chapter 15 IX C 1).

   (1) **Primary hemochromatosis** is a genetic disorder in which the intestinal absorption of iron increases despite normal or increased iron stores. **Secondary hemochromatosis** results from iron overloading, as from repeated blood transfusions.

   (2) In primary hemochromatosis, iron is first deposited as **hemosiderin** within hepatocytes; whereas in secondary hemochromatosis, hemosiderin deposits are seen first in reticuloendothelial cells of the liver, spleen, and bone marrow. In both disorders, hemosiderin subsequently can be deposited in the skin, gonads, heart, and endocrine glands.

STUDY QUESTIONS

Directions: Each of the numbered items or incomplete statements in this section is followed by answers or by completions of the statement. Select the **one** lettered answer or completion that is **best** in each case.

1. Vitamin B_{12} deficiency can result from all of the following disorders EXCEPT

(A) total gastrectomy
(B) Crohn's disease
(C) esophageal carcinoma
(D) infestation with *Diphyllobothrium latum*
(E) celiac disease

2. Malnutrition can result in all of the following conditions EXCEPT

(A) numerous infections
(B) emaciation
(C) fatty liver
(D) gastric carcinoma
(E) anorexia

Directions: The group of items in this section consists of lettered options followed by a set of numbered items. For each item, select the **one** lettered option that is most closely associated with it. Each lettered option may be selected once, more than once, or not at all.

Questions 3–7

Match each disorder with the associated nutrient or vitamin deficiency or excess.

(A) Dietary protein
(B) Thiamine
(C) Iron
(D) Copper
(E) Niacin

3. Beriberi

4. Hemochromatosis

5. Pellagra

6. Wilson's disease

7. Kwashiorkor

1-C   4-C   7-A
2-D   5-E
3-B   6-D

ANSWERS AND EXPLANATIONS

1. The answer is C *[IV B 2 e]*.
Esophageal carcinoma is not likely to interfere with the site or mechanism of absorption of vitamin B_{12}. Vitamin B_{12} deficiency can result from loss of intrinsic factor in the stomach, which occurs with total gastrectomy. In diseases of the small intestine, such as Crohn's disease or celiac disease, the vitamin B–intrinsic factor complex cannot be absorbed, so vitamin B_{12} deficiency occurs. Similarly, the fish tapeworm, *Diphyllobothrium latum,* can interfere with absorption of vitamin B_{12} by competing for the vitamin.

2. The answer is D *[III B]*.
Malnutrition has no known relationship to gastric carcinoma. The results of malnutrition obviously include emaciation. Because malnutrition depresses cellular and humoral immunity, numerous infections may occur. Malnutrition often results in fatty liver, which also may be associated with anorexia.

3–7. The answers are: 3-B *[IV B 2 a]*, **4-C** *[V B 6]*, **5-E** *[IV B 2 c]*, **6-D** *[V B 5]*, **7-A** *[III B]*.
Beriberi is a deficiency of thiamine (vitamin B_1). The major organs affected are the nervous system and the heart, with manifestations of peripheral neuropathy, muscle weakness, and cardiac failure.

Hemochromatosis is a disorder of iron metabolism and occurs as two forms. Primary hemochromatosis is a genetic disorder in which intestinal absorption of iron increases. Secondary hemochromatosis results from an exogenous overload of iron given directly into the blood stream, as in repeated blood transfusions. Iron is deposited in various organs. Deposition in the liver can cause cirrhosis; in endocrine glands, various endocrine deficiencies; and in the myocardium, cardiac failure.

Pellagra is a disorder associated with niacin deficiency and is manifested by the classic four Ds: dermatitis, diarrhea, dementia, and death.

Wilson's disease is a genetic disorder in which an abnormality in copper metabolism causes copper to be deposited in excessive amounts in the liver, the brain, and the cornea.

Kwashiorkor is a disease of severe malnutrition caused by marked deficiency of dietary protein. Usually seen in children, it is manifested by hepatosplenomegaly, with fatty liver and ultimately cirrhosis.

6

Immunopathology

John E. Tomaszewski

I. INTRODUCTION. The past decade has been a period of exponential gain in knowledge regarding the immune system. At the same time, the number of disease states identified as having a fundamental immunologic abnormality also has increased. Epidemic diseases such as AIDS are dominated by immunologic aberrations. For these reasons, immunopathologic research has assumed a major role in the search for a better understanding of disease.

II. CELLS AND OTHER ELEMENTS INVOLVED IN THE IMMUNE RESPONSE

A. Lymphocytes and their products

1. **T lymphocytes,** or **T cells,** are the thymus-derived lymphocytes that are found mainly in the interfollicular and paracortical areas of lymph nodes as well as in the periarteriolar sheaths of the spleen. T cells constitute 70% to 80% of circulating peripheral blood lymphocytes.

   a. T cells recognize antigens in their environment through an antigen-specific T-cell receptor (TCR).

   (1) About 95% of T cells have a TCR composed of two disulfide-linked polypeptide chains, α and β, which are noncovalently bound to the CD3 molecular complex (Figure 6-1). Antigen binds the variable region of the TCR. Postrecognition steps leading to T-cell activation appear to be a function of the CD3 complex.

   (2) About 5% of T cells have a TCR composed of two other distinct chains, γ and δ. These cells do not have either CD4 or CD8 on their surface (see also II A 1 b).

   (3) Antigenic diversity of the TCR develops through a process of gene rearrangements analogous to those found in immunoglobulin (Ig) synthesis (see also II A 2).

   b. T-cell subtypes. Multiple subpopulations of T cells exist (see also Chapter 1 II F 2 a).

   (1) Cytotoxic T cells are capable of antigen-directed killing. They are important in delayed hypersensitivity reactions, rejection of solid organ transplants, immunity to certain bacteria and viruses, and, possibly, tumor immunity. Monoclonal antibodies that react with cell-surface glycoproteins of these cells are designated CD8, and the T-cell subtype is referred to as **CD8⁺**.

   (2) Helper T cells are regulatory cells that help B cells and other T cells to respond appropriately to antigen. Monoclonal antibody markers for these cells are designated CD4, and the T-cell subtype is referred to as **CD4⁺**.

   (3) Suppressor T cells act to suppress antibody production by B cells and, thus, partially control the T- and B-cell immune response. These cells also are designated **CD8⁺**.

   c. T-cell products. A variety of substances known as **lymphokines** are produced and secreted by T cells and play important roles in cell-mediated immunologic activities. Examples of lymphokines that regulate lymphocyte activities follow.

   (1) Interleukin-2 (IL-2) is a T-cell growth factor that is important for long-term proliferation of activated T cells.

   (2) Interleukin-3 (IL-3) stimulates differentiation of bone-marrow stem cells.

   (3) Interleukin 4 (IL-4) acts as a growth factor for activated T cells, B cells, and mast cells. IL-4 up-regulates class II **major histocompatibility complex (MHC)** expression on B cells.

   (4) Interleukin 5 (IL-5) aids in differentiation of B cells into antibody-producing plasma cells.

   (5) Interleukin 6 (IL-6) aids in maturation of T cells and B cells, stimulates growth of hematopoietic precursor cells, and inhibits fibroblasts.

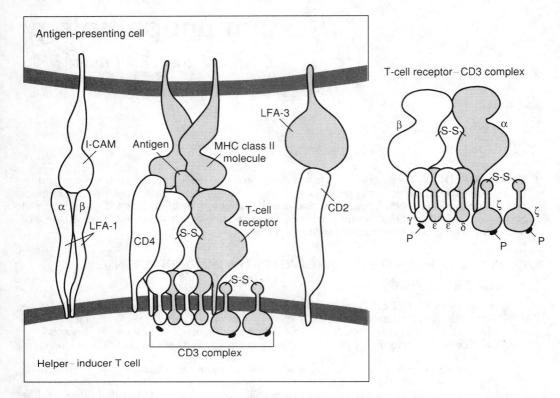

Figure 6-1. The figure shows the T-cell receptor (TCR)–CD3 complex and the accessory immune molecules CD4, CD2, and LFA-1, which are present on helper T cells. The TCR is formed as a heterodimer also linked by disulfide bridges. In most CD4 cells, α and β chains form the heterodimer, although in a smaller population, γ and δ chains are employed. The CD3 complex is spatially related to the TCR and has six membrane-associated proteins. Phosphorylation of the cytoplasmic domain may control signal transduction. The TCR of CD4 T cells binds antigen, which is "presented" in association with the major histocompatibility complex (MHC) II molecule displayed on the surface of antigen-presenting cells. CD4 stabilizes the interaction between the antigen-presenting cell and the helper T cell. Accessory immune molecules LFA-1 and I-CAM, plus LFA-3 and CD2, act as adhesion molecules that strengthen the attachment of the antigen-presenting cell and the helper T cell and allow the TCR–MHC antigen interaction. (Adapted from Terhorst C, David J: Antigens, antibodies, and T cell receptors. In *Scientific American: Medicine*. New York, Scientific American, 1989, section 6, subsection II, p 21.)

    (6) Gamma interferon (INF-γ) is one of a family of interferons that are proteins with diverse functions. INF-γ has antiviral activity, activates macrophages, promotes B-cell differentiation, suppresses hematopoietic precursor cells, and induces the expression of class II MHC on many cell types.

  2. B lymphocytes, or **B cells,** constitute up to 15% of circulating peripheral blood lymphocytes and typically are defined by the presence of endogenously produced **immunoglobulins**.
    a. Origin, maturation, and differentiation of B cells
      (1) Origin. B cells are derived from lymphoid progenitor cells, which are believed to differentiate in the fetal liver and spleen and in the adult bone marrow, although the exact origin in humans is unknown. Once formed, B cells come to reside in the blood, the germinal centers and superficial cortex of lymph nodes, the lymphoid follicles of the white pulp in the spleen, and the bone marrow.
      (2) Maturation. B cells normally pass through a maturation sequence characterized by gene rearrangements that produce distinct phenotypes and enormous diversity in the B-cell repertoire [see also II A 2 b (2)].
        (a) Pre–B cells contain cytoplasmic mu (μ) heavy chain but no surface immunoglobulin.
        (b) Immature B cells have surface immunoglobulin M (IgM).

(c) With further gene rearrangement, B cells acquire surface IgD and then proceed to "switch" heavy-chain isotypes to express IgG, IgA, or IgE.

(3) Differentiation. Competent B cells recognize antigen through their surface immunoglobulin receptors. B-cell responses are expanded with the help of T cells and macrophages.

   (a) If antigen stimulation persists, B cells differentiate into their final stage—the antibody-synthesizing **plasma cell**.

   (b) If not, the activated B cells return to a resting, or "memory," stage.

b. B-cell products: immunoglobulins. Immunoglobulins are globular proteins produced by B cells or plasma cells in response to exposure to a particular antigen. The immunoglobulins react specifically to (i.e., bind to) that antigen. Five isotypes of immunoglobulins—IgG, IgA, IgM, IgD, and IgE—are identified by structural differences. The basic structure and functional properties of immunoglobulins are the same for all isotypes.

   (1) Structure (Figure 6-2). The basic structural unit (**monomer**) of immunoglobulins consists of two identical heavy polypeptide chains and two identical light polypeptide chains covalently linked by disulfide bonds. Each heavy and light chain of the immunoglobulin molecule is divided into two regions.

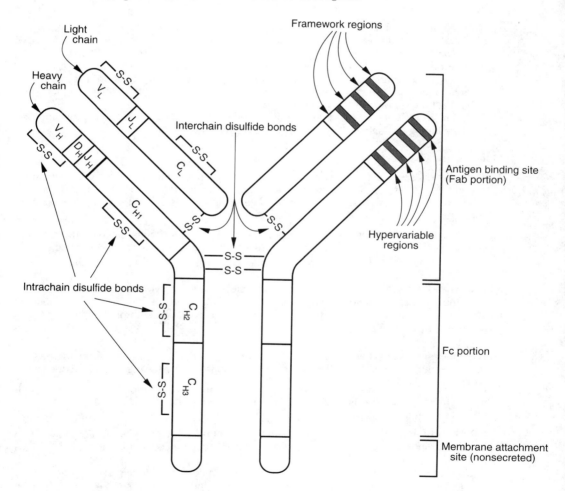

Figure 6-2. The basic structural unit (monomer) of immunoglobulin molecules consists of two identical heavy polypeptide chains and two identical light polypeptide chains linked covalently by disulfide bonds. In two immunoglobulin subclasses, IgM and IgA, the basic units are linked by a short polypeptide, the J chain, to form pentamers and dimers, respectively. V = variable region; J = joining region; C = constant region; D = diversity region; H = heavy chain; L = light chain; S-S = disulfide bond. (Reprinted from Besa EC, Catalano PM, Kant JA, et al: NMS *Hematology*. Malvern, PA, Harwal Publishing, 1992, p 160.)

        (a) The **variable regions** of immunoglobulins are highly heterogeneous and are the sites responsible for binding antigen. These regions are contained within the **Fab fragments** that are produced following pepsin degradation of the molecule (see Figure 6-2).

        (b) The **constant regions** of immunoglobulins control other functions, such as the binding of complement and cytotropic reactions. The constant regions of the heavy chains are found in the **Fc fragment** that is produced following papain degradation of the molecule. (The constant regions of light chains are in the Fab fragment.)

    (2) Genetic regulation

        (a) Certain genes control the various regions on the heavy and light chains of the immunoglobulin. For functional immunoglobulin to be encoded, these genes must undergo rearrangement, bringing the individual regions into continuous sequence (Figures 6-3 and 6-4). This process of gene rearrangement yields an enormous number of combinations. (The mammalian immune system is capable of producing roughly 10^9 different antibodies.)

        (b) This heterogeneity happens through rearrangements of the immunoglobulin heavy and light chains and accounts for the enormous diversity found in the B-cell repertoire.

3. Null cells are a population of cytotoxic lymphocytes that are large, possess cytoplasmic granules, and are negative for TCRs and surface immunoglobulin. Their name reflects this lack of traditional T- or B-cell markers.

    a. Natural killer (NK) cells represent the majority of null cells. NK cells possess cytolytic activity against a variety of targets in the absence of purposeful immunization. Their cytotoxic activity does not seem to be restricted by the MHC (see II F). NK cells require cell–cell contact for killing, which is enhanced by interferon and IL-2.

    b. Killer (K) cells are a related population of null cells, which possess Fc receptors and mediate killing through antibody-dependent mechanisms.

B. Mononuclear phagocytes

    1. Mononuclear phagocytes are widely distributed in the body; they are given different names depending on their location. In connective tissue, they are called **histiocytes;** in blood, **monocytes;** in bone marrow, **macrophages;** in the liver, **Kupffer cells;** and in the lung, **alveolar macrophages**.

    2. Mononuclear phagocytes in all of these sites show common properties that make them critical components of inflammatory and immune reactions. The functions of mononuclear phagocytes are discussed in Chapter 1 II E 2–4.

C. Mast cells and basophils are granulocytes whose electron-dense cytoplasmic granules contain many of the chemical mediators of inflammation, including histamine, heparin, and chemotactic factors (see also Chapter 1 III). Secretion of these products is mediated through type I hypersensitivity mechanisms (see III A 1).

D. The complement system is a plasma-based system of proteins that play a major role in host defense (both specific and nonspecific), in the inflammatory response, and in the mediation of tissue injury.

    1. Functions. Activated complement components regulate a variety of biologic activities, including chemotaxis, opsonization, phagocytosis, and cytolysis. They also promote smooth muscle contraction and vascular permeability.

    2. Pathways of activation. Complement is activated sequentially in a cascading manner such that a protein is activated only by the protein that directly preceded it in the sequence. Two pathways are possible.

    a. Classic pathway. This pathway requires all nine major complement components.

        (1) Activation occurs by direct binding of **C1** to an antibody (most often IgG or IgM) in the form of an antigen–antibody complex.

        (2) Activated C1 cleaves C4 and C2 to form the bimolecular complex **C4b2a**. This compound has enzymatic properties and is referred to as **C3 convertase**.

        (3) **C3** then splits under the influence of C3 convertase to form C3a and C3b.

            (a) **C3a** is a small fragment that, along with other low-molecular-weight peptides generated later in the cascade, causes the release of vasoactive amines and lysosomal

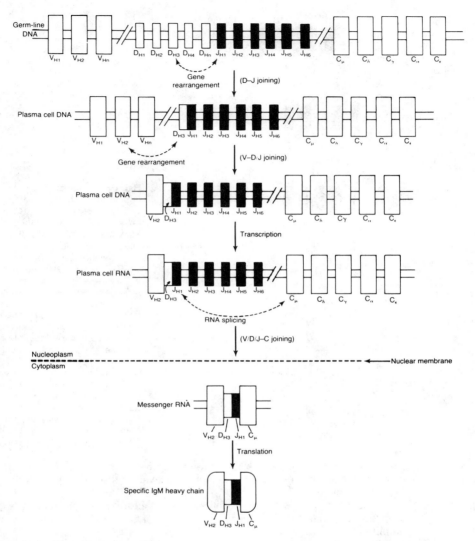

Figure 6-3. Human μ heavy chain gene organization. The potential for variety in heavy chains, as in light chains, is due to somatic recombination in the DNA and to RNA splicing. As the B-cell precursor differentiates into a mature B cell, DNA deletion brings one of the variable (V_H) genes , one of the diversity (D_H) genes, and one of the joining (J_H) genes together—in this example, V_{H2}, D_{H3}, and J_{H1}. This unit and the remaining J genes are separated from the constant (C) region by an intervening sequence of DNA. The plasma cell DNA is transcribed into nuclear RNA, which is spliced to form messenger RNA (mRNA). In this process, the C_μ gene is selected and joined to the $V_{H2}/D_{H3}/J_{H1}$ complex, and the entire unit is ready for translation into a μ chain. (Reprinted from Hyde RM: NMS *Immunology*, 2nd ed. Malvern, PA, Harwal Publishing, 1991, p 40.)

        enzymes. C3a also causes enhanced vascular permeability and smooth muscle contraction.

    (b) **C3b** acts as an opsonin and also binds with C4b2a to form **C5 convertase**.

  (4) Cleavage of **C5** by C5 convertase generates **C5a** (an important chemotactic factor) and **C5b**, which binds with the last components of the complement cascade to form the **membrane attack complex**.

  b. Alternate pathway. In this pathway, the early components (C1, C4, and C2) are bypassed, and C3 is activated directly.

    (1) C3b (generated from C3 by **C3 priming convertase**) is activated by substances such as bacterial lipopolysaccharides (endotoxin), aggregated globulins (IgA and some IgG),

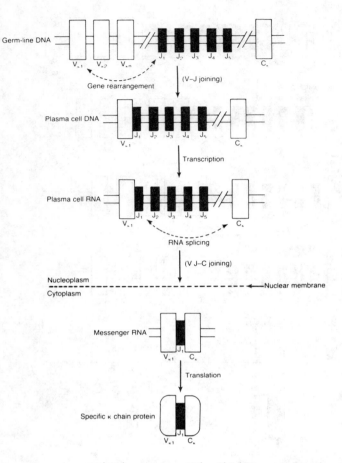

Figure 6-4. Human κ light chain gene organization. The potential for a large variety of light chains exists due to somatic recombination in the DNA and RNA splicing. As the B cell precursor differentiates into a mature B cell, DNA deletion brings one of the variable (V_κ) genes next to one of the joining (J) genes—in this example, $V_{\kappa 1}$ and J_1. This unit and the remaining J genes are separated from the constant (C_κ) region by an intervening sequence (intron) of DNA. The $V_{\kappa 1}/J_1$ unit codes for one of the numerous possible κ chain variable exons. The plasma cell DNA is transcribed into nuclear RNA, which is spliced to form messenger RNA (mRNA) with $V_{\kappa 1}$, J_1, and C_κ messages joined and ready for translation into the κ chain. (Reprinted from Hyde RM: NMS *Immunology*, 2nd ed. Malvern, PA, Harwal Publishing, 1991, p 38.)

and cobra venom. C3b, which is continuously present in small amounts in the circulation, is deposited on the surfaces of these activator substances and is "protected" from degradation.

(2) This surface-bound, protected C3b interacts with **factor B** in the presence of Mg^{2+} to form **C3b,B**. **Factor D** then cleaves a portion of B to form **C3b,Bb** (also called **amplification C3 convertase**).

(3) C3b,Bb can cleave large amounts of C3 and activate the terminal (membrane attack) sequence. Cleavage of C3 also generates additional C3b, which further amplifies the loop.

E. Other mediators of the immune reaction

1. Plasma factors. The **kinin system** and **coagulation cascade** are additional plasma protein systems that augment the inflammatory reaction by producing factors that increase vascular permeability and chemotaxis. The kinin system is described in more detail in Chapter 1 III B 1; the coagulation cascade is discussed in Chapter 8 II A 2.

2. Vasoactive amines stored in mast cells, basophils, and platelets are important in the early inflammatory reaction of IgE-mediated (type I) hypersensitivity reactions (see III A 1). Vasoactive amines are described in more detail in Chapter 1 III A.

3. Arachidonic acid metabolites and platelet-activating factor

a. Prostaglandins and **leukotrienes** are products of the cyclooxygenase and lipoxygenase pathways, respectively, of arachidonic acid metabolism. These compounds are described in more detail in Chapter 1 III C.

b. Platelet-activating factor is derived from antigen-stimulated IgE-sensitized basophils. It causes platelet aggregation and release of vasoactive amines, leading to modulation of vascular tone and permeability.

F. Histocompatibility antigens. In humans, the major histocompatibility genes are located on the short arm of chromosome 6. These genes code for the histocompatibility antigens termed **human leukocyte antigens (HLAs)**. HLAs are products of genes of the **MHC**, which is a highly polymorphous set of membrane-associated glycoproteins that are critical for the recognition of self during cell–cell immunologic reactions. Two broad categories of MHC antigens are described.

1. **Class I MHC antigens**
   a. Class I MHC antigens are composed of two noncovalently linked polypeptide chains. The smaller chain is a superficial protein termed β_2-**microglobulin**. The heavy chain is a **transmembrane protein** that bears the antigenic determinants for the alleles of the three major class I loci, which are designated **HLA-A, HLA-B,** and **HLA-C**. The alleles of this antigen system are codominant.
   b. Class I antigens are expressed on the surface of essentially all cells and are recognized by cytotoxic T cells. Thus, CD8$^+$ T cells are said to be "restricted" in their activity by class I MHC antigens. The class I MHC antigens "present" foreign antigens to CD8$^+$ T cells in a groove that resides at the surface of the molecule (Figure 6-5). Class I antigen is an important antigenic target in transplant rejection.

2. **Class II MHC antigens**
   a. Class II MHC antigens are composed of two noncovalently linked glycoproteins; however, both are transmembrane proteins. Class II antigens are encoded by the HLA-D gene, which is divided into three major loci designated **HLA-DP, HLA-DQ,** and **HLA-DR**.
   b. Class II antigens are located mostly in macrophages, B cells, activated T cells, endothelial cells, and dendritic cells.* Helper T cells recognize foreign antigen in the context of class II MHC antigens. Thus, CD4$^+$ T cells are said to be "restricted" in their activity by class II antigens. Class II antigen is critical to the process of foreign antigen recognition by T cells.

III. IMMUNOLOGIC MECHANISMS OF TISSUE DAMAGE. Although the immune system generally is protective, the same mechanisms that protect the host may at times cause tissue damage so severe that death results. Gell and Coombs have classified these damaging immune reactions (sometimes referred to as **hypersensitivity reactions**) into four types.

A. Type I reaction: immediate hypersensitivity. This local or generalized response occurs within minutes of reexposure to an antigen to which the host has been previously sensitized.

1. **Pathogenetic mechanism.** Type I reactions are initiated by antigens reacting with cell-bound antibody—usually IgE.
   a. The first step is initial exposure to the antigen, which stimulates IgE production. Mast cells and basophils are strongly attracted to IgE and bind the antibody through Fc receptors. This cytotropic antibody persists for weeks.
   b. Upon reexposure, the antigen binds to the cell-bound IgE at its Fab portion. When adjacent IgE molecules become bound (bridged) by the antigen, the mast cells and basophils are activated to release a variety of substances that mediate the hypersensitivity response. Mast cells also can be activated directly by C3a and C5a.
   c. The mediators of immediate hypersensitivity include histamine, chemotactic factors for eosinophils (ECF) and neutrophils (NCF), platelet-activating factor, enzymes, leukotrienes, and prostaglandins. Their effects include smooth muscle contraction, vasodilation, increased vascular permeability, and proteolytic destruction.

2. **Clinical features.** Immediate hypersensitivity reactions can manifest in many ways, depending on the target tissue. Type I reactions range from life-threatening systemic anaphylaxis to the more minor conditions of allergic rhinitis (hay fever), atopic dermatitis, and food allergies.
   a. Local signs include swelling, erythema, edema, pruritus, and urticaria; scaling, papular, or lichenoid lesions may be seen in atopic dermatitis.
   b. Generalized symptoms may include bronchoconstriction (which may be severe and progress to asphyxia), nausea and vomiting, hypotension, and circulatory collapse.

****Dendritic cells** are characterized by long cytoplasmic processes and large amounts of surface class II MHC antigen. These cells exist in a variety of tissues and are believed to be important antigen-presenting cells. In the skin, dendritic cells are known as **Langerhans' cells**.

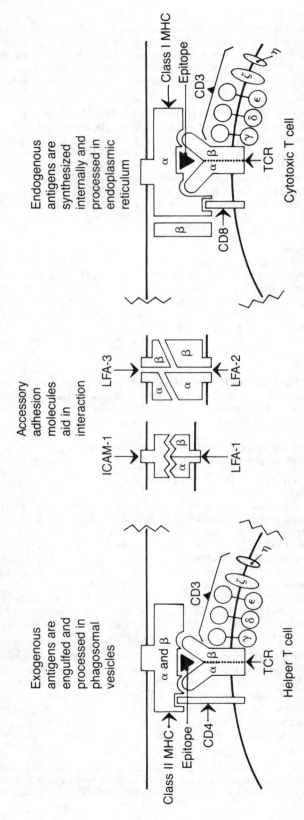

Figure 6-5. Interaction between major histocompatibility complex (MHC) class I and II antigens and the T-cell receptor (TCR) are illustrated. Exogenous antigens, which have been engulfed and processed in acidic lysosomes, are "presented" at the cell surface in association with MHC II. CD4 binds MHC II during antigen presentation, and the TCR of CD4 cells recognizes the MHC II–antigen complex. Endogenous antigens are processed in the endoplasmic reticulum and are displayed in association with MHC I. During the presentation of this type of antigen, CD8 cells bind MHC I. TCR engages the MHC I–antigen complex, causing recognition. Thus CD4 cells are said to be "restricted" by MHC II, and CD8 cells are restricted by MHC I. (Reprinted from Hyde RM: NMS *Immunology*, 2nd ed. Malvern, PA, Harwal Publishing, 1991, p 72.)

B. Type II reaction: antibody-mediated cytotoxicity. In this type, antibody reacts with a normal or altered cell-surface component, leading to subsequent destruction or inactivation of the target cell.

1. **Pathogenetic mechanism.** Type II reactions are initiated by cytotoxic antibodies—usually IgM or IgG. When such antibody binds to antigen on a cell surface or in connective tissue, one of two antibody-mediated cytotoxic reactions occurs.

   a. **Complement-mediated cytotoxicity.** In this reaction, the binding of antibody with cell surface antigen causes complement to be activated via the classic pathway. This results in activation of the terminal complement components (the **membrane attack complex**), which can directly lyse cell membranes. C3b also enhances cytotoxicity by functioning as an opsonin.

   b. **Antibody-dependent cell-mediated cytotoxicity (ADCC).** Antibody also may affect cytotoxicity through complement-independent mechanisms. In this reaction, target cells coated with antibody are lysed by K cells, which possess Fc receptors.

2. **Clinical features.** Examples of antibody-mediated cytotoxic reactions include:

   a. **Transfusion reactions,** in which transfusion of a mismatched blood type results in an immediate antibody reaction to nonself blood-group antigens, with resultant intravascular homolysis

   b. **Autoimmune hemolytic anemia,** in which patients produce antibodies to their own red cell antigens, with resultant intravascular hemolysis

C. Type III reaction: immune complex disease. In this type of reaction, circulating antigen–antibody (immune) complexes (which normally are removed by the reticuloendothelial system) are deposited in tissues, leading to complement activation and further tissue injury. Immune complexes also may develop in situ (i.e., antibodies are directed against antigens that are endogenous to the tissues or have been planted there), thus triggering localized tissue damage.

1. **Pathogenetic mechanism**

   a. **Immune complex formation.** Immune complexes are formed in the presence of antigen—which may be exogenous (e.g., drugs, hormones, infectious agents) or autogenous (e.g., tumors, rheumatoid factor, altered DNA)—and antibody. The concentration and duration of exposure to the antigen as well as the quantity and type of antibody are important in determining the quantity and chronicity of complex formation and deposition.

   b. **Inflammatory mechanisms.** Once formed, immune complexes incite a variety of inflammatory processes.

      (1) They can interact with complement, leading to the activation of C3a and C5a, with resultant release of vasoactive amines, increase in vascular permeability, and attraction of neutrophils. Neutrophils, through release of lysosomal enzymes, produce local tissue injury.

      (2) Immune complexes also interact with platelets, leading to the formation of microthrombi and further increase in vascular permeability due to the release of vasoactive amines from the activated platelets.

2. **Clinical features.** Immune complex diseases typically are characterized by multisystem involvement, reflecting that immune complexes are deposited in various tissues (e.g., the vessels, kidneys, joints, skin, muscle). Two important examples of type III reactions—systemic lupus erythematosus (SLE) and polymyositis—are described in IV B and IV E, respectively.

D. Type IV reaction: cell-mediated hypersensitivity. Cell-mediated hypersensitivity reactions do not require the presence of antibody and, characteristically, are delayed anywhere from about 24 hours to 2 weeks. Three interrelated mechanisms are recognized, all of which involve activated T cells.

1. **Delayed-type hypersensitivity** may be of the tuberculin or granulomatous type.

   a. **Tuberculin-type hypersensitivity.** A subcutaneous injection of soluble protein antigen (tuberculin) will elicit an inflammatory reaction composed of lymphocytes and mononuclear phagocytes. This reaction, characterized by induration and swelling at the injection site, becomes most intense within 1 to 2 days.

      (1) In this reaction, protein antigen is taken up and processed by macrophages, then presented in the cell membrane of the macrophage in conjunction with class II MHC antigen. Antigen-specific T cells recognize this complex and become activated.

      (2) Through lymphokine and monokine signals, recruitment and proliferation of additional T cells, macrophages, and fibroblasts yield an amplified inflammatory reaction. If antigen is not cleared, the reaction may present as granulomatous inflammation.

   b. **Granulomatous hypersensitivity** is clinically the most significant form of type IV reaction; **sarcoidosis** is an example of this type of reaction.
      (1) Granulomatous hypersensitivity results from the presence of a persistent antigen within macrophages. Usually, this antigen is the infectious agent, although granulo-mas may form in the presence of immune complexes or particulate matter (e.g., talc) or for no apparent reason (e.g., in sarcoidosis, which is of idiopathic origin).
      (2) The characteristic morphologic pattern of granulomatous inflammation is discussed in Chapter 1 V B 2 b.
   2. **Cell-mediated cytotoxicity.** The targets of cytotoxic T cells may include MHC antigen, as is the case in organ transplantation rejection as well as in immunity to viral antigens in certain tumors. Cytotoxic T cells may kill by disrupting ionic flux in target cells.
      a. In cell-mediated cytotoxic reactions, helper (CD4$^+$) T cells recognize target cell antigen in the context of class II MHC antigen. Cells naturally expressing class II MHC molecules (e.g., mononuclear phagocytes, endothelial cells, dendritic cells), thus, are important in the initiation of this inflammatory pathway. CD4$^+$ T cells become activated, proliferate, and release lymphokines (IL-2), which amplify the proliferation.
      b. Cytotoxic (CD8$^+$) T cells recognize target cell antigen in the context of class I MHC glyco-protein. Antigen-specific CD8$^+$ T-cell populations are expanded under the influence of IL-2.
   3. **NK-cell cytotoxicity.** As described in II A 3 a, NK cells recognize a variety of cellular targets and are not restricted by MHC molecules. NK activity is thought to be important in immune reactions aimed at viral or tumor targets.

IV. AUTOIMMUNE DISEASE

   A. **General concepts: immunologic tolerance and autoimmunity.** An immune response generated against self antigens is an aberrancy that implies a loss of immunologic ability to distinguish be-tween self and nonself. The normal status of immunologic nonresponsiveness to self is termed **tolerance**. Tolerance probably represents an active process involving continuous generation of cellular and humoral inhibitory regulators. Loss of tolerance to self antigen is referred to as **au-toimmunity**. The mechanisms by which tolerance is generated and lost are poorly understood. **Theories of autoimmunity** include:

   1. Recognition of previously hidden or sequestered antigen

   2. Diminution of suppressor T-cell function

   3. Increase in helper T-cell activity

   4. T-cell–independent polyclonal B-cell activation by complex antigens

   5. Modification of self antigens by drugs or microorganisms

   6. Cross-reactivity between autologous antigens and microbial antigens

   B. **SLE** (often referred to simply as **lupus**) is the classic multisystem autoimmune disease.
   1. **Etiology.** No single cause of lupus has been identified, although environmental, genetic, and hormonal influences are suspected.
      a. **Environmental factors** may include viruses, drugs, or toxins that interfere with T-cell func-tion, allowing the disease to be expressed.
      b. **Genetic factors.** Family studies of lupus show an association with certain HLAs (HLA-DR2, -DR3, -A1, and -B8). Lupus also is associated with deficiencies of **complement compo-nents C2 and C4**. Abnormalities in the immune response genes located near the HLA and complement genes may be important.
      c. **Hormonal factors.** The fact that lupus occurs primarily in women of childbearing age sug-gests a role for hormones, although this is unlikely to be causative.
   2. **Pathogenesis**
      a. **Autoantibodies.** Antibodies against a variety of nuclear and cytoplasmic antigens are the hallmark of lupus. **Antinuclear antibodies (ANA)** may be against double- or single-stranded DNA, RNA, RNA-associated proteins, histones, nucleoli, and a soluble nuclear antigen known as the Sm antigen. Although many of these antibodies can be found in other diseases, antibody to native double-stranded DNA is highly diagnostic for lupus.
      b. **Immune complex formation.** The antibodies usually are not directly cytotoxic but, rather, participate in the development of immune complexes that trigger inflammatory reactions. Thus, lupus is a prototypical type III hypersensitivity reaction.

    c. Lymphocyte dysfunction. Defects in suppressor T-cell function or prolonged polyclonal B-cell activation are two mechanisms by which the pronounced antibody response may occur.

3. Clinical features. Lupus is characterized by prominent constitutional features (i.e., fever, weight loss, fatigue) as well as a variety of organ-specific manifestations of immune complex deposition.

4. Pathology

    a. Skin. Immune complexes are deposited at the dermoepidermal junction in erythematous areas but also are found in uninvolved skin. Immune complexes incite an inflammatory reaction including liquefactive degeneration of the basal layer of the dermis, perivascular mononuclear inflammation, fibrosis, and occasional fibrinoid necrosis of the vessel walls.

    b. Joints. Joint involvement almost always is a feature of lupus. In acute lupus arthritis, there is an exudative reaction with neutrophils and fibrin and a perivascular mononuclear infiltrate. Unlike the synovitis in rheumatoid arthritis, the synovitis in lupus is nonerosive.

    c. Kidneys. Immune complex deposition in the kidney can lead to a variety of glomerular interstitial and vascular changes (see also Chapter 16 III D 1 b).

    d. Serosal surfaces. The pericardium, pleura, and peritoneum may be affected by an acute inflammation with a fibrinous exudate, a mix of neutrophilic and mononuclear inflammation, edema, and focal vasculitis. With resolution, fibrosis and a lymphoplasmacytic infiltrate predominate.

    e. Heart. Small, nonbacterial vegetations are found on the mitral and tricuspid valves, along surfaces exposed to forward flow as well as behind the cusps (Libman-Sacks endocarditis). Microscopically, the vegetations are fibrin and inflammatory debris overlying an area of fibrinoid necrosis. Arterioles in the heart also may show fibrinoid necrosis and vasculitis; however, focal myocardial necrosis occurs in only the most severe cases.

    f. Vessels. Immune complex deposition in capillaries and small arteries leads to variable cellular infiltration and the formation of inflammatory lesions. Vasculitis is an important pathologic feature of lupus and is responsible for much of the tissue damage seen in the disease.

    g. Other changes. Hyperplasia of the lymph nodes and spleen, inflammatory reactions of the lung and liver, and immune-mediated cytopenias (e.g., hemolytic anemia, leukopenia, thrombocytopenia) also are seen in lupus.

5. Prognosis. The clinical course is quite variable. Renal failure and infectious complications are common causes of death in lupus patients.

C. Sjögren's syndrome is an idiopathic autoimmune disorder with characteristic organ and exocrine glandular features (especially lacrimal and salivary gland destruction), which may occur in association with another autoimmune disease (e.g., rheumatoid arthritis, lupus).

1. Pathogenesis

    a. Sjögren's syndrome involves both antibody-mediated (type II) and cell-mediated (type IV) immune reactions. The inflammatory reaction is characterized by a dense infiltrate of T cells (both $CD4^+$ and $CD8^+$) and some B cells.

    b. A variety of antibodies can be found in the serum of affected patients, including ANA and antibody to salivary duct cells. Antibody to the extractable RNA protein, SS-B, is found in 60% to 70% of patients with Sjögren's and is believed to be highly specific. Antibody SS-B binds with Epstein-Barr virus (EBV) RNA.

2. Clinical features

    a. Dry mouth (xerostomia), **dry eyes** (keratoconjunctivitis sicca), and variable **salivary gland enlargement** result from the lymphocytic infiltration. These abnormalities may be isolated or occur in association with abnormalities in other organs [e.g., skin, lungs, kidneys, gastrointestinal system, central nervous system (CNS)] due to a concurrent autoimmune disease such as lupus, rheumatoid arthritis, vasculitis, scleroderma, or polymyositis.

    b. Patients with Sjögren's syndrome are at increased risk for developing **lymphoid malignancies.**

3. Pathology

    a. The earliest finding is that of a dense, periductal lymphocytic infiltrate composed of small and large lymphocytes and plasma cells. Duct destruction is seen.

    b. Later, atrophy, fibrosis, and fatty replacement may occur.

    c. Differentiation of acute-phase Sjögren's syndrome from lymphoma may be difficult when the infiltrate is intense.

D. Scleroderma (also known as **progressive systemic sclerosis**) is characterized by small-vessel destruction and fibrosis of the skin and multiple internal organs.

1. **Pathogenesis.** The pathogenesis of scleroderma is poorly understood, although vascular endothelial cell damage is believed to trigger the connective tissue overgrowth.
   a. Possible mechanisms of endothelial injury include serum cytotoxic factors, cellular or humoral autoimmunity, and toxins.
   b. Fibroblast proliferation occurs, perhaps by the same mechanisms that cause endothelial injury. T-cell sensitization to collagen and humoral hypersensitivity have been postulated.
   c. A variety of autoantibodies are found in scleroderma patients, including antibodies to smooth muscle, rheumatoid factor, ANA, and antibodies to nucleolar components.
      (1) **Antinucleolar antibodies** are highly specific for scleroderma. Another specific autoantibody associated with scleroderma is **antibody to Scl-70** (a nonhistone nuclear protein).
      (2) **Antibody to centromere** is highly associated with the more benign and much less progressive variant of scleroderma known as **CREST syndrome** (calcinosis, Raynaud's phenomenon, esophageal dysfunction, syndactyly, and telangiectasia).

2. **Clinicopathologic features.** The salient feature in scleroderma is the development of fibrosis in multiple organs. Vascular sclerosis with myxoid change and focal fibrinoid necrosis also are seen. The following is a brief discussion of the characteristic clinical and pathologic features seen in commonly involved organs.
   a. **Skin.** Early in the disease, there are edema, perivascular lymphoid infiltrates, and a degenerative change of the dermal collagen. Later, dense dermal sclerosis occurs, with atrophy of the epidermis and adnexal structures. Arterioles may be hyalinized. These changes account for the skin "tightness" that is characteristic of clinical scleroderma.
   b. **Gastrointestinal tract** involvement occurs in about 50% of patients. The lower two-thirds of the esophagus develops fibrosis of the submucosal muscularis, with associated motility dysfunction. Fibrosis also may be seen in the small bowel and colon, with similar associated motility problems.
   c. **Kidney** involvement is characterized by slowly progressive, interlobular arterial intimal proliferation and periarterial fibrosis, which may be clinically silent. However, acute collapse of renal blood flow, with consequent renal cortical ischemia and malignant hypertension, can be associated with fibrinoid necrosis of the microvasculature and result in acute renal failure (the leading cause of death in scleroderma patients).
   d. **Lung.** The picture is very similar to the one for idiopathic pulmonary fibrosis with diffuse interstitial fibrosis. Variable thickening of the pulmonary vessels also is seen. Symptoms may be limited to progressive dyspnea on exertion.
   e. **Musculoskeletal system.** Joints may show a nonerosive mildly inflammatory synovitis. Tendon sheath involvement is not unusual, with **carpal tunnel syndrome** as a possible outcome. In skeletal muscle, edema and perivascular mononuclear inflammation appear early. In more established disease, interfascicular fibrosis has occurred.

3. **Prognosis.** Changes usually are slowly progressive. Cardiac, renal, and pulmonary involvement and the presence of intervening malignant hypertension are poor prognostic signs.

E. Polymyositis and dermatomyositis. Polymyositis is an idiopathic disease characterized by prominent proximal muscle weakness and chronic inflammatory myopathy; when a characteristic skin rash accompanies these features, the disorder is known as dermatomyositis.

1. **Classification.** A variety of disease subsets are described. These include:
   a. Adult polymyositis
   b. Adult dermatomyositis
   c. Polymyositis or dermatomyositis associated with malignancy
   d. Childhood dermatomyositis (associated with immune complex deposition and vasculitis)
   e. Polymyositis or dermatomyositis associated with other autoimmune disease

2. **Pathogenesis.** The basic cause of polymyositis is unknown. Lymphocyte-mediated muscle cell damage is thought to be the underlying mechanism. Also, autoantibodies to extractable nuclear antigens PM_1 and JO-1 are said to be most specific for this disease.

3. **Clinicopathologic features**
   a. **Striated muscle**
      (1) Symmetrical, proximal, upper and lower extremity muscle weakness is characteristic.

      (2) Microscopically, edema and a scant mononuclear infiltrate appear early in the disease. Later, a prominent mononuclear infiltrate occurs in conjunction with interstitial fibrosis and myofiber degeneration.

  b. Skin

      (1) An erythematous, sometimes scaling rash occurs in the malar region and is similar to that seen in lupus. However, it also is found on the upper chest, neck, forehead, and shoulders. **Heliotrope rash,** a lilac discoloration on the upper eyelids, is said to be pathognomonic.

      (2) Microscopically, edema, a perivascular infiltrate, and liquefactive degeneration of the dermoepidermal junction are similar to those seen in lupus.

F. Mixed connective tissue disease is a syndrome characterized by clinically overlapping features of lupus, polymyositis, and scleroderma in association with high serum levels of antibody to an extractable nuclear ribonucleoprotein. Whether mixed connective tissue disease represents an overlap with other autoimmune disorders or is a unique entity is unclear.

G. Bullous disease of the skin. In several of the bullous skin diseases, such as pemphigus vulgaris, bullous pemphigoid, and dermatitis herpetiformis, there is evidence of immunoglobulin and complement deposition, serum autoantibodies, or both (see also Chapter 24 IV).

H. Graves' disease (primary hyperthyroidism) is associated with the production of autoantibodies to thyroid-stimulating hormone (TSH) receptor. These antibodies bind to TSH receptor and stimulate thyroid growth and hypersecretion.

  1. Pathogenesis. Isolated defects that allow the generation of such antibody include:

    a. Cross-reaction with infectious antigens similar to TSH

    b. Recognition of neoantigen in the form of a TSH–HLA-DR complex induced by aberrant class II MHC antigenic expression on thyroid epithelial cells

    c. Alterations in antiidiotypic antibody networks

  2. Pathology. The pathologic and clinical features of Graves' disease are described in Chapter 20 III B 5.

V. IMMUNODEFICIENCY DISORDERS may be genetically determined (i.e., primary), or they may be secondary to infection, malnutrition, aging, irradiation, or chemotherapy. Immunodeficiency states classically have been divided according to the predominant deficient factor. Although this description is an oversimplification (many elements may be aberrant in each syndrome), such a categorization does provide a useful heuristic framework.

A. B-cell deficiency disorders

  1. Bruton's (X-linked) agammaglobulinemia

    a. In 1952, Bruton described an X-linked deficiency in immunoglobulin production. These patients suffered from recurrent bacteria-related bronchitis, otitis, and skin infection. Infections usually began at about age 6 months, as circulating maternal antibodies in the infants subsided. All immunoglobulins were either markedly decreased or absent. Circulating mature B cells also were absent.

    b. It is now recognized that pre–B cells are present in patients with Bruton's agammaglobulinemia, and there seems to be a defect in the B-cell maturation sequence. Morphologically, there are no germinal centers in lymph nodes, the spleen, and the tonsils. Plasma cells are absent.

  2. Transient hypogammaglobulinemia of infancy is characterized by diminished levels of immunoglobulin but the ability to produce certain antibody. The disorder appears to be related to an abnormally long delay in the production of serum immunoglobulin. (Maternal antibodies normally decline in the infant over the first 6 months of life.) Defects in helper T-cell function are thought to be responsible.

  3. Common variable immunodeficiency is a somewhat poorly defined entity characterized by hypogammaglobulinemia despite normal numbers of circulating B cells. In most cases, there is no clear-cut genetic predisposition. Patients range in age from very young to elderly, although young adults are most commonly affected.

a. Clinical features. The hypogammaglobulinemia is not as severe as in Bruton's; however, recurrent infection (e.g., pneumonia) does occur. These patients also suffer from gluten hypersensitivity (celiac disease), with associated malabsorption. Giardiasis also is common. Idiopathic noncaseating granulomas of the liver, spleen, lung, and skin also have been reported.

b. Pathology. Microscopically, B-cell lymphoid areas are hyperplastic, but no plasma cells are seen.

c. Immunologic defects. A number of defects have been suggested.

(1) In some patients there is abnormal glycosylation of immunoglobulin heavy chain. In others, there is a deficiency of 5′ nucleotidase.

(2) Some young patients with common variable immunodeficiency show a failure to switch from IgM isotype to IgG or IgA. Thus, serum levels of IgM are normal, whereas IgG and IgA levels are depressed.

(3) Abnormalities of T-cell regulatory function also have been described.

4. Selective IgA deficiency is the most common immunodeficiency disorder, occurring in about 1 in 700 people.

a. Clinical features. Recurrent sinopulmonary infections, an increased incidence of IgE-mediated allergies and of celiac and inflammatory bowel disease (IBD), and a high association with autoimmune disorders are the clinical characteristics of selective IgA deficiency.

b. Immunologic defects. Serum IgA levels are low, but the numbers of circulating IgA cells are normal. However, these IgA cells possess an immature phenotype that coexpresses IgD and IgM. Thus, the defect seems to be in the maturation of IgA-bearing cells. Similar selective deficiencies in IgM are reported but rare.

B. T-cell immunodeficiency disorders

1. DiGeorge syndrome is a selective deficiency of T cells. This lack results from failure of the third and fourth pharyngeal pouches to develop and become thymus and parathyroid glands. DiGeorge syndrome is thought to be the result of an early intrauterine growth defect. It is not genetically linked.

a. Clinical features and immunologic defects. Affected infants have total absence of T-cell immunity, in association with hypocalcemia and tetany. All lymphocytes are B cells. Plasma cells are present in normal numbers. T-cell areas, such as paracortical areas of lymph nodes and periarteriolar sheaths, are depressed.

b. Treatment. Patients may be treated with thymic hormone or with transplantation of fetal thymus.

2. Chronic mucocutaneous candidiasis is a selective defect of T-cell immunity characterized by recurrent candidal infections involving the skin and mucous membranes. The remainder of T-cell functions are intact, as is B-cell immunity. The defect may be inherited as an autosomal recessive gene. Chronic mucocutaneous candidiasis is associated with endocrinopathies. Hypoparathyroidism is most common. Addison's disease, hypothyroidism, diabetes mellitus, and pernicious anemia also are seen. This association suggests a multiorgan endocrinopathy with selective thymic dysfunction.

C. Severe combined immunodeficiency (SCID) is a severe disorder characterized by near total absence of both T-cell and B-cell immunity. Infants present early with recurrent opportunistic infections. SCID may be transmitted as either an X-linked or autosomal recessive trait.

1. Pathology. Morphologically, there is a virtual absence of lymphoid tissue in the form of lymph nodes, spleen, and tonsils. The thymus gland fails to descend from the neck into the mediastinum and lacks lymphoid cells and Hassall's corpuscles.

2. Pathogenesis. These patients appear to have a stem-cell defect. A deficiency in the enyzme adenosine deaminase (ADA) is found in the cells of many patients with the autosomal recessive form of SCID. ADA converts adenosine to inosine or deoxyadenosine to deoxyinosine. Without this enzyme, there is an accumulation of adenosine, deoxyadenosine, and deoxyadenosine triphosphate (dATP). This latter compound inhibits ribonucleotide reductase, causing depletion of deoxyribonucleotide triphosphates and abnormal lymphocyte function. SCID with ADA deficiency may be diagnosed prenatally by amniocentesis.

3. Treatment. Patients with SCID may benefit from bone marrow transplantation or gene replacement therapy.

D. AIDS. Acquired immunodeficiency, in its broadest sense, may be secondary to a variety of causes, including infectious agents, malnutrition, aging, immunosuppressive agents, autoimmune disease, uremia, and malignancy. In the 1980s, however, acquired immunodeficiency has come to be associated with human immunodeficiency virus (HIV) infection.

1. **Epidemiology.** HIV is transmitted by inoculation of blood products, through sexual contact, and transplacentally. Populations at high risk for HIV infection include homosexual and bisexual men, intravenous drug users, hemophiliacs, and sexual partners of these groups as well as infants born to HIV-infected mothers.

2. **Pathogenesis**
   a. The agent of AIDS, HIV, is a retrovirus that is tropic for **helper T cells**.
      (1) The virus most likely enters helper T cells through receptor-mediated endocytosis accomplished via interaction of the CD4 receptor on T cells with a glycoprotein (termed **GP120**) on the viral envelope. The genomic RNA of the virus is transcribed into DNA through reverse transcriptase, and this DNA, then, is either circularized or integrated into the host genome.
      (2) With mitogenic, antigenic, or allogeneic stimulation of the host T cell, transcription of the viral genome occurs, followed by protein synthesis. Viral proteins and genomic RNA are assembled at the cell surface. A burst of budding virions from the cell surface may cause sufficient disruption of the cell membrane to cause cell lysis.
      (3) In culture, infected T cells fuse with uninfected cells via GP120, CD4 binding. Fused cells form syncytia, with subsequent ballooning of the cell cytoplasm and cell death.
   b. Since CD4$^+$ T cells are central to many immune functions, a depletion of this pivotal cell leaves the host immunosuppressed and susceptible to a variety of infections and secondary malignancies.

3. **Clinical features**
   a. **Acute infection** may present as a mononucleosis-like illness, with subsequent seroconversion for HIV antibody. This phase often is clinically inapparent. An asymptomatic period usually follows the acute infection.
   b. **Persistent generalized lymphadenopathy** may either follow the acute illness or appear without any preceding clinical disease. Fatigue, fever, and malaise usually are mild. Depression of CD4 cells is mild.
   c. **AIDS-related complex (ARC)** is described in patients with fever of over 3 months' duration, weight loss, and diarrhea. CD4 cells are markedly decreased.
   d. The term **AIDS** is reserved for a patient who is positive for HIV antibody and who has had at least one life-threatening opportunistic infection, Kaposi's sarcoma, or lymphoma, and no other identifiable reason for profound immunodeficiency.

4. **Pathology**
   a. **Infections.** A large variety of infections may develop in AIDS patients. Infectious agents include:
      (1) Protozoans (*Pneumocystis, Toxoplasma, Cryptosporidium*)
      (2) Fungi (*Candida, Cryptococcus, Histoplasma, Coccidioides, Aspergillus*)
      (3) Mycobacteria (*M. tuberculosis, M. avium-intracellulare*)
      (4) Other bacteria (pyogenic bacteria, Enterobacteriaceae)
      (5) Viruses [cytomegalovirus (CMV), EBV, herpes simplex and zoster viruses, hepatitis B virus (HBV), human papilloma virus (HPV)]
   b. **Neoplasms**
      (1) **Kaposi's sarcoma** (see also Chapter 24 VII D) is an angioproliferative lesion most frequently found in mucocutaneous sites. Prior to the AIDS epidemic in the United States, Kaposi's sarcoma was most commonly found in older men. However, the epidemiology of Kaposi's has changed; approximately one-third of AIDS patients, who generally are young, develop Kaposi's.
         (a) **Pathogenesis.** Kaposi's sarcoma is a multifocal neoplasm of endothelial cells. It has been postulated that depressed cellular immunity combines with activation of growth factors specific for endothelial cells to permit the development of this neoplasm.
         (b) **Macroscopically,** Kaposi's has the appearance of multiple red-to-purple tumor nodules, which most frequently are found in mucocutaneous sites.
         (c) **Microscopically,** dilated and irregularly shaped vascular spaces are lined by thin endothelial cells, a surround of interweaving fascicles of spindle-shaped cells, and an extravasation of erythrocytes. Kaposi's also may be found in lymph nodes and visceral organs.

(2) Lymphoma
(a) Non-Hodgkin's lymphoma also is increased among AIDS patients. These lymphomas usually are of B-cell origin. Portions of the EBV genome can be found in these lymphomas, suggesting that this virus plays a major role in the pathogenesis of AIDS-related lymphoma.
(b) Cases of Hodgkin's disease also have been observed but are less frequent.
(3) Oral and anorectal carcinoma. Squamous cell carcinoma (SCC) of the tongue and cloacogenic carcinoma of the inner rectum are increased in AIDS patients.
c. HIV-associated lymphadenopathy. As mentioned, a phase of persistent generalized lymphadenopathy may occur as a prodrome to AIDS.
(1) Three histologic patterns are associated with ARC and AIDS:
(a) Follicular hyperplasia with increased plasma cells
(b) A mixed pattern of follicular hyperplasia and interfollicular depletion.
(c) Follicular involution, generalized lymphoid depletion, medullary fibrosis, and vascular proliferation
(2) Since the early stages are more common in ARC patients and the later patterns are more common in full-blown AIDS, these pictures probably represent progressive lymphoid depletion.

STUDY QUESTIONS

Directions: Each of the numbered items or incomplete statements in this section is followed by answers or by completions of the statement. Select the **one** lettered answer or completion that is **best** in each case.

1. Which autoantibody is most specific for scleroderma?

(A) Antinuclear antibody
(B) Antinucleolar antibody
(C) Antibody to double-stranded DNA
(D) Antibody to histone
(E) Antibody to Sm

2. Which immunodeficiency state is most common?

(A) Bruton's agammaglobulinemia
(B) DiGeorge syndrome
(C) Selective immunoglobulin A (IgA) deficiency
(D) Common variable immunodeficiency
(E) Severe combined immunodeficiency (SCID)

3. Human immunodeficiency virus (HIV) has a special affinity for infecting which type of cell?

(A) $CD8^+$ T cell
(B) $CD4^+$ T cell
(C) Natural killer (NK) cell
(D) Dendritic cell
(E) B cell

4. Which description is true of the class II major histocompatibility complex (MHC)?

(A) It includes human leukocyte antigen (HLA) loci A, B, and C
(B) It consists of a single transmembrane glycoprotein chain
(C) It "restricts" the expansion of $CD8^+$ T cells
(D) It includes HLA loci DR, DP, and DQ
(E) It has β_2-microglobulin as part of its glycoprotein structure

5. Which statement describes systemic lupus erythematosus (SLE)?

(A) Organ damage is predominantly mediated by natural killer (NK) cells
(B) Autoantibodies are restricted to antibodies against native double-stranded DNA
(C) The condition is associated with deficiencies of complement components C2 and C4
(D) Immune complex deposition is sparse
(E) The patterns of clinical disease are very limited

6. Which is the predominant immunologic mechanism in atopic dermatitis?

(A) Antibody-mediated cytotoxicity
(B) Immune complex disease
(C) Immediate hypersensitivity
(D) Cell-mediated cytotoxicity
(E) Delayed-type hypersensitivity

7. The predominant immunologic mechanism in autoimmune hemolytic anemia is

(A) antibody-mediated cytotoxicity
(B) immune complex disease
(C) immediate hypersensitivity
(D) cell-mediated cytotoxicity
(E) delayed-type hypersensitivity

8. Which autoantibody is highly specific for Sjögren's syndrome?

(A) Antinuclear antibody (ANA)
(B) Anti-Scl-70
(C) Anti-SS-B
(D) Anti-JO-1
(E) Anti-Sm

9. Antibody to centromere is associated with

(A) systemic lupus erythematosus (SLE)
(B) Sjögren's syndrome
(C) progressive scleroderma
(D) polymyositis
(E) CREST syndrome

1-B	4-D	7-A
2-C	5-C	8-C
3-B	6-C	9-E

10. DiGeorge syndrome involves all of the following features EXCEPT

(A) hypocalcemia
(B) tetany
(C) absent thymus
(D) absent plasma cells
(E) absent parathyroid glands

ANSWERS AND EXPLANATIONS

1. The answer is B *[IV D 1 c].*
Although many autoantibodies have been discovered in patients with scleroderma, antibodies to nucleolar antigens and antibody to Scl-70 (a nonhistone nuclear protein) are said to be specific for progressive systemic sclerosis. Antibody to centromere is highly associated with the more benign and less progressive form of scleroderma known as CREST (calcinosis, Raynaud's phenomenon, esophageal dysfunction, syndactyly, and telangiectasia) syndrome. Autoantibodies also are a common finding in lupus patients; the most specific is antibody to native double-stranded DNA.

2. The answer is C *[V A 4].*
Selective immunoglobulin A (IgA) deficiency, although not generally a life-threatening condition like the others, is quite common. It occurs in about 1 in 700 people. Serum levels of IgA are low, but the numbers of circulating IgA cells are normal. Affected patients are prone to recurrent sinopulmonary infections, IgE-mediated allergies, and celiac and inflammatory bowel disease (IBD).

3. The answer is B *[V D 2].*
Human immunodeficiency virus (HIV) is a retrovirus that is tropic for helper T cells. HIV infection begins with the binding of the virus to the CD4 receptor on the helper T cells, via a glycoprotein on the viral envelope. The affinity of HIV for this pivotal cell of the immune system helps to make HIV infection a lethal entity.

4. The answer is D *[II F 2].*
The major histocompatibility complex (MHC) is a group of antigens that are critical for the recognition of self during cell–cell interactions of the immune response. The class II MHC antigen is encoded by the human leukocyte antigen (HLA)-D gene, which is divided into three major loci designated HLA-DR, HLA-DP, and HLA-DQ. The class II MHC antigen is composed of two noncovalently linked transmembrane glycoproteins. Helper T cells recognize foreign antigen in relationship to self class II MHC antigen; thus, helper (CD4$^+$) T cells are said to be "restricted" in their activity by class II antigens.

5. The answer is C *[IV B 1–2].*
Systemic lupus erythematosus (SLE) is a multisystem autoimmune disease with no clear-cut etiology or pathogenesis, although environmental, genetic, and hormonal influences are suspected. A genetic link is suggested by studies showing an association with certain HLAs; there also is an association with deficiencies of complement components C2 and C4. Lupus is characterized by the generation of multiple autoantibodies. Many of these antibodies are directed against nuclear components. Multiorgan deposition of immune complex material also is recognized. In severe cases of lupus, multiple organ systems are involved.

6. The answer is C *[III A].*
Atopic dermatitis is a clinical manifestation of type 1 hypersensitivity reaction mediated by immunoglobulin E (IgE). Other clinical expressions of type 1 (immediate) hypersensitivity are anaphylaxis, allergic rhinitis, and food allergies.

7. The answer is A *[III B].*
In autoimmune hemolytic anemia, autoantibody binds to self red blood cells, causing direct cytotoxicity. Transfusion reaction is a similar process caused by autoantibody.

8. The answer is C *[IV C].*
In Sjögren's syndrome, a variety of autoantibodies can be found. Antibody to extractable RNA protein, SS-B, is found in 60% to 70% of cases with Sjögren's and is highly specific for this disease. Anti-SS-B binds with Epstein-Barr virus (EBV) RNA.

9. The answer is E *[IV D].*
Patients with scleroderma experience a more benign and less progressive disease variant associated with CREST syndrome (**c**alcinosis, **R**aynaud's phenomenon, **e**sophageal dysfunction, **s**yndactyly, and **t**elangiectasia). Antibody to centromere is associated with this variant.

10. The answer is D *[V B 1 a].*
DiGeorge syndrome is caused by failure of the thymus and parathyroid glands to develop. The defect in parathyroid tissue leads to hypocalcemia and tetany. The B-cell areas are intact in DiGeorge syndrome; thus, plasma cells are present in normal numbers. The absence of thymus leads to absence of T-cell immunity.

7
Transplantation
John E. Tomaszewski

I. BASIC IMMUNOLOGIC MECHANISMS

A. General concepts. Normal tissue that is transferred between genetically different individuals from the same species is referred to as an **allograft**. Allogeneic transplantation results in an immune reaction which can involve type II, type III, or type IV hypersensitivity. Two different reactions can occur following allogeneic transplantation.

1. **Host-versus-graft reaction (rejection).** In this response, the recipient's immune system recognizes the donor tissue as foreign and mounts an immunologic attack on the graft. Rejection is a dominant process in solid organ transplantation.

2. **Graft-versus-host (GVH) reaction.** In this response, an immunocompetent graft mounts an immunologic attack on a host whose immune system has been therapeutically eradicated. GVH reaction is a major consideration in bone marrow transplantation (BMT).

B. Immune mechanisms in rejection

1. **Sensitization**
   a. The **dominant allogeneic antigens** in organ transplantation are those of the **human leukocyte antigen (HLA)** system, the human branch of the **major histocompatibility complex** (MHC).
   b. **Foreign (donor) HLA antigens** are presented to the host immune system either within the allograft or by leukocytes carried with the allograft and transferred to regional host lymphoid tissue.
      (1) **Antigen-presenting cells** may include monocytes, endothelial cells, dendritic cells, and even epithelial cells.
      (2) Antigen presentation requires the presence of HLA class II antigens (i.e., HLA-DP, HLA-DQ, or HLA-DR) at the surface of the antigen-presenting cells. Foreign antigens (either major or minor histocompatibility antigens) are presented to host helper T cells (CD4$^+$) in association with HLA class II antigens.
   c. **Cytotoxic T-cell (CD8$^+$)** precursors recognize antigen in the context of HLA class I antigens (i.e., HLA-A, HLA-B, or HLA-C).
   d. Secondary **signaling mechanisms** and complex **cytokine networks** may up-regulate the expression of HLA class I and class II antigens on the allograft.

2. **T-cell reactions**
   a. Sensitized **helper T cells** (CD4$^+$) are expanded under the autocrine and paracrine influences of interleukin-2 (IL-2) and by IL-1 (a product of macrophages).
   b. Sensitized **CD4 cells** secrete gamma interferon (INF-γ) and other lymphokines that may increase HLA antigen expression on the allograft.
   c. Sensitized **CD8$^+$ cells,** under the influence of IL-2, undergo postantigeneic differentiation and expansion.
   d. CD8$^+$ cells attack HLA targets on the allograft. **Target lysis,** which is mediated through cytotoxic T lymphocytes, is an example of type IV hypersensitivity.
   e. T cells may also participate with macrophages to produce **graft damage via granulomatous type IV hypersensitivity reaction.**

3. **Antibody-mediated damage**
   a. Antibodies to both major and minor HLA histocompatibility antigens may be preformed

and secondary to sensitization that occurred prior to engraftment, or their formation may be part of the host response to foreign alloantigen.
  b. Preformed antibody in the recipient may cause immediate graft damage and lead to hyperacute rejection (see III A 3).
  c. Antibodies developed after engraftment may initiate damage via at least two mechanisms:
    (1) Complement-dependent cytotoxicity
    (2) Antibody-dependent cell-mediated cytotoxicity
  d. Antibody-mediated damage is often morphologically evidenced by vascular damage.
  e. Complement-dependent tissue injury and coagulation cascades are secondary mediators of antibody-initiated damage.

4. **Tolerance** is a poorly understood process. Rejection may be considered a breakdown in the mechanisms supporting tolerance.

II. PATHOLOGIC FEATURES COMMON TO SOLID ORGAN ALLOGRAFT REJECTION

A. Acute cellular rejection. T-cell–mediated damage predominates in acute cellular rejection, which is characterized by an infiltrate of mononuclear cells.

1. Medium and small lymphocytes predominate and are admixed with transformed lymphocytes, macrophages, occasional plasma cells, and neutrophils. Responding host cells are recruited from the microvasculature and infiltrate the allograft parenchyma.

2. Cytotoxic lymphocytes are morphologically characterized by their geographic juxtaposition to damaged allograft structures.

3. The severity of the acute cellular rejection may vary from mild to severe, depending on the density of the infiltrate and the extent of parenchymal damage.

B. Acute vascular rejection. In acute vascular rejection, the microvasculature of the organ is a primary target. Both cell- and antibody-mediated mechanisms are at work.

1. **Early acute vascular rejection** shows endothelial hypertrophy and vacuolation, with neutrophils, lymphocytes, and monocytes in the subendothelial space.

2. In the **intermediate stage of acute vascular rejection,** fibrin thrombi and transmural inflammation are present. Intimal proliferation is moderate.

3. In **severe acute vascular rejection,** small vessel walls show fibrinoid necrosis. Intimal proliferation is severe.

C. Chronic rejection. In all solid organs, chronic rejection is the end result of uncontrolled cellular or vascular rejection. Fibrosis is the constant pathologic feature.

1. Destroyed allograft parenchyma is replaced by fibrous tissue.

2. In the microvasculature, dense intimal fibrosis leads to allograft ischemia and further dysfunction.

III. ORGAN-SPECIFIC TRANSPLANTATION

A. Renal allografts

1. **Donor kidney.** Both cadaveric and living related donors are clinically screened for preexisting renal disease, however, subclinical pathology may be present in the donated organ prior to engraftment.
  a. Approximately 40% of donor kidneys show nonspecific pathology such as patchy interstitial fibrosis and hyaline arteriolar sclerosis.
  b. Approximately 15% of donor kidneys show specific lesions such as glomerulosclerosis, glomerulonephritis, atheroembolism, or intravascular coagulation.

2. **Harvest injury**
  a. About 50% of time-zero biopsies show evidence of "harvest damage." **Pathologic lesions** include tubular dilatation, tubular epithelial vacuolation, and frank tubular epithelial necrosis. The changes are related to **cold ischemia time** and the **mode of donor death.**

    b. From 30% to 40% of allograft recipients suffer from **"primary nonfunction,"** which is a variable period of anuria after engraftment. A significant proportion of primary nonfunction is secondary to harvest injury. Other possible causes of primary nonfunction include infection, thrombotic microangiopathy, toxic acute tubular necrosis (ATN), hyperacute rejection, or preexisting disease.

    c. The significance of **glomerular neutrophilia** in a time-zero biopsy is controversial. Some authors have associated this finding with poor graft function and rejection.

3. Hyperacute rejection is a form of type II hypersensitivity reaction.

    a. Hyperacute rejection occurs in the first 72 hours following engraftment and is the result of preformed antibody in the recipient directed against some antigen on the donor kidney.

    b. The process of hyperacute rejection is represented histopathologically by acute vascular damage, arterial thrombosis, capillary neutrophilia, interstitial hemorrhage, and edema.

4. Acute cellular rejection is the most frequent form of rejection. It occurs most often in the first 3 months after engraftment, but is generally responsive to immunosuppression therapy.

    a. Acute cellular rejection is mediated by allogeneically restricted cytotoxic T cells (CD8$^+$) and thus represents an example of type IV hypersensitivity. In some cases, antibody-dependent, cell mediated cytotoxicity may also play a role.

    b. The **pathology** of acute cellular rejection in the kidney includes an interstitial infiltrate of small and transformed lymphocytes, monocytes, neutrophils, and, occasionally, plasma cells. The mononuclear cells transgress the tubular basement membrane and come to lie in direct contact with the tubular epithelium, resulting in "tubulitis." Lymphocytic glomerulitis may also be prominent in a minority of cases.

    c. Acute cellular rejection can be graded as mild, moderate, or severe depending on the intensity of the inflammation and the amount of tubular damage.

5. Acute vascular rejection

    a. Acute vascular rejection may be mediated by either antibody-dependent or cell-dependent immune mechanisms.

    b. The **pathologic features** are those of vascular damage. Changes may be focal.

        (1) In mild (grade I) acute vascular rejection, there is endothelial hypertrophy and a subintimal accumulation of lymphocytes, monocytes and neutrophils.

        (2) In moderate (grade II) acute vascular rejection, there are grade I lesions as well as more extensive intimal proliferation, focal fibrinoid necrosis of vessel walls, and medial and perivascular infiltration by mononuclear cells. Focal patches of acute interstitial hemorrhage may also be found.

        (3) In severe acute vascular rejection, lesions are the same as those in grade II, but they are more extensive.

    c. Acute vascular rejection is frequently associated with deposits of immunoglobulin and complement in the arterioles and glomeruli.

    d. Moderate or severe acute vascular rejection responds poorly to immunosuppression and suggests a poor prognosis.

6. Chronic rejection results when acute cellular or vascular rejection is resolved by parenchymal scarring.

    a. Chronic rejection is characterized pathologically by fibrosis in various compartments.

        (1) In the interstitium, chronic rejection is represented by fibrosis, tubular atrophy, and tubular basement membrane thickening.

        (2) The vessels in chronic rejection show intimal fibrosis and medial thickening.

        (3) The glomerular compartment in chronic rejection shows global glomerulosclerosis, diffuse tuft collapse, or the changes of so-called "posttransplant glomerulopathy."

            (a) The glomerulopathy is the result of chronic vascular rejection. Glomerular capillary loops are thickened by mesangial matrix interposed into the capillary lumen.

            (b) This reaction is thought to be, at least in part, a reaction to intravascular coagulation.

    b. The **prognosis** for allograft function is poor in patients with chronic rejection.

7. Cyclosporine nephrotoxicity

    a. Cyclosporine is a nephrotoxin. Toxicity is dose-dependent, although individual sensitivity to the drug varies widely. Thus, toxicity may occur with a lower dose or at trough levels in a very susceptible patient.

b. The four categories of cyclosporine nephrotoxicity damage are functional, tubular, acute vascular–interstitial, and chronic vascular–interstitial.

(1) Functional toxicity in cyclosporine nephrotoxicity involves a decreased glomerular filtration rate (GFR) and renal plasma flow (RPF). No pathologic change occurs. Abnormal hemodynamics may be the result of excess thromboxane A_2 (TXA_2).

(2) Tubular toxicity shows epithelial damage, with isometric tubular vacuolation, giant mitochondria and lysosomes, and mitochondrial calcifications.

(3) Acute vascular–interstitial toxicity is morphologically similar to hemolytic-uremic syndrome and usually occurs soon after transplantation. Capillaries are occluded by fibrin thrombi.

(4) Chronic vascular–interstitial toxicity occurs after months to years of therapy. Renal dysfunction and hypertension usually progress slowly.

(a) Pathologic changes include glomerular and arteriolar sclerosis—sometimes with focal fibrinoid arteriopathy, tubular atrophy, and stripped interstitial fibrosis.

(b) Distinction from hypertension or diabetic arteriopathy can be very difficult, and clinical correlation is critical.

8. Recurrent disease. Almost every disease that can occur in native kidneys has been described as recurrent disease in renal allografts.

a. The frequency of recurrent disease is approximately 2% to 3%. Most recurrent disease occurs after 6 months of engraftment.

b. Morphological changes of recurrent disease occur more frequently than the clinical dysfunction that can be attributed directly to the disease; however, 50% of patients who develop recurrent disease do eventually lose the allograft.

9. De novo glomerulonephritis is quite rare. De novo membranous glomerulopathy, anti-glomerular basement membrane (GBM) disease, and acute serum sickness are the most frequent forms.

B. Liver allografts

1. Acute rejection

a. In the liver, acute rejection is predominantly of the **cellular variety**. It is morphologically characterized as a mixed portal inflammation, with lymphocytes (both small and activated) and some eosinophils. This inflammation produces "ductitis" and endotheliitis in the portal space. Interestingly, lobular inflammation is slight in rejection.

b. Acute rejection secondary to humoral mechanisms has rarely been reported. Patients with documented donor-specific antibodies may show hemorrhagic necrosis of liver parenchyma and fibrinoid necrosis of vessels.

2. Chronic rejection occurs in 3% to 17% of liver allografts.

a. In the liver, chronic rejection is characterized by a progressive loss in the number of bile ducts. "Ductopenia" leads to cholestasis.

b. Chronic rejection in the liver may also show vasculopathy, with accumulation of subintimal foam cells and luminal narrowing.

3. Biliary obstruction

a. Extrahepatic biliary obstruction may be secondary to anastomotic insufficiency or ischemia in the large intrahepatic bile ducts. Extrahepatic biliary obstruction can cause changes in the hepatic parenchyma. In the portal tract, findings include a proliferation of ductules, a neutrophilic infiltrate, and cholestasis.

b. Functional cholestasis in the absence of anatomic biliary tract obstruction can occur in the first 2 to 3 weeks after transplantation. Findings include lobular cholestasis and hepatocellular swelling without any significant inflammation. This change is attributed to the cold ischemia time of the allograft and is the morphologic manifestation of "harvest injury."

4. Vascular compromise

a. Pathology associated with vascular compromise is most often seen in the first 2 months after engraftment.

b. Obstruction may occur in either the arterial or venous hepatic systems.

c. Ischemia secondary to arterial obstruction is characterized by centrilobular necrosis.

d. Venous obstruction secondary to stenosis of the vena cava anastomosis causes centrilobular hemorrhage. Budd-Chiari syndrome may be associated with ascites.

5. **Recurrent disease**
   a. Hepatitis B, C, and D are capable of causing recurrent disease in the allograft. For hepatitis B, the recurrence rate is more than 50%.
   b. Recurrent hepatitis shows a pattern of lobular hepatitis or chronic active hepatitis. Immunohistochemical localization of viral antigens in the allograft can aid in the diagnosis.
   c. Other primary hepatic diseases, such as autoimmune hepatitis or primary biliary cirrhosis, may recur in the allograft; however, the morphologic distinction from the rejection process may be difficult.

C. **Heart transplantation.** The diagnosis of **cardiac allograft rejection** cannot be substantiated using clinical parameters such as laboratory tests or electrocardiogram (ECG) findings. Patient monitoring with endomyocardial biopsy is the method of choice for identifying rejection.

1. In the heart, acute cellular rejection is the **best recognized pattern**.
   a. **Mild acute cellular rejection** shows a mild perivascular and interstitial lymphoid infiltrate without myocyte destruction.
   b. **Moderate acute cellular rejection** shows a more extensive interstitial infiltrate with focal myocyte destruction.
   c. **Severe acute cellular rejection** shows very dense infiltrate composed of lymphocytes, eosinophils, and neutrophils. Myocyte destruction is extensive.

2. **Acute humorally mediated rejection** in heart allografts is poorly described. Some authors have suggested that extensive interstitial immunoglobulin deposition may be a feature of this process.

3. **"Harvest damage"** results from the cold ischemia time. Necrobiosis of myocytes without substantial inflammation is diagnostic. Allografts may also suffer ischemic damage prior to harvesting as a result of marginal perfusion or a pressor effect.

4. **Prior biopsy site effect** is suggested by geographic necrosis with granulation tissue. This condition must be distinguished from severe rejection.

5. The term **"quilty effect"** refers to a subendocardial infiltrate of lymphocytes. The etiology is unknown; however, the effects of cyclosporine, Epstein-Barr virus (EBV) infection, or even early lymphoproliferative disorder have been postulated.

6. **Chronic rejection** in cardiac allografts shows variable degrees of fibrosis. More specifically, in chronic cardiac allograft rejection, there is coronary artery sclerosis, with an accumulation of lipid-laden macrophages. Because of its pathologic similarity to atherosclerotic injury, the condition has been termed "accelerated atherosclerosis."
   a. This process is believed to be predominantly the result of an allogeneic tissue reaction.
   b. Chronic rejection is unusual prior to 1 to 2 years after engraftment.

D. **Lung transplantation**

1. Lung transplantation is a relative newcomer to the field. Worldwide experience is limited to about 1500 patients. Lung transplantation may be performed as a combined **heart–lung transplant, single-lung block,** or a **double-lung block**.

2. Lung allografts may suffer from rejection, but they are also particularly **susceptible to infection**. Opportunistic infections are described in IV.

3. **Acute rejection**
   a. The following schema for categorizing pulmonary rejection has recently been adopted as a working formulation by the International Society for Heart and Lung Transplantation.
      (1) **Minimal acute rejection.** Focal perivascular, arteriolar, and venular cuffing by lymphocytes, macrophages, plasma cells and neutrophils is present, but not easily seen at low magnification.
      (2) **Mild acute rejection.** More frequent perivascular infiltrates often occur with increased neutrophils and eosinophils. Lymphocytic endotheliolitis frequently appears. The infiltrate is easily seen at low magnification.
      (3) **Moderate acute rejection.** The infiltrate extends into the interalveolar septae and the alveolar spaces. Neutrophils are more frequent.
      (4) **Severe acute rejection.** Confluent interstitial and intraalveolar infiltrate may result in hemorrhage, necrosis, and hyaline membrane formation.

    b. Each grade of rejection may be accompanied by **lymphocytic bronchitis** or **bronchiolitis**. These inflammations should be distinguished from inflamed airways with fibrous scarring, or obliterative bronchiolitis (OB), although such lesions may represent precursors to OB.

  4. Obliterative bronchiolitis (OB)
    a. OB is a progressive fibrosing lesion of the membranous and respiratory bronchioles.
      (1) Pathologically, there is a concentric, eccentric, or obliterative fibrosis of the submucosa in these airways.
      (2) OB may be inactive (i.e., without inflammation) or active (i.e., with inflammation).
    b. The many causes of OB include rejection, infection, GVH disease, and airway ischemia.
    c. OB needs to be differentiated from chronic organizing pneumonia, which is characterized by fibrosing granulation tissue in alveolar spaces.

  5. Chronic rejection in the lung is morphologically represented by a fibrosing intimal occlusion of the microvasculature. This change correlates with accelerated atherosclerosis of the coronary arteries in combined heart–lung grafts.

  6. GVH disease. The transplanted lung carries donor lymphoid tissue and may put the host at risk for GVH disease (see III E 5).

E. Bone marrow transplantation (BMT)

  1. Transfer of marrow. BMT refers to the transfer of marrow precursor elements.
    a. Allogeneic BMT takes place between unrelated but partially HLA-matched individuals.
    b. Syngeneic BMT takes place between HLA-identical individuals.
    c. BMT may be **autologous** (i.e., harvested marrow undergoes in vitro treatment to destroy malignant cells and, after therapy, is reinfused into the same patient).

  2. Applications. BMT is usually performed in the therapy of patients with hematopoietic malignancies, marrow aplasia, or metastatic carcinoma (e.g., metastatic breast cancer).

  3. Bone marrow pathology in BMT. Examination of the bone marrow after engraftment is an important gauge of marrow reconstitution.
    a. The bone marrow on day 0, immediately after obliterative radiochemotherapy, shows fat and scattered residual lymphocytes, plasma cells, or mast cells. No hematopoietic precursors are found.
    b. At 1 week, isolated erythroblasts and myeloblasts are seen.
    c. At 2 weeks, small aggregates of precursors in the erythropoietic, granulopoietic, and megakaryocytic series are observed. Dysplastic changes in the erythroid series, such as abnormal mitoses, nuclear pyknosis, and megaloblastic changes, also are seen at this time. These changes are transient and it has been suggested that they parallel fetal hematopoiesis.
    d. By week 3 or 4, precursor cells have reconstituted almost all allogeneic transplants. In autologous transplants, recovery is slower.
    e. Clusters of granulocytes are seen from day 28. Neutrophils predominate. Dysgranulopoiesis (including pseudo–Pelger-Huet anomaly, degranulation, and cytoplasmic vacuolation) are transient.

  4. Bone marrow rejection. The changes are nonspecific but include disappearance of marrow elements, with fat necrosis, edema, hemorrhage, lymphocytosis, plasmacytosis, and microgranulomas.

  5. GVH disease and **infection** are the two major complications of BMT. GVH disease is caused by sensitized immunocompetent donor lymphocytes that attack host (recipient) tissues. The major sites of damage in GVH disease are the skin, gastrointestinal tract, and liver. GVH disease may be either acute or chronic.
    a. Acute GVH disease
      (1) Skin
        (a) The early (**grade I**) changes include focal epidermal basal cell vacuolation and a mild lymphocytic infiltrate cuffing superficial dermal vessels. There is also a mild lymphocytic epidermal infiltrate.
        (b) Grade II acute GVH disease shows the same changes as are seen in grade I, but with scattered necrotic (apoptotic) keratinocytes.
        (c) In grade III, there is confluent damage to the basal cell layer, with extensive keratinocyte necrosis.
        (d) In grade IV acute GVH disease, there is dermal–epidermal clefting with bulla formation.

(2) **Gastrointestinal tract**
  (a) Between 30% and 60% of patients with allogeneic bone marrow transplants develop GVH disease in the gastrointestinal tract. Lower tract symptoms include diarrhea, abdominal pain, and ileus. Upper tract symptoms are dyspepsia, nausea, and vomiting.
  (b) In the **colon,** the pathologic change of GVH disease is crypt cell necrosis, with intraepithelial lymphocytes. In low-grade (grade I) GVH disease, there is cell crypt necrosis of individual cells; in grade II, crypt abscess; in grade III, dropout of whole crypts; and in grade IV, total denudation of the epithelium.
  (c) Changes in the **small intestine** and **stomach** also include individual cell necrosis.
  (d) Changes of acute GVH disease in the intestine are closely mimicked by the **radiochemotherapy effect** in the **bowel.** Changes secondary to therapy, however, are present only in the first 20 days after transplantation.
(3) Liver. Acute GVH disease in the liver usually occurs after skin or intestinal involvement.
  (a) Clinical laboratory changes include cholestasis and an increase in serum transaminases.
  (b) Biopsies show damage to interlobular bile ducts, with cytoplasmic swelling and vacuolation, segmental nuclear loss, a mild lymphocytic infiltrate within the ducts, and regenerating nuclear atypia. The hepatocytes show ballooning degeneration, isolated hepatocellular necrosis, and cholestasis.
  b. **Chronic GVH disease.** The constant feature of chronic GVH disease is a **loss of parenchymal structures** damaged by the inflammatory reaction of acute GVH disease.
(1) Chronic GVH disease in the skin develops more than 100 days after BMT.
  (a) It may be generalized or localized.
  (b) In its well-developed form, chronic GVH disease of the skin shows an atrophic epidermis, with prominent fibrotic changes in the dermis. Changes are reminiscent of scleroderma.
(2) **Gastrointestinal chronic GVH disease** in the intestine and stomach shows fibrosis of the lamina propria, submucosa, and serosa, with hyalinization of blood vessels. In the esophagus, there is a desquamative esophagitis.
(3) **Hepatic chronic GVH disease** shows extensive bile duct damage, with marked bile duct dropout. Fibrosis of portal tracts and cholestasis are also present.

IV. COMPLICATIONS OF TRANSPLANTATION

A. Infections

1. **Viral.** All immunosuppressed allograft recipients are at increased risk for viral infection. Infections may be **primary or reactivated**.
  a. **Cytomegalovirus (CMV)** is a common pathogen in all transplants, particularly in the first few months after engraftment. Recipients with no prior immunity to CMV may be at high risk for infection by donor tissue.
    (1) Almost any organ may be infected, but the lungs and gastrointestinal tract are particularly susceptible.
    (2) CMV may be recognized histopathologically by a characteristic cytopathic effect that includes cell enlargement, with nuclear and cytoplasmic inclusions. Immunohistochemistry (IHC) and in-situ hybridization (ISH) for viral antigen, nucleic acids, or both can increase diagnostic sensitivity.
  b. **Herpes simplex virus (HSV)** may produce localized infection or it may be disseminated.
    (1) Sites of infection include the skin, conjunctiva, pharynx, eosphagus, bronchi, lungs, and central nervous system (CNS).
    (2) Cowdry type A intranuclear inclusions are the characteristic cytopathic effect in HSV. Infected cells may show nuclear molding to form polykaryons.
  c. **EBV** infection produces a spectrum of lymphoproliferative disorders (see IV B).

2. **Parasitic**
  a. *Pneumocystis carinii* may present as pneumonitis in heavily immunosuppressed recipients. In pneumocystis pneumonitis, lung biopsy tissue shows a frothy intraalveolar exudate. Cysts appear as small cup-shaped structures that stain black with methenamine silver.
  b. **Toxoplasmosis** is an intracellular parasite that primarily infects heart transplant patients.

The myocardium is infected in the acute phase. ***Toxoplasma*** cysts are seen in the myocardium, but they do not induce an inflammatory reaction.

  c. Other parasitic infections which may involve the gastrointestinal tract (particularly in BMT patients) include ***Giardia lamblia*** and ***Coccidia*** species.

3. Fungal

  a. ***Candida*** is a common infection in transplantation. It is often found in association with other infections, such as CMV. *Candida* infection may be localized or disseminated. Diagnosis is made by recognizing tissue-invasive yeast and pseudohyphae on silver stains.

  b. ***Aspergillus*** infection may be a problem in any transplant situation, but it is a particular issue in lung transplantation. In the lung, *Aspergillus* may colonize large airways or it may become invasive. Local invasion is common at anastomotic lines and may lead to dehiscence. When *Aspergillus* invades lung parenchyma, it has a tendency to involve vascular structures, leading to hematogenous dissemination.

B. Posttransplant lymphoproliferative disorder (PTLD) is a spectrum of clinical conditions involving an **atypical expansion of lymphocytes,** usually B cells. PTLD occurs in 1% to 2% of allografts.

  1. Etiology. PTLD is almost always associated with **EBV infection**. The EBV infection in these patients may be **primary or reactivated**.

  a. Transplant patients are immunosuppressed and have low levels of T cells, which are necessary for controlling virally infected cells, such as **B lymphocytes** infected with EBV.

  b. EBV also stimulates B-lymphocyte growth, perhaps through activation of the cell surface antigen CD-23.

  2. Types

  a. Early populations of proliferating B cells in PTLD are morphologically heterogeneous and consist of small lymphocytes, plasma cells, and immunoblasts. These proliferations are termed **polymorphous PTLD**. If immunosuppression is reduced at this stage, T-cell control may be reestablished. The EBV infection is then controlled, and the atypical B-cell proliferation usually subsides.

  b. If EBV infection is not controlled, unopposed B-cell proliferation provides a fertile field for genetic mishaps. Under the influence of an altered genome, B-cell malignancy may evolve. These more advanced proliferations usually have a monotonous morphology consistent with large-cell lymphoma and are termed **monomorphous PTLD**. Monomorphous PTLD is **often fatal**.

STUDY QUESTIONS

Directions: Each of the numbered items or incomplete statements in this section is followed by answers or by completions of the statement. Select the **one** lettered answer or completion that is **best** in each case.

1. A biopsy of a renal allograft shows fibrinoid necrosis of small vessels. Which one of the following immune mechanisms is most likely at work?

(A) Cell-mediated cytotoxicity
(B) Antibody- and complement-mediated damage
(C) CD8–mediated damage
(D) Natural killer cell–mediated cytotoxicity
(E) Type IV hypersensitivity

2. In hepatic allografts, the damaging lymphocytic inflammation is directed against

(A) bile ducts
(B) hepatocytes
(C) Kupffer cells
(D) Ito cells
(E) sinusoids

3. A renal allograft recipient fails to produce urine after 48 hours. A biopsy is performed. Tubules show loss of brush border, loss of nuclei, and tubular cast formation. There are no other changes. What is the most likely etiology for this patient's "primary nonfunction"?

(A) Acute cellular rejection
(B) Hyperacute rejection
(C) Chronic rejection
(D) Acute tubular necrosis (ATN)
(E) Recurrent disease

4. Cyclosporine nephrotoxicity includes all of the following features EXCEPT

(A) isometric tubular vacuolization
(B) vascular sclerosis
(C) stripped fibrosis
(D) dense interstitial lymphocytic inflammation
(E) capillary loop thrombosis

Directions: The group of items in this section consists of lettered options followed by a set of numbered items. For each item, select the **one** lettered option that is most closely associated with it. Each lettered option may be selected once, more than once, or not at all.

Questions 5–9

For each condition, select the associated pathologic finding.

(A) Graft-versus-host (GVH) disease
(B) Cytomegalovirus (CMV) infection
(C) Bone marrow biopsy immediately after engraftment
(D) Hepatic rejection
(E) Adenovirus infection
(F) Posttransplant lymphoproliferative disorder (PTLD)
(G) Graft-versus-host (GVH) reaction
(H) Recurrent disease

5. Atypical expansion of lymphocytes

6. Lymphocytic dermatitis with keratinocyte necrosis

7. Fat, plasma cells, absent hematopoietic precursors

8. Lymphocytic cryptitis

9. Enlarged cells with nuclear inclusions

1-B	4-D	7-C
2-A	5-F	8-A
3-D	6-A	9-B

ANSWERS AND EXPLANATIONS

1. The answer is B *[III A 5 b (2), c].*
Fibrinoid necrosis of vessels is seen in acute vascular rejection. When the vessels are examined by immunofluorescence, immunoglobulin and complement can be identified. Acute vascular rejection is frequently secondary to alloantibody directed against an antigen found in the vasculature. This antibody fixes complement and incites an inflammatory reaction.

2. The answer is A *[III B 1].*
The bile ducts and microvasculature in the liver are the primary targets of acute cellular rejection. Morphologically, acute cellular rejection is represented by bile "ductitis" and small-vessel endotheliitis. In chronic rejection bile ducts disappear as the damaged structures are replaced by collagen.

3. The answer is D *[III A 2 b, 3 a, 4, 6, 8 a].*
Isolated changes of tubular damage are more consistent with acute tubular necrosis (ATN), which, in this setting, is usually secondary to "harvest injury." Acute cellular rejection, chronic rejection, and recurrent disease may be excluded as etiologies for this patient's "primary nonfunction" on the basis of the amount of time that has elapsed. Hyperacute rejection is a possible etiology, but this type of rejection is secondary to the presence of preformed antibody in the recipient that has specificity for donor antigen. Hyperacute rejection is pathologically characterized by vascular thrombosis with neutrophilia and tissue infarction.

4. The answer is D *[III A 7 b (2)–(4)].*
Cyclosporine nephrotoxicity may be either acute or chronic. In acute cyclosporine nephrotoxicity, there is tubular damage, with small uniform vacuoles in the cytoplasm (isometric vacuolation). Occasional cases of acute cyclosporine nephrotoxicity may show thrombotic microangiopathy. In chronic cyclosporine nephrotoxicity (usually after months to years of therapy), vascular sclerosis, glomerulosclerosis, and stripped interstitial fibrosis appear. A dense interstitial cellular infiltrate is a feature of acute cellular rejection and is rarely seen in cyclosporine nephrotoxicity.

5–9. The answers are: 5-F *[IV B]*, **6-A** *[III E 5 a (1)]*, **7-C** *[III E 3 a]*, **8-A** *[III E 5 a (2) (b)]*, **9-B** *[IV A 1 a (2)].*
Posttransplant lymphoproliferative disorder (PTLD) is an expansion of B cells which occurs in Epstein-Barr virus (EBV)–infected immunocompromised hosts. EBV infection, in the absence of T-cell control, drives B-cell expansion.

Graft-versus-host (GVH) disease is a reaction of immunocompetent donor T lymphocytes against host antigens in an immunocompromised recipient. Common sites of GVH disease include the skin and gastrointestinal tract. In the skin, a lymphocytic inflammation shows variable degrees of keratinocyte necrosis. In the gastrointestinal tract, lymphocytic inflammation and destruction of crypts are common.

Bone marrow transplantation (BMT) is most often done for neoplastic disease. Prior to engraftment, the native marrow and tumors are ablated with high-dose radiochemotherapy. This treatment leaves the marrow space empty, with only fat and scattered plasma cells but no hematopoietic elements. This aplasia continues for the first few weeks after engraftment; then, reconstitution with transplanted cells proceeds.

Infection is a common complication in transplantation. Cytomegalovirus (CMV) infection is the most common viral pathogen. CMV is recognized in tissue by the large cells (cytomegaly) with intranuclear and intracytoplasmic inclusions. Inclusions are aggregates of virions. The diagnosis of CMV may be difficult; combined serologic, culture, histopathologic, immunohistochemical (IHC), and molecular techniques may be necessary to make the diagnosis.

I. DISORDERS OF RED BLOOD CELLS

A. Anemia

1. **General concepts.** Anemia is a reduction in the amount of circulating hemoglobin, red blood cells, or both.
   a. It occurs when a loss of red blood cells or hemoglobin from the circulation surpasses the body's ability to replace these elements, or when hematopoietic tissues are malfunctioning or replaced. Basically, then, there are two **mechanisms of anemia**:
      (1) Excessive blood turnover (with increased reticulocyte count)
      (2) Failure of blood production (with decreased reticulocyte count)
   b. **Morphologic classification of anemias.** The morphologic categorization of anemias into macrocytic, microcytic, normocytic, hypochromic, and normochromic normocytic can lead the clinician to the appropriate etiology.
      (1) **Macrocytic, microcytic,** and **normocytic** refer to red cell **size,** a relatively objective measurement.
      (2) **Hypochromic** and **normochromic normocytic** refer to hemoglobin content as determined by red cell **color** differences, a very subjective measurement. Decreased iron and, thus, decreased hemoglobin would result in a hypochromic anemia.
   c. **Symptoms of anemia** vary with the degree of anemia and its rate of development.
      (1) Common to moderate and severe acute anemias are pallor of the skin and mucous membranes, increased pulse rate, shortness of breath, palpitations, dizziness, and fatigue. The symptoms result from a decreased oxygen supply to the affected organs. Heart failure may occur. Examples include traumatic rupture of an internal organ or a reaction to mismatched blood unit.
      (2) If anemia develops slowly, compensation occurs, so few symptoms and signs may be present. Examples include iron deficiency and hemolysis.

2. **Anemias due to excessive blood turnover**
   a. **General concepts**
      (1) Excessive blood turnover occurs through **hemorrhage** (blood loss to the outside of the vascular system) and **hemolysis** (red cell destruction within the body). If red cells are lost (through bleeding) or destroyed too rapidly, **red cell production** in the marrow is stimulated. The stem cells are transformed along erythroid lines.
      (2) **Common to hemorrhage and hemolysis** is the evidence of attempted compensation by the marrow: erythroid hyperplasia in the bone marrow and **increase of reticulocytes** (young red blood cells) in the peripheral blood.
      (3) To **distinguish between hemorrhage and hemolysis,** several tests may be used.
         (a) In **acute situations** of excessive blood turnover, one can measure **serum haptoglobin,** a plasma protein whose usual function is to conserve the iron elaborated from the small amount of hemoglobin that is normally in the plasma.
            (i) If hemolysis is acute, haptoglobin binds the released hemoglobin in the plasma. The formed complex is cleared from the circulation by the reticuloendothelial system; and within a matter of hours after the acute hemolytic episode, serum haptoglobin is unmeasurable.
            (ii) Thus, if haptoglobin is present, the diagnosis is hemorrhage; if absent, acute hemolysis has occurred.

(b) In **chronic excessive blood turnover,** in order to differentiate hemorrhage from hemolysis, knowledge of **iron metabolism** is necessary. Iron, which is found predominantly in red cells, decreases in the serum and in the reticuloendothelial cells of the marrow only during blood loss to the outside. In any other type of anemia, the marrow shows increased iron stores. Thus, a bone marrow aspirate or biopsy is helpful in making this distinction.

b. Blood loss

(1) **Acute blood loss** usually results in a **normochromic normocytic anemia,** which is dramatic and often traumatic. The dominant clinical picture is one of decreased blood volume and **shock,** with tachycardia, hypovolemia, and hypotension.

(2) A **prolonged low rate of bleeding** nearly always results in a deficiency of iron, which, when severe, is characterized by a **hypochromic anemia**. The **cause** of chronic hemorrhage is usually gastrointestinal (ulcer, cancer, or polyp), genitourinary (cancer or stone), or gynecologic (excessive menstrual flow).

c. Hemolysis, whether acute or chronic, can be of two **types:** an intrinsic erythrocyte defect or an abnormal marrow or systemic environment.

(1) An **intrinsic red cell defect** is congenital. Effects are manifested in childhood, and a family history of anemia is common.

(2) An **abnormal marrow or systemic environment** is an acquired abnormality (the red cell itself is normal). In acquired defects, the patient's family history is normal, and often the onset of the anemia can be pinpointed.

d. Congenital hemolytic anemias. These disorders can result from a defect in hemoglobin structure, in red cell metabolism, or in hemoglobin synthesis. Complications of these various congenital defects include jaundice, bilirubinate gallstones, iron overload (hemosiderosis), and the effects of chronic anemia (fatigue, weakness, and cardiac enlargement and failure).

(1) **Hemoglobinopathies** are hemolytic anemias caused by a hereditary **abnormality in the hemoglobin molecule**. Differences that can be demonstrated by electrophoresis are in the globin portion of the molecule.

(a) **General concepts**

(i) **Types of hemoglobin.** Hemoglobin A (Hb A), which is normal adult hemoglobin, consists of two α and two β chains and is written as $\alpha_2\beta_2$. Although α chains are unique, both γ and δ chains can substitute for β chains. Thus, Hb F is $\alpha_2\gamma_2$, and Hb A_2 is $\alpha_2\delta_2$. The type of hemoglobin is genetically controlled.

(ii) **"Trait" versus disease.** When abnormal hemoglobin occurs in the **heterozygous state** along with normal adult hemoglobin, a nonsymptomatic **trait** condition usually results. When abnormal hemoglobin is present in the **homozygous state** or when a person is heterozygous for two abnormal hemoglobin types, a **clinical disease** characterized by hemolysis usually occurs.

(b) **Sickle cell anemia** is the prototype of the congenital hemoglobinopathies. Its cause is a single amino acid substitution in the β chain, namely, valine for the normal glutamic acid at position 6; the designation for the abnormal hemoglobin is **Hb S**.

(i) This autosomal dominant gene defect predominantly affects blacks. It occurs as the **sickle cell trait** in 8% to 10% of black persons in the United States. The disease itself, which develops in the homozygous state, occurs in about 0.2% of blacks in the United States.

(ii) The biochemical anomaly in the β chain alters the solubility of hemoglobin. At low pH and with decreased oxygen tension, Hb S precipitates out of solution in the red cells, and the cells become sickle-shaped. Such red cells get stuck in the small blood vessels, with consequent vascular obstruction, occlusion, and then hemolysis of red cells.

(iii) Although sickle cell trait is usually asymptomatic, **sickle cell anemia** leads to severe disease. Vascular occlusions account for most of the symptoms and signs, which include leg ulcers, bone pain from microscopic infarcts, hematuria from necrosis of renal papillae, and splenic autoinfarction, eventuating in splenic atrophy in adults, hepatomegaly, hepatic dysfunction, cholelithiasis, pulmonary thrombi, and stroke. Unusual infections (e.g., salmonellal osteomyelitis, pneumococcal meningitis) can also occur.

(iv) Sickle cell crisis is a painful and dramatic expression of vascular occlusion and may result in sudden death. The initiating factor in sickle cell crisis is unknown. Febrile episodes from infection seem to predispose a patient to crisis. Portal circulations in which oxygen tension is low, such as those in the liver and kidneys, seem to be at particular risk.

(2) Disturbances of red cell metabolism affect red cell membrane structure or intracellular enzymes.

(a) Hereditary spherocytosis, the classic example of a red cell membrane defect, is inherited as an autosomal dominant trait.

(i) A genetically determined abnormality occurs in a membrane polypeptide called **spectrin,** a component of the membrane skeleton. The degree of deficiency correlates with the degree of spherocytosis. The red cells that have a decreased diameter and an abnormal shape are sequestered selectively by the reticuloendothelial cells of the spleen and then destroyed.

(ii) The **red cell indices** [mean corpuscular volume (MCV), hemoglobin (MCH), and hemoglobin concentration (MCHC)] are usually normal, but some smaller-than-normal, hyperchromatic spherocytes are visible on the peripheral smear.

(b) Glucose-6-phosphate dehydrogenase (G6PD) deficiency is a red cell enzyme defect. About 10% of American blacks carry this X-linked, incompletely dominant trait; it is also relatively common among people of Mediterranean heritage. Affected persons are often women who are susceptible to drugs or other compounds with oxidative activity (e.g., sulfonamides, nitrofurantoins, antimalarial drugs, fava beans). The ingestion of such compounds can lead to massive acute hemolytic episodes. In actuality, infections are a common precipitating cause of hemolysis.

(3) Defects in hemoglobin synthesis. β Thalassemia, the prototype, is an autosomal dominant abnormality that occurs predominantly in patients from the Mediterranean region. A failure or decrease in synthesis of the β chain of hemoglobin results in abnormal hemoglobins that are functionally inadequate. The red cells are deformed and **hypochromic.**

(a) Thalassemia major (Cooley's anemia), the **homozygous** form of the disease, is fatal in early life because intercurrent infection or hemosiderosis leads to liver or heart failure.

(b) Thalassemia minor, the **heterozygous** form, results in a mild anemia but is compatible with a normal life span.

e. Acquired hemolytic anemias

(1) Autoimmune destruction of red cells provides the basis for most of these disorders. Antibodies, usually of the immunoglobulin G (IgG) class, are directed against red cells and may lyse the cells directly or may react with red cell membrane antigens, altering their susceptibility to destruction in the spleen. The hemolytic process may be idiopathic or secondary to some underlying disease, such as lymphoma [e.g., chronic lymphocytic leukemia (CLL), Hodgkin's disease], carcinoma, sarcoidosis, or one of the collagen disorders.

(2) Blood group incompatibilities are classic examples of immune—but not autoimmune—hemolysis.

(a) In **fetomaternal incompatibility** at Rh locus D, the D-negative mother, after contact with D-positive red cells, may produce an IgG anti-D antibody, which crosses the placenta, attacks fetal red cells, and destroys them. The fetus is jaundiced **(erythroblastosis fetalis).** ABO incompatibilities are more common but milder in effect.

(b) When a patient receives an **incompatible blood transfusion,** a devastating sequence of acute intravascular hemolysis occurs within minutes.

(3) Microangiopathic hemolytic anemia is due to **mechanical injury** of the red cell. It is characterized by the appearance of bizarre **fragmented** erythrocytes on a peripheral smear and by signs of hemolysis. The erythrocyte can withstand moderate deformation and twisting, but it breaks up when subjected to strong stretching or shearing forces. Stress of this magnitude occurs in jets produced by deformed aortic valves, arteriovenous shunts, ventricular septal defects, or older cardiac valvular prostheses.

(4) Malaria is a disease that causes red cell destruction by direct infection of red cells.

3. **Anemias due to failure of blood production.** These anemias can be caused by nutritional deficiencies, by marrow aplasia, by myelophthisis (marrow replacement), and by systemic disorders.

   a. **Anemias due to nutritional deficiencies** (see also Chapter 5 IV B 2 and V B 6). Iron, folic acid, or vitamin B_{12} deficiencies produce the nutritional anemias seen most commonly in clinical practice. Anemia may also result from severe protein deficiency.

      (1) Iron deficiency results when the diet does not provide enough iron for normal erythropoiesis. It also can result from a chronic low-grade blood loss (e.g., gastrointestinal malignancy). The red cells are **hypochromic and microcytic,** with decreased MCV and MCH in more severe anemias. Serum ferritin and iron concentrations are low; the serum iron-binding capacity is high; the transferrin saturation is low—16% (normal is about 30%). This situation is due to the small amount of iron on the binding protein, transferrin, which is, therefore, not saturated, but has a binding capacity that is now greater than normal.

      (2) Folic acid and vitamin B_{12} deficiencies produce a megaloblastic anemia. Associated with this condition are glossitis, lingual atrophy, and, with B_{12} deficiency, neurologic abnormalities. The red cells are normochromic but **macrocytic.**

         (a) **Pernicious anemia** is an autoimmune disorder characterized by the absence of parietal cells in the gastric fundus, with consequent achlorhydria and gastric mucosal atrophy. **Intrinsic factor,** produced by the fundus and required for the absorption of dietary vitamin B_{12}, is absent.

         (b) Pernicious anemia patients may show circulating antibodies to parietal cells; they are likely to have other **autoimmune disorders,** especially idiopathic hypoadrenalism (Addison's disease), and they are prone to develop gastric cancer.

   b. **Anemias due to marrow aplasia (normochromic, normocytic)**

      (1) **Inciting or causative agents** may be radiation, drugs (especially benzene derivatives), certain antibiotics (especially chloramphenicol), viruses (especially non-A, non-B hepatitis virus), or unknown agents. Not only the marrow but also other sites of hematopoiesis reflect injury to the stem cells. The marrow spaces are occupied only by fat; no erythroid hyperplasia is seen.

      (2) Some cases of aplasia involve only one hematopoietic line, as in **Diamond-Blackfan syndrome,** a congenital defect involving erythroid hypoplasia. Certain tumors, such as **thymomas,** are associated with pure red cell aplasia.

   c. **Myelophthisic anemias.** In these conditions, the marrow is replaced by foreign "invaders" (e.g., carcinomas, leukemias, granulomas). Extramedullary hematopoiesis, particularly in the spleen (as in the fetal period), is found. **Primary bone marrow myelofibrosis** (Figure 8-1) also induces this type of anemia by replacing marrow with fibrosis of unknown cause.

   d. **Anemias due to systemic disorders.** Endocrine diseases, such as hypothyroidism, hypopituitarism, and hypoadrenalism, are associated with low blood counts. Poor marrow function and anemia can be seen in uremia, chronic low-grade infection, and malignancy. It is not known whether these systemic conditions produce anemia via deficiency states or via production of specific substances that are toxic to marrow stem cells or their maturation.

B. **Polycythemia.** Erythrocytosis and an increased red cell mass may be **marrow-based** (primary polycythemia) or a **reaction to hypoxia** (secondary polycythemia).

   1. **Primary polycythemia (polycythemia rubra vera).** This **myeloproliferative disorder** is characterized by **panmyelopathy** (proliferation of all bone marrow cell lines—red cells, white cells, and platelets). An absolute increase in red cell mass dominates the clinicopathologic syndrome.

      a. **Pathogenesis.** Cytogenetic and karyotypic studies indicate that polycythemia vera is a clonal disorder, suggesting a neoplastic transformation in this disease.

      b. **Clinical features.** Polycythemia vera is an uncommon disease, chiefly affecting persons in the sixth to eighth decade of life.

         (1) The disorder is often insidious in onset, and its diagnosis may result from an incidental laboratory finding. However, patients may present with symptoms of vascular occlusion, headache, and itching.

         (2) The total erythrocyte count is usually between 7 and 10 million, resulting in a high hematocrit. In contrast to findings in secondary polycythemia, patients have normal erythropoietin levels and high transcobalamin III levels.

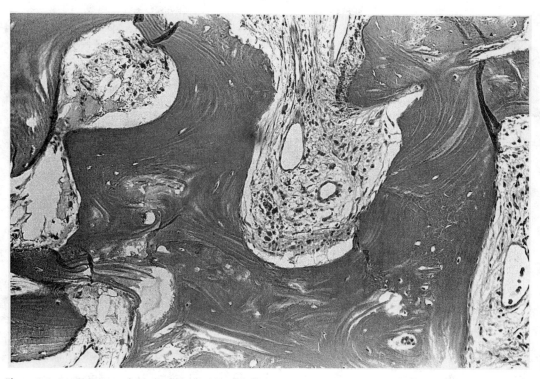

Figure 8-1. Agnogenic myeloid metaplasia with myelofibrosis. Bone marrow biopsy shows prominent fibrosis of marrow spaces with sparsely isolated residual marrow elements. The bone also is thickened [hematoxylin and eosin (H and E) stain; high power].

      (3) About 20% of patients develop myelofibrosis with spent marrows and anemia, and about 10% develop leukemia. Both complications are considerably more common in patients treated with alkylating agents or radioactive phosphorus. The associated thrombocytosis may produce local capillary or venule occlusion, causing ischemia and infarction. Gangrene of the extremities may occur.

      (4) The disease runs a chronic course, with median survival times of 10 to 20 years. Important causes of death include heart failure, myocardial infarction, stroke, hemorrhage, and the sequelae of leukemia or myelofibrosis.

    c. Pathology. The bone marrow demonstrates trilineage hyperplasia. Abnormal platelet precursors may be seen. Myelofibrosis with increased reticulin and collagen fibers is common and progresses during the course of the disease. Extramedullary hematopoiesis is found in the spleen, liver, and lymph nodes.

  2. Secondary polycythemia. A variety of hypoxic conditions, such as impaired pulmonary ventilation and heart disease, may lead to elevations of red cell count. In such disorders, erythropoietin is elevated and stimulates marrow stem cells to produce erythrocytes. Other marrow elements are normal in number, function, and morphology; no marrow fibrosis is found.

II. DISORDERS OF COAGULATION AND HEMOSTASIS (HEMORRHAGIC DISORDERS)

  A. General concepts. Important to the **process of hemostasis** are the actions of **platelets (thrombocytes)** and of **coagulation factors** from plasma, platelets, and other cells. Also important are the **counterbalancing mechanisms** that keep the clotting process within bounds and prevent thrombosis or disseminated intravascular coagulation (DIC).

    1. Platelets provide an **initial plug** to limit bleeding from an injured vessel.

      a. When the vascular endothelium is broken, the exposed collagen causes **platelet adhesion**.

      b. The platelets, activated by the collagen, become irregular in shape, send out pseudopods, and become sticky, so that **platelet aggregation** occurs.

  c. The activated platelets secrete adenosine diphosphate (ADP) and thromboxane A_2 (TXA_2), which, along with thrombin, augment platelet **aggregation** and make it **irreversible**.

  d. The platelets also produce a phospholipid (**platelet factor 3**) that serves in coagulation and fibrin clot formation.

2. The **coagulation sequence,** or **coagulation cascade** (Figure 8-2), activates a series of **coagulation factors** to produce **thrombin,** the enzyme needed for the formation of an insoluble fibrin clot.

  a. The **coagulation factors** are proenzymes that become activated enzymes (Table 8-1).

  b. The sequence may proceed via an **extrinsic pathway** (which is triggered by **thromboplastin,** the "tissue factor") or via an **intrinsic pathway** (which is triggered by **factor XII,** the **Hageman factor**).

  c. Each **reaction step** in the sequence involves:

   (1) An enzyme (the factor activated in the prior step)

   (2) A substrate (the factor to be activated in this step)

   (3) A cofactor (which accelerates the reaction)

  d. Most steps in the sequence require **calcium ion;** and factors II, VII, IX, and X are vitamin K–dependent.

  e. **Prothrombin activation** requires a phospholipid, platelet factor 3; its location on the platelets forming the platelet plug helps to keep the clotting process localized.

3. The **fibrinolytic system** controls clotting, limiting it to the injury site. Fibrinolysis begins almost as soon as clots begin to form.

  a. An important **mechanism** is the **generation of plasmin (fibrinolysin):**

$$\text{proactivator} \rightarrow \text{plasminogen activators} \rightarrow \text{plasminogen} \rightarrow \text{plasmin}$$

   (1) **Plasminogen activators** include tissue plasminogen activator (t-PA), urokinase, and streptokinase. Activated coagulation factor XII can also act in the conversion of plasminogen to plasmin.

   (2) Plasmin degrades the fibrin clot, through proteolysis, into **fibrin split products** (fibrin

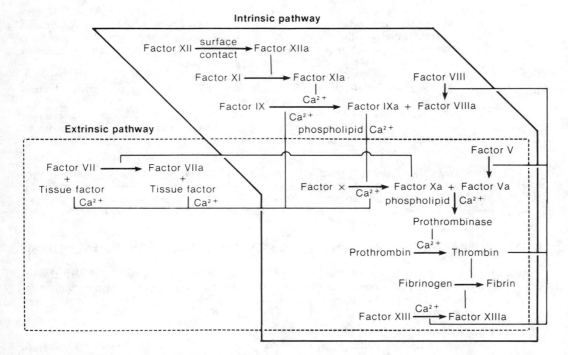

Figure 8-2. The coagulation cascade. The reactions enclosed by the *dark solid lines* are those of the intrinsic pathway. The reactions enclosed by the *dark dashed lines* are those of the extrinsic pathway. (Adapted from Williams WJ: Mechanisms of coagulation. In *Hematology,* 4th ed. Edited by Williams WJ, et al. New York, McGraw-Hill, 1990, p 1295.)

Table 8-1. Coagulation Factors and Their Functions

	Factor	Function
I	Fibrinogen	Fibrin precursor protein
II	Prothrombin	Thrombin precursor*
III	Tissue thromboplastin (tissue factor)	Activates extrinsic clotting system
IV	Calcium	Required in several steps
V	Labile factor (proaccelerin)	Required in prothrombin activation stage
VI	(No name)	Regarded as activated form of factor V
VII	Proconvertin (stable factor)	Important in extrinsic clotting system*
VIII	Antihemophilic factor (related to von Willebrand's factor)†	Important in intrinsic clotting system
IX	Christmas factor (plasma thromboplastin)	Involved only in intrinsic clotting system*
X	Stuart-Prower factor (thrombokinase)	Pivotal step in extrinsic and intrinsic clotting systems*
XI	Plasma thromboplastin antecedent	Involved in intrinsic system activation
XII	Hageman factor (contact factor)	Initial step in cascade of intrinsic factor system
XIII	Fibrin stabilizing factor	Stabilizes fibrin clot

*Vitamin K–dependent.
†Produced by endothelial cells.

degradation products), which are able to inhibit platelet aggregation and coagulation. Plasmin also lyses fibrinogen and factors V and VIII.

   b. Other mechanisms also have roles in **regulating coagulation**.

     (1) Antithrombin III, aided by heparinlike molecules, inactivates thrombin and several key enzymes in the coagulation sequence.

     (2) When thrombin binds to the endothelial cell receptor **thrombomodulin,** its clotting actions are strongly inhibited. Moreover, thrombomodulin binding also activates two vitamin K–dependent proteins, **protein C** and its cofactor **protein S,** which then can lyse factors V and VIII.

B. Coagulation disorders. Because the coagulation sequence is complex, a deficiency of any of the coagulation factors, or defects in their synthesis, function, or composition, would interfere with proper clotting. Individuals with coagulation defects must receive an injury before they bleed.

   1. Hereditary disorders of all the coagulation factors are known. The prototype is **hemophilia A,** caused by defective or deficient factor VIII. This X-linked disorder occurs in about 1 in 20,000 live births. Diagnosis reflects the clinical picture, family pedigree, and the factor VIII level in serum.

   2. Acquired clotting disorders occur more often than hereditary clotting disorders. The causes can be grouped roughly into three classes—by origin and behavior.

     a. Vitamin K deficiency can be identified by a decrease in serum levels of prothrombin and factors VII, IX, and X, combined with normal levels of factors V, VIII, and fibrinogen. Vitamin K deficiency can result from malnutrition, malabsorption (e.g., sprue), and obstructive jaundice. Vitamin K–dependent factors can also be decreased by vitamin K antagonists (e.g., drugs such as warfarin).

     b. Liver disease. Decreases in factors V, VII, IX, and X, prothrombin, and fibrinogen point to liver disease so severe that these substances cannot be produced.

     c. Disseminated intravascular coagulation (DIC, defibrination syndrome, consumption coagulopathy) is identified by decreases in factors V and VIII, fibrinogen, and prothrombin.

       (1) This disorder occurs acutely in incompatible blood transfusion, in the peripartum period with premature separation of the placenta, and in endotoxic shock. Although the coagulation cascade is invoked, in acute DIC the consequence is usually a **bleeding diathesis** because the clotting factors are rapidly degraded and fibrinolysis is activated.

       (2) Chronic DIC usually involves metastatic malignancies and is more likely to produce thrombotic effects.

       (3) In both forms, fibrin is deposited widely in vessels, the fibrinolytic mechanism is activated, and fragments of fibrinogen and fibrin (**fibrin split products**) are found in the plasma. Moreover, platelets are decreased because they are trapped in areas of clotting. This situation further perpetuates the bleeding tendencies.

C. **Platelet disorders.** A decrease in the number of platelets (**thrombocytopenia**), thrombocytosis, or abnormal platelet function can lead to a hemorrhagic disorder. It should be remembered that platelet dysfunction can occur despite a normal or even an elevated platelet count.

1. **Thrombocytopenia**
   a. **Clinical features**
      (1) The clinical features vary according to the etiology and the presence or absence of pancytopenia. The hallmark of thrombocytopenia is the presence of petechiae; but if the platelet count is very low, a purpura, mucosal bleeding, and even deep tissue bleeding may occur.
      (2) Drug history is important since many classes of drugs can produce thrombocytopenia by idiopathic, idiosyncratic, or allergic reactions. Folate deficiency, whether dietary or drug-induced (e.g., by methotrexate), can result in thrombocytopenia.
      (3) Patients may exhibit anemia, neutropenic infection, connective tissue disease, or a lymphoma.
   b. **Abnormalities of platelet production.** A hypoplastic marrow in which the total cellularity is reduced implies **aplastic anemia**. A marrow that is fibrosed (myelofibrosis) or infiltrated with leukemic or other malignant cells is **myelophthisis**. A marrow showing normal cellularity and maturation with decreased numbers of apparently normal megakaryocytes suggests **ingestion of a drug** that specifically affects the megakaryocytic precursor cells.
   c. **Accelerated removal of platelets**
      (1) When a patient has thrombocytopenia despite an abundance of normal megakaryocytes in the marrow, it is likely that the **mechanism** of thrombocytopenia is accelerated removal of platelets. Systemic lupus erythematosus (SLE), lymphoma, or Coombs'-positive acquired hemolytic anemia is usually the underlying problem.
      (2) **Idiopathic thrombocytopenic purpura.** This disorder typically appears in young women without a relevant history of drug ingestion. The marrow shows abundant megakaryocytes, many of which are young; and erythroid and myeloid precursors remain normal. In the serum of about 70% of these patients, an **antiplatelet antibody** coats and damages platelets, which are selectively removed by the spleen.
      (3) **Platelet sequestration** causes a relatively modest thrombocytopenia (platelet counts of 40,000 to 870,000/μl) in patients with **marked splenomegaly (hypersplenism),** which can be due to a variety of disorders.

2. **Thrombocytosis (thrombocythemia)**
   a. **Reactive (secondary) thrombocytosis** is an elevated platelet count (above 500,000/μl) that occurs as a secondary response to a variety of clinical disorders (e.g., chronic inflammatory diseases, acute infections, neoplasms).
   b. **Essential (primary) thrombocythemia** is a **myeloproliferative disorder** in which a clonal stem cell abnormality causes a marked increase in platelet production. The platelet count can vary from 1,000,000 to 3,000,000/μl or more, and tests of platelet function are frequently abnormal. There appears to be an enhanced propensity for hemorrhage, thromboembolism, or thrombosis.

3. **Platelet function defects**
   a. Some drugs, most notably aspirin, certain antibiotics (penicillin derivatives, cephalosporins), and antihistamines, can lead to **hemorrhage** because of interference with platelet function.
   b. Patients with **von Willebrand's disease** have defects that involve von Willebrand's factor (VWF), a glycoprotein synthesized by endothelial cells and megakaryocytes and released into the circulation. The factor aids in platelet adhesion to endothelium, and patients present with episodes of bleeding diathesis. Factor VIII may also be deficient. This autosomal dominant disease has various subtypes, and treatment involves cryoprecipitate (with VWF and factor VIII), a type of vasopressin, or combinations, depending on the subtype.
   c. The myeloproliferative disease, essential thrombocythemia, also can cause **platelet dysfunction**. Megakaryocytes frequently are abnormal. Abnormal platelet morphology is present sometimes.

D. **Vascular anomalies**

1. **General features.** Patients whose vessel walls are fragile and do not withstand normal pressures have a history of **purpura** (**petechiae,** which are small, often pinhead-sized; hemorrhages or aneurysms in the skin or mucosae; and **ecchymoses,** which are larger areas of

hemorrhage). Tests of platelet number and function and tests of coagulation factors are normal. Individuals with vascular fragility need no injury before they bleed.

2. **Hereditary hemorrhagic telangiectasia** is transmitted as an autosomal dominant trait and appears clinically with epistaxis or gastrointestinal bleeding.

3. **Scurvy** , which is due to vitamin C deficiency, is very rare in the United States. It can cause skin, gingival, and mucosal bleeding with petechiae.

4. **Corticosteroid excess,** whether from endogenous or exogenous causes, produces cutaneous hemorrhages, which probably are due to corticosteroid-induced catabolism of the protein in vascular supportive tissues.

5. **Drug allergies** can cause a vasculitic purpura.

6. **Senile purpura** presumably represents an age-dependent deterioration of the vascular supportive tissues. Patients have cutaneous hemorrhages on the dorsum of the hands, the wrists, the upper arms, and occasionally the calves. Serious bleeding does not occur.

III. NONNEOPLASTIC WHITE BLOOD CELL DISORDERS

A. Leukocytopenia

1. **Neutropenia.** A decrease in the absolute neutrophil count below 500/μl is associated with a significant incidence of infection. The causes of neutropenia include inadequate production (aplastic marrow), toxic reactions and drug effects, immune (autoimmune) diseases, and increased removal and redistribution of neutrophils as in hypersplenism. Neutropenia is now seen most commonly in cancer patients on chemotherapy.

2. **Lymphocytopenia.** A decrease in the absolute lymphocyte count below 1500/μl is found in steroid-treated patients, in patients with certain malignancies—after treatment with radiation therapy, in patients with uremia, and in those with marrow aplasia.

B. Leukocytosis. Nonneoplastic elevation of the white cell count (WBC) usually reflects infection.

1. In some severe infections, the **neutrophil** count is very high (**leukemoid reaction**). Specific elevation of **eosinophils** is found in parasitic infestations, especially with worms, and in allergic reactions (asthma, hay fever, drug allergies).

2. **Monocytosis** can be found in patients with infections that elicit a chronic inflammatory response (e.g., tuberculosis, fungal infections, listeriosis).

3. **Lymphocytosis** can be found in tuberculosis and viral infections (e.g., infectious mononucleosis, measles).

IV. LEUKEMIA

A. General considerations

1. **Pathophysiology**
   a. Leukemia is a condition in which leukocytes proliferate uncontrollably in the peripheral blood, in the bone marrow, and in other lymphoreticular tissues (e.g., lymph nodes, spleen) and may infiltrate any organ. The leukemic population of cells may arise from granulocytic, monocytic, or lymphocytic precursors.
   b. Leukemia is characterized by the proliferation of an abnormal hematopoietic cell clone that responds poorly to normal regulatory mechanisms. The leukemic cell tends to have a diminished capacity for normal cell differentiation, tends to expand at the expense of normal myeloid or lymphoid lines, and, possibly, has the ability to suppress or impair normal myeloid cell growth.
   c. The growing cell population infiltrates the marrow and renders it functionally aplastic, leading to death by infection or hemorrhage through the depletion of normally functioning white cells and platelets. Leukemic cells also can infiltrate other areas, chiefly the liver, spleen, lymph nodes, and meninges, and cause organ dysfunction.

2. Classification (Table 8-2)

a. Leukemias generally are divided into **acute** and **chronic** types. The terms are predictive in that most chronic leukemias follow an insidious course, whereas acute leukemias kill rapidly unless there is aggressive therapeutic intervention. Paradoxically, cures may be achieved in acute leukemias—in a variable percentage (20% to 50%) depending on the type, whereas chronic leukemias cannot be cured.

(1) Acute leukemias are characterized by precursor cells (**blasts**) that proliferate without undergoing the normal maturation process. Thus, the leukemic cells are large and primitive in appearance.

(a) The primitive cells fill and replace the normal marrow and then spill over into the peripheral blood. They often comprise over 90% of the circulating leukocytes.

(b) Monoblasts, myeloblasts (the precursors of granulocytes), and lymphoblasts may be distinguished by various morphologic criteria and by cytochemical and immunohistochemical techniques.

(2) In **chronic leukemias,** there are mature elements; the proliferating neoplastic cells are able to undergo normal or nearly normal maturation. However, the proliferative process advances without the control mechanisms that normally operate to limit production. Thus, the abnormal cell line fills the bone marrow space.

b. The second way of classifying leukemias is by their **cell of origin** (or the normal marrow cell that they most resemble). Hence, there are lymphocytic leukemias, granulocytic or myelocytic leukemias, monocytic types, and even combinations, such as myelomonocytic leukemias.

c. The most important distinction for clinical therapy is the classification of acute leukemias into **acute lymphocytic leukemia** (ALL) and acute myelogenous, or acute nonlymphocytic, leukemia (AML, or ANLL).

3. Etiology

a. Animal leukemias are caused by RNA **viruses,** but a viral etiology for human leukemias has not been proved.

b. Human leukemias can occur after exposure to ionizing **radiation** or to **radiomimetic agents** (e.g, antimetabolites, chloramphenicol, benzene) that produce marrow aplasia.

c. The genetic makeup of the host influences the incidence of both animal and human leukemias. Specifically, certain **chromosomal abnormalities** show an increased incidence of ALL.

(1) One example is Down syndrome, which is **trisomy of chromosome 21**.

(2) Chromosomal translocations are found in a number of leukemias (see Table 8-2); in most cases, these translocations occur at or near the site of a cellular oncogene. The **Philadelphia chromosome** is diagnostic of chronic myelogenous leukemia (CML); the other examples in Table 8-2 are listed mainly for interest but are also important diagnostically.

4. Diagnosis

a. The diagnosis of leukemia rests on cytologic and morphologic evidence: the finding of abnormal cells in the peripheral blood and the presence in a marrow smear of an infiltrate of abnormal cells replacing normal marrow elements.

b. Biopsies of bone marrow, liver, spleen, or skin lesions also can provide the diagnosis through showing infiltration by the abnormal cells.

Table 8-2. Chromosomal Translocations and Associated Oncogenes Found in Various Leukemias

Type of Leukemia	Translocation	Associated Oncogene (and Chromosome Site)
Chronic myelogenous (CML)	t(9;22)*	c-*abl* (9)
Acute myelogenous (AML)[+]	t(8;21)	c-*ets* (8)
Acute promyelocytic (APL)	t(15;17)	c-*erb* (17)
Acute lymphocytic (ALL), T-cell type	t(11;14)	
Acute lymphocytic (ALL), B-cell type	t(8;14 or 8;22)	c-*myc* (8)

*The Philadelphia chromosome.
[+]In some forms only.

B. Myelogenous leukemias

1. **CML** is a marrow-derived neoplasm composed principally of granulocytic cells in **various stages of maturation**. WBCs are usually greater than 50,000/µl. The **Philadelphia chromosome** (see Table 8-2) is present in bone marrow cells in 90% of the cases.

  a. **Clinical features.** The typical patient is an adult who has peripheral blood and marrow granulocytosis with a shift to the left with myelocytes and scattered blasts. Fever, splenomegaly, and fatigue are common symptoms.

  b. **Laboratory test.** The leukocyte alkaline phosphatase (LAP) test is one way to distinguish a reactive leukocytosis from CML.

    (1) A blood smear is made and substrate added; if the enzyme is present in a cell, the cell is colorized by the detection system. The number and degree of positive (0–4) cells per 100 cells are counted.

    (2) In reactive leukocytosis, over 25% leukocytes are positive (high score: 100–200). By contrast, the cells of CML are defective, and only a small number of positive cells are seen (low score: 10–40).

  c. **Course and prognosis.** More patients with CML enter an accelerated phase (increase in blasts with differentiation) or **blast crisis** (pure blastic proliferation) in which the predominant cells resemble blast cells of primitive myeloid, monocytic, or lymphoid cells. In many cases, death is the result of a blast crisis. Recently, **bone marrow transplantation (BMT)** has altered the prognosis—with improved length of survival.

2. **AML**

  a. **Acute myelomonocytic leukemia** is a marrow-derived neoplasm composed of blasts and cells differentiating into early granulocytes. The marrow is infiltrated by blasts and promyelocytes (Figure 8-3).

    (1) **Clinical features.** AML affect adults mainly and is preceded by a few days to weeks of weakness, bleeding, and fever. Physical examination shows petechiae, sternal tenderness, and sometimes thickened gums, adenopathy, splenomegaly, and hepatomegaly. Infection is evident often. Occasionally, the leukemia presents as a mass lesion composed of blast cells (**granulocytic sarcoma or chloroma**) in the head, neck, and bowel.

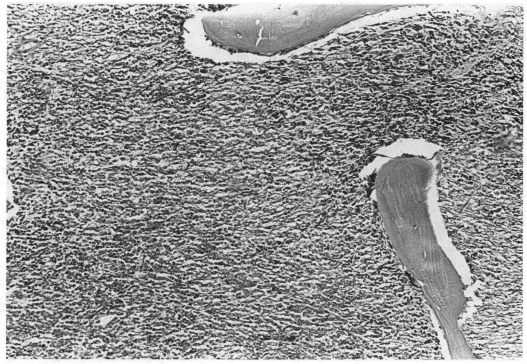

Figure 8-3. Marrow spaces replaced by leukemic blasts in acute myelogenous leukemia (AML); no fat remains (H and E stain; high power).

(2) **Laboratory data.** The blood picture is characterized by anemia, thrombocytopenia, and an elevated leukocyte count in which the predominant cell is a blast. The bone marrow shows a myeloblastic infiltrate replacing all marrow (see Figure 8-3). On a bone marrow aspirate, abnormal blasts may show the **Auer rod,** an abnormal granule.

(3) **Course and prognosis.** Untreated, this form of leukemia causes death within 1 to 3 months, usually as a result of infection or hemorrhage. With current therapeutic regimens, about half of the patients achieve a complete remission. BMT has increased the chances for cure.

   b. Acute promyelocytic leukemia is characterized by prominent primary cytoplasmic granules, as seen in the normal promyelocyte. It accounts for about 10% of all cases of AML.

(1) **Clinical features.** Due to the release of a procoagulant factor, with thromboplastin activity by the granules, 75% of patients either present with a significant bleeding diathesis or develop bleeding during therapy. This bleeding results in either cutaneous or mucosal hemorrhage and may progress to frank DIC.

(2) **Course and prognosis.** As with other forms of AML, many patients with acute promyelocytic leukemia have an initial response to therapy. With this form, however, a better survival rate (50%) is the rule; again, transplantation has improved the chance of survival.

C. Lymphocytic leukemias

1. General considerations
   a. The advent of specific tumor markers for specific stages of T-cell and B-cell differentiation has aided greatly in the understanding of lymphoproliferative processes.
   b. Lymphomas may become leukemic, and sometimes the distinction between lymphoma and leukemia is obscured.

2. Chronic lymphocytic leukemia (CLL) is a lesion of the mature small lymphocyte and has a low proliferative rate. Fully 98% of cases are of B-cell origin; lesions of T-cell origin are more aggressive.
   a. Clinical features. A common form of leukemia, CLL affects the elderly. Patients present with splenomegaly and symptoms related to anemia. Occasionally, patients are asymptomatic.
   b. Laboratory data. While most patients have a marked lymphocytosis (above 20,000/μl, some have only a mild absolute lymphocytosis (defined as a lymphocyte count above 4000/μl. The marrow shows focal or diffuse lymphocytic infiltration.
   c. Course and prognosis. The length of survival is most closely related to total tumor burden.

(1) Since many cases are diagnosed early, **longevity** is not necessarily affected by the presence of CLL, and patients often die of other diseases of the elderly. Patients presenting with profound anemia have bulky disease and survive an average of 2 years.

(2) As the disease progresses, infiltrates in organs occur. Rarely, patients develop **Richter's syndrome,** in which transformation to a large cell type signals aggressive preterminal disease with tumor nodules in various sites.

3. Acute lymphocytic (lymphoid, lymphoblastic) leukemia (ALL). In this form of leukemia, an immature (blastic) lymphoid precursor proliferates at a high rate. Fully 80% are of B-cell origin (early pre-B, pre-B, or B). Because of the good chance for cure of ALL with specific therapy, it is important to distinguish it from AML.
   a. Clinical features. ALL occurs most often in children, in whom it represents the most common form of leukemia. For patients with B-cell types, the average age at diagnosis is 4 years; for those with T-cell ALL, the average age is 7 years. Adult ALL occurs in the same age group as AML.
   b. Laboratory data. The bone marrow shows complete replacement by leukemia cells. Very high lymphocyte counts (above 50,000/μl) and a mediastinal mass are seen more frequently in T-cell ALL.
   c. Course and prognosis. In childhood ALL, the cure rate is greater than 50% and appears to be approaching 75%. Patients are treated aggressively and given drugs that differ from those used for AML.

4. Hairy cell leukemia (formerly called **leukemic reticuloendotheliosis**) has been shown to be a low-grade clonal proliferation of a type of B lymphocyte. Oddly enough, patients often present with **pancytopenia,** although others may have overt leukemia.
   a. Clinical features. The typical patient is a man over 40 or 50 years of age with symptoms

related to anemia (weakness), thrombocytopenia (easy bruisability), or leukopenia (proneness to infection). Splenomegaly is nearly always present, and about one-third of patients have hepatomegaly.

b. Laboratory data. In all cases, peculiar lymphoid cells with prominent cytoplasmic projections—**"hairy" cells**—can be identified in a smear of the buffy coat with characteristic enzyme histochemistry. The bone marrow is replaced to variable degrees and shows nonoverlapping lymphoid cells with clear cytoplasm and increased reticulin. Splenic pathology is also characteristic: Cells replace the red pulp in sheets and produce "blood lakes."

c. Course and prognosis. In the past, the clinical course was often prolonged, and splenectomy was the primary therapy. However, hairy cell leukemia has uniformly shown a marked response to interferon-α (INF-α): Hematologic values return to normal, and hairy cells decrease in the blood and marrow. INF-α therapy plus splenectomy is expected to significantly improve long-term survival for many patients and, possibly, cure some patients.

V. HODGKIN'S DISEASE

A. General features. Hodgkin's disease is a neoplastic process that primarily affects the lymph nodes (Figure 8-4).

1. **Cells of origin.** The malignant cells of Hodgkin's disease are called **Reed-Sternberg cells** when binucleate and **Reed-Sternberg variants** when mononuclear or multinucleate. These cells have been shown to be aneuploid and clonal, but their origin is still the subject of considerable debate.

   a. When the cells were shown to lack the surface markers of B and T lymphocytes, speculation centered around their derivation from either true histiocytes or interdigitating reticulum cells.

   b. Today, a lymphocyte origin is again considered a possibility on the basis of recent (though conflicting) gene rearrangement data.

2. Hodgkin's disease is, nonetheless, clearly **different from the non-Hodgkin's lymphomas** in the following ways.

   a. Manner of spread

   (1) **Hodgkin's disease** spreads in a logical, step-by-step fashion to **contiguous lymph node regions,** usually proceeding from the neck (in 90% of cases) to mediastinum to celiac nodes and from there to the spleen, the liver, and the bone marrow.

   (2) By contrast, **non-Hodgkin's lymphomas** frequently involve **many node groups** at presentation—due to an unseen circulating population.

   b. Histology

   (1) **In Hodgkin's disease,** the cell population is **polymorphic,** and most are reactive cells: small lymphocytes, plasma cells, eosinophils, and macrophages. The malignant cells are vastly outnumbered.

   (2) **Other lymphomas** are **monomorphic,** and the malignant cells comprise most of the proliferation.

   c. Age at onset. Hodgkin's disease occurs mainly in the **young** (under age 30); **non-Hodgkin's lymphomas** are seen mainly in **older age groups** (over age 40).

   d. Prognosis. In about 80% of patients with Hodgkin's disease, virtual cure is possible. Small cell lymphomas are currently incurable. A proportion of other lymphomas are curable—but at lower frequencies.

3. **Immunologic deficit.** Hodgkin's disease is accompanied by early and profound immunologic dysfunction. T-cell–mediated immunologic responses are most severely depressed. Patients with Hodgkin's disease are, therefore, particularly susceptible to viral, mycobacterial, and fungal infections.

B. Clinical features and pathology. Hodgkin's disease is divided into four **histopathologic subtypes,** each of which has particular clinicopathologic correlations (Table 8-3). The four types show a rough correlation with the number of Reed-Sternberg cells (lymphocyte depletion > mixed cellularity > nodular sclerosis > lymphocyte predominance). In the past, this number also correlated roughly with the prognosis—best in lymphocyte predominance with the fewest Reed-Sternberg cells; worst in lymphocyte depletion with the most Reed-Sternberg cells.

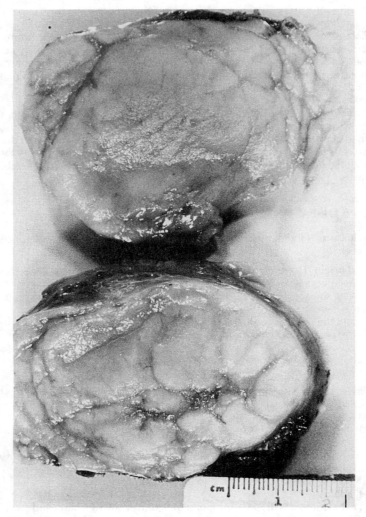

Figure 8-4. Axillary lymph node involved by Hodgkin's disease, nodular sclerosis variant. Note large size and nodular configuration.

1. **Nodular sclerosis** comprises about 60% of all cases of Hodgkin's disease.
   a. **Clinical features.** This form is most common in adolescents and young adults and is the only type that shows a female predominance. Involvement of the anterior mediastinum (thymus) is common.
   b. **Pathology.** Histologically, fibrous connective tissue bands demarcate involved tissues into nodules that contain the tumor cells, along with benign lymphocytes, plasma cells, and eosinophils. Distinctive mononuclear Reed-Sternberg variants—called **lacunar cells**—are present in the nodules (Figure 8-5); lacunar cells are not seen in other Hodgkin's disease types.
   c. **Prognosis.** Nodular sclerosis is an indolent neoplasm, and results of current therapy are excellent.

2. **Lymphocyte predominance** comprises about 5% of all cases of Hodgkin's disease and has the best prognosis. Patients range in age from young adults to elderly individuals, and they generally present with early-stage disease. **Histologically,** the involved nodes demonstrate very few Reed-Sternberg cells dispersed in a lymphocytic and macrophagic immunologic reaction. It may be an unusual form of B-cell lymphoma.

Table 8-3. Subtypes of Hodgkin's Disease

Subtype	Frequency (%)	Patients	Extent	R-S Cells	Comments
LP (lymphocyte predominant)	5	All ages	Localized	+/−	Excellent course; may be a B-cell disease
NS (nodular sclerosis)	60	Young females	Localized	+ + +	Very good survival
MC (mixed cellularity)	30	Middle aged	Localized and systemic	+ + +	Very good survival
LD (lymphocyte depleted)	1–2	Elderly	Systemic	+ + + +	Poor survival

3. **Mixed cellularity** comprises about 30% of all cases and is most common in middle-aged adults. **Histologically,** numerous Reed-Sternberg cells are distributed in a lymphocytic infiltrate in which eosinophils, histiocytes, and plasma cells are prominent.

4. **Lymphocyte depletion** comprises only 1% of cases. It is most common in elderly persons who present with disseminated disease, which has a rather poor prognosis.
   a. **Histologically,** numerous Reed-Sternberg cells grow in sheets with few lymphocytic elements and little inflammatory reaction.
   b. Importantly, many cases originally diagnosed as lymphocyte depletion have now been reclassified as **large cell lymphoma.** One must be skeptical of this diagnosis: It exists but is very rare.

VI. NON-HODGKIN'S LYMPHOMAS. Malignant lymphomas are common neoplasms, comprising approximately 10% of all malignant tumors. Second only to acute leukemia as the most common form of cancer in children and young adults, lymphomas occur more frequently in middle-aged and elderly adults and are increasing in incidence.

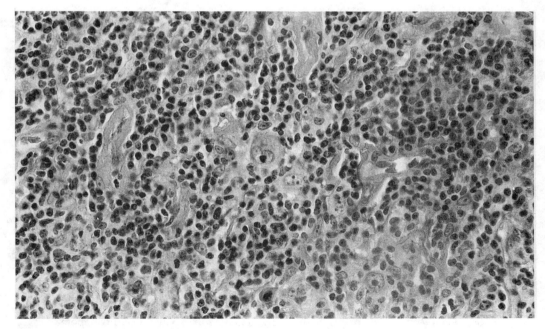

Figure 8-5. Hodgkin's disease, nodular sclerosis pattern, showing mononuclear malignant Reed-Sternberg variant cells (lacunar cells) in *center* (high power).

A. Etiologic factors

1. The etiology of non-Hodgkin's lymphomas is unknown, but an increased incidence is associated with alteration in **immunoregulatory control mechanisms**.
   a. Patients with **congenital immunologic defects** (e.g., ataxia telangiectasia, Wiskott-Aldrich syndrome) may have up to 50 times the incidence of malignant lymphomas in normal individuals.
   b. Patients with **acquired immunologic disorders** (e.g., Sjögren's syndrome, SLE, rheumatoid arthritis, Hashimoto's disease, AIDS) show an increased incidence of lymphomas, as do aging patients and those with altered immunologic function induced by drug therapy (e.g., immunosuppression for transplantation).

2. Certain **viruses and chemicals** have been implicated in the etiology of lymphomas.
   a. **Epstein-Barr virus (EBV)**, which is probably not intrinsically oncogenic, is a potent polyclonal stimulator for B-cell proliferation. It is etiologically implicated (though unproven) in African cases of **Burkitt's lymphoma** and immunoblastic large cell lymphomas, both **B-cell lymphomas.**
   b. Certain **chemicals,** including the drug phenytoin, alter the surface membranes of certain lymphocytes, interfering with immunoregulatory control and promoting cellular proliferation in a manner favoring the development of lymphomas.

3. Specific **chromosomal changes** occur in certain lymphomas. These changes seem to occur at sites of cellular **proto-oncogenes,** a fact that may be etiologically significant. In **Burkitt's lymphoma,** there is a translocation between chromosome 8 (the site of **proto-oncogene c-myc**) and one of the chromosomes carrying genes for portions of the **immunoglobulin molecule**.
   a. In 90% of patients with Burkitt's lymphoma, the translocation involves chromosome 14, which carries the heavy-chain gene.
   b. In 10% of patients with Burkitt's lymphoma, the translocation involves either chromosome 22, which carries the λ-chain gene, or chromosome 2, which carries the κ-chain gene.
   c. In other types of B-cell lymphomas, the preceding chromosomes also are often involved.

4. **Infectious complications.** The immunoregulatory changes predispose lymphoma patients to infectious diseases. **B-cell lymphomas** generally predispose patients to **bacterial disease** because they show increased catabolism of immunoglobulins and suppression of all B-cell function. **T-cell lymphomas** frequently predispose patients to **viral, mycobacterial,** or **fungal infections**.

B. General concepts

1. The lymphomas represent **clonal expansions** of lymphocytic elements **blocked** at particular stages of B-cell and T-cell differentiation. The cells of these tumors recapitulate the morphologic and functional characteristics of the normal analog.

2. **Classification of lymphomas** is changing as more is learned about neoplasms of the lymphoid system.
   a. The various classifications take into account such features as:
      (1) Presumed cell of origin: B cell; T cell
      (2) Cell size and morphology: small; small cleaved; large; mixed small and large
      (3) Pattern of nodular involvement: diffuse infiltration; nodular (follicular) aggregates
      (4) Degree of differentiation: well differentiated; poorly differentiated; undifferentiated
      (5) Grade and prognosis: low grade (favorable prognosis); intermediate grade (intermediate prognosis); high grade (unfavorable prognosis)
   b. Regardless of T- or B-cell origin, the natural history of lymphomas is easier to understand if three major **categories** (Table 8-4) are considered and if three concepts are kept in mind: **proliferation rate, cell mobility,** and **neoplastic progression** or transformation. Note that the spread of non-Hodgkin's lymphomas is unlike that of Hodgkin's disease.
   c. In the **International** Panel **Working Formulation** (IWF) for Clinical Usage (Table 8-5), lymphomas are categorized into low grade (see category 1 in Table 8-4), intermediate grade (category 2 and other variations), and high grade (category 3 and others). Treatment follows from this classification and is more aggressive for the higher grades.

C. Lymphomas of B-cell type comprise about 65% of all non-Hodgkin's lymphomas.

1. **Small cell [small lymphocytic; well-differentiated lymphocytic (WDL)] lymphoma**
   a. This form is the node-based **counterpart of CLL** and, indeed, may enter a leukemic phase. Patients are elderly, and most have multiple involved node groups and bone marrow disease.

Table 8-4. Characteristics of the Non-Hodgkin's Lymphomas

Morphologic Type	Proliferation Rate	Cell Mobility	Neoplastic Progression
1. Small cell "lymphocytic" types (e.g., B cell: small and small cleaved lymphocytic lymphoma; T cell: mycosis fungoides)	Low	High	Older adults; cells gradually accumulate, but mobility results in dissemination (late stage) at presentation; incurable, probably due to low level of cell division; may transform to large cell type; otherwise, long survival time (8 to 10 years)
2. Large cell types (T cell, B cell, and true histiocyte types)	High	Low at first, then increases	Older adults; localized (early stage) at presentation, but cells rapidly divide and disseminate in months; curable in > 50%; otherwise, brief survival time
3. Primitive or blastic types (e.g., B cell: Burkitt's lymphoma; T cell: lymphoblastic lymphoma)	High	High	Young patients; present with rapidly growing masses that quickly disseminate and often have a leukemic phase; curable in > 50%; otherwise, brief survival time

    b. Pathologically, the cell is small with a round nucleus, and the pattern of nodal involvement is diffuse. In some cases, plasmacytoid differentiation is seen (in Waldenström's macroglobulinemia); these tumors produce an IgM spike in serum and may cause amyloidosis.
    c. Average length of survival is 8 to 10 years.
  2. Small cleaved cell [poorly differentiated lymphocytic (PDL)] lymphoma
    a. This type is derived from a cell normally present in a follicle or germinal center of a lymph node. Therefore, this type and related types (mixed and large cell) are called **follicular center cell lymphomas;** together, they comprise nearly half of all lymphomas.

Table 8-5. International Working Formulation of Lymphomas

Grade	Cell Type	Cell Differentiation
I. Low grade		
A. Small lymphocytic	B	Mature
B. Follicular, small cleaved	B	Mature
C. Follicular, mixed	B	Mature
II. Intermediate grade		
A. Follicular, large cell	B	Transformed*
B. Diffuse, small cleaved	B or T	Transformed
C. Diffuse, mixed	B or T	Transformed
D. Diffuse, large cell	B or T	Transformed
III. High grade		
A. Immunoblastic (diffuse large cell subtype)	B or T	Transformed
B. Small noncleaved		Immature
1. Burkitt's	B	Blastic[†]
2. Non-Burkitt's	B	Blastic
C. Lymphoblastic	T	Blastic

This table is an abridged version of the 1992 International Working Formulation (IWF); some T-cell lymphomas and other types are classified as "miscellaneous" in the original table.
*A large lymphoid cell results from a transformation of a small cell (normally by antigenic stimulus).
[†]A blastic cell is similar to a stem cell, or an immature progenitor cell.

    (1) Due to their origin, these lymphomas may recapitulate the **normal germinal center structure** and have a follicular (nodular) growth pattern.

    (2) The **follicular pattern** can be seen only in a B-cell lymphoma, such as the small cleaved cell type; it is never seen in T-cell tumors. However, some B-cell tumors are not follicular center cell in origin and are, therefore, diffuse rather than follicular in pattern; the point is of prognostic significance. Follicular lymphomas are more favorable and have a lower grade than diffuse lymphomas.

   b. Pathologically, small cleaved cell lymphomas have cells with small, indented ("cleaved") nuclei (Figure 8-6). Most patients have disseminated nodal, splenic, and marrow involvement, since the cells "home" to all the germinal centers of the dispersed lymphoid tissue. These organs show subtle infiltration rather than masses.

   c. Paradoxically, this low-grade lymphoma is **incurable**. However, relatively long survival (8 to 10 years) is the rule unless patients develop a transformation to a large cell type.

3. Mixed small and large cell lymphomas. Some lymphomas have mixtures of cell types. If follicular in pattern, they also are low grade.

4. Large cell lymphomas. These more aggressive tumors are usually **diffuse** (with a poorer prognosis) but may be follicular in pattern. Thus, only some large cell B-cell lymphomas are follicular center cell in origin.

   a. Large cell lymphomas may **arise de novo** or may **result from transformation** of a small cell type. The tumors usually begin in one place, such as the neck or axilla, but spread to form large tumor masses in the spleen, liver, and elsewhere.

   b. Morphologically, the cells have large nuclei with nucleoli. The nuclei may be **cleaved or noncleaved** (Figure 8-7). Most tumors are intermediate grade, but some have cells that show a similarity to immunoblasts with plasmacytoid cytoplasm and are classified as high-grade neoplasms. These tumors, termed **immunoblastic large cell lymphomas,** occur in association with abnormal immune disorders, such as Sjögren's syndrome.

   c. The **prognosis** for large cell B-cell lymphomas was formerly dismal, but chemotherapy now cures over 50% of the patients.

5. Burkitt's lymphoma. This B-cell lymphoma occurs most frequently in Africa. Most patients are children. Its associations with EBV and with a chromosomal translocation are discussed in VI A 2, 3.

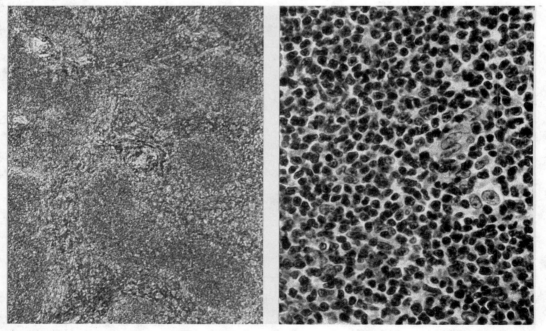

Figure 8-6. Malignant lymphoma of follicular center cells (B-cell neoplasm). The pattern is follicular or nodular (*left*). The predominant cell is a small cleaved lymphocyte (*right*) [H and E stain; high power].

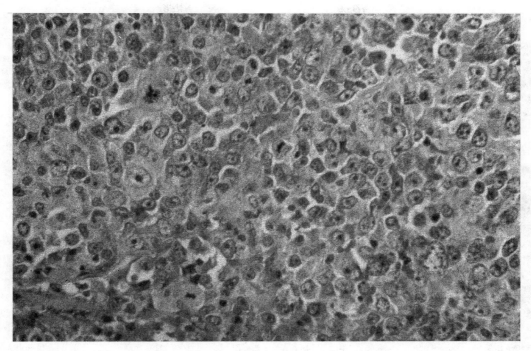

Figure 8-7. Non-Hodgkin's lymphoma, diffuse large cell B-cell type. Cells with round (noncleaved) nuclei and prominent nucleoli grow in a diffuse pattern (H and E stain; high power).

    a. This primarily extralymphatic tumor in its typical African form arises in the jawbones, but it also has a **predilection** for abdominal viscera, ovaries, breasts, the epidural space, and meninges. Bone marrow involvement causes peripheral blood manifestations (i.e., leukemia).

    b. Burkitt's lymphoma probably arises from small transformed follicular center cells. **Microscopically,** the neoplastic cells are small, transformed lymphocytes, uniform in size and shape but slightly larger than true small lymphocytes. The nuclei have finely dispersed chromatin, as do primitive lymphoid cells. Mitoses and macrophages are abundant, with the macrophages producing a characteristic "starry sky" appearance.

    c. In its advanced forms, the disorder is rapidly fatal, but over half of the patients are highly responsive to chemotherapy.

D. Lymphomas of T-cell type comprise about 30% of all non-Hodgkin's lymphomas. **All T-cell lymphomas are diffuse** in pattern. Older patients have skin-based or node-based disease; whereas in younger patients with the lymphoblastic type, the thymus is involved (Figure 8-8).

    1. Cutaneous T-cell lymphoma (mycosis fungoides). This low-grade, **epidermotropic disease** is caused by a neoplasm of helper T cells (CD4$^+$ cells; see Chapter 1 II F 2 a), which are small in size and have irregular nuclei.

      a. The **skin lesion** initially appears as a reddish patch, which then expands to a thickened plaque, followed by the development of diffuse erythroderma, affecting the whole body and face. Characteristic groups of intraepidermal cells **(Pautrier's abscesses)** are present in skin biopsies.

      b. Besides its epidermotropic spread, **other changes** take place over the course of the disease.

        (1) Lymph node involvement becomes apparent.

        (2) More and more large cells with a cerebriform shape accumulate.

        (3) Frank leukemia (**Sézary syndrome**) may develop preterminally.

      c. This incurable tumor has an average 4-year course. Recently, treatment by **removal of peripheral blood lymphocytes** has shown some success, with temporary disappearance of skin disease. Radiotherapy and topical nitrogen mustard also are used to palliate the symptoms.

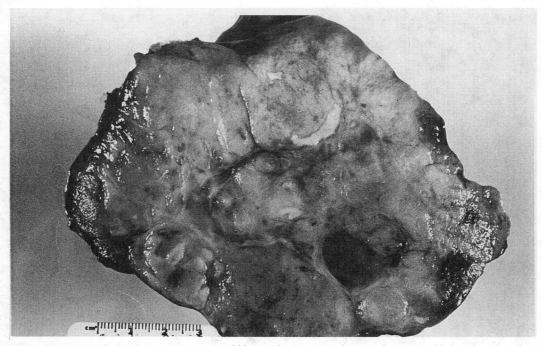

Figure 8-8. Huge mediastinal mass in a 14-year-old boy with respiratory distress. This mass is likely to be a lymphoblastic lymphoma arising in the thymus.

2. **Node-based T-cell lymphomas.** The **range of types** includes lymphomas with predominantly small cells and others with a mixed or mainly large cell pattern. On the whole, these tumors may be more aggressive than their B-cell counterparts.

3. **Lymphoblastic lymphoma.** The majority of tumors with this morphology are of primitive T-cell origin. Patients are typically young (age 15 to 25 years) and present with a mediastinal mass in 50% of cases (see Figure 8-8). Thus, a relationship to the thymus was long suspected.
   a. The tumors grow rapidly, and there often is quick progression to a **leukemia phase,** at which point this lymphoma appears identical clinically and histologically to childhood ALL.
   b. **Histologically,** small cells (somewhat larger than the resting small lymphocyte and about the size of Burkitt cells) are seen. These cells have primitive nuclei and dispersed chromatin. Numerous mitoses are present.
   c. **Untreated cases** show dissemination to many body sites, including the central nervous system (CNS), and death occurs in 2 months. However, the high growth fraction bespeaks a high rate of response to chemotherapy, and a large percentage of patients (about 70%) are cured.

E. **Ki-1 lymphoma, or anaplastic large cell lymphoma (ALCL).** A recent addition to the lymphoma family, this aggressive type can be seen in both children and adults.

   1. **Clinical features.** Patients may present with localized or systemic disease with fever, as with other lymphomas.

   2. **Pathology.** Because of the presence of large cells with abundant cytoplasm, often in lymph node sinuses, this tumor mimics metastatic carcinoma. Also, it typically contains cells resembling Reed-Sternberg cells, thus mimicking Hodgkin's disease.

   3. **Cytogenetics.** Many cases show a characteristic translocation t(2;5) setting them apart from other lymphomas.

   4. **Cell of origin.** ALCL can be of either B- or T-lymphocyte origin, but is a clinicopathologic entity.

   5. **Course.** While initially reported cases were highly aggressive, more recent data show a good response to chemotherapy in a high percentage of patients.

VII. PLASMA CELL DISORDERS. Besides the disorders discussed in this section benign monoclonal gammopathy is present in 5% of elderly patients, the majority of whom never develop a plasma cell malignancy.

A. Multiple myeloma is a clonal plasma cell neoplasm primarily involving the bone marrow, with minimal significant extension to extraosseous sites.

1. **Clinical features.** Most patients are middle-aged to elderly and present with anemia, infection, bone fractures, and hypercalcemia. Punched-out (lytic) bone lesions are typical.

2. **Pathology**
   a. If the malignant clone retains the capacity to produce complete immunoglobulin molecules, the patient demonstrates the classic serum **immunoglobulin spike** (para-protein), consisting of **M component (M protein)**—monoclonal immunoglobulin molecules of a single light-chain class and a single heavy-chain class (e.g., IgM κ, IgG λ).
   b. The production of normal immunoglobulins is suppressed, as though the malignant plasma cells had replaced the normal B cells and their function, predisposing the patient to **infection**.
   c. **Histologically,** massive replacement of marrow by homogeneous sheets of plasma cells is diagnostic of multiple myeloma (Figure 8-9). In the kidney, tubules are often plugged with immunoglobulin precipitates, resulting from excretion of the M component as Bence Jones protein in the urine.
   d. Occasionally, **transformation** to an aggressive histology resembles large cell B-cell immunoblastic lymphoma, termed **anaplastic myeloma**. Tumors are formed in soft tissues and organs in this preterminal phenomenon.

3. **Prognosis.** Life expectancy in myeloma is usually a few years. Death may result from infection, the consequences of renal involvement, the development of amyloidosis, or transformation to the aggressive form.

B. Solitary plasmacytoma. Occasionally, clonal plasma cell neoplasms develop in the lung or other sites; however, they are solitary, and no bone marrow disease is present. A high proportion are cured by excision, radiotherapy, or both, but some will progress to multiple myeloma.

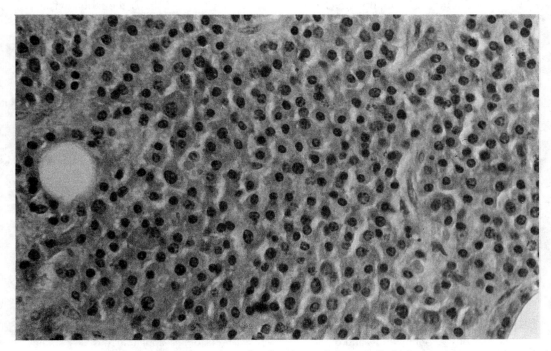

Figure 8-9. Multiple myeloma showing sheets of plasma cells (high power).

C. Amyloidosis is a condition that occurs in a group of diseases, all having the localized or gener-alized deposition of amyloid in common.

1. **General concepts. Amyloid** is a fibrillar protein with a peculiar configuration, namely, the β-pleated sheet, which gives amyloid the property of polarized birefringence and the ability to stain with Congo red dye. Amyloid has several **forms**.

   a. **AL (amyloid light chain)** is made of immunoglobulin light chains, usually λ and less often κ.

   b. **AA (amyloid associated)** is believed to come from serum amyloid-associated (SAA pro-tein), an acute-phase reactant that is the apoprotein of a high-density lipoprotein.

   c. **AE (amyloid endocrine)** is a hormonal polypeptide.

   d. **AS (amyloid senile)** is related to prealbumin.

2. **Localized amyloidosis** may occur in two forms: in the **heart** (senile cardiomyopathy, with dep-osition of AS) or in **endocrine tumors,** such as medullary carcinoma of the thyroid (with AE deposition here related to calcitonin).

3. **Systemic (generalized) deposition of amyloid** also occurs in two different forms, with different organ distributions and deposition of different amyloid substances.

   a. **Immunocyte-associated amyloidosis** is characterized by the deposition of AL.

      (1) In some cases, this condition is due to either a lymphoma or a plasma cell dyscrasia (e.g., plasmacytoma or myeloma). However, most patients do not have a recognizable B-cell neoplasm. Practically all patients, however, have a serum or urine paraprotein.

      (2) This form of amyloidosis (primary) mainly affects the so-called mesenchymal organs (heart, tongue, skin, gastrointestinal tract, nerves). However, other organs may also be involved; for example, in myeloma, renal tubular amyloid casts can cause renal fail-ure. Indeed, the same organs affected by secondary amyloidosis may also be affected by this form.

   b. **Reactive systemic (secondary) amyloidosis** is characterized by the deposition of AA. This form is secondary to prolonged chronic diseases, such as rheumatoid arthritis, tubercu-losis, osteomyelitis, and, occasionally, nonlymphoid tumors. It tends to lead to the most severe systemic involvement, characteristically affecting the kidneys, liver, spleen, lymph nodes, adrenals, and thyroid gland.

4. **Laboratory tests for amyloid.** When a physician suspects that a patient has amyloidosis, the diagnostic test is a biopsy, which may be of the rectum, tongue or lip, or the abdominal fat pad (the favored location in recent literature).

   a. **Histochemical tests.** Amyloid deposits around blood vessels are detected with the **Congo red** stain, which stains them **orange**. If the slide is then viewed under ultraviolet light, the **apple-green** part represents the birefringence.

   b. **Immunohistochemical tests**. The use of monoclonal antibodies to each of the preceding amyloid proteins now allows diagnosis of the specific type of amyloidosis on a biopsy spec-imen.

VIII. DISORDERS AFFECTING HISTIOCYTES (THE MONOCYTE—MACROPHAGE SYSTEM)

A. Histiocytosis X is a collective term for several disorders characterized by a proliferation of **Langerhans-type histiocytes.** In addition to specific cell markers, these cells have an ultrastruc-tural hallmark, the so-called Birbeck or **Langerhans granule,** which aids in diagnosis. This granule sets this distinct cell type apart from other types of histiocytes. Recent data suggest that the his-tiocyte proliferation represents a neoplastic accumulation.

1. **Eosinophilic granuloma** occurs in all age groups but is more common in the first decade of life. The disorder may affect one or more bones or may present in the skin or lymph nodes. Bones most commonly involved are the skull, ribs, and femur.

   a. **Histologically,** the lesions consist of accumulations of Langerhans-type histiocytes with eosinophils and scattered giant cells; necrosis may be present.

   b. The **prognosis** is excellent, with good response to therapy (curettage and radiotherapy in most cases). Lesions often regress spontaneously.

2. **Hand-Schüller-Christian disease** occurs mainly in older adults and is characterized by bone lesions, exophthalmos, and diabetes insipidus. The histologic appearance is very similar to that of eosinophilic granuloma.

3. **Letterer-Siwe disease** occurs in infants less than 3 years old and is more common in males. It is a systemic visceral disease from its onset and has an acute, usually fatal course. Skin rash and hepatosplenomegaly usually are present initially. **Pathologically,** lesions may be found in bones, lymph nodes, skin, liver, lungs, and spleen. These show a diffuse growth of histiocytes but do not contain eosinophils or giant cells.

B. Lipid storage diseases (lipidoses)

1. **General concepts**
   a. In the hereditary lipidoses, a biochemical abnormality in a lysosomal enzyme impairs the catabolism of a complex glycolipid, ganglioside, or globoside. The incompletely degraded metabolite accumulates in the reticuloendothelial system (i.e., the histiocytes in lymph nodes, spleen, and liver).
   b. The consequence is a clinical disorder whose characteristics depend on the biochemical nature of the abnormal metabolite. Many of the lipidoses are inherited as autosomal recessive traits and show an increased prevalence among Ashkenazi Jews.

2. **Gaucher's disease** is due to deficiency of the enzyme **glucocerebrosidase,** with a resultant accumulation of the sphingolipid glucocerebroside.
   a. The **proliferation of histiocytes** leads to hepatosplenomegaly and erosion of the cortices of long bones. Anemia and thrombocytopenia are due mainly to hypersplenism, with a possible element of decreased production due to cellular infiltration of the bone marrow.
   b. Diagnosis is made by identification of the **Gaucher's cells** (histiocytes with linear streaks) in bone marrow or spleen aspirates (Figure 8-10).

3. **Niemann-Pick disease** is due to deficiency of the enzyme **sphingomyelinase**. "Foamy histiocytes," containing both sphingomyelin and ceroid (a brown pigment), proliferate in the liver, spleen, lymph nodes, and occasionally skin. Affected infants usually show hepatosplenomegaly and neurologic deterioration.

4. **Tay-Sachs disease** is due to a defect in **hexosaminidase A**. Gangliosides accumulate in various organs, predominantly in the brain. Affected infants suffer from blindness and mental retardation and die before age 3.

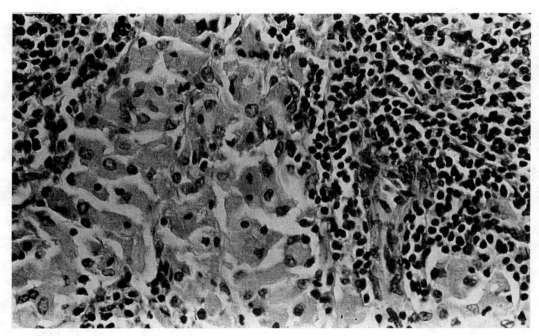

Figure 8-10. Gaucher's cells in the spleen. Large cells with clear cytoplasm are the diagnostic elements (H and E stain; high power).

C. Malignant histiocyte disorders

1. Malignant histiocytosis

a. Clinical features

(1) Malignant histiocytosis may occur at any age, but the **average age at onset** is in the fourth decade. Most series show that men are affected almost twice as often as women.

(2) Malignant histiocytosis is often confused with other hematopoietic or lymphoid malignancies. **Presenting features** include fever, lymphadenopathy, hepatosplenomegaly, skin lesions, and pancytopenia. The disorder is almost invariably fatal.

(3) Many previous cases have been reclassified as T-cell lymphomas with benign histiocytes.

b. Pathology

(1) There is a proliferation throughout hematopoietic and lymphoid tissues of histiocytes with nuclear atypia. The cells range in maturation; importantly, the most differentiated cells exhibit characteristic **phagocytosis of blood cells** (red cells, white cells, and platelets), which probably causes the cytopenias.

(2) Nodal lymphoid tissues characteristically show partial or complete **filling of** medullary and subcapsular **sinusoids,** with masses of noncohesive neoplastic cells. The overall architecture is preserved, however, and only rare areas of infiltration of cortical or capsular tissue are found.

2. True histiocytic lymphomas.
Rare lymphomas display the cell markers of histiocytes and are large cell lymphomas. They cannot be distinguished clinically or histologically from other (T, B) large cell lymphomas, and the course is as aggressive as it is for other large cell lymphomas.

3. Fibrous histiocytomas
(see Chapter 25 III B 2). Despite the nomenclature, the cells of these soft tissue tumors are probably facultative fibroblasts and have no relation to the bone marrow—derived true histiocyte–monocyte–macrophage system.

IX. BENIGN LYMPHADENOPATHIES OF DIVERSE ETIOLOGIES

A. Toxoplasmosis,
caused by the protozoan *Toxoplasma gondii,* is characterized by lymphadenopathy in its acquired (as opposed to congenital) form.

1. **Clinical features.** Most patients with the mild lymphatic form of toxoplasmosis are asymptomatic, but some have fever and sore throat. Posterior cervical nodes in young adults are typically involved.

2. **Pathology.** The overall architecture of nodes is preserved, and follicles (germinal centers) are usually prominent. Capsulitis is noted, with cellular proliferation in the capsule and the subcapsular sinus. Diagnostic evidence of toxoplasmosis is the presence of epithelioid histiocytes in clusters, both in the interfollicular areas and in the follicular (germinal) centers; however, these histiocytes can be seen in Hodgkin's disease also. Rarely, toxoplasma cysts may be identified.

B. Syphilis.
The lymphadenopathy of syphilis usually affects the inguinal nodes, but generalized adenopathy may be present in secondary syphilis. **Histologically,** capsular inflammation and fibrosis are striking. (This feature is similar to nodular sclerosing Hodgkin's disease.) The architecture of the nodes is preserved, and follicular centers are very active. Plasmacytosis is noted in the interfollicular areas and capsule. Necrotizing granulomas may be seen. Spirochetes may be demonstrated by silver stain.

C. Infectious mononucleosis.
Lymphadenopathy is a typical manifestation of this viral infection. **Histologically,** variable distortion of the architecture is noted, with some follicular centers obscured. The sinusoids of the nodes generally are preserved and often are packed with cells. Usually, there are large numbers of transformed lymphocytes (**immunoblasts**) in portions of all of the nodes; this situation can cause diagnostic confusion with malignant lymphomas. Immunoblasts also are seen in other viral lymphadenopathies (e.g., herpes).

D. Dermatopathic lymphadenitis
is a fairly common disorder associated with a variety of chronic skin diseases. Hyperplasia of the follicles and interfollicular histiocytes are present. Ill-defined foci of histiocytes, containing fat and melanin, extend between the follicles.

E. Angiofollicular hyperplasia (lymphoid hamartoma, Castleman's disease) is a rare disorder associated with the production of solitary asymptomatic masses up to 7 cm in size; these masses are usually located in the mediastinum. **Histologically,** follicular centers contain centrally placed arterioles with a whorling of the follicular center cells, producing an appearance resembling Hassall's corpuscles or splenic follicles. Occasional cases have shown monoclonality in this lesion with a benign course. Systemic involvement is a life-threatening disease.

F. Sarcoidosis. The cause of this systemic granulomatous disease is unknown; it may have several heterogeneous causes. In the United States, patients are usually young blacks.

   1. Clinical features. Lungs, lymph nodes, and less commonly the liver, spleen, marrow, skin, eyes, and phalangeal bones are affected. Pulmonary dysfunction is common.

   2. Pathology. The typical pattern is small, noncaseating granulomas evenly distributed throughout the tissues, particularly the enlarged lymph nodes.

G. Tuberculosis is a frequent cause of granulomatous adenopathy, which differs pathologically from sarcoid adenopathy in that the granulomas of tuberculosis are caseating or necrotizing. Organisms may be difficult to detect in the tissues.

H. Cat-scratch disease. Often axillary lymphadenopathy will occur after a scratch by a feline. Necrotizing granulomas also are seen in this condition. Recently, causative small, gram-negative bacilli have been identified by means of a silver stain.

I. AIDS

   1. Patients with **AIDS-related complex (ARC)** may have persistent generalized lymphadenopathy. **Histologically,** the germinal centers (follicles) are markedly hyperplastic and enlarged, and the node shows a considerable plasmacytosis.

   2. In patients with **full-blown AIDS,** the nodal histology can be characteristic though variable and nonpathognomonic.
      a. A sequential, time-dependent spectrum has been suggested. In this situation, early follicular hyperplasia is followed by follicular lysis, progressing to follicular depletion (absence of germinal centers and loss of many lymphocytes in other areas of the node).
      b. Importantly, inapparent mycobacterial infection may be present. Special staining procedures always must be performed to search for this possibility since, in these immunosuppressed patients, a true granulomatous reaction usually is not present.
      c. Occasionally, lymph nodes in patients with AIDS may show Kaposi's sarcoma.

J. Immunoblastic adenopathy (angioimmunoblastic lymphadenopathy) is considered to be a **T-cell deficiency disorder** (possibly drug-induced).

   1. Clinical features
      a. Adults of both sexes are affected in middle or late life; the median age at onset is 60 years. In the typical case, patients have fever, sweats, generalized lymphadenopathy, and hepatosplenomegaly, often with an associated skin rash, which may be severely pruritic. Some patients have had recent exposure to drugs.
      b. Immunoblastic adenopathy is a true precancerous state: Some patients progress to a full-blown lymphoma. In some patients with the same presentation, a true T-cell lymphoma is mimicking immunoblastic adenopathy, both clinically and histologically. Specific marker studies or gene rearrangement analysis are required to make this distinction.

   2. Pathology. Although clinically distinct, the condition often has been confused with Hodgkin's disease. There are proliferations of arborizing small vessels. Immunoblasts, plasma cells, and often an amorphous, acidophilic, interstitial material also are present.

   3. Course and prognosis. A few patients respond well to cytotoxic chemotherapy, but most do poorly and die of infections.

X. DISORDERS OF THE SPLEEN

A. Hypofunction

   1. Etiology. Congenital immunodeficiency states, radiation, chemotherapy, and steroids interfere with splenic function, as does autoinfarction of the spleen in sickle cell anemia. Surgical removal of the spleen (e.g., in cases of trauma) also leads to asplenism or hypofunction. Infiltrative diseases (e.g., granulomas, neoplasms, amyloidosis) can destroy sufficient splenic tissue to cause hyposplenism.

2. Clinical features. Most patients who suffer solely from hyposplenism or asplenia (especially after surgery) show an increased incidence of gram-positive bacterial infections (particularly pneumococcal) but apparently compensate well in regard to other splenic functions.

B. Disorders of the white pulp. The white pulp of the spleen is part of the **lymphoid system** and, consequently, reacts like germinal centers elsewhere. Thus, it shows **hyperplasia and hyperfunction** in certain **autoimmune disorders** (e.g., SLE); **hypoplasia** in **immunodeficiency disorders;** and **histologic changes** common to all germinal centers in the **lymphomas**.

C. Disorders of the red pulp. The red pulp of the spleen is part of the **reticuloendothelial system;** it also serves as a blood bank and even, at times, as an extramedullary hematopoietic organ. **Diseases involving the splenic cords** produce cord widening by the accumulation of abnormal blood cells (red cells and platelets) or by the infiltration of neoplastic or reactive cells (e.g., histiocytes).

1. Hereditary spherocytosis [see 1 A 2 d (2) (a)] results in cord widening because the abnormal red blood cells cannot traverse the maze of the splenic cords. This stagnation and retention of red cells lead to their premature destruction.

2. In **portal hypertension,** widened cords occur because of congestion, leading to histiocytic proliferation and fibrosis and resulting in red cell stagnation.

3. The **lipidoses** produce similar functional defects in the red pulp by accumulations of histiocytes.

4. Leukemias characteristically infiltrate the red pulp.

D. Splenomegaly. Causes of splenomegaly include hemolytic disorders, portal hypertension, infiltrative disorders, and neoplasms—lymphocytic, myeloid, or histiocytic. **Clinically,** in addition to the problems of the disease producing it, splenomegaly can lead to left upper quadrant pain, gastric discomfort, and—most serious and life-threatening—spontaneous rupture of the spleen. **Hypersplenism** is any situation in which the spleen destroys excessive quantities of blood cells (red cells, white cells, or platelets).

1. Clinical features. In hypersplenism, the spleen usually is enlarged and frequently palpable on physical examination.

2. Pathogenesis. Hypersplenism may result from **abnormal blood cells** and their increased sequestration by the spleen, **antibodies** that coat the blood elements and make them easy prey for splenic phagocytes, or **stagnation and hemoconcentration of blood cells,** leading to their increased vulnerability to splenic phagocytes.

E. Cysts and tumors of the spleen

1. Benign cysts of the spleen may represent parasitic (*Echinococcus*) disease or mesothelial-lined (peritoneal inclusion) cysts. More commonly encountered in the United States are **"false" cysts** without recognizable lining cells; they represent encapsulated hematomas and probably are always the result of trauma.

2. Primary tumors of the spleen are rare, and examples are hemangioma or a primary non-Hodgkin's lymphoma. Some patients with malignant hematopoietic diseases may present with splenomegaly, and the diagnosis of a malignant lymphoma or hairy-cell leukemia may be made initially from examination of the spleen.

3. The spleen is commonly involved in Hodgkin's disease and non-Hodgkin's lymphomas, in the leukemias (both chronic and acute), in the myeloproliferative disorders, and in histiocytic neoplasms. Lymphomas will preferentially involve the **white pulp,** and leukemias, the **red pulp**.

STUDY QUESTIONS

Directions: Each of the numbered items or incomplete statements in this section is followed by answers or by completions of the statement. Select the **one** lettered answer or completion that is **best** in each case.

1. Which provides for a definitive diagnosis of hemolytic anemia?

(A) Red blood cell antibodies
(B) Red blood cell destruction
(C) Red blood cell enzyme deficiency
(D) Marrow erythroid hyperplasia
(E) Abnormal hemoglobin

2. Which statement about sickle cell anemia in adults is true?

(A) It occurs in 20% of the black population of the United States
(B) It produces splenomegaly
(C) It results from decreased hemoglobin synthesis
(D) It is accompanied by iron deficiency
(E) It protects against malaria

3. A deficiency of the red cell membrane component spectrin causes

(A) pernicious anemia
(B) hereditary spherocytosis
(C) sickle cell anemia
(D) thalassemia major
(E) Diamond-Blackfan syndrome

4. Nonimmune hemolytic anemia occurs in patients with

(A) systemic lupus erythematosus (SLE)
(B) malarial infection
(C) chronic lymphocytic leukemia (CLL)
(D) Hodgkin's disease
(E) Rh incompatibility

5. Which disorder most often causes iron deficiency anemia?

(A) Severe liver disease
(B) Cardiomyopathy
(C) Peptic ulcer
(D) Pancreatitis
(E) Renal failure

6. In blood coagulation, which coagulation factor links fibrin monomers to stabilize the early fibrin clot?

(A) Ia
(B) III
(C) VIII
(D) Xa
(E) XIIIa

7. In the process of fibrinolysis, which substance splits the fibrin molecule into products of varying molecular size?

(A) Proactivator
(B) Activator
(C) Plasminogen
(D) Plasmin
(E) Antiplasmin

8. Which coagulation factor is reduced or absent in classic hemophilia (hemophilia A)?

(A) I
(B) III
(C) VIII
(D) X
(E) XIII

9. For 2 weeks, a 36-year-old man has complained of purpura and bleeding of the gums. On examination, he is pale and his temperature is 39° C. This clinical picture is compatible with

(A) chronic lymphocytic leukemia (CLL)
(B) acute lymphocytic leukemia (ALL)
(C) chronic myelogenous leukemia (CML)
(D) acute myelogenous leukemia (AML)
(E) infectious mononucleosis

10. The similarity between thalassemia major and thalassemia minor is

(A) severity of anemia
(B) incidence of infection
(C) life span
(D) familial occurrence
(E) homozygous form

1-B	4-B	7-D	10-D
2-E	5-C	8-C	
3-B	6-E	9-D	

11. Which coagulation factor may be affected by vitamin K deficiency?

(A) Fibrinogen
(B) Labile factor (V)
(C) Stable factor (VII)
(D) Hageman factor (XII)
(E) Plasmin

12. If a person has documented anemia but is asymptomatic, the physician can eliminate all of the following causes EXCEPT

(A) trauma resulting in ruptured spleen
(B) a sulfa drug given to a patient with glucose-6-phosphate dehydrogenase (G6PD) deficiency
(C) ruptured abdominal aortic aneurysm
(D) iron deficiency anemia
(E) mismatched blood unit

13. Myelophthisic anemia can occur in patients with any of the following conditions EXCEPT

(A) miliary tuberculosis
(B) carcinomatosis
(C) myelofibrosis
(D) multiple myeloma
(E) uremia

14. Patients with polycythemia vera show all of the following characteristic findings EXCEPT

(A) high platelet count (thrombocytosis)
(B) high hematocrit
(C) high erythropoietin level
(D) high mean age at presentation
(E) higher than average chance of stroke or myocardial infarction

15. All of the following etiologic associations with human acute leukemia have been proved valid EXCEPT

(A) viruses
(B) irradiation
(C) antibiotics
(D) antineoplastic drugs
(E) benzene compounds

16. Transformation to acute leukemia may occur during the course of all of the following disorders EXCEPT

(A) polycythemia vera
(B) chronic myelogenous leukemia (CML)
(C) chronic lymphocytic leukemia (CLL)
(D) Hodgkin's disease
(E) myelofibrosis

17. Thrombocytopenia is commonly caused by all of the following EXCEPT

(A) folate deficiency
(B) myelofibrosis
(C) chronic leukemia
(D) marked splenomegaly
(E) platelet sequestration

11-C   14-C   17-C
12-D   15-A
13-E   16-D

Directions: The group of items in this section consists of lettered options followed by a set of numbered items. For each item, select the **one** lettered option that is most closely associated with it. Each lettered option may be selected once, more than once, or not at all.

Questions 18–22

For each disease process listed, select the associated histologic characteristic of the lymph nodes.

(A) Fibrosis
(B) Epithelioid histiocytes
(C) Necrotizing granulomas
(D) Immunoblastic proliferation
(E) Melanin

18. Toxoplasmosis

19. Herpes

20. Syphilis

21. Dermatopathia

22. Cat-scratch disease

18-B   21-E
19-D   22-C
20-A

ANSWERS AND EXPLANATIONS

1. The answer is B *[I A 2 a, e]*.
Only evidence of actual destruction of red cells is diagnostic. Red blood cell antibodies, red blood cell enzyme deficiency, abnormal hemoglobin, and erythroid hyperplasia all may occur in or cause hemolytic anemia, but hemolysis does not necessarily result. Erythroid hyperplasia in the marrow is a general response to anemia of any type. Red blood cell antibodies or enzyme deficiencies may be innocuous and not cause hemolysis.

2. The answer is E *[I A 2 d (1) (b)]*.
Sickle cell anemia occurs in only 1% or less of the black population of the United States, although sickle cell trait may occur in up to 10%. In adults, the tiny spleen is due to autoinfarction. The anemia results from production of abnormal hemoglobin and the subsequent hemolysis of the red blood cells containing the hemoglobin; it is not the result of decreased hemoglobin synthesis. Since the hemolyzed cell products release iron, there is excess, rather than deficient, iron. In parts of the world where malaria is endemic, individuals with sickle cell anemia fare better.

3. The answer is B *[1 A 2 d (1)–(3), 3 a (2), b (2)]*.
Hereditary spherocytosis is a classic example of a red cell membrane defect. There is a genetically determined abnormality in a membrane polypeptide called spectrin. The degree of deficiency correlates with the degree of spherocytosis. Pernicious anemia is caused by conditions or dietary deficiencies that result in low vitamin B_{12} or folate. Sickle cell anemia has a single amino acid substitution in the β chain of hemoglobin, and thalassemia is caused by decreased production of the β chain. Diamond-Blackfan syndrome is a type of aplastic anemia.

4. The answer is B *[I A 2 e (4)]*.
Of the disorders listed, only malarial infection causes a nonimmune hemolysis. Autoantibodies that lyse red cells can be demonstrated in systemic lupus erythematosus (SLE), Hodgkin's disease, and in chronic lymphocytic leukemia (CLL). In Rh incompatibility, maternal antibodies lyse fetal red cells. In malaria, hemolytic anemia results from parasitic invasion of erythrocytes.

5. The answer is C *[I A 2 b (2), 3 a (1)]*.
Peptic ulcer leads to chronic blood loss and, therefore, loss of iron. Although severe liver disease may produce upper gastrointestinal bleeding (varices), the bleeding is usually acute, not chronic. The anemia of renal failure is due to toxic damage to the marrow; the iron stores are normal. Cardiomyopathy and pancreatitis are not normally associated with anemia.

6. The answer is E *[II A 2 a; Table 8-1]*.
Coagulation factor XIII—fibrin stabilizing factor—is activated by the enzymatic action of thrombin and becomes factor XIIIa (transglutaminase), which binds to fibrin monomers and forms cross-links between the γ and α chains of the polymerizing fibrin molecules. Patients with factor XIII deficiency have a mild bleeding tendency, particularly following trauma. Delayed wound healing and irregular scar formation are also common in these individuals.

7. The answer is D *[II A 3 a]*.
Plasmin, derived from plasminogen, degrades both fibrinogen and fibrin. Once the fibrin is cross-linked, however, the breakdown process is slower because plasmin cannot gain access to the stable fibrin polymer as readily as it can to the unstable, non–cross-linked fibrin mesh. The proteolysis caused by plasmin produces the various fibrin split products that can be detected in serum by immunologic methods.

8. The answer is C *[II B 1]*.
The coagulation factor VIII complex is under the control of the X chromosome and is reduced or absent in classic hemophilia, which is an X-linked disorder. Factor VIII is also reduced in von Willebrand's disease, an autosomal dominant disorder characterized by an abnormality in a plasma protein (von Willebrand's factor) that is a component of the factor VIII complex and also functions in platelet adherence.

9. The answer is D *[IV B, C]*.
The short history of the symptoms and the signs of anemia, infection, and thrombocytopenia in the patient described indicate acute myelogenous leukemia (AML). The duration of symptoms excludes both chronic

lymphocytic leukemia (CLL) and chronic myelogenous leukemia (CML). Acute lymphocytic leukemia (ALL) rarely is present beyond the pediatric age. Purpura, evidence of anemia, and thrombocytopenia are unlikely to occur in mononucleosis.

10. The answer is D *[I A 2 d (3)]*.
The only similarity between thalassemia major and thalassemia minor is that both conditions are determined genetically. Whereas anemia is marked in thalassemia major, it may be mild or nonexistent in thalassemia minor. Infection is a common complication only in thalassemia major; most patients with this disease die in young adulthood or before, whereas thalassemia minor is compatible with a normal life span. Only thalassemia major is homozygous.

11. The answer is C *[II A 2 a, d, B 2 a, b; Table 8-1]*.
A vitamin K deficiency, either from severe liver disease or a nutritional lack of the fat-soluble vitamins (A, D, E, K), affects the production of coagulation factors II, VII, IX, and X. Fibrinogen and plasmin are not coagulation factors.

12. The answer is D *[I A 2 b, c, 3 a (1)]*.
Only slowly developing anemias are asymptomatic; thus, all causes of acute blood loss or hemolysis can be eliminated. These causes include traumatic events (e.g., ruptured spleen or aorta) and the acute hemolytic episodes due to mismatched blood and drug reactions in glucose-6-phosphate dehydrogenase (G6PD) deficiency. In contrast, a gradual impairment of blood production or blood loss that is caused by or results in iron deficiency would be asymptomatic. A workup for a gastrointestinal malignancy should be done for such a patient.

13. The answer is E *[I A 3 c]*.
Myelophthisis is a reduction in the productive capacity of the bone marrow through the presence of space-occupying lesions. Granulomas replace the marrow in tuberculosis. Metastatic carcinoma and myeloma produce mass lesions, replacing and destroying marrow. Likewise, in myelofibrosis, the marrow cavity is also replaced, but by a fibrous proliferation, resulting in a loss of marrow elements. The anemia of uremia, however, is not related to space-occupying lesions; rather, a toxic effect results in marrow depression.

14. The answer is C *[I B 1]*.
Polycythemia vera patients, who are typically elderly, may present with vascular thrombotic episodes affecting the brain or heart and may have thrombocytoses in addition to high hematocrits. In addition, these patients have normal erythropoietin levels, in contrast with patients with secondary polycythemia whose erythropoietin levels are high; this diagnostic distinction in important.

15. The answer is A *[IV A 3]*.
Although viruses have been shown to be associated with leukemia in animals, this association has not been proved in humans. Irradiation has been linked with the subsequent development of leukemia, probably as a result of marrow stem cell damage, leading to chromosomal aberrations and subsequent malignancy. Certain antibiotics and benzene compounds, which share specific chemical configurations, have also been associated with leukemia development. Finally, chemotherapeutic agents, by causing marrow damage, have been implicated.

16. The answer is D *[I B 1 b (4); IV B 1 c, C 2 c (2)]*.
Polycythemia vera and myelofibrosis are chronic conditions in which dysplastic marrow elements occur. Each carries a risk of acute leukemia, although the risk in polycythemia vera is lower than that in myelofibrosis. Both chronic myelogenous (CML) and chronic lymphocytic leukemia (CLL) can undergo transformation to acute leukemia; however, this change occurs more commonly in the myeloid type. Although some lymphomas (e.g., small cleaved and small cell types) may undergo leukemia transformation, Hodgkin's disease essentially never does.

17. The answer is C *[II C 1]*.
Thrombocytopenia is characterized by a decrease in the number of platelets. The clinical features vary according to the etiology, which may include folate deficiency, myelofibrosis, acute leukemia, and splenomegaly. The hallmark of thrombocytopenia is petechiae, which are also a typical presentation of acute, but not chronic, leukemia. Folate deficiency, whether dietary or drug-induced, can affect red cell and platelet production. Myelofibrosis, a type of myeloproliferative syndrome, causes thrombocytopenia through a replacement of marrow precursors with fibrosis; it also results in anemia. Sequestration of platelets in a very enlarged spleen is another cause.

18–22. The answers are: 18-B, 19-D, 20-A, 21-E, 22-C *[IX A–D, H].*
Small collections of epithelioid histiocytes are seen in the sinusoids and nodal substance of nodes affected by toxoplasmosis. Histologically, the lymph nodes show prominent capsular fibrosis in syphilitic lymphadenitis. Histiocytes containing melanin are characteristic of excoriative dermatopathia. The mature lesion of cat-scratch disease is a granuloma with central necrosis. Characteristic of changes seen in some viral infections (including those of herpesvirus) is the formation of numerous immunoblasts in the involved lymph node.

9
Heart

Scott H. Saul

I. NORMAL CARDIAC STRUCTURE

A. Anatomy

1. **Location, dimensions, and function of the heart**
   a. The heart, lying in the middle mediastinal compartment, is enclosed within the pericardial sac. The pericardial sac, lined with a serosal membrane, contains up to 30 ml of clear serous fluid, which acts as a lubricant.
   b. Normally, the heart is roughly the size of a fist and weighs about 250 to 300 g in women and 300 to 350 g in men; this weight varies, however, with age, body size, nutritional status, and the amount of epicardial fat deposits.
   c. The heart functions as a muscular pump for the distribution of blood and fluid nutrients throughout the body and for the collection of waste products and carbon dioxide to be excreted from the body.

2. **Chambers of the heart.** The heart is divided into right and left sides, with two chambers (an **atrium** and a **ventricle**) on each side.
   a. Blood that has circulated through the body enters the **right atrium,** passes into the **right ventricle,** and then is delivered to the pulmonary circulation, where it is oxygenated.
   b. After oxygenation, blood returns to the heart, entering at the **left atrium**. Blood then passes into the **left ventricle** and then to the aorta, from which it circulates to the tissues of the body.
   c. The ventricular chambers vary greatly in thickness. The left ventricle normally is about 15 mm thick, whereas the right ventricle is about 3 mm thick.

3. **Valves of the heart.** The heart has two **atrioventricular (AV) valves,** which direct the flow of blood between the atria and ventricles, and two other **valves,** which direct the flow of blood from the ventricles to the systemic and pulmonary circulations. The latter two sometimes are called semilunar valves because of the crescent-moon shape of their leaflets.
   a. The **tricuspid valve** directs right atrial blood flow anteriorly and to the left into the right ventricle. Normally, the tricuspid valve has three leaflets, which are of unequal size.
   b. The **mitral valve** has two major leaflets to direct blood flow from the left atrium into the left ventricle.
   c. The **aortic valve** is a semilunar valve that directs blood from the left ventricle to the aorta. Normally, the aortic valve has three fibrous leaflets.
   d. The **pulmonic valve** is a semilunar valve that directs blood from the right ventricle to the pulmonary arterial trunk. This valve also has three leaflets.

4. **Blood supply to the heart.** This blood supply is provided chiefly by the two major **coronary arteries**.
   a. The **left coronary artery** originates from the aorta in the sinus of Valsalva, behind the left coronary leaflets. Shortly after its origin, the left coronary artery divides into two main branches.
      (1) The first branch, the **left anterior descending coronary artery,** commonly supplies the left ventricular apex, the medial half of the anterior surface of the left ventricle, a portion of the medial anterior wall of the right ventricle, and the anterior portion of the interventricular septum.
      (2) The other branch, the **left circumflex coronary artery,** supplies blood to the anterolateral wall of the left ventricle and a portion of the posterior wall of the left ventricle.

    b. The **right coronary artery** originates from the aorta, behind the right coronary leaflet. It supplies a large part of the right ventricle as it passes to the right and then posteriorly along the posterior–inferior heart surface. The right coronary artery commonly provides circulation to the posterior portion of the interventricular septum, to adjacent parts of the posterior left ventricle, and sometimes to the apex of the left ventricle.

    c. **"Dominance"** of the coronary circulation is determined by the coronary artery that supplies the **posterior descending coronary artery**. The coronary arteries are arranged in a right dominant distribution in 70% to 80% of cases.

    d. **Collateral blood flow.** Because the coronary artery "watersheds" are highly variable, coronary blood flow distribution may be slightly different from one person to the next. This distribution becomes important in considering potential pathways for collateral blood flow in coronary artery atherosclerotic diseases.

5. Conducting system of the heart. The conducting system consists of specialized cardiac muscle cells that are responsible for the initiation and conduction of the heartbeat.

    a. The heartbeat begins in the **sinoatrial (SA) node**—the pacemaker of the heart—which is located near the junction of the superior vena cava and right atrium.

    b. The impulse then travels through the **AV node** to the AV bundle, or **bundle of His**—a small band of modified cardiac muscle fibers.

    c. The bundle of His branches into **left and right bundle branches** (leading to the left and right ventricles, respectively) and terminates at the **Purkinje fibers,** which transmit the impulse to the myocardial cells.

B. Histology. The cardiac wall has three layers.

1. Endocardium. The endocardium, which lines the inner surface of the heart, consists of a single, thin layer of endothelium overlying a continuous basement membrane. The bulk of the endocardium is in the connective tissue of the subendothelial region, which merges with the connective tissue of the myocardium.

2. Myocardium

    a. The myocardium, the intermediate layer, consists of a unique form of striated muscle termed **cardiac muscle,** which is embedded in a connective tissue framework with numerous capillaries.

    b. Each myocardial cell has a central nucleus and many **myofibrils,** which have the **sarcomere** as their integral unit. The cells are bound to each other by intercellular junctions called **intercalated disks**. These junctions allow the individual myofibers to function as a unit.

3. Epicardium. The epicardium (also called the **pericardium**) is the outermost cardiac layer. It is lined by a thin layer of mesothelium that rests on a layer of connective tissue, which merges with the connective tissue of the myocardium.

II. CONGESTIVE HEART FAILURE (also called **heart failure** or **pump failure**) is a symptom complex, not a disease entity, that can result from a variety of cardiac disorders. The syndrome is characterized by inability of the heart to pump enough blood to keep pace with the body's circulatory demands.

A. Etiology and pathophysiology

1. The heart can fail because of **impaired pump function** (e.g., due to decreased myocardial contractility or decreased compliance) or **increased cardiac work demands** (e.g., due to pressure or volume overload). In some cases, both mechanisms may be responsible.

2. Several physiologic mechanisms help the heart try to compensate for its decreased pump function or increased work load. One is the **Frank-Starling mechanism:** Increased stroke volume and, hence, cardiac output occur in response to the increased diastolic muscle fiber length caused by increased end-diastolic pressure or volume.

3. Over time, chronic pressure or volume overload can lead to **myocardial hypertrophy** or **ventricular dilatation,** respectively.

B. Classification. Congestive heart failure is classified in two ways for clinical purposes.

1. **Backward versus forward failure** (i.e., classification according to the mechanism of clinical manifestations)
   a. **Backward failure** emphasizes the role of elevated cardiac filling pressures and, thus, venous congestion ("damming up" of blood behind the failing ventricle) in the evolution of clinical manifestations.
   b. **Forward failure** refers to the manifestations caused by decreased cardiac output of the failing ventricle and, thus, inadequate organ perfusion.

2. **Left-sided versus right-sided failure** (i.e., classification according to the ventricle that is failing)
   a. **Left-sided failure** refers to the signs and symptoms caused by failure of the left ventricle or excessive pressure in the left atrium (i.e., clinical features of pulmonary congestion).
   b. **Right-sided failure** refers to the signs and symptoms caused by failure of the right ventricle or excessive pressure in the right atrium (i.e., clinical features of systemic venous congestion).
   c. **Biventricular failure** (i.e., failure of both ventricles) usually is not simultaneous but develops over time due to the increased stress placed on the remaining ventricle.

C. Clinical features

1. **Clinical manifestations of left-sided failure** are the most common because relatively common disorders (e.g., ischemic heart disease, hypertension) cause left ventricular damage.
   a. The most common **symptoms** are dyspnea, orthopnea, paroxysmal nocturnal dyspnea, cough, and hemoptysis. These features result from passive pulmonary congestion, which leads to edema of the alveolar septa and, finally, fluid in the alveolar spaces, or **pulmonary edema**. With chronic left-sided failure, the sputum may be rust-colored because of the many hemosiderin-laden alveolar macrophages (heart-failure cells).
   b. The most prominent **signs** are pulmonary rales, cardiac enlargement, an S_3 gallop, and pulsus alternans.

2. **Clinical manifestations of right-sided failure** in most cases are caused by left-sided failure, although **cor pulmonale** (i.e., right ventricular enlargement due to pulmonary hypertension)* is another important cause.
   a. The most common **signs** are related to systemic venous congestion, including jugular venous distention, enlarged and tender liver and spleen, ascites, and peripheral edema.
   b. Less significant are **symptoms** such as fatigue and weakness, anorexia, decreased tissue mass, and cyanosis.

III. ISCHEMIC HEART DISEASE (also called **coronary artery disease**) is a collective term for various diseases characterized by inability of the coronary arteries to deliver adequate oxygen to meet the needs of the myocardium. The degree of coronary insufficiency, the rapidity of onset, and the degree of collateral circulation determine the nature of the resulting disease; that is, chronic ischemic heart disease, angina pectoris, myocardial infarction, or sudden death.

A. Mortality. Ischemic heart disease is by far the most common form of cardiac disease in the industrialized world, where it is the number one cause of death. It is uncommon, however, in less developed areas of the world, such as Africa and China.

1. Ischemic heart disease accounts for 80% to 90% of all mortality related to heart disease in the United States. In 1985, roughly 534,000 deaths were due to ischemic heart disease; this total represented nearly 25% of deaths from any cause.

2. The mortality rate associated with ischemic heart disease has improved dramatically. Since 1965, when the mortality rate peaked at 215 per 100,000 population, the age-adjusted death rate has declined steadily to 127 per 100,000 population in 1985, representing a 40% decrease. The relative contributions of individual factors (e.g., prevention efforts, improved general health measures, improved treatment measures) to this fall in mortality rate have not been defined.

---

*Acute cor pulmonale, which causes abrupt onset of right ventricular dilatation, is due to massive pulmonary embolism. Chronic cor pulmonale causes right ventricular hypertrophy, often with subsequent dilatation.

B. Etiology and risk factors

1. **Atherosclerosis** of the coronary arteries is by far the leading cause of ischemic heart disease. The risk factors identified for atherosclerosis essentially are the risk factors for ischemic heart disease. Table 9-1 lists the modifiable and unmodifiable risk factors.

2. **Other causes** of ischemic heart disease include:
   a. **Thromboemboli** derived from valvular vegetations or mural thrombi dislodged either from the left ventricle overlying an aneurysm or from the left atrial appendage in patients with atrial fibrillation
   b. **Coronary artery spasm** (i.e., spasm of morphologically normal coronary arteries), which may result in variant angina [see III D 2 a (3)]
   c. **Coronary arteritis** (usually caused by polyarteritis nodosa), **luetic aortitis** (which causes obliteration of the coronary orifice), and other inflammatory conditions that significantly impair coronary artery perfusion
   d. **Conditions that increase cardiac work load and oxygen demand** (e.g., increased heart rate, hyperthyroidism, catecholamine treatment) **or decrease oxygen delivery to the heart** (e.g., anemia, hypotension, carbon monoxide poisoning)
   e. **Anomalous origin of left coronary artery**
   f. **Chest trauma**

C. Pathogenesis.
Regardless of the eventual outcome, ischemic heart diease almost always begins with atherosclerotic changes in the coronary circulation.

1. Atherosclerosis of the coronary arteries develops like that of other large arteries of the body (see Chapter 10 I B 1 b).

2. Severe or fatal disease often involves a 70% or greater decrease in the diameter of at least one of the major coronary vessels (usually more than one), which correlates with a 90% reduction of its normal cross-sectional area and, thus, a critical decrease in blood flow. Typically, the most severe narrowing occurs in the proximal 2 cm of the left anterior descending coronary artery followed by the anterior right and left circumflex coronary arteries.

3. Sudden thrombotic occlusion, probably due to rupture of an atheromatous plaque, appears to be the precipitating event of most acute myocardial infarcts. Endothelial injury and platelet aggregation play a central role in most cases.

D. Clinicopathologic entities

1. **Chronic ischemic heart disease,** the most common clinical form of the disease, is caused by slowly developing ischemic damage.
   a. **Clinical features.** Although often initially clinically silent, chronic ischemic heart disease eventually may lead to the insidious onset of congestive heart failure, with predominantly left-sided manifestations.
   b. **Pathology.** The pathologic features are those of diffuse coronary artery atherosclerosis in association with diffuse left ventricular myocardial fibrosis and small, patchy myocardial scars.
      (1) The heart varies in size; it may be small because of progressive muscle loss or large because of compensatory hypertrophy.

Table 9-1. Risk Factors for Ischemic Heart Disease (IHD)

Unmodifiable Risk Factors	Modifiable Risk Factors
Older age (peak ages 65 to 74 years)*	Hypertension
Male gender (prior to age 74 years)*	Cigarette smoking
Family history of premature IHD	Hypercholesterolemia
	Diabetes mellitus
	Obesity**
	Physical inactivity**
	Psychosocial factors ("type A personality")**

*Data from Framingham study of 5127 patients
**The influence of these less significant factors is controversial.

(2) Any extensive scarring indicates prior acute myocardial infarcts, and fibrocalcific deposits may be present on the mitral valve annulus and within the aortic valve sinuses.

2. Angina pectoris is a syndrome of episodic, paroxysmal, substernal or precordial chest pain resulting from the inability of diseased coronary vessels to provide adequate blood for myocardial oxygenation.

   a. Clinical features. The pain of angina pectoris usually is described as a heaviness or tightness in the substernal or precordial region; radiation to the back, neck, jaw, or left arm is not uncommon. ST segment abnormalities may be found on electrocardiograms (ECGs). Three distinct forms of angina pectoris have been described.

   (1) In **stable angina,** attacks of chest pain are of limited duration (usually no longer than 15 to 20 minutes) and are predictably induced by exertion (i.e., a temporary increase in demands on the heart). The pain usually is relieved by decreasing the cardiac metabolic level (i.e., rest from exertion) or by administration of nitroglycerin. ST segment depression often is found on the ECG.

   (2) In **unstable angina,** the clinical syndrome has manifestations intermediate between stable angina and acute myocardial infarction. Patients with chronic stable angina may develop a progressive increase in the frequency and severity of pain. The anginal pain may be more easily provoked and may occur at rest. Unstable angina is more difficult to treat with traditional measures and requires hospitalization to rule out myocardial infarction.

   (3) In **variant angina** (also known as **Prinzmetal's angina**), chest pain occurs at rest and is associated with ST segment elevation on ECG. Coronary artery spasm appears to be an important mechanism in this disorder since the coronary vessels are angiographically normal in 20% of cases. If prolonged, variant angina may result in myocardial infarcts, arrhythmias, or death.

   b. Pathology. Angina pectoris alone provides no pathologic evidence of myocardial infarction. However, the presence of patchy myocardial fibrosis indicates prior (usually clinically silent) ischemic episodes. Severe coronary artery atherosclerosis usually is found.

3. Acute myocardial infarction refers to irreversible myocardial injury from prolonged ischemia. The result is coagulative necrosis of the myocardial fibers, with loss of the normal conductive and contractile properties of the affected myocardial tissue. Infarction most frequently involves the left ventricle because its work load is greater than that of the other heart chambers. When right ventricular infarction occurs, it almost always represents an extension of severe left ventricular infarction.

   a. Clinical features

   (1) Myocardial infarction most often is characterized by a sudden onset of chest pain that is similar to the pain of angina but more severe and prolonged, generally lasting more than 15 or 20 minutes, and is unrelieved by nitroglycerin. The discomfort may occur when the patient is relatively inactive and even may awaken the patient from sleep. Sweating, nausea, and vomiting often are present. In many patients, a period of unstable angina precedes acute myocardial infarction.

   (2) In some cases, myocardial infarction may be clinically silent or associated with only mild discomfort—particularly in diabetics and in patients who have undergone cardiac transplantation.

   b. Diagnosis. With acute myocardial infarction, usually two out of three of the following are present: impressive clinical history of chest pain, ischemic ECG abnormalities, and elevated cardiac enzymes.

   (1) ECG. The presence of significant (pathologic) Q waves (Q-wave infarct) usually indicates transmural myocardial infarction. ST-segment and T-wave changes are also present in Q-wave infarcts; their presence without pathologic Q waves (non–Q-wave infarcts) often indicates a subendocardial infarct.

   (2) Isoenzyme studies aid in the diagnosis of acute myocardial infarction and can be helpful in estimating the size of the infarct.

   (a) The serum level of the **MB isoenzyme of creatine kinase (CK)** is a highly specific and sensitive marker for acute myocardial infarction, if elevated in serial measurements taken within 48 to 72 hours from the onset of symptoms. CK peaks at 12 to 24 hours after infarction. The number of hours needed to peak correlates with infarct size.

   (b) Changes in the serum levels of **lactic dehydrogenase (LDH) isoenzymes** also are helpful.

(i) The isoenzyme LDH_1, found in highest concentrations in the heart, normally is present in relatively low quantities in the serum. With acute myocardial infarction, LDH_1 levels increase out of proportion to LDH_2 levels, leading to a "reverse" LDH_1/LDH_2 ratio.

(ii) The serum LDH_1 level remains elevated after the serum MB CK level has subsided and, thus, is a useful diagnostic marker in patients whose symptoms began later than 72 hours prior to admission.

c. **Classification.** Myocardial infarcts commonly are described in two ways: according to the degree of ventricular wall involvement and according to the location within the heart or the specific artery involved.

(1) **Depth of mural involvement**

(a) Most infarcts are **transmural,** involving at least one-third to half of the ventricular wall thickness. Transmural infarcts usually correspond with the distribution of one of the major coronary vessels, often with associated coronary thrombosis, and they may result in shock, the formation of aneurysms, or cardiac rupture.

(b) Infarcts that involve the inner one-third to half of the ventricular wall are described as **subendocardial,** or **nontransmural.** Subendocardial infarcts usually are circumferential; often result from hypoperfusion states (e.g., shock); and rarely result in aneurysms, pericarditis, or rupture. Although severe coronary atherosclerosis usually is present, thrombosis generally is absent.

(2) **Location/coronary artery involvement.** According to this classification, a myocardial infarct may be described as an "anterior wall left ventricular infarct," a "left anterior descending coronary infarct," and so on.

(a) Infarcts involving the left anterior descending coronary artery are most common (accounting for 40% to 50% of infarcts), followed by infarcts of the right coronary artery (30% to 40%) and the left circumflex coronary artery (15% to 20%). Infarcts may involve the distribution of more than one coronary artery.

(b) The development of collateral blood vessels can cause **infarcts at a distance** (ectopic infarction), as in an acute thrombosis of the left anterior descending coronary artery that leads to an infarct in the right coronary artery distribution because myocardium distal to the right coronary artery depends on blood flow from the left anterior descending artery.

d. **Pathology.** Some investigators define a myocardial infarct as being at least 2.5 cm in diameter, whereas others do not assign a lower limit for size. The morphologic features of infarcts are similar regardless of location. In large infarcts, zones of necrosis farthest from viable interstitial blood vessels may persist for weeks.

(1) **Appearance during the first week postinfarction**

(a) **Macroscopic appearance**

(i) The first grossly visible change—pallor of myocardium—is visible about 15 to 24 hours postinfarction. Hemorrhage may be prominent in patients treated with thrombolytic therapy.

(ii) At 2 to 3 days, the infarct becomes mottled and more circumscribed.

(iii) From 3 to 7 days postinfarction, the necrotic area becomes progressively more apparent, with a soft, yellow-brown central area and a hyperemic border.

(b) **Microscopic appearance** (Figure 9-1)

(i) The first histologic sign of infarction, seen at 5 to 12 hours, is the appearance of coagulation necrosis, including loss of cross-striations, cytoplasmic hyaline change and eosinophilia, clumping of nuclear chromatin (nuclear pyknosis), and karyorrhexis. "Wavy myocardial fibers" may be found earlier.

(ii) At 12 to 24 hours, intercellular edema and focal hemorrhages appear, and neutrophils are first seen at the periphery of the infarct. Contraction band necrosis (myofibrillar degeneration), which consists of thick irregular eosinophilic bands in the myocyte cytoplasm, often is seen at the periphery of the infarct.

(iii) Over the next several days, coagulative necrosis becomes more extensive as does the neutrophilic infiltrate.

(iv) At 3 to 7 days, the neutrophilic infiltrate abates, and the number of mononuclear cells progressively increases. Macrophages engulf and destroy the necrotic myocytes.

(v) At the end of the first week, new capillaries and fibroblasts (granulation tissue) are seen at the periphery of the infarct.

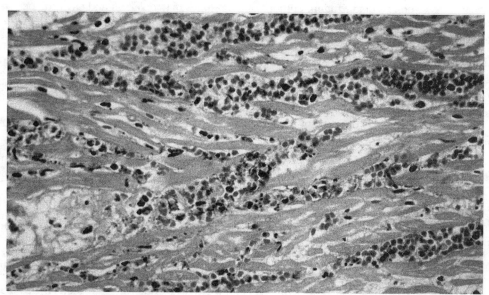

Figure 9-1. Photomicrograph of an acute myocardial infarct during the first week postinfarction. Coagulative necrosis of myocardial fibers is apparent. Edema and focal hemorrhage have caused separation of individual myofibers. The dark nuclei of leukocytes, which have entered the zone of infarction, are seen between individual myocardial fibers.

    (c) Electron microscopic appearance. Changes in myocardial cells, including swelling of the mitochondria and endoplasmic reticulum, nuclear pyknosis, and early degeneration of the sarcolemma, can be seen within 1 hour after the onset of ischemia when examined with an electron microscope.

  (2) Appearance at 2 and 3 weeks postinfarction. Removal of necrotic muscle fibers continues. Macrophages in the necrotic zone contain abundant lipofuscin granules from phagocytosis of necrotic myocytes and erythrocytes. Collagenation of the infarct continues.

  (3) Appearance at 7 weeks postinfarction. The entire infarct has been transformed into a fibrous scar. Occasional viable myofibers may be seen in the scar.

 e. Complications of myocardial infarction that produce histologic findings also may produce clinical manifestations. Other complications, such as ventricular arrhythmias, do not demonstrate histologic findings.

  (1) Arrhythmias, the most common complications, may result from ischemia, hypoxia, sympathetic and parasympathetic stimulation, lactic acidosis, hemodynamic abnormalities, or electrolyte imbalances. Several types of arrhythmias may follow myocardial infarction. The most serious, **ventricular arrhythmias,** probably are the most common cause of sudden cardiac death in the first hour after infarction.

  (2) Heart failure develops when the infarct involves 20% to 25% of the left ventricle. Scar tissue over the infarcted area results in decreased contractility and abnormal ventricular wall motion, with subsequent reduction of cardiac output. Infarction involving 40% or more of the left ventricle leads to **cardiogenic shock,** which is the most common cause of death among hospital patients with acute myocardial infarcts.

  (3) Rupture of the myocardium at the site of infarction can occur at any time within about 3 weeks after onset of the infarct, but it tends to occur most frequently between 2 and 10 days postinfarction, when the infarcted zone has minimal structural strength. After cardiogenic shock and arrhythmias, cardiac rupture is the most common cause of death postinfarction, being responsible for up to 20% of all fatal infarcts.

    (a) Intrapericardial hemorrhage can result, leading to **cardiac tamponade,** if the rupture is through any portion of the ventricular wall other than the septum.

    (b) Rupture of the ventricular septum can cause a left-to-right intracardiac shunt.

    (c) Rupture of the papillary muscle of the left ventricle results in mitral insufficiency.

  (4) Thromboembolism. Mural thrombi can form on the disrupted endocardial surface over areas of myocardial infarction. Because these thrombi are quite friable prior to fibrous organization, portions of a thrombus may break off and enter the peripheral circulation as **emboli**. They most frequently lodge in arterial vessels that supply the brain, kidneys, spleen, intestine, and extremities and may result in infarction.

(5) **Fibrinous pericarditis** can develop soon after infarction in the region overlying the necrosis, or it may become generalized. Clinically evident in 7% to 15% of cases, it is characterized by a pericardial friction rub heard on auscultation. Total resolution or conversion to inconsequential fibrous adhesions may occur. **Dressler's syndrome**, characterized by pericarditis, pericardial effusion, and fever, may develop within 2 weeks to several months postinfarction. Its cause is unknown.

(6) **Ventricular aneurysm** is a late complication that occurs in 12% to 20% of patients. It develops when the fibrous scar that forms after infarction has insufficient structural strength to withstand the intraventricular chamber pressure. The scar stretches, resulting in extreme thinning of the ventricular wall with progressive convex deformity of the external cardiac surface. Stasis of blood within the aneurysm results in mural thrombi in 50% of patients, because the affected segment of myocardium cannot contract in phase with the remaining normal ventricle.

f. **Prognosis and treatment**

(1) **Prognosis.** Most patients who develop an acute myocardial infarct have an uncomplicated course. The advent of optimal emergency ambulance systems has reduced the prehospital mortality rate due to ventricular arrhythmias by 25% to 30%. Currently, the overall mortality rate for patients who reach the hospital is 3% to 30%. Among patients who develop cardiogenic shock, the mortality rate is greater than 70%.

(2) **Treatment.** Therapeutic intervention within a few hours after an acute myocardial infarct is indicated to limit infarct size, thereby reducing complications and the risk of death. Early **thrombolytic therapy** appears to be an important treatment modality. Other potential treatment modalities include bypass grafting, percutaneous transluminal coronary angioplasty, and the administration of drugs to reduce myocardial oxygen demand.

IV. SYSTEMIC HYPERTENSION* is a disorder characterized by sustained elevation of systemic arterial blood pressure, usually above a diastolic level of 90 mm Hg and a systolic level of 140 mm Hg. This disorder is the most significant risk factor for cardiovascular disease and a major cause of heart failure, renal failure, and stroke.

A. Classification. Hypertension can be classified according to the etiology or to the course and extent of the disease.

1. **Etiologic classification**
   a. **Primary hypertension** (also known as **essential hypertension**) has an unknown etiology, although the renal mechanisms that affect blood pressure (see IV C 1) are believed to play a role. Also, risk factors for atherosclerosis have been implicated in the development of primary hypertension (see III B 1).
   b. **Secondary hypertension** has a specific underlying cause, which often is a renal disease (e.g., renal vascular or parenchymal disease, renin-secreting tumor) or an endocrine disease (e.g., primary aldosteronism, Cushing's disease, pheochromocytoma).

2. **Clinical course of hypertension**
   a. **Benign hypertension** is a chronic and relatively mild increase in systemic arterial blood pressure (to a diastolic level not higher than 110 to 120 mm Hg), which may or may not have an underlying cause. Although the secondary effects of hypertension may not be clinically evident for a long time, benign hypertension may progress to serious end-organ effects.
   b. **Malignant (accelerated) hypertension** involves a profound and acute elevation of blood pressure (to a diastolic level higher than 130 to 140 mm Hg), which can develop de novo or as a complication of benign hypertension. It is a true medical emergency. In malignant hypertension, end-organ effects of hypertension develop in a brief period of time. Papilledema, retinal hemorrhage, encephalopathy, angina, and cardiac and renal failure may all complicate malignant hypertension.

---

*Coauthored by John E. Tomaszewski.

B. Incidence and epidemiology

1. **Primary (essential) hypertension** accounts for about 90% of cases of elevated blood pressure. In about 5% to 10% of patients with secondary benign hypertension, an underlying cause can be identified.

   a. Essential hypertension is more common in adults than in adolescents and is rare in children. Men are affected more often than women.

   b. Essential hypertension is more common among blacks than among whites.

2. **Malignant hypertension** is a rare form of high blood pressure that can complicate the course of both essential and secondary hypertension; rarely, it is the initial manifestation of high blood pressure. Persons at high risk include patients with renovascular hypertension, glomerulonephritis, chronic renal failure, or scleroderma and pregnant women with toxemia.

C. Pathogenesis.

Hypertension represents an imbalance in the factors that control cardiac output, peripheral resistance, and sodium homeostasis. The renal vasculature may be the primary source of kidney disease as it contributes to a renal cause for hypertension (called **renovascular hypertension;** see Chapter 16 VI) as well as to the acceleration of other forms of vascular disease (e.g., thrombosis, embolization, infarction). The kidney influences blood pressure through several mechanisms.

1. The **renin–angiotensin–aldosterone system** is a major pressor mechanism. Activation of the system results in an increase in systemic blood pressure. The system works as follows.

   a. Renin is released by the juxtaglomerular cells under the stress of decreased afferent arteriolar pressure, decreased sodium delivery to the distal tubule, or direct sympathetic stimulation.

   b. Renin cleaves angiotensinogen, a circulating α_2-globulin produced in the liver, to form **angiotensin I,** which is further modified by converting the enzyme (in a single passage through the lungs) to the potent vasoconstrictor **angiotensin II.** Angiotensin II is a potent stimulus for the production of aldosterone by the zona glomerulosa of the adrenal cortex. It also stimulates renin release by increasing the activity of the sympathetic nervous system.

   c. Adrenal secretion of aldosterone, in response to renin stimulation, results in increased renal absorption of sodium.

2. **Atrial natriuretic factor,** a hormone secreted by specialized cells in the cardiac atria, antagonizes the effect of the renin–angiotensin–aldosterone system, counteracts the vasoconstrictive action of angiotensin II, and increases the urinary excretion of sodium. Secretion of atrial natriuretic factor may be induced by atrial distention secondary to increased vascular volume.

3. **Other renal agents** (e.g., prostaglandins, elements of the kallikrein–kinin system) also have antihypertensive effects, which are likely to be more local than systemic.

D. Pathology.

The long-term effects of sustained hypertension are most significant in the heart, kidneys, and cerebral blood vessels. The morphologic features of hypertensive heart disease are discussed here. (Renal changes are discussed in Chapter 16 VI, and cerebrovascular changes are discussed in Chapter 21 II A 1, D 2.)

1. **Macroscopic features.** The major morphologic feature of hypertensive heart disease is an enlarged heart, characterized by **concentric hypertrophy** of the left ventricle with hypertrophied papillary muscles and trabeculae carneae cordis. Endocardial fibrous thickening occasionally may be present.

   a. The left ventricular wall may increase from a normal thickness of 13 to 15 mm to a thickness of 25 mm or more. This hypertrophy correlates with a twofold to fourfold increase in the weight of the heart.

   b. The volume of the ventricular cavity is decreased by the cardiac hypertrophy. The degree of elevation of blood pressure often is poorly correlated with the degree of hypertrophy.

   c. Cardiac hypertrophy can be seen on echocardiogram, ECG, or chest x-ray.

2. **Microscopic features.** No microscopic findings are unique to hypertensive heart disease, although individual myofiber hypertrophy often is seen.

E. Clinical manifestations and complications

associated with hypertensive heart disease are discussed here. (See Chapter 16 VI B–D, and Chapter 21 II D 2, for these features of renovascular and cerebrovascular hypertension, respectively.)

1. When the heart no longer can compensate for its increased work load by hypertrophy alone, cardiac dilatation and failure may occur (in about 40% of cases). **Congestive heart failure** is the most important cause of death in hypertensive patients.

2. **Coronary atherosclerosis,** which is exacerbated by the hypertension, increases the risk for cardiac ischemia and infarction and for heart failure.

V. INFLAMMATORY DISEASES OF THE HEART may involve any or all of the anatomic layers of the heart and may produce severe deformity of one or more of the heart valves. Chronic valvular disease may become the most important clinical feature of inflammatory heart disease.

A. Rheumatic heart diease is the most important manifestation of **acute rheumatic fever** because it alone can cause severe parenchymal injury or death. Rheumatic fever is a systemic, nonsuppurative inflammatory complication of untreated pharyngeal infection with group A β-hemolytic streptococci, which is characterized by inflammatory lesions primarily involving the heart, joints, and subcutaneous tissue. Acute rheumatic carditis develops in 40% to 50% of patients with a first attack of acute rheumatic fever.

1. **Epidemiology.** Overall, less than 1% of untreated cases of group A streptococcal pharyngitis develops into acute rheumatic fever. Patients who do develop rheumatic fever are susceptible to recurrent attacks and risk greater cardiac effects with each attack.
   a. Rheumatic fever typically occurs in children between the ages of 5 and 15 years; however, any age-group may be affected. Males and females are equally susceptible.
   b. Worldwide in distribution, rheumatic fever most frequently occurs in developing countries and in lower socioeconomic groups; it is believed to be the cause of 25% to 40% of all cardiovascular disease in the Third World. In the United States and Western Europe, the incidence of rheumatic fever has decreased dramatically over the past five decades, although small outbreaks are still reported.

2. **Etiology and pathogenesis.** Although the precise mechanism of rheumatic fever is unknown, it appears that an autoimmune reaction is involved. In patients with rheumatic fever, antibodies to several streptococcal antigens (e.g., antibodies to the group A streptococcal M protein and carbohydrate) have been found to cross-react with cardiac antigens. Although the specific cross-reacting antigens are unknown, myocardial myosin and sarcolemmic and vascular intimal structures are probably important. Heredity also may play a role.

3. **Pathology**
   a. **Acute rheumatic carditis** is a **pancarditis** (i.e., all heart layers are affected); typically, the myocardium is most severely involved. The gross appearance of the heart is relatively unremarkable, with only modest dilatation and mural softening. Characteristic microscopic features of the carditis are as follows.
      (1) **Myocarditis.** The presence of well-developed **Aschoff bodies** is the pathognomonic feature of acute rheumatic carditis, although a **diffuse nonspecific myocarditis** associated with a variable amount of myocyte necrosis and chronic inflammation often is present as well. Although classically found in the interstitial fibrous regions of the heart, Aschoff bodies also may be identified in the joints, tendons, and other connective tissues. They may be found in the heart long after the clinical signs of disease have resolved. There are three histologic phases in the development of Aschoff bodies.
         (a) The **early phase** (exudative stage) occurs within 4 weeks after the onset of carditis and is characterized by a focus of swollen, eosinophilic, perivascular collagen fibers (fibrinoid necrosis) associated with an inflammatory infiltrate of neutrophils (primarily) and chronic inflammatory cells (to a lesser degree).
         (b) In the **intermediate phase** (proliferative or granulomatous stage), which extends from 4 to 13 weeks after the onset of carditis, the central focus of fibrinoid necrosis is surrounded by chronic inflammatory cells and fibroblasts. This cellular zone also contains large mesenchymal cells known as **Anitschkow cells,** which may be multinucleate (**Aschoff giant cells**) and are believed to be derived from fibroblasts. Anitschkow cells are identified by their characteristic nuclei, which have a "caterpillar" appearance when cut longitudinally and an "owl-eye" appearance when cut transversely. The intermediate phase is **the only pathognomonic phase for acute rheumatic fever** (Figure 9-2).

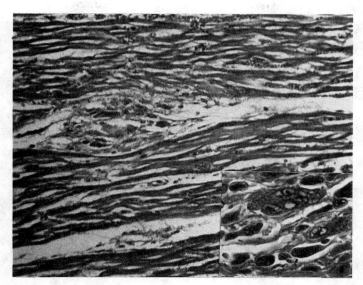

Figure 9-2. The Aschoff body of acute rheumatic fever in its distinctive granulomatous phase. Note its location in the interstitial fibrous region of the heart. Also shown (*inset, lower right*) are a large multinucleate Aschoff giant cell and smaller Anitschkow cells. (Courtesy of Giuseppe Pietra, M.D., Director of Anatomic Pathology, Hospital of the University of Pennsylvania.)

        (c) In the **late phase** (healed or fibrous stage), which extends from 3 to 4 months after the onset of carditis, the Aschoff body appears as a nonspecific hyalinized scar.

    (2) Endocarditis is the most characteristic and potentially damaging effect of rheumatic fever. Typically, the valvular endothelium demonstrates numerous small (1 to 2 mm), rubbery verrucae (i.e., warty vegetations) composed of fibrinoid material along the lines of leaflet closure. These vegetations arise over foci of ulcerated endocardium, which may demonstrate mesenchymal proliferation similar to that of an Aschoff body.

    (3) Pericarditis. A prominent fibrinous pericarditis often is present, which may lead to fibrous organization that is of little significance.

  b. Chronic rheumatic heart disease refers to the late valvular effects (i.e., stenosis, insufficiency, or both) of rheumatic fever (Figure 9-3). About half of the cases involve only the mitral valve. The remaining cases involve (in decreasing order of frequency) the mitral and aortic valves; the aortic valve only; the mitral, aortic, and tricuspid valves; the tricuspid valve only; and the pulmonic valve.

    (1) Valvular effects. The valve leaflets become quite thickened and deformed by fibrosis, the commissures often are fused, and valvular calcification frequently is noted (see Figure 9-3). Neovascularization is often present. The chordae tendineae become thickened, shortened, and fused. The atrial surface of the mitral valve may acquire a "fish-mouth" appearance. Focal fibrotic thickenings of the left atrial mural endocardium located just above the mitral valve, termed **MacCallum's plaques,** represent jet lesions related to mitral regurgitation.

    (2) Secondary effects
      (a) Marked **left atrial dilatation** may result from severe mitral stenosis or insufficiency. In about 40% of cases, this condition is complicated by the formation of **mural thrombi,** which most often are found in the left auricular appendage.
      (b) Cor pulmonale (see II C 2) may develop as a consequence of secondary pulmonary hypertension induced by severe mitral valve disease.

4. Clinical features and diagnosis. Diagnosis of the initial attack of rheumatic fever is based on the **modified Jones criteria** and requires the presence of at least two major or one major and two minor clinical manifestations as well as supportive evidence of prior streptococcal infection (Table 9-2). Individuals with a history of rheumatic fever are at high risk for recurrence when reinfected with group A streptococci.

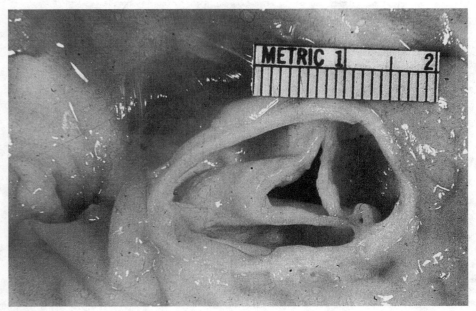

Figure 9-3. Photograph of a thickened aortic valve demonstrating partial fibrotic fusion of the commissures that has occurred as a late complication of rheumatic fever.

5. Course and prognosis

  a. Although death during the acute phase of rheumatic fever (usually due to intractable myocarditis) is quite rare, the long-term sequelae of chronic valvular disease (i.e., congestive heart failure, bacterial endocarditis, peripheral embolism) remain important causes of morbidity and mortality in these patients. Valve replacement may become necessary. An increased risk for developing chronic valvular disease is seen in those patients who demonstrate clinical evidence of carditis during the acute attack of rheumatic fever and in those who suffer recurrent attacks.

Table 9-2. Diagnosis of the Initial Attack of Acute Rheumatic Fever: The Modified Jones Criteria (1992 Update)

Major manifestations
Carditis
Polyarthritis
Chorea
Erythema marginatum
Subcutaneous nodules

Minor manifestations
Arthralgia
Fever
Elevated serum acute phase reactants
Prolonged PR interval on ECG

Proof of previous (group A) streptococcal infection
Increased or rising levels of antistreptococcal antibodies
Positive throat culture or rapid streptococcal antigen test
Recent scarlet fever

Modified from the special writing group of the Committee on Rheumatic Fever, Endocarditis, and Kawasaki Disease in the Young of the American Heart Association. *JAMA* 268:2070, 1992.

ARF = Acute rheumatic fever; ECG = electrocardiogram; RHD = rheumatic heart disease.

    b. Primary prevention consists of antibiotic treatment of streptococcal pharyngitis; however, rheumatic fever arises after clinically inapparent infections in about one-third of cases.

B. Endocarditis is an inflammation of the inner lining of the heart, or endocardium. It usually involves an infection of the heart valves.

    1. Infective endocarditis is a serious infection characterized by the deposit of vegetations on the endocardium, particularly the heart valves. The vegetations may contain bacteria, fungi, or—rarely—rickettsiae. As bacteria are the most frequent pathogens, the term bacterial endocarditis often is used. The **mitral** and **aortic** valves are most frequently involved.

        a. Clinical course. Clinically, bacterial endocarditis has been classified as acute or subacute.*

            (1) Acute endocarditis has a rapid and severe onset of symptoms that are of rather short duration. The vegetations typically occur on previously normal valves and are caused by a virulent organism, such as *Staphylococcus aureus.* Valve perforation may occur.

            (2) Subacute endocarditis has an insidious onset. Vegetations frequently occur on a previously damaged valve and are caused by less virulent organisms, such as α-hemolytic (viridans) streptococci. Perforation is uncommon.

        b. Etiology

            (1) Of all cases of **infective endocarditis involving native heart valves,** about 65% are caused by various streptococci—particularly α-hemolytic (viridans) streptococci—and 25% are caused by *S. aureus. S. aureus* is responsible for up to 75% of acute bacterial endocarditis on native valves.

            (2) Prosthetic valve endocarditis frequently is caused by staphylococci, either *S. aureus* or *S. epidermidis.* Gram-negative bacilli and fungi also are important causes of infectious endocarditis in patients with prosthetic heart valves as well as in immunocompromised patients and **intravenous drug abusers**.

        c. Pathogenesis

            (1) Subacute endocarditis typically occurs on an **abnormal valve**. Clinically significant infection usually is not present elsewhere in the body, with minor trauma to the oral, intestinal, or bladder mucosa providing a portal of entry.

                (a) The underlying cause of the valvular heart disease includes mitral valve prolapse (currently most common), rheumatic heart disease (previously most common), congenital heart disease, degenerative (calcific) lesions of the aortic and mitral valves, previous cardiac surgery, and intravenous drug abuse.

                (b) It appears that endothelial damage, typically on the surface of a damaged valve, leads to the formation of sterile platelet fibrin thrombi (called **nonbacterial thrombotic endocarditis;** see V B 2). When these foci are colonized by circulating bacteria, subacute bacterial endocarditis results. Vegetations developing at sites where a regurgitant jet of blood strikes and damages the endothelium of a cardiac chamber are called **jet lesions**.

            (2) Acute endocarditis typically occurs on a normal valve in the setting of well-defined bacteremia (the source of infection).

                (a) Persons at risk for acute endocarditis include those with debilitating illness, immunocompromised patients, and chronic alcoholics.

                (b) The toxic agents of acute endocarditis are responsible for the initial damage to the heart valves. Once damaged, the valves are predisposed to thrombus formation and subsequent infection as in subacute cases.

        d. Pathology

            (1) The vegetations consist of fibrin, inflammatory cells (particularly neutrophils), and the offending organism. They typically are friable and somewhat bulky and may grow large enough to interfere with valve closure.

            (2) The location of the vegetations depends on the nature of the predisposing heart condition. In the general population, the left-sided valves are affected more often, whereas the right-sided valves are involved more frequently in intravenous drug abusers.

        e. Complications and prognosis

            (1) Patients may develop signs of **septic emboli,** which originate from the valvular vegetation and which may result in septic infarct in the brain, heart, kidneys, and spleen.

---

*Antibiotic treatment has dramatically altered the natural history of bacterial endocarditis, such that traditional classification into acute and subacute types has fallen into disfavor.

Embolization to the extremities may result in gangrene. Mycotic aneurysms may result. Other complications include **focal glomerulitis** or **diffuse proliferative glomerulonephritis,** which probably results from immune complex deposition.

    (2) Infective endocarditis always is fatal if not treated. Bacteriologic cure can be achieved in most patients with bacterial endocarditis. This statement is not true, however, in the uncommon cases involving resistant gram-negative bacilli or fungi. In spite of bacteriologic cure, the 5-year survival is only 60% to 70% because of valvular damage occurring prior to treatment.

  2. Noninfective endocarditis

    a. Nonbacterial thrombotic endocarditis (i.e., **marantic endocarditis**)

      (1) This form of endocarditis is characterized by small (1- to 5-mm), sterile, fibrin–platelet vegetations randomly distributed along the line of valve closure; the mitral, aortic, or—rarely—tricuspid valve may be involved. Nonbacterial thrombotic endocarditis can be the source of systemic emboli and, thus, lead to organ infarcts, and it may serve as the nidus for the development of bacterial endocarditis.

      (2) Nonbacterial thrombotic endocarditis typically is found in patients with disorders associated with a **hypercoagulable state,** most frequently disseminated intravascular coagulation or carcinoma (particularly adenocarcinoma). Although there is an association with debilitating disorders in general, this form of endocarditis occasionally is found in previously healthy patients.

    b. Nonbacterial verrucous endocarditis (i.e., **Libman-Sacks disease**)

      (1) This form of endocarditis is characterized by the presence of one or more small, warty vegetations of any of the surfaces of the cardiac valves in a patient with **systemic lupus erythematosus.** Although the vegetations may occur on the valve surface exposed to the forward flow of blood, their presence on the undersurface of the valve is a distinctive feature of this disorder.

      (2) **Microscopically,** these lesions are similar to the endocardial lesions seen in acute rheumatic carditis [see V A 3 a (2)].

C. Syphilitic (luetic) heart disease, one of the manifestations of tertiary syphilis, currently is quite rare in the United States. Although myocardial **gummas** may be associated with cardiac dysfunction in rare cases, syphilitic carditis usually is a complication of the much more common **syphilitic aortitis**.

  1. Pathogenesis and pathology

    a. Obliterative endarteritis of the vasa vasorum, particularly of the ascending portion of the thoracic aorta, leads to ischemic medial necrosis and fibrosis of the media and adventitia. Secondary atherosclerosis adds to the injury, which results in the formation of a **thoracic aortic aneurysm**.

    b. Proximal extension of this process leads to scarring and dilatation of the aortic valve ring, fibrosis of the valve leaflets, and narrowing of the coronary ostia. The resultant **aortic insufficiency** may lead to massive dilatation and hypertrophy of the left ventricle, with the weight of the heart being as much as 1000 g (a condition called **"cor bovinum"**).

  2. Clinical course and prognosis. Patients die of cardiac failure or myocardial infarction because of the increased work load and myocardial ischemia caused by the combined effects of the aortic insufficiency and the narrowed coronary ostia.

D. Myocarditis is a nonspecific term used to describe inflammation of the myocardium.

  1. Etiology. Although primary myocarditis does occur, secondary involvement of the myocardium in generalized disease is more common.

    a. Previously, most cases of myocarditis were considered to be idiopathic; however, **viruses** now are considered to be the most common causes of myocarditis in the United States and Western Europe. This change probably reflects the greater availability of serologic tests to make the appropriate diagnosis. Other infectious agents also may cause myocarditis (e.g., bacteria, fungi, certain protozoa). Many cases continue to be idiopathic.

    b. Less commonly, myocarditis may be produced by physical agents (e.g., radiation), chemical agents, metabolic derangements (e.g., uremia), hypersensitivity and immunologically mediated disorders (e.g., acute rheumatic fever, lupus), and various idiopathic conditions (e.g., sarcoidosis). Myocarditis of varied etiology has been described in 50% of AIDS patients.

2. Clinical patterns

    a. Acute viral myocarditis can occur in severel common viral infections. The most common viral cause of clinically significant myocarditis is Coxsackie B virus, although Coxsackie A virus, echoviruses, and rubella (in utero) also are important.

        (1) Clinical features. Although often asymptomatic, viral myocarditis can lead to debilitating loss of cardiac function, particularly in children and young adults.

        (2) Pathogenesis

            (a) Acute infection of the heart by enteroviruses (i.e., Coxsackie A and B viruses, echoviruses) appears to be the result of viremia after initial replication in the gastrointestinal tract. During the acute illness, the virus can be cultured from the myocardium.

            (b) In chronic infection, the lesions may have an immunopathologic basis, and the virus cannot be isolated.

    b. Other forms of infectious myocarditis are found in areas endemic for specific organisms.

        (1) Chagas' disease is the most common form of heart disease in parts of South America where *Trypanosoma cruzi* is endemic. More than 7 million persons are affected, usually men in the third or fourth decade of life.

        (2) Echinococcal myocarditis is found in regions of the world where sheep-raising is a common occupation, such as Uruguay, Australia, New Zealand, and some Mediterranean countries.

        (3) Trichinosis is the most common helminthic infection in the world, and myocarditis is its most serious and frequent complication.

3. Pathology

    a. Macroscopically, the heart appears pale and flabby but otherwise is not distinctive in appearance. Four-chamber dilatation is common. Small granulomas may be seen in myocarditis due to tuberculosis, tularemia, brucellosis, sarcoidosis, mycosis—or as a nonspecific finding.

    b. Microscopically, most cases of myocarditis (viral as well as idiopathic) are characterized by a **nonspecific inflammatory infiltrate** consisting of variable numbers of chronic and acute inflammatory cells. The amount of interstitial edema is variable, being marked in rickettsial myocarditis. Myofiber degeneration and necrosis vary from minimal to marked. Infections caused by pyogenic bacteria (e.g., staphylococci, streptococci), filamentous bacteria (e.g., actinomyces), or fungi (e.g., blastomyces) may be associated with **abscess formation**. Myocardial healing is accompanied by a variable amount of interstitial fibrosis. Dilated cardiomyopathy may result from prior myocarditis.

E. Pericarditis represents an inflammatory disorder of the visceral or parietal pericardium, with or without associated myocardial disease.

1. Etiology

    a. Similar to myocarditis, pericarditis is of varied etiology. It may be of infectious or noninfectious etiology (including that due to metastatic neoplasms), or it may be idiopathic. Most frequently, pericarditis is secondary to extracardiac disease (e.g., direct spread from adjacent pulmonary infection), represents a component of a systemic illness (e.g., lupus), or is idiopathic.

    b. Currently in the United States and Western Europe, the most severe type of pericarditis—constrictive pericarditis—usually is idiopathic or is due to neoplastic infiltration, radiotherapy, trauma, or a connective tissue disease. Tuberculosis and pyogenic bacterial infection also can cause constrictive pericarditis; however, these disorders are less frequent causes than in the past.

2. Clinical features. Although pericarditis often is only an incidental autopsy finding, it can cause **severe chest pain** that simulates a myocardial infarction. A **pericardial friction rub** is a pathognomonic clinical sign but is not always present.

3. Pathology

    a. Acute pericarditis often is classified by the morphologic pattern of inflammation.

        (1) Fibrinous inflammation is characterized by shaggy, granular fibrin deposits ("bread and butter" pericarditis) and suggests acute rheumatic fever, uremia, or lupus as a cause, among others.

        (2) Purulent inflammation suggests bacteria (e.g., staphylococci) or fungi as a cause.

        (3) Caseating granuloma suggests tuberculosis.

(4) Prominent hemorrhage typically is associated with malignant cells that have metastasized to the pericardium.

b. Occasionally, accumulation of fluid in the pericardial sac, or **pericardial effusion,** is so massive that it impedes venous return to the heart, resulting in cardiac tamponade.

c. In most cases, acute pericarditis resolves completely or develops into mild fibrosis, which may cause the pericardium to adhere to adjacent structures (**adhesive pericarditis**).

d. Diffuse organization may lead to dense fibrous thickening and, sometimes, calcification of the pericardium, a condition known as **constrictive pericarditis**. The pericardial fibrosis impairs ventricular filling in diastole, resulting in decreased cardiac output. Both atria have elevated filling pressures, which results in congestion of both the pulmonary and systemic venous circulations.

VI. CONGENITAL HEART DISEASE refers to any structural abnormality of the heart or great vessels

present at birth as a result of incomplete or faulty embryonic or fetal development. This group of disorders represents the most common form of cardiac disease encountered in children, occurring in up to 1% of live births. In most instances, environmental factors interact with a genetic predisposition to produce the abnormality. The defects may exist alone or in conjunction with other defects. Congenital heart disease can be classified into three types of defects: those initially involving left-to-right shunting of blood, those involving right-to-left shunting of blood, and those not involving shunts.

A. **Defects with initial left-to-right shunts.** Patients with these anomalies initially are acyanotic, since they have a larger than normal volume of blood delivered to the lungs. However, pulmonary hypertension typically results, causing a shunt reversal (**Eisenmenger complex**) and, therefore, cyanosis.

1. **Patent ductus arteriosus (PDA)** accounts for 15% to 20% of congenital heart anomalies and may be associated with **maternal rubella** in early pregnancy.

   a. **Pathology and pathophysiology**

      (1) The ductus connects the main or left pulmonary artery with the aorta in the fetus, so that fetal blood bypasses the developing lungs as oxygenation occurs in the placenta. After birth, pulmonary expansion causes an increase in arterial oxygen saturation, leading to contraction and (within 2 months) conversion of the ductus into a fibrous cord.

      (2) If closure does not occur, a pressure gradient is established, and blood flows from the aorta into the pulmonary circulation, thus depriving the systemic circulation.

   b. **Treatment and prognosis.** Surgical closure of an isolated PDA usually is successful. Current therapy with drugs such as inhibitors of prostaglandin synthesis (e.g., indomethacin) can facilitate closure in many instances prior to the development of a right-to-left shunt and may obviate the need for surgery.

2. **Atrial septal defect (ASD),** the most common defect seen in adults, accounts for 10% to 15% of congenital heart disease.

   a. **Pathology.** ASD is characterized by incomplete separation of the atria. **Ostium secundum defect** (i.e., incomplete closure at the level of the fossa ovalis) is responsible for 90% of ASD. **Lutembacher's syndrome** is characterized by an ostium secundum defect in association with mitral stenosis. The sinus venosus defect (located high in the atrial septum) and the ostium primum defect (located low in the atrial septum) comprise the remainder of the forms of ASD.

   b. **Pathophysiology**

      (1) ASD results in a pressure gradient from the left to the right atrium. Although the fossa ovalis remains patent in 25% of all adults, the greater pressures in the left atrium keep it functionally closed.

      (2) Shunt reversal may result in **paradoxical emboli** (i.e., thromboemboli from the right side of the circulation pass through the ASD and cause systemic infarction of organs).

   c. **Treatment and prognosis.** ASD must be surgically corrected prior to development of irreversible pulmonary hypertension. Once treated, patients generally survive into adulthood, although life expectancy is shortened.

3. **Ventricular septal defect (VSD)** is the most frequent form of congenital heart disease, accounting for 25% to 30% of all cases.

   a. **Pathology and pathophysiology.** VSD is characterized by an abnormal opening in the muscular or membranous portion of the ventricular septum, which allows blood to shunt from the left to the right ventricle.

b. Course, treatment, and prognosis

   (1) As with other disorders in this group, the volume of the left-to-right shunt often determines the prognosis. Large left-to-right shunts may cause death in infancy if they are not immediately corrected.

   (2) Infective endocarditis on the margins of the defect or at the site of bloodstream impact on the right ventricle can lead to **septic emboli**.

   (3) Surgical closure in childhood is now common, and the prognosis often is excellent.

B. Defects with permanent right-to-left shunts are less common statistically but include some of the more complicated anomalies. Cyanosis, clubbing of the fingers, and dyspnea are common clinical findings. The most common of these defects is **tetralogy of Fallot,** which accounts for 6% to 15% of all cases of congenital heart disease.

   1. Pathology and pathophysiology. The following structural abnormalities constitute tetralogy of Fallot:

   a. VSD

   b. Dextroposition of the aorta (so as to override the ventricular septum), causing the aorta to receive blood from both ventricular chambers

   c. Pulmonic stenosis, usually due to infundibular muscular hypertrophy (less often valvular stenosis is present, with or without an infundibular defect)

   d. Right ventricular hypertrophy

   2. Course, treatment, and prognosis

   a. The course and prognosis for tetralogy of Fallot depend on the severity of the pulmonic stenosis.

   b. Cerebral infarction, brain abscess, and infective endocarditis are important complications.

   c. This disorder is fatal unless surgical correction (to close the VSD and relieve the pulmonic stenosis) is performed.

C. Defects not involving shunts

   1. Transposition of the great vessels represents 5% to 10% of all congenital heart disease and is characterized by development of the aorta in the anterior position that normally is occupied by the main pulmonary artery. The aorta, thus, arises from the right ventricle and the pulmonary artery from the left ventricle.

   2. Coarctation of the aorta accounts for about 5% of all congenital heart disease and is characterized by a discrete narrowing of the distal segment of the aortic arch. In 50% of cases there is an associated bicuspid aortic valve. The postductal (adult) type is most common.

   a. Clinical features. When the aortic constriction is sufficient to cause symptoms, they are related to hypertension proximal to the obstruction (e.g., dizziness, headaches) and relative hypotension of the lower extremities (e.g., weakness, pallor, coldness). Blood pressure in the arm is greater than in the leg.

   b. Complications, prognosis, and treatment. Complications include congestive heart failure, infective endarteritis at the point of aortic narrowing, dissecting aortic aneurysm, and ruptured cerebral berry aneurysms. Death from coarctation occurs prior to middle age if the condition is not surgically corrected.

   3. Aortic stenosis is responsible for about 5% of all congenital heart disease. It can occur in three forms, all of which cause functional obstruction of left ventricular outflow.

   a. Aortic valvular stenosis (the most common form) usually is characterized by only one commissure in the aortic valve, resulting in a **bicuspid valve.** This anomaly may cause left ventricular hypertrophy with left ventricular decompensation in infancy, or it may be silent until adult life, when dystrophic calcification following fibrosis leads to rigidity of the valve. Severe valvular stenosis may be the underlying abnormality of the **hypoplastic left-heart syndrome**.

   b. Subvalvular aortic stenosis and **supravalvular aortic stenosis** are the two other forms that cause functional obstruction. Poststenotic dilatation of the aorta and coarctation are common associated conditions.

   4. Isolated pulmonic stenosis usually is caused by fusion of the valve cusps. Patients become cyanotic and symptoms worsen with closure of the ductus arteriosus.

   5. Ebstein's anomaly involves displacement of the tricuspid valve into the right ventricle, dividing the chamber into upper (atrialized) and lower (functional) portions. Marked right ventricular dilatation, heart failure, and arrhythmias result.

6. **Endocardial fibroelastosis,** which results in cardiomegaly and chamber dilatation, may occur alone or in association with other anomalies, such as aortic atresia or aortic coarctation. An association with antibody to mumps virus has been reported.

VII. OTHER CLINICALLY SIGNIFICANT CARDIAC CONDITIONS

A. **Mitral valve prolapse** (also called **floppy mitral valve, click-murmur syndrome,** or **Barlow syndrome**) is a disorder characterized by prolapse of one (particularly the posterior leaflet) or both cusps of the mitral valve into the left atrium. It currently is the most common cause of **mitral regurgitation**. Although most cases are sporadic, a familial pattern as well as an increased frequency in patients with Marfan syndrome have been described.

1. **Clinical features.** Echocardiography has demonstrated mitral valve prolapse in up to 10% of the adult population; it is most frequently found in young adult women. Most patients are asymptomatic, but palpitations, fatigue, chest pain, and psychiatric symptoms (e.g., panic attacks) may be presenting manifestations. The characteristic finding on physical examination is a systolic click associated with a mid- to late-systolic murmur. Infective endocarditis and sudden death may occur.

2. **Pathology**
   a. **Macroscopically,** the affected leaflets are redundant and often slightly thickened, resulting in the **parachute deformity.** The chordae tendineae usually are elongated and thinned, although they may be thickened or ruptured.
   b. **Microscopically,** the mucopolysaccharide component of the valve spongiosa expands and replaces a variable portion of the valve fibrosa. This condition sometimes is called **myxoid degeneration.**

B. **Cardiomyopathy** is the term generally used to indicate a disorder of the heart muscle in the absence of ischemic, hypertensive, congenital, valvular, or pericardial mechanisms of myocardial disease. Cardiomyopathy may be classified according to etiology or pathology, with some overlap in the two classification systems. **Overall, the most common type is idiopathic dilated cardiomyopathy.** Cardiac transplantation is an important treatment modality for patients with end-stage disease.

1. **Etiologic classification**
   a. **Primary (idiopathic) cardiomyopathy** refers to a disorder of the heart muscle that has no known cause.
   b. **Secondary cardiomyopathy** refers to myocardial damage that occurs in association with any of the following conditions:
      (1) Chemical toxicity [e.g., alcohol, adriamycin, cobalt ("beer-drinker's cardiomyopathy")]
      (2) Infections (e.g., viral diseases, Chagas' disease)
      (3) Hypersensitivity or immunologically mediated diseases (e.g., lupus)
      (4) Metabolic diseases (e.g., hyperthyroidism, myxedema, beriberi, amyloidosis, hemochromatosis)
      (5) Neuromuscular diseases (e.g., Friedreich's ataxia, some muscular dystrophies)
      (6) Storage diseases [e.g., glycogen storage disease type II (Pompe's disease), Hurler syndrome, Fabry's disease]
      (7) Pregnancy (peripartum and postpartum cardiomyopathy)
      (8) Neoplastic diseases (e.g., leukemia)

2. **Pathologic classification and pathologic features**
   a. **Dilated (congestive) cardiomyopathy** is the most common type (90% of all cases). The insidious onset of cardiac failure typically occurs. Cardiac transplantation is an important treatment option.
      (1) **Macroscopic findings** include **cardiomegaly, symmetrical biventricular hypertrophy,** and **four-chamber cardiac dilatation.** Marked ventricular dilatation may lead to relative thinning of the ventricular walls. Mural thrombi are found in the left ventricle in 75% of cases.
      (2) **Microscopic and ultrastructural findings** are nonspecific and include **interstitial fibrosis, myofiber hypertrophy and vacuolization,** and **mitochondrial abnormalities.**
   b. **Hypertrophic cardiomyopathy** (also called asymmetric septal hypertrophy or idiopathic hypertrophic subaortic stenosis) indicates cardiomegaly without ventricular dilatation. An

autosomal dominant or familial pattern of inheritance has been reported in many cases. Heart failure is the end result, with or without **aortic outflow obstruction**.

    (1) Macroscopic findings include cardiomegaly, with small or normal-sized ventricular cavities. The most distinctive and nearly universal macroscopic feature of this disorder is the **disproportionate hypertrophy of the ventricular septum as compared to the free wall**.

    (2) Microscopic findings include marked disarray of the myofibers with loss of their normal parallel arrangement, particularly in the ventricular septum. Mitral valve thickening and endocardial thickening in the region of the left outflow tract are common.

  c. Restrictive cardiomyopathy is quite uncommon. The increased wall stiffness results from infiltrative disorders such as amyloidosis, hemochromatosis, leukemia, or storage diseases. **Eosinophilic endomyocardial disease,** which is characterized by peripheral blood and tissue eosinophilia, myocardial necrosis, mural thrombi, and extensive endomyocardial fibrosis, is an important idiopathic cause of restrictive cardiomyopathy. Impaired ventricular filling leads to cardiac failure.

C. Tumors and cysts of the heart

  1. Primary tumors of the heart are extremely rare. They arise from the cells that form the various tissues that comprise the heart. Roughly 75% of primary cardiac tumors are benign and 25% are malignant. The more common tumors of this group are mentioned here.

    a. Myxoma is the most common primary cardiac tumor, accounting for about 40% of the benign tumors and 25% of all cardiac tumors. These tumors generally are considered to be benign neoplasms derived from primitive mesenchymal or endothelial cells, although some investigators feel that they represent organized hematomas. About 75% of myxomas are found in the **left atrium**.

      (1) Clinical features. Clinically, myxomas most commonly simulate mitral valve disease. Cardiac murmurs often are of changing intensity. Effects of systemic emboli are the second most frequent cause of clinical manifestations.

      (2) Pathology

        (a) Macroscopically, myxomas are seen as broad-based masses that are friable, polypoid, and usually attached to the atrial septum.

        (b) Microscopically, they consist of a myxoid matrix with a high content of acid mucopolysaccharide, in which are embedded stellate and spindle cells arranged singly and in clusters as well as vascular channels.

    b. Rhabdomyomas are the most common primary cardiac tumors in infants and children, accounting for 40% of all tumors in this age-group. They probably represent **fetal hamartomas** derived from embryonic cardiac myoblasts. About one-third of patients have associated **tuberous sclerosis**. In most patients (90%), rhabdomyomas are large and multiple, virtually always arising within the ventricular myocardium. Blood flow obstruction may result if the tumors bulge into the cardiac lumen. The tumors consist of large cells that contain abundant glycogen and focally demonstrate cross-striations.

    c. Pericardial cysts account for nearly 20% of all cardiac tumors and, in most cases, are asymptomatic. Pericardial cysts are derived from the parietal pericardium. They are lined by a uniform layer of mesothelium and are uniformly benign.

    d. Malignant tumors. The most common primary malignant tumor of the heart is the **angiosarcoma**. Other, less common, examples of cardiac malignancies include rhabdomyosarcoma, mesothelioma, and fibrosarcoma.

  2. Metastatic tumors are the most frequently encountered cardiac tumors; they are identified (usually as incidental findings) in 10% to 20% of autopsies performed on patients with metastatic malignancies. Virtually any type of malignancy can metastasize to the heart; carcinomas from the lung and breast are the most common solid tumors to do so, although leukemias and lymphomas also may involve the heart. Clinical manifestations may include pericarditis, pericardial effusion, arrhythmias, or cardiac failure.

STUDY QUESTIONS

Directions: Each of the numbered items or incomplete statements in this section is followed by answers or by completions of the statement. Select the **one** lettered answer or completion that is **best** in each case.

1. Which coronary artery most commonly supplies blood to the posterior portion of the interventricular septum?

(A) Left main coronary artery
(B) Left anterior descending coronary artery
(C) Left circumflex coronary artery
(D) Proximal marginal coronary artery
(E) Right coronary artery

2. Which statement about heart failure is true?

(A) Forward failure refers to the motion of the heart pushing against the chest wall when the ventricular chambers are dilated
(B) Dyspnea is a result of stasis of blood in the extremities
(C) Right-sided failure may result in hepatomegaly
(D) Cor pulmonale usually is due to severe pulmonic stenosis
(E) The clinical manifestations of heart failure most commonly reflect right-sided failure

3. The modified Jones criteria are used to diagnose which cardiac disease?

(A) Secondary hypertension
(B) Secondary cardiomyopathy
(C) Acute rheumatic fever
(D) Cyanotic heart disease
(E) Syphilitic carditis

4. "Cor bovinum" is a Latin term that describes the appearance of a heart affected by which disease?

(A) Viral myocarditis
(B) Long-standing hypertension
(C) Syphilitic carditis
(D) Alcoholic cardiomyopathy
(E) Atherosclerosis

5. The most common cause of myocarditis in the United States is

(A) trypanosomiasis
(B) echinococcal infection
(C) trichinosis
(D) viral infection
(E) granulomatous myocarditis

6. A patient who suffers from dizziness, occasional dyspnea, and intermittent claudication of the legs when running is most likely to have which congenital heart defect?

(A) Tetralogy of Fallot
(B) Coarctation of the aorta
(C) Eisenmenger complex
(D) Ventricular septal defect
(E) Atrial septal defect (ASD)

7. Which statement about ventricular aneurysm following acute myocardial infarction is true?

(A) The cardiac silhouette on chest radiograph often appears to be reduced in size
(B) Renal infarction may result
(C) Mural thrombi rarely form
(D) Hemorrhagic pneumonia is a common complication
(E) The aneurysm wall consists of amyloid with little collagen

8. A congenital heart defect that initially causes cyanosis is

(A) patent ductus arteriosus (PDA)
(B) coarctation of the aorta
(C) atrial septal defect (ASD)
(D) tetralogy of Fallot
(E) bicuspid aortic valve

1-E   4-C   7-B
2-C   5-D   8-D
3-C   6-B

9. Which statement about cardiomyopathy is true?

(A) The most common type is idiopathic dilated cardiomyopathy
(B) Hypertrophic cardiomyopathy is characterized by very large ventricular cavities
(C) Cardiac transplantation cannot be performed for patients with end stage disease
(D) Restrictive cardiomyopathy typically results from viral infection or ethanol abuse
(E) Patients with hypertensive or valvular related myocardial disease form an important subgroup

10. Which type of inflammation is most characteristic of acute rheumatic fever?

(A) Endocarditis
(B) Myocarditis
(C) Pericarditis
(D) Pancarditis
(E) Vasculitis

11. The classic histologic lesion of acute rheumatic fever is the

(A) Mallory's body
(B) Aschoff body
(C) psammoma body
(D) Negri body
(E) Anitschkow cell

12. All of the following statements about infective endocarditis are correct EXCEPT

(A) it is most commonly caused by gram-negative bacilli
(B) it most often involves a previously damaged valve
(C) valve perforation may occur
(D) it is fatal if not treated
(E) damage to the left-sided valves is more common in the general population

13. True statements regarding nonbacterial thrombotic endocarditis include all of the following EXCEPT

(A) there is a common association with a hypercoagulable state
(B) the inflammation frequently, but not always, is due to viral infection
(C) it may contribute to the formation of bacterial endocarditis
(D) the mitral and aortic valves are involved most commonly
(E) systemic emboli are an important complication

14. Histologic findings present in chronic ischemic heart disease include all of the following EXCEPT

(A) diffuse myocardial fibrosis
(B) fibrocalcific valvular changes
(C) small patchy myocardial scars
(D) endocardial fibroelastosis
(E) coronary artery atherosclerosis

15. Morphologic examination of a heart diseased by pericarditis may reveal all of the following EXCEPT

(A) fibrinous exudate
(B) calcification
(C) fibrosis
(D) malignant cells
(E) hemochromatosis

16. Mitral valve prolapse (floppy mitral valve) is characterized by all of the following EXCEPT

(A) prolapse of the mitral valve leaflets into the left ventricular cavity
(B) an excess of mucopolysaccharide in the valve spongiosa, which progressively replaces the valve fibrosa
(C) thinning of the chordae tendineae
(D) a systolic click or murmur
(E) a frequency of 5% to 10% in the general population when examined by echocardiography

9-A   12-A   15-E
10-D   13-B   16-A
11-B   14-D

17. Cardiac anatomic abnormalities associated with tetralogy of Fallot include all of the following EXCEPT

(A) dextroposition of the aorta
(B) ventricular septal defect (VSD)
(C) right ventricular hypertrophy
(D) atrial septal defect (ASD)
(E) pulmonic stenosis

18. All of the following agents contribute to the kidney's regulation of systemic blood pressure EXCEPT

(A) renin–angiotensin system
(B) aldosterone
(C) prostaglandins
(D) kallikrein–kinin system
(E) lymphokines

Directions: The group of items in this section consists of lettered options followed by a set of numbered items. For each item, select the **one** lettered option that is most closely associated with it. Each lettered option may be selected once, more than once, or not at all.

Questions 19–23

Match each phrase describing a feature of inflammatory heart disease with the disease it characterizes.

(A) Acute rheumatic fever
(B) Chronic rheumatic heart disease
(C) Acute endocarditis
(D) Subacute endocarditis
(E) Libman-Sacks endocarditis

19. Fusion of the commissures

20. Infection by group A β-hemolytic streptococci

21. Infection by α-hemolytic (viridans) streptococci

22. Infection by *Staphylococcus aureus*

23. Warty vegetations on the undersurface of the mitral valve

---

17-D	20-A	23-E
18-E	21-D	
19-B	22-C	

ANSWERS AND EXPLANATIONS

1. The answer is E *[I A 4 b]*.
In most humans, the right coronary artery arises from the right aortic sinus and passes along the right aortic sulcus onto the diaphragmatic ventricular surfaces. From the base of the ventricles to the cardiac apex, the right coronary artery is known as the posterior descending interventricular branch. Penetrating branches of the right coronary artery usually supply the posterior part of the interventricular septum. "Dominance" of the coronary circulation is determined by the artery that supplies the posterior descending branch. The coronary arteries are arranged in a right dominant pattern in 70% to 80% of cases. The anterior part of the interventricular septum receives its blood supply from penetrating branches of the left anterior descending coronary artery.

2. The answer is C *[II B, C]*.
In heart failure, there is an imbalance between the body's circulatory demands and the heart's ability to keep pace with them. Right-sided failure results in systemic venous congestion, including an enlarged and tender liver. The term "forward failure" is used to indicate decreased cardiac output and inadequate organ perfusion, whereas the term "backward failure" is used to emphasize the increased cardiac filling pressures and venous congestion that occur as a consequence of cardiac failure. Manifestations of left-sided failure include dyspnea, orthopnea, and paroxysmal nocturnal dyspnea, which are consequences of pulmonary congestion. Cor pulmonale represents right ventricular enlargement due to pulmonary hypertension.

3. The answer is C *[V A 4; Table 9-2]*.
The diagnosis of an initial attack of acute rheumatic fever must fulfill the modified Jones criteria, which require the presence of at least two major manifestations or one major and two minor manifestations plus supportive evidence of a prior streptococcal infection. The major clinical manifestations include carditis, polyarthritis, chorea, erythema marginatum, and subcutaneous nodules; the minor manifestations include arthralgia, fever, elevated serum acute-phase reactants, and prolonged PR interval on electrocardiogram (ECG). Supportive evidence of a prior streptococcal infection includes increased serum antistreptococcal antibodies, positive throat culture, or positive rapid streptococcal antigen test.

4. The answer is C *[V C 1 b]*.
Syphilitic (luetic) carditis occurs as a consequence of the spread of the causative spirochetes from mediastinal lymph nodes into the adventitia of the aorta. This results in the formation of an aneurysm, typically in the ascending aorta, which leads to dilatation and scarring of the aortic valve ring and subsequent aortic insufficiency and ventricular dilatation. In order to compensate for this, the left ventricle hypertrophies, sometimes to massive proportions, approaching the size of a bovine ventricle ("cor bovinum").

5. The answer is D *[V D 1 a]*.
Myocarditis is a nonspecific term that refers to inflammation of the myocardium, regardless of etiology. The frequency of myocarditis due to specific agents varies with the population studied. Currently in the United States and Western Europe, viruses are considered to be the most common causes of myocarditis. Coxsackie B virus probably is the most important viral cause of clinically significant myocarditis; however, Coxsackie A virus, enteroviruses, and rubella viruses are other important viral causes of myocarditis. Many cases of myocarditis in the United States are idiopathic.

6. The answer is B *[VI C 2]*.
Coarctation of the aorta is characterized by a discrete narrowing of the distal segment of the aortic arch, which may be proximal to, at, or just distal to the ductus arteriosus; in about 50% of cases, the defect is associated with a bicuspid aortic valve. Postductal coarctation, the more common form (especially in adults), is clinically characterized by a significant difference between the systolic blood pressure in the upper extremities (which is elevated) and the systolic pressure in the lower extremities (which is decreased). Many patients have typical symptoms of mild to severe hypertension, such as dizziness. Claudication occurs when there is insufficient lower extremity blood flow to meet the metabolic needs of the leg muscles.

7. The answer is B *[III D 3 e]*.
Ventricular aneurysms are found as late complications in 12% to 20% of patients who have experienced a myocardial infarction. Portions of mural thrombi may break off, embolize, and cause infarction at various sites, most notably the kidneys, brain, spleen, intestines, and extremities. If the aneurysm-distorted

ventricular segment forms one of the heart margins seen on a chest radiograph, the cardiac silhouette may appear enlarged. Mural thrombi are associated with ventricular aneurysms in 50% of cases, because the akinesia and dyskinesia of the thin fibrotic aneurysm wall cause stasis of blood. The wall of the aneurysm consists primarily of fibrous tissue; amyloid is absent. Hemorrhagic pneumonia is not a complication of ventricular aneurysm.

8. The answer is D *[VI A 1, 2, B].*
Tetralogy of Fallot is one of the more common congenital heart defects to produce cyanosis, the bluish discoloration of the skin and mucous membranes. This condition is the clinical manifestation of an increased amount of incompletely oxygenated blood in the systemic circulation. Cardiac disorders that allow blood to bypass the pulmonary circulation (by way of a right-to-left shunt) result in cyanosis. Eisenmenger complex can be produced by a variety of heart defects that initially are associated with a left-to-right shunt. The increased pulmonary blood flow across the shunt results in pulmonary hypertension, and the left-to-right shunt then reverses to a right-to-left shunt, producing cyanosis. Patients with patent ductus arteriosus (PDA) or atrial septal defect (ASD) initially are acyanotic because these defects are associated with initial left-to-right shunts; cyanosis only occurs when there has been shunt reversal. Patients with coarctation of the aorta and bicuspid aortic valve do not have shunts.

9. The answer is A *[VII B].*
Cardiomyopathy refers to any disorder of the heart muscle that occurs without underlying ischemic, hypertensive, congenital, valvular, or pericardial disease. Most cases of cardiomyopathy are idiopathic and are characterized by biventricular dilatation (dilated or congestive cardiomyopathy). Hypertrophic cardiomyopathy indicates cardiomegaly without ventricular dilatation. Restrictive cardiomyopathy is uncommon; the increased wall stiffness results from infiltrative disorders such as amyloidosis, hemochromatosis, storage diseases, and leukemia. Idiopathic cardiomyopathy and ischemic heart disease are the most common disorders for which cardiac transplantation is performed.

10. The answer is D *[V A 3 a].*
The cardiac inflammation that results during first attacks of acute rheumatic fever characteristically is a pancarditis (i.e., the inflammation involves the endocardium, myocardium, and pericardium).

11. The answer is B *[V A 3 a (1)].*
The well-developed Aschoff body is the pathognomonic histologic feature of acute rheumatic fever. Although characteristically found in the interstitial fibrous regions of the heart, Aschoff bodies also may be found in the subendocardial region and at extracardiac sites (most typically, the joints and subcutaneous tissue). The well-developed Aschoff body has a granulomatous appearance. Anitschkow cells are large mesenchymal cells that probably are derived from fibroblasts and are not cardiac muscle cells, although their origin is controversial. Mallory's bodies characteristically are found in the cytoplasm of hepatocytes in alcoholic liver disease. Negri bodies characteristically are seen in the cytoplasm of neurons infected with the rabies virus. Psammoma bodies are calcific deposits seen in papillary epithelial tumors.

12. The answer is A *[V B 1].*
Although an uncommon cause of infective endocarditis on native valves, gram-negative bacilli are important causes in cases involving prosthetic valves and in immunocompromised patients and patients with a history of intravenous drug abuse. Infective endocarditis is infection of the endocardium, particularly the valves; in most cases, it is caused by bacteria and, therefore, often is referred to as bacterial endocarditis. Of cases involving native heart valves, about 65% are caused by streptococci (particularly the α-hemolytic type) and 25% are caused by *Staphylococcus aureus*. Infective endocarditis sometimes is clinically classified as acute or subacute. The acute form may be associated with valve perforation; the subacute form typically involves a previously damaged valve. The disease is always fatal if not treated. Damage to the left-sided valves is more common in the general population, whereas the right-sided valves are affected more often in disease that occurs in intravenous drug abusers.

13. The answer is B *[V B 2 a].*
Nonbacterial thrombotic endocarditis has no particular relationship to viral disorders. The sterile, fibrin–platelet vegetations of nonbacterial thrombotic endocarditis occur primarily on the mitral and aortic valves (rarely the tricuspid valves) in patients who often have some disorder associated with a hypercoagulable state. The vegetations of nonbacterial thrombotic endocarditis (similar to those of infective endocarditis) may result in peripheral embolization as well as serve as breeding grounds for the subsequent development of infective endocarditis.

14. The answer is D *[III D 1 b]*.
Endocardial fibroelastosis is a condition characterized by left ventricular dilatation and a thick fibroelastic coating over the endocardium. It is seen alone or in combination with other congenital heart defects but is not a feature of chronic ischemic heart disease. Chronic ischemic heart disease is the result of slowly developing damage to the heart muscle due to insufficient blood supply to meet its metabolic needs. Microscopic examination of the heart in this diseased state reveals the presence of small patchy myocardial scars as well as larger scars, indicating prior infarction. Fibrocalcific deposits on the mitral valve annulus and within the sinuses of the aortic valve also may be found.

15. The answer is E *[V E 3]*.
Hemochromatosis is not associated with pericarditis although it may cause dilated or restrictive cardiomyopathy. Pericarditis is an inflammatory disorder of the visceral or parietal pericardium. Although of varied causes (infectious or noninfectious), pericarditis typically is the result of an extracardiac disorder rather than a primary cardiac disease. The varied causes of pericarditis are reflected by the different morphologic patterns of inflammation that are seen during the acute phase of pericarditis. This late sequela of pericarditis is characterized by dense fibrous thickening and, in some cases, calcification of the pericardium.

16. The answer is A *[VII A]*.
In mitral valve prolapse, one or both leaflets of the mitral valve prolapse into the left atrium. Mitral valve prolapse (also called floppy mitral valve, click-murmur syndrome, or Barlow syndrome) most frequently is detected in young women who are asymptomatic. In this disorder, one or both leaflets of the mitral valve prolapse into the left atrium.

17. The answer is D *[VI B 1]*.
Atrial septal defect (ASD) is not a component of tetralogy of Fallot, but is the most common congenital heart defect seen in adults. Tetralogy of Fallot is a relatively uncommon form of congenital heart disease characterized by four cardiac anatomic defects. These include an aortic root that overrides a large ventricular septal defect (VSD), right ventricular hypertrophy, and anatomic obstruction of the pulmonary outflow tract. The pulmonic stenosis usually is due to infundibular muscular hypertrophy rather than isolated valvular stenosis.

18. The answer is E *[IV C]*.
Lymphokines (T-cell products) primarily are mediators of inflammation; they do not contribute to the kidney's regulation of systemic blood pressure.

19–23. The answers are: 19-B *[V A 3 b (1)]*, **20-A** *[V A 2]*, **21-D** *[V B 1 c (2) (b)]*, **22-C** *[V B 1 a]*, **23-E** *[V B 2 b]*.
Chronic rheumatic heart disease refers to the long-term cardiac complications (especially valvular) of acute rheumatic fever. Typically, the mitral and aortic valve leaflets become thickened and deformed by fibrosis, with commissural fusion. The damaged valves represent a fertile ground for the development of infective endocarditis (subacute type).

Chronic rheumatic heart disease is a complication of rheumatic fever, which is a nonsuppurative systemic disorder related to an untreated pharyngitis caused by group A β-hemolytic streptococci. Although the precise mechanism of acute rheumatic fever is unknown, the presence of antistreptococcal antibodies that cross-react with heart antigens in these patients suggests an autoimmune basis for this disorder.

Subacute bacterial endocarditis most commonly is caused by α-hemolytic (viridans) streptococci, an organism that is a normal component of the oral flora. Typically, the organism gains entry to the circulation with minor oral trauma, and a transient bacteremia ensues. The bacteria then colonize a platelet–fibrin thrombus that has formed on a valve previously damaged by chronic rheumatic heart disease, mitral valve prolapse, previous cardiac surgery, or some other cause.

The acute form of bacterial endocarditis, in contrast to the subacute form, typically involves a normal heart valve in the setting of a well-defined bacteremia. In this case, the infectious agent usually is a virulent organism (e.g., *Staphylococus aureus*) that causes the initial damage to the valves by way of a toxin.

Libman-Sacks endocarditis (also known as nonbacterial verrucous endocarditis) may occur as a complication of systemic lupus erythematosus. This disorder is characterized by the presence of warty endocardial vegetations along the valve margins and, most distinctively, on the undersurface of the valves.

10
Vascular System
John E. Tomaszewski

I. ARTERIES

A. Normal structure. Anatomic and histologic classification of the arteries is important to the study of arterial diseases, because each class of artery tends to have its own characteristic types of lesions.

1. **Large elastic arteries** (also called **conducting arteries**) are the arterial trunks, such as the aorta and its branches, which are characterized by their large size and elasticity. The wall of these arteries is composed of three histologically defined layers.
   a. The **tunica intima** is composed of endothelial cells, myointimal cells, collagen, and longitudinally arranged elastic fibers forming a feltlike support layer.
   b. The **tunica media** is the muscular layer that contains elastic fibers interspersed with fibrous connective tissue. The external limit is defined by the condensed layer of elastin fibers that form the **external elastic membrane**.
   c. The **tunica adventitia** is a poorly defined connective tissue layer. The outermost layer contains nerve fibers and the small, thin-walled **vasa vasorum,** which supply blood to the artery.

2. **Muscular arteries** (also called **distributing arteries**) are medium-sized vessels that deliver blood to specific organ systems. Like the large elastic arteries, the muscular arteries have walls that contain three layers.
   a. The inner layer, the **tunica intima,** is more clearly defined than in large elastic arteries because of its compact **internal elastic membrane**. Increased amounts of elastic tissue often reflect the abnormal stress of hypertension.
   b. The **tunica media** contains prominent smooth muscle cells arranged in concentric layers.
   c. The **tunica adventitia** contains more extensive neural innervation than the large arteries, reflecting the role of the muscular arteries in autonomic regulation of blood flow.

3. **Small arteries,** usually less than 2 mm in diameter, are defined histologically by the progressive loss of, first, the external elastic membrane and then the internal elastic membrane. These small arteries and the still smaller arterioles are located predominantly within organs and tissues.

4. **Arterioles** are richly supplied by the autonomic nervous system and, thus, constitute the major focus for autonomic control of blood flow.

B. Arteriosclerosis is the generic term for three different patterns of arterial disease that produce narrowing of the lumina, thickening of arterial walls, and loss of elasticity.

1. **Atherosclerosis** is characterized by the formation of elevated plaques, called **atheromas,** in the intima. Atheromas narrow arterial channels, damage the underlying tunica media, and may progress to calcification, ulceration with thrombosis, and intraplaque hemorrhage.
   a. **Epidemiology and risk factors.** Atherosclerosis is a disorder chiefly of developed countries; it is common in North America, Europe, and Russia and may be related to diet and other cultural factors. Atherosclerosis contributes to significant morbidity and mortality from cardiovascular disease, myocardial infarction, and stroke. The incidence of atherosclerosis is higher in men than in women and increases with advancing age. However, the most important risk factors for the development of atherosclerotic vascular disease are hyperlipidemia, hypertension, cigarette smoking, and diabetes mellitus.
      (1) **Hyperlipidemia.** Significant evidence links atherosclerosis to hyperlipidemia, particularly **hypercholesterolemia**. Not all atherosclerotic patients have hyperlipidemia, which suggests that other factors must be involved in the development of the disease.

(a) Classification of lipids. Lipids that circulate in the blood do so in the form of lipoprotein complexes that contain a core of neutral lipids including cholesteryl esters and triglycerides, surrounded by a layer of polar lipids (i.e., cholesterol and phospholipids) and apoproteins. Five classes of lipoproteins are distinguished on the basis of density (Figure 10-1).

  (i) Chylomicrons are large particles produced by the intestines for the purpose of carrying exogenous triglycerides. The major apoproteins are C, A1, A11, and B48. Normally, chylomicrons are depleted of their triglyceride components (by the action of lipoprotein lipase) and then are cleared rapidly from the body. If lipolysis is impaired, chylomicron metabolism is decreased, and remnants accumulate in the plasma.

  (ii) Very low-density lipoproteins (VLDLs) are formed in the liver as by-products of chylomicron lipolysis. VLDLs carry 10% to 15% of the total circulating cholesterol and consist mainly of triglycerides of hepatic origin. The major apoproteins in VLDL are C, E, and B48.

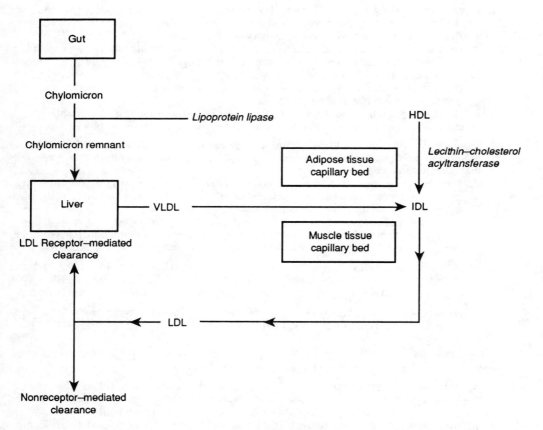

Figure 10-1. Dietary cholesterol and triglycerides are transported across the intestinal mucosa as chylomicrons. Under the action of lipoprotein lipase in the endothelium, triglyceride is released from chylomicrons. Cholesterol-enriched chylomicron remnants are taken up by the liver. Triglyceride-enriched very low–density lipoprotein (VLDL) is synthesized by the liver. VLDL is metabolized in capillaries of fat and muscle tissue to intermediate-density lipoprotein (IDL). IDL has reduced triglyceride and increased cholesterol. IDL has two fates: It may be cleared by receptor-mediated endocytosis in the liver through the action of low-density lipoprotein (LDL) receptors; IDL can also be converted to cholesterol-rich LDL. Two-thirds of LDL is cleared by the liver and other tissues through LDL receptor–mediated endocytosis. The remaining one-third of LDL is cleared by nonreceptor-mediated mechanisms, including scavenging by mononuclear phagocytes. Cholesterol from cell membrane turnover is transported as high-density lipoprotein (HDL), and, under the action of lecithin–cholesterol acyltransferase, is converted to IDL.

      (iii) **Intermediate-density lipoproteins (IDLs)** also are by-products of chylomicron metabolism. These particles result from the interaction of VLDL and lipoprotein lipase. IDLs are the precursors of LDLs. The major apoproteins in LDL are E and B100.

      (iv) **Low-density lipoproteins (LDLs)** transport about 60% to 70% of the circulating cholesterol. The major apoprotein is B100.

      (v) **High-density lipoproteins (HDLs)** carry 20% to 25% of the total serum cholesterol as well as transporting phospholipids and fatty acids. The major apoproteins are A1 and A11.

(b) **Classification of hyperlipidemia** typically is based on the type of lipoprotein involved. Elevated serum HDL levels are correlated with a decreased incidence of atherosclerosis, whereas very low serum HDL levels may be associated with premature atherosclerosis. Five major types of **familial hyperlipoproteinemias** have been identified.

      (i) **Type I** is associated with increased levels of circulating chylomicrons and markedly elevated triglyceride levels but normal cholesterol levels. This type involves a deficiency of lipoprotein lipase levels.

      (ii) **Type II** is associated with increased LDL levels and hypercholesterolemia. Atherosclerosis is common, especially in young persons; some affected patients may die of coronary artery disease in childhood.

      (iii) **Type III** is characterized by increased abnormal VLDL and VLDL remnant particles (i.e., IDLs). Serum cholesterol is markedly elevated, and triglyceride levels are moderately elevated.

      (iv) **Type IV** is the most common type of hyperlipoproteinemia. VLDL levels are elevated, and moderate to severe hypertriglyceridemia is accompanied by normal serum cholesterol levels.

      (v) **Type V,** which is rare, is characterized by elevated levels of both VLDLs and chylomicrons. Affected patients may have bouts of pancreatitis, abnormal glucose tolerance, and hepatosplenomegaly.

(c) **Correlations.** Most hyperlipidemia in the United States is not related to defined familial pedigrees, but probably is the expression of combined environmental and polygenic influences. Hypercholesterolemia is a major risk factor in the development of atherosclerosis. The closest association with ischemic heart disease is in hypercholesterolemia secondary to elevated LDL levels. Hypertriglyceridemia with increased levels of VLDL also increases risk. Serum levels of HDL are inversely correlated to risk. Diets high in omega-3 fatty acids (found in fish and fish oils) may impart an antiatherogenic effect.

(2) **Hypertension.** High blood pressure is strongly correlated with an increased risk for the development of atherosclerosis as well as ischemic heart disease. Epidemiologic studies appear to indicate that the role of hypertension in the pathogenesis of atherosclerosis is most significant in older persons. For further discussion of systemic hypertension, see Chapter 9 V.

b. **Pathogenesis.** The pathogenesis of atherosclerosis is not completely known. Several theories have been proposed.

(1) **Lipid infiltration theory.** This theory postulates that lipid accumulates in the intima as the result of either increased influx or decreased catabolism of serum lipoprotein. A source of controversy concerns how lipid might enter the wall. Transport via receptor-mediated uptake of lipoprotein or engulfment by macrophages are two possible mechanisms.

(2) **Thrombogenic theory.** This theory suggests that atherosclerosis is the end product of multiple episodes of intramural thrombosis, with subsequent organization of thrombi producing an atheroma (see also II B 1).

(3) **Smooth muscle hypothesis.** Many investigators have focused on smooth muscle proliferation as part of atherogenesis.

    (a) **Reaction-to-injury theory.** Vascular smooth muscle proliferates in response to growth factors released at the site of injury. **Platelet-derived growth factor** is a mitogenic polypeptide secreted by platelets, which stimulates smooth muscle growth in tissue culture.

(b) **Monoclonal hypothesis.** Many atheromatous plaques demonstrate monoclonal proliferation of smooth muscle. Atherogenesis may be the result of abnormal growth of vascular smooth muscle, similar to that which occurs in smooth muscle neoplasms.

(c) **Intimal cell mass hypothesis.** Focal proliferation of smooth muscle cells in the intima of certain vessels, particularly at branch points, has also been postulated as an alternative to the fatty streak as the initial lesion of atherosclerosis.

c. **Clinical features.** The clinical presentation of atherosclerosis usually is reflected in **ischemic injury** of the organs supplied by the diseased arteries, in **embolic injury** resulting from the "downstream" flow of components of an atheroma, or in local compromise of the circumferential strength of an artery, resulting in **aneurysm** formation.

d. **Pathology. Fatty streaks and atheromas** are two of the classic lesions of atherosclerotic vascular disease. Many investigators believe that fatty streaks are the initial lesions of atherosclerosis.

(1) **Fatty streaks**

(a) **Macroscopically,** fatty streaks are slightly elevated, poorly demarcated, yellow intimal lesions, which usually are localized to the thoracic aorta and coronary arteries.

(b) **Microscopically,** fatty streaks are composed of lipid-containing cells, some extracellular lipid pools, and variable amounts of collagen, elastic fibers, and proteoglycans.

(2) **Atheromas**

(a) **Macroscopically,** atheromas are fibrous, fibromuscular, or fibrofatty intimal plaques that appear as elevated, white–yellow lesions. Atheromas characteristically are found in the abdominal aorta, coronary arteries, lower thoracic aorta, carotid arteries, and circle of Willis. Atheromas have a tendency to occur at points of arterial branching and around ostia of primary branches of the aorta.

(b) **Microscopically,** atheromas are composed of smooth muscle cells, fibrous tissue, and lipid deposits. The three components are present in varying proportions, depending on the age of the lesion (Figure 10-2).

(3) **Complicated plaques** are produced when atheromas undergo calcification, ulceration, superficial thrombosis, or intraplaque hemorrhage. These processes may cause either total occlusion in the smaller coronary and cerebral arteries or aneurysms, particularly in the aorta, when the tunica media receives sufficient damage.

2. **Mönckeberg's arteriosclerosis** (also called **medial calcific sclerosis**), a much less common histologic pattern of arteriosclerosis, is characterized by bandlike calcifications within the tunica media of medium-sized and small muscular arteries. Medial calcific sclerosis and atherosclerosis may occur in the same patient—even in the same artery—but these two disease processes are thought to be distinct entities.

a. **Epidemiology.** Medial calcific sclerosis shows no sex predilection and is rare before the fifth decade.

b. **Pathology.** The lesion of medial calcific sclerosis is **circumferential calcification** of the tunica media, with no associated inflammatory response. The endothelium remains intact, and the lesions of the tunica media do not encroach on the lumen of affected arteries to cause obstruction of blood flow. The lesions of medial calcific sclerosis occasionally undergo ossification, so that bone and bone marrow may be found within the arterial wall.

3. **Arteriolosclerosis,** the third form of arteriosclerosis, is characterized by proliferative fibromuscular and endothelial thickening of the walls of small arteries and arterioles. Two subtypes have been described: hyaline arteriolosclerosis and hyperplastic arteriolosclerosis.

a. **Epidemiology.** Both forms of arteriolosclerosis show a relationship with hypertension. Hyaline arteriolosclerosis also is found in diabetic patients who are normotensive.

b. **Clinicopathologic subtypes**

(1) **Hyaline arteriolosclerosis** commonly affects older patients with long-standing, mild to moderate hypertension.

(a) **Clinical features.** These patients have a long history of hypertension and may have signs and symptoms of hypertension-associated diseases, such as atherosclerotic heart disease and congestive heart failure. Hyaline arteriolosclerosis also may be seen in diabetes.

(b) **Pathology.** Hyaline arteriolosclerosis appears as a homogeneous, pink (when stained with hematoxylin and eosin), acellular thickening of the walls of arterioles,

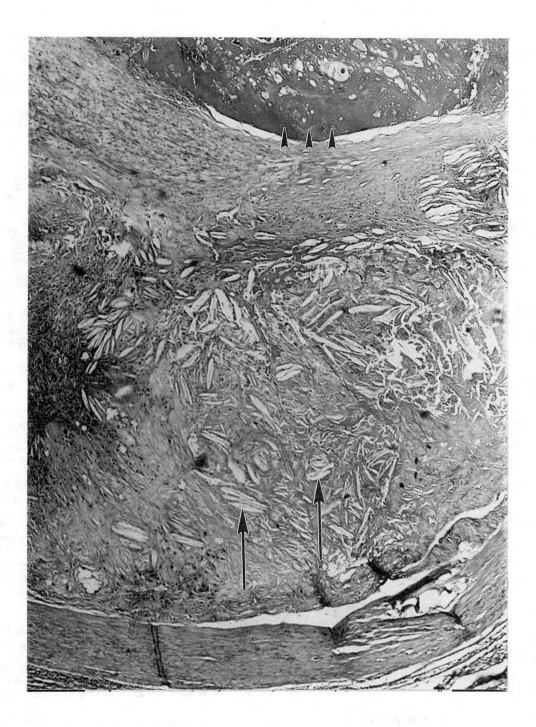

Figure 10-2. Complicated atherosclerotic plaque. *Long arrows* indicate needlelike spaces of cholesterol debris. *Arrowheads* mark organizing thrombus.

with an apparent loss of structural detail and narrowing of the lumen. The result is decreased blood flow to the tissues that are downstream from the lesion. This process is seen best in the kidneys; hyaline arteriolosclerosis is a major morphologic characteristic of nephrosclerosis, which produces symmetrically contracted fibrotic kidneys as the result of renal ischemia.

(2) Hyperplastic arteriolosclerosis occurs in patients who have malignant hypertension, which may appear de novo or be superimposed on preexisting mild to moderate hypertension.

(a) Clinical features. The clinical presentation of these patients usually reflects cardiac decompensation or central nervous system (CNS) disturbances. Patients with malignant hypertension also may present with oliguric acute renal failure.

(b) Pathology. Hyperplastic arteriolosclerosis appears as an onionlike, concentric, laminated thickening of arteriolar walls with resultant narrowing of the lumen. Frequently, these hyperplastic changes are accompanied by fibrinoid deposits and necrosis of the wall of the arterioles—termed **necrotizing arteriolitis.**

C. Arteritis refers to a variety of inflammatory or immunologically mediated diseases that are primary lesions of the arteries. Focal inflammation of an artery due to spread of a contiguous inflammation, such as occurs in an abscess, is not considered an arteritis. Arteritis includes a number of entities, each with incompletely understood pathogenetic mechanisms. The more common forms are briefly described next.

1. Polyarteritis nodosa refers to a group of systemic necrotizing vasculitides that have a widespread distribution of arterial lesions, with involvement of multiple organ systems and signs of widespread ischemic tissue injury. These lesions often result in the formation of microaneurysms in affected vessels. The common thread among the polyarteritis nodosa group is the presence of necrotizing lesions of medium-sized and small muscular arteries.

2. Giant cell arteritides include temporal arteritis and Takayasu's arteritis. The inflammatory lesion in both diseases usually contains multinucleate giant cells. However, the presence of giant cells is not required for either histologic diagnosis.

a. Temporal arteritis usually involves branches of the carotid artery, particularly the temporal artery, but the disease can be systemic and may affect any medium-sized or large artery. It occurs most frequently in elderly women.

(1) Clinical features. The symptoms of temporal arteritis are variable and depend on the site of arterial involvement. Sometimes, the only complaints are weakness, malaise, low-grade fever, and weight loss. More specific symptoms include headache with pain radiating to the neck, jaws, or tongue; intermittent claudication of the jaw is quite characteristic. The scalp may be exquisitely sensitive to pressure, and, if the ophthalmic artery is involved, vision disturbances occur.

(2) Pathology. Microscopic examination reveals partial destruction of the artery wall by an infiltrate of inflammatory cells, including multinucleate giant cells of both the Langhans' type (peripheral nuclear necklace) and foreign-body type (random distribution of nuclei). Phagocytic cells may contain fragments of the disrupted internal elastic lamina. The lesions often involve long segments of the artery, with interspersed normal segments ("skip areas"), which can lead to false-negative temporal artery biopsies.

b. Takayasu's arteritis sometimes is called **"pulseless disease"** because of the weakness of the pulse in the upper extremities of affected patients. This process produces a pronounced irregular thickening of the wall of the aortic arch, the proximal segments of the great vessels, or both. In nearly half the cases, the main pulmonary artery also is involved.

(1) Clinical features

(a) Early symptoms are nonspecific (e.g., malaise, low-grade fever, weight loss, nausea) and may include some cardiopulmonary effects, such as palpitations and shortness of breath.

(b) The characteristic clinical feature is the weakening of upper-extremity pulses with increased pressure in the lower extremities.

(c) Dizziness, syncope, paresthesia, and vision disturbances as well as heart failure develop with progressive involvement of the aortic branches.

(2) Pathology. Microscopic examination initially reveals a mononuclear cell infiltrate surrounding the vasa vasorum in the tunica adventitia. This infiltration is followed by diffuse polymorphonuclear leukocyte infiltration and subsequent mononuclear cell influx into the tunica media. As in temporal arteritis, giant cells of both types may be seen. Temporal arteritis appears to begin in the tunica media, whereas Takayasu's arteritis seems to appear first at the junction of the adventitia and media.

3. **Thromboangiitis obliterans** (also called **Buerger's disease**) is a recurrent inflammatory disorder of arteries that is characterized by thrombosis of medium-sized vessels, especially the radial and tibial arteries. Although the arteries are the primary sites of inflammation, adjacent veins and nerves can become involved.
   a. **Epidemiology.** Thromboangiitis obliterans occurs almost exclusively in cigarette smokers and is prevalent in men between the ages of 25 and 50 years. It is extremely rare in nonsmoking men and in women, although as more women smoke cigarettes, this pattern may change.
   b. **Etiology and pathogenesis.** The strong epidemiologic association with cigarette smoking suggests that this factor plays a role in the pathogenesis of Buerger's disease. The exact mechanism, however, is unknown.
   c. **Clinical features.** Affected patients initially may present with recurrent episodes of patchy thrombophlebitis of superficial veins. Once the actual arterial lesion develops, these patients usually complain of pain in the affected extremity, brought on at first by exercise and eventually present even at rest. Ischemia may cause tissue ulcerations and gangrene. Because individual thrombi can recanalize, the symptoms may abate until a new thrombus forms and ischemia returns.
   d. **Pathology.** Microscopic examination shows occlusion of the involved arterial segment by a thrombus with varying degrees of organization, recanalization, or both. The thrombus contains microabscesses. A nonspecific inflammatory infiltrate is found at first in the adjacent arterial wall; but as the disease advances, both inflammation and subsequent fibrosis extend through the tunica adventitia to envelop adjacent veins and nerves. This fibrous encasement of artery, vein, and nerve is the histologic hallmark of thromboangiitis obliterans.

4. **Other vasculitic disorders.** Several other disorders are characterized by a necrotizing vasculitic component. These conditions include Wegener's granulomatosis, systemic lupus erythematosus, rheumatoid arthritis, hypersensitivity vasculitis, and allergic granulomatosis of Churg and Strauss. These disorders are discussed in other chapters, because the vasculitis is just one aspect of the conditions.

D. **Aneurysms** are abnormal dilatations of either arteries or veins. Because aneurysms of arteries are much more common and clinically significant than venous aneurysms, only arterial aneurysms are discussed in this chapter. Arterial aneurysms are classified according to etiology or anatomic form.

1. **Etiologic classification.** Etiologic (i.e., functional) groupings of arterial aneurysms include several types.
   a. **Atherosclerotic aneurysms,** the most common type, usually are located in the abdominal aorta below the origin of the renal arteries. The common iliac arteries often are involved as well. The complex atheromas that form in these areas lead to destruction of the tunica media, allowing aneurysm formation. Mural thrombi are common. Atherosclerotic aneurysms may dissect or thrombose to occlude renal artery blood flow, blood flow to the lower extremities, or both.
   b. **Syphilitic aneurysms** are not as common as in the past because of the decreased incidence of tertiary syphilis in today's population.
      (1) **Clinical features.** The clinical presentation of patients with syphilitic aneurysms is varied but can include respiratory difficulty due to compression of lungs, major bronchi, or both; dysphagia secondary to compression of the esophagus; persistent cough if there is pressure on the recurrent laryngeal nerve; possible bone pain caused by pressure erosion of ribs, vertebral bodies, or both; and aortic valvular disease secondary to dilatation of the aortic valve ring.
      (2) **Pathology**
         (a) Syphilitic aortitis nearly always is confined to ascending and transverse portions of the thoracic aorta. Secondary atherosclerotic change often is superimposed.
         (b) Advanced syphilis occludes the vasa vasorum of the aorta through a proliferative endarteritis, including perivascular cuffing by plasma cells and gumma formation. The resulting ischemic injury of the aortic wall permits aneurysmic dilatation, which may extend to involve the aortic valve ring and the ostia of the coronary arteries.
   c. **Dissecting aneurysms** from **idiopathic cystic medial necrosis** result from multifocal destruction of elastic and muscular components of the tunica media of the aorta. Hemorrhage within the medial layer can cause longitudinal dissection until external rupture occurs.

(1) Etiology and pathogenesis. Studies suggest that hypertension may be a cause of dissecting aneurysms. Enzymatic defects in connective tissue metabolism also may be a cause. Medial necrosis is more common in patients with Marfan syndrome than in the general population and has been experimentally produced in the condition known as **lathyrism**.

(2) Clinical features. Symptoms usually develop only after aortic dissection has started, with affected patients complaining of episodic chest pain similar to that experienced in myocardial infarction. Sensory and motor functions of the lower body become abnormal when vertebral arteries are compromised; hematuria and renal failure occur when the renal arteries are obstructed; and myocardial infarction can follow obstruction of the coronary arteries.

(3) Pathology
- **(a)** Dissection usually begins in the ascending aorta and extends both toward the heart and distally along the aorta. Typically, the plane of hemorrhagic dissection separates the outer one-third of the tunica media from the inner two-thirds. If both proximal and distal intimal tears occur, a double-barreled aorta is formed; however, rupture usually is directed toward the outside of the aorta, with subsequent hemorrhage.
- **(b)** Histologic examination of an affected aorta shows irregular clefts devoid of normal elastic tissue within the tunica media. There is no associated inflammatory process. These clefts contain metachromatic acid mucopolysaccharides, which can be identified using special staining techniques.

d. Cirsoid aneurysms are aneurysmic arteriovenous fistulas in the form of a tangled mass of intercommunicating vessels. These aneurysms predispose to possible rupture with hemorrhage and can cause heart strain because of arteriovenous shunting of blood.

2. Anatomic classification
- **a. Saccular aneurysms** are balloonlike arterial dilatations on one side of an artery; the orifice may be small compared to the diameter of the aneurysm. Because the blood usually is stagnant in these aneurysms, the lumen can contain a thrombus.
- **b. Fusiform aneurysms** are spindle-shaped dilatations of an artery; they need not be symmetric around the long axis of the affected artery. Fusiform aneurysms increase in size gradually to their maximum diameter and then taper back to the diameter of the normal portion of the artery. Thrombosis is variable.
- **c. Cylindroid aneurysms** are abrupt, cylindrical dilatations of an artery (Figure 10-3). Again, symmetry and mural thrombosis are variable.
- **d. Berry aneurysms** are small saccular aneurysms, 0.5 cm to 2 cm in diameter, which resemble berries. They often are congenital and commonly are present in the smaller cerebral arteries, particularly in the circle of Willis (see also Chapter 21 II C 1).

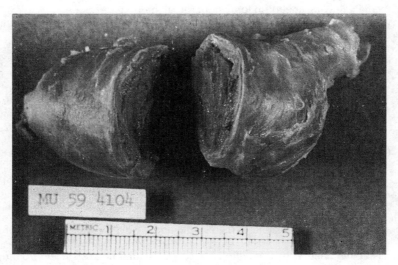

Figure 10-3. Cylindroid aneurysm of the femoral artery, showing mural thrombosis.

II. VEINS

A. Normal structure. Veins are not as precisely characterized by size as arteries.

1. Unlike the arteries, large veins, particularly those in the extremities, have **valves** formed by endothelial folds. These valves help to buttress the column of blood within the large veins, thereby reducing the hemodynamic load.

2. **Histologic examination** of veins shows relatively thin-walled vessels without the well-defined layers that are found in arteries. The tunica intima in veins is mainly an endothelial lining covering a scant layer of connective tissue. Only the largest veins have an internal elastic membrane or much supporting muscle and elastic tissue in the tunica media. Because so little normal supporting structure is present, veins are vulnerable to dilatation, compression, and easy penetration by neoplastic and inflammatory processes.

B. Venous thrombosis refers to the formation of **thrombi** within the veins. **Thrombophlebitis** (i.e., thrombus formation with associated venous inflammation) and **phlebothrombosis** (i.e., thrombus formation without associated inflammation) are the most significant clinical problems affecting the venous system. Thrombophlebitis of the deep veins is called **deep venous thrombosis**.

1. **Etiology and pathogenesis**
   a. **Predisposing conditions.** Venous thrombi apparently can form in veins without preceding endothelial damage. Although the exact pathogenetic mechanism is unknown, certain factors are thought to predispose to thrombus formation, including:
      (1) **Venous stasis** (e.g., due to prolonged immobility or congestive heart failure), which increases the tendency for blood to clot
      (2) **Hypercoagulable states** (e.g., due to dehydration, blood dyscrasias, or certain malignancies), which cause hemoconcentration
   b. **Thrombus formation.** The proposed formation sequence includes blood stasis, blood coagulation, and then thrombus formation. A thrombus formed by the clotting system attaches at some point along the vascular wall. Most venous thrombi form in the deep veins of the legs, often near venous valves.
   c. **Thrombus progression.** The outcome may be enzymatic dissolution, organization with recanalization, or detachment as thromboemboli.
      (1) Further clotting may result in propagation of the thrombus along the vascular lumen, as in **deep venous thrombosis**.
      (2) Venous thrombi may dislodge and become emboli, which may come to rest in various locations (e.g., the lung in **pulmonary embolism**).
         (a) Although most emboli are dislodged thrombi (**thromboemboli**), some are composed of other solids, including fat, bone marrow (as may occur from the ribs during resuscitation), or fragments of a tumor.
         (b) Gaseous emboli may form in decompression sickness or from injection of air into vessels.

2. **Clinical features**
   a. **Superficial thrombophlebitis** causes fibrosis of the involved vein, with extreme tenderness and erythema of the tissues overlying the inflamed area. Generalized edema and venous engorgement generally are absent.
   b. **Deep venous thrombosis** may be clinically silent, causing only nonspecific symptoms (most typically in the calf or thigh). Swelling and aching in the involved extremity occur with enlargement of the thrombus. Deep venous thrombosis is the most frequent cause of pulmonary embolism, which is sometimes a life-threatening presenting feature.

3. **Complications.** The most common serious complication of venous thrombosis is embolization to the pulmonary arteries. Occlusion of veins by thrombi also can cause skin ulcerations distal to the blockage.

C. Varicose veins are persistently dilated, tortuous veins, which are thought to result from chronically increased intraluminal pressure complicated by the loss of adequate structural support of the veins. Superficial veins of the lower extremities are the most frequently involved, probably because of a high venous pressure resulting from upright posture and the relatively little support these veins receive from surrounding tissues.

1. **Epidemiology.** Elderly women with a positive family history are predisposed to varicose veins. Persons whose occupations require prolonged standing also seem to be predisposed.

2. **Clinical features**
    a. Initially, the involved veins do not produce any clinical manifestations, but are visible as dark, twisted, and prominent veins of the legs.
    b. The typical pattern of increasing intraluminal venous pressure, with resultant poor return blood flow, leads to edema and congestion of distal tissues, with associated aching and a feeling of heaviness in the calves. Dystrophic tissue changes, stasis dermatitis, skin ulceration, and cellulitis may result.
    c. Special clinical problems occur with varicosities of the hemorrhoidal vein plexus at the anorectal junction and with esophageal varices, which can result from portal hypertension induced by cirrhosis of the liver.

3. **Pathology.** Varicose veins have nodular or fusiform distentions and outpouchings with variable wall thickness. Valvular deformities and intraluminal thrombi are common. Adjacent zones along the vein may have a compensatory wall hypertrophy with increased smooth muscle content and subintimal fibrosis. In larger veins, degeneration of the elastic tissue and focal calcifications (**phlebosclerosis**) are commonly found.

III. LYMPHATICS

A. **Normal structure.** The lymphatics are essentially endothelial-lined spaces or canals through which lymph flows. Only the major lymphatic ducts have a small amount of smooth muscle and valves formed by endothelial folding.

B. **Primary disorders** of lymphatics are extremely uncommon; all result in dilated lymphatics, with increased intraluminal pressure and, thus, increased interstitial fluid pressure. The increased pressure, in turn, leads to interstitial fibrosis, particularly of the subcutaneous tissues, and can predispose to ulceration and cellulitis. Three primary forms have been described.

1. **Simple congenital lymphedema** occurs as an isolated limb abnormality, presumably because normal lymphatics have failed to develop.

2. **Milroy's disease,** or **heredofamilial lymphedema,** is a similar defect, but its occurrence follows a familial inheritance pattern.

3. **Lymphedema praecox** does not manifest until the second or third decade of life, usually occurs in women, and can result in progressive massive edema of one or both lower extremities with eventual involvement of the trunk.

C. **Secondary disorders** of lymphatics causing lymphedema are much more common than any of the primary forms. Again, cellulitis, interstitial fibrosis, skin changes, and incapacitation of affected limbs can occur. Various causes include the following:

1. Postinflammatory fibrosis of lymphatics following soft tissue infections

2. Obstruction of lymphatics or lymph nodes by spread of metastatic tumors

3. Surgical disruption of lymphatics, particularly with excision of lymph node groups (e.g., radical mastectomy with axillary lymph node dissection)

4. Postirradiation fibrosis with lymphatic obstruction

5. Filariasis, in which parasites enter through the skin, find their way to regional lymph nodes, and cause obstructive fibrosis of lymphatics and nodes, resulting in edema of the extremity (**elephantiasis**)

IV. TUMORS OF THE ARTERIES, VEINS, AND LYMPHATICS are considered together, as the morphology and outcome associated with these tumors often are the same regardless of their exact origin.

A. **Angiomas** are benign tumors composed of either cavernous spaces or serpentine, capillarylike channels containing blood or lymph.

1. **Cavernous hemangiomas** commonly affect the skin or mucosal surfaces, but can occur in deep tissues. These lesions generally are red–blue, spongelike tumors, which may be several centimeters in diameter and have sharply defined margins. Histologic examination shows cavernous spaces lined by normal endothelium, which contain liquid blood, a thrombus, or both.

Von Hippel-Lindau disease is a syndrome of multiple cavernous hemangiomas involving the cerebellum, brain stem, eyes, pancreas, and liver in association with renal cell carcinoma and cerebellar hemangioblastoma.

2. **Cavernous lymphangiomas** (cystic hygromas) are masses of lymphatic channels containing clear lymph fluid. They usually are located in the neck or axilla and, rarely, in the retroperitoneum. Although benign, these tumors grow by budding and expand into surrounding tissues, making total surgical excision difficult.

3. **Capillary hemangiomas** are unencapsulated skeins of capillaries separated by scant amounts of connective tissue. These tumors can occur in any tissue or organ but are common in the skin and mucous membranes. Because these vascular mazes contain liquid or clotted blood, they can vary from bright red to dusky blue in color. Clinical problems occur only if traumatic ulceration of these lesions causes bleeding.

4. **Capillary lymphangiomas** are the very uncommon lymphatic counterparts of capillary hemangiomas. The two tumors are differentiated by the absence of blood cells in the capillary lymphangioma. Presumably, only lymph is present in the fluid-containing spaces of lymphangiomas.

B. **Glomangiomas** (glomus tumors) are benign tumors composed of vascular channels in a connective tissue stroma that is surrounded by nests of glomus cells. These tumors originate from a neuromyoarterial glomus—an arteriovenous shunt that is richly supplied with nerve fibers. The glomus body has a function in temperature regulation. The typical location for glomangiomas is in the subungual part of a digit, but others occur in soft tissues and in the stomach wall. Subungual glomus tumors are quite painful because of their rich nerve supply and frequent contact trauma.

C. **Telangiectases** are abnormal dilatations of preexisting small vessels—not true neoplasms. Often the lesions consist of a small central dilated vessel surrounded by radiating fine capillaries; in these cases, the condition is termed "spider telangiectasia." These lesions are common during pregnancy and with chronic liver disease. Telangiectases may be caused by altered estrogen levels. The hereditary form of multiple aneurysmal telangiectasia is called **Rendu-Osler-Weber disease**.

D. **Angiosarcomas.** Malignant neoplasms of vascular tissues are termed angiosarcomas when they arise from the endothelial cells of vessels. These tumors grow as freely anastomosing, communicating channels lined by atypical endothelial cells (see also Chapter 25 III D 8).

STUDY QUESTIONS

Directions: Each of the numbered items or incomplete statements in this section is followed by answers or by completions of the statement. Select the **one** lettered answer or completion that is **best** in each case.

1. The most common serious complication of lower extremity thrombophlebitis is

(A) cerebral infarction
(B) kidney infarction
(C) myocardial infarction
(D) pulmonary infarction
(E) intestinal infarction

2. Thromboangiitis obliterans occurs predominantly in people with

(A) congenital cardiac atrial defects
(B) atherosclerotic heart disease
(C) diets high in saturated fats
(D) heavy cigarette-smoking habits
(E) low exercise tolerance

3. Glomus tumors (glomangiomas) originate in structures that are responsible for which function?

(A) Blood pressure regulation
(B) Temperature regulation
(C) Taste sensation
(D) Tactile sensation
(E) Temperature sensation

4. Lymphedema of an extremity can be the result of infestation by which parasite?

(A) *Plasmodium vivax*
(B) *Entamoeba histolytica*
(C) *Strongyloides stercoralis*
(D) *Schistosoma mansoni*
(E) *Filaria bancrofti*

5. Which statement describing Takayasu's arteritis is true?

(A) The vessels affected are predominantly in the lower extremities
(B) The vessels affected are predominantly intraabdominal
(C) The inflammatory infiltrate begins first in the intima
(D) The inflammatory infiltrate begins first at the junction of media and adventitia
(E) The histopathology is that of necrotizing arteriolitis

6. Which statement describing the dissecting aneurysm of idiopathic cystic medial necrosis is true?

(A) The plane of dissection is between intima and media
(B) Dissections are most common in the lower extremity
(C) The plane of dissection is within the tunica media
(D) Dissections are associated with a brisk acute inflammatory reaction in the tunica media
(E) The characteristic isolated finding is absent pulses in the upper extremities

7. All of the following statements about angiomas (vascular tumors) are true EXCEPT

(A) cavernous hemangiomas are dilated vascular spaces often found in the skin and mucosal surfaces
(B) cavernous lymphangiomas usually are located in the neck
(C) capillary hemangiomas are lined by endothelial cells and filled with blood
(D) capillary hemangiomas have a high frequency of malignant degeneration to angiosarcoma
(E) cavernous hemangiomas are a component of von Hippel-Lindau disease

1-D	4-E	7-D
2-D	5-D	
3-B	6-C	

Directions: The group of items in this section consists of lettered options followed by a set of numbered items. For each item, select the **one** lettered option that is most closely associated with it. Each lettered option may be selected once, more than once, or not at all.

Questions 8–12

For each vascular layer described, select the correct histologic name.

(A) Tunica intima
(B) Tunica media
(C) Tunica adventitia
(D) Internal elastic membrane
(E) External elastic membrane

8. The layer in large elastic arteries that contains the bulk of the smooth muscle fibers

9. The arterial layer that contains the vasa vasorum

10. The arterial layer classically damaged in Mönckeberg's arteriosclerosis

11. The arterial layer that shows the earliest signs of atherosclerosis

12. The venous layer that forms the valves in peripheral veins

8-B   11-A
9-C   12-A
10-B

ANSWERS AND EXPLANATIONS

1. The answer is D *[II B 3]*.
When thrombi form in the veins of the lower extremities and embolize, the emboli travel to the right side of the heart and enter the pulmonary arterial tree. Pulmonary emboli can cause pulmonary infarction, leading to necrosis of the lung tissue that is served by the occluded branch of the pulmonary artery. These emboli could not cause infarction of the brain, kidney, heart, or intestines unless a right-to-left shunt is present to allow emboli access to the systemic circulation.

2. The answer is D *[I C 3]*.
Although the exact pathogenesis of thromboangiitis obliterans (Buerger's disease) is unclear, the association with heavy cigarette smoking is inescapable. The disease occurs much more frequently in men than in women, and the onset of symptoms typically is before the age of 35 years. At least one study has shown that these patients may be hypersensitive to tobacco components.

3. The answer is B *[IV B]*.
Glomus tumors are benign tumors that originate in a structure known as the neuromyoarterial glomus, which is an arteriovenous structure rich in autonomic nerves. The cutaneous glomus organ has a function in temperature regulation.

4. The answer is E *[III C 5]*.
Filariasis is the common name for bancroftian filariasis, which is caused by infestation by the parasite *Wuchereria (Filaria) bancrofti*. The larvae enter the dermal lymphatics when a person is bitten by a carrier mosquito. The adult worms often take up residence in the regional lymphatics and nodes of the lower extremities. The inflammatory and fibrotic reaction to the dead worms causes lymphatic obstruction, with lymphedema sometimes so extensive as to progress to elephantiasis.

5. The answer is D *[I C 2 b]*.
Takayasu's arteritis appears first at the junction of the adventitia and media of affected patients. Takayasu's arteritis sometimes is called pulseless disease because of the characteristic weakness in the pulses in the upper extremities. The process produces irregular thickenings of the aortic arch and pulmonary artery. Microscopically, the aortic changes show a mononuclear infiltrate surrounding the vasa vasorum in the tunica adventitia. This infiltrate is later followed by a diffuse neutrophilic infiltrate and subsequent mononuclear infiltrate into the tunica media.

6. The answer is C *[I D 1 c]*.
Idiopathic cystic medial necrosis is caused by destruction of the elastic and muscular components of the tunica media in the aorta. Dissecting aneurysms in cystic medial necrosis show a plane of separation between the outer one-third and inner two-thirds of the tunica media. These aneurysms usually begin in the ascending aorta, with no associated inflammatory process. Affected patients present with complaints of chest pain similar to that experienced in acute myocardial infarction, as well as sensory and motor defects in the lower body and hematuria.

7. The answer is D *[IV A 1–4]*.
Angiomas are benign vascular tumors that may be composed of either cavernous or capillary-like channels containing blood or lymph. Capillary and cavernous hemangiomas are blood-filled tumors that are common in the skin and mucous membranes. Cavernous hemangiomas are found in the cerebellum in von Hippel-Lindau disease. The cavernous lymphangioma is a mass of lymphatic channels filled with lymph fluid, which usually is located in the neck. Capillary lymphangiomas are the uncommon lymphatic counterparts of capillary hemangiomas; only lymph is present in the fluid-containing spaces of these tumors.

8–12. The answers are: 8-B *[I A 1 b]*, **9-C** *[I A 1 c]*, **10-B** *[I A 1 b, B 2]*, **11-A** *[I A 1 a, B]*, **12-A** *[I A 1 A; II A 1]*.
The tunica media in both large elastic arteries and medium-sized muscular arteries contains most of the smooth muscle fibers found in the arterial wall. These smooth muscle fibers are arranged in concentric layers. The tunica media is not exclusively smooth muscle, however; it also has elastic fibers and fibrous connective tissue elements.

The tunica adventitia is the outermost connective tissue layer of the large arteries and contains not only the vasa vasorum but also nerve fibers. The vasa vasorum are the small nutrient blood vessels that perfuse the thick walls of the larger arteries.

Mönckeberg's medial sclerosis is a type of arteriosclerosis that classically produces lesions in the tunica media of the muscular arteries. The lesions of Mönckeberg's arteriosclerosis are bandlike calcifications that involve the entire circumference of the artery. These lesions often are complicated by atherosclerotic lesions, since the two diseases can occur together.

Although several lesions are seen in atherosclerosis, the primary damage seems to be inflicted on the tunica intima. Fatty streaks, atheromas, and the complicated plaques all primarily involve the tunica intima.

Although veins are without the precisely defined layers seen in the larger arteries, they do have internal structure. The largest veins can have an internal elastic membrane and some smooth muscle and elastic tissue in a tunica media. Infoldings of the tunica intima form valves within the lumen of the larger veins to aid in supporting unidirectional blood flow in these vessels.

11
Lung
Maria J. Merino

I. NORMAL ANATOMY AND PHYSIOLOGY OF THE LUNG

A. Respiratory anatomy

1. The bronchial tree

a. The segmental (tertiary) bronchi arise from a lobar (secondary) bronchus. Each segmental bronchus branches into numerous bronchioles.

b. The terminal (lobular) bronchioles subdivide into respiratory (alveolar) bronchioles, which blend into alveolar ducts and terminate in the alveoli (alveolar sacs).

2. Functional anatomy

a. The **conducting portion** of the respiratory system includes the trachea and bronchi as far as the terminal bronchioles.

b. The **respiratory portion** consists of the respiratory bronchioles, alveolar ducts, and alveoli.

c. The **acinus** (sometimes called the **secondary lobule**) constitutes the basic unit of lung function. It includes all of the structures distal to the terminal bronchiole; that is, the respiratory bronchioles, the alveolar ducts and sacs (which together constitute a **primary lobule**), and a capillary bed that derives from the pulmonary artery.

d. The **alveolar septa** are well structured to allow gas exchange. They consist of a thin lining of type I alveolar cells, endothelium, and interstitial cells.

B. Histology and function of pulmonary cells

1. Type I alveolar cells (membranous pneumonocytes; squamous alveolar cells; small alveolar cells) are the basic alveolar lining cells. They are flat, with a long nucleus and a thin cytoplasm that extends around the entire surface of the alveolus; and they adjoin adjacent type I cells. This thinness is optimal for gas diffusion and exchange.

2. Type II alveolar cells (granular pneumonocytes; great alveolar cells) are rounder than type I cells and have large, somewhat circular, central nuclei. They have cytoplasmic extensions (microvilli) and contain osmiophilic secretory lamellar bodies (cytosomes), which appear granular on light microscopy. Type II cells secrete a **pulmonary surfactant** and serve as repair cells after alveolar membrane damage.

3. Cells of the interstitium. The interstitial compartment consists of mesenchymal cells that resemble elongated fibroblasts, elastic fibers, and connective tissue types I, III, and V.

4. Alveolar macrophages belong to the mononuclear phagocyte system and are derived from peripheral blood monocytes. They are recognized instantly by the phagocytosed foreign matter (e.g., carbon particles) in their cytoplasm.

a. Alveolar macrophages have a role in immunity besides their phagocytic properties (see Chapter 1 II E 3).

b. **Pores of Kohn** are minute openings in the alveolar septae of adult lungs, through which alveolar macrophages pass from one alveolar space to adjacent spaces.

c. Diffuse alveolar injury is reflected by proliferation of alveolar macrophages and type II pneumonocytes.

5. Endothelial cells of the alveolar septal capillary are involved in the metabolism of bradykinin, serotonin, acetylcholine, norepinephrine, and angiotensin I.

6. Cells of the bronchi and bronchioles
   a. The bronchi are lined by pseudostratified ciliated **columnar epithelial cells,** with intervening mucus-secreting **goblet cells.**
      (1) The mucus moistens the inspired air and traps inspired foreign particles; the cilia move the mucus and particles upward toward the larger airways.
      (2) Viral infections or inhalation of tobacco smoke and toxins may compromise the ciliary function of the respiratory epithelium. Injury to the ciliated columnar epithelium results in reversible squamous metaplasia.
   b. The bronchioles are lined by columnar cells and nonciliated **secretory (Clara) cells** ,which have numerous electron-dense core granules. They are thought to be involved in the secretion of fluid by the bronchiolar lining.

C. Pulmonary vasculature
   1. The **respiratory portion** of the lung is supplied by branches of the **pulmonary artery,** which bring hypooxygenated venous blood from the right ventricle to the acini.
   2. After gaseous exchange, the **pulmonary veins** return oxygenated blood to the left atrium.
   3. The **conducting (nonrespiratory) airways** are supplied with oxygenated blood by the **bronchial arteries,** which emanate from the aorta.
   4. The dual blood supply of the lungs can have a limited protective effect in the event of occlusion, since anastomoses can develop between the bronchial arteries and the pulmonary circulation to provide a secondary blood source for the acini.

II. CONGENITAL PULMONARY ABNORMALITIES

A. Congenital lobar emphysema is due to bronchial obstruction that is caused by either a congenital absence or hypoplasia of bronchial cartilage. The absence of cartilage may be focal or diffuse and results in a flaccid wall that collapses easily. The resultant trapping of air in the affected lobe causes hyperinflation of the lobe during the expiratory phase. It presents as respiratory distress occurring at birth or shortly thereafter.

B. Pulmonary sequestration refers to a mass of isolated, nonfunctioning lung tissue, complete with alveoli and bronchi. The sequestration most often is present in the left lower lobe, but may occur behind the lung proper and in or below the diaphragm. Blood supply is aberrant, coming from the aorta or from subclavian, intercostal, or diaphragmatic arteries.

C. Congenital adenomatoid malformation is frequently associated with **hydrops fetalis** and **polyhydramnios** and causes respiratory distress of the newborn and recurrent infections in the older child. Varying degrees of cystic change consist of microscopic tubular malformations lined by cuboidal epithelium and admixed broad bands of smooth muscle.

D. Bronchogenic cysts arise from accessory lung buds and are lined by bronchial epithelium. Cartilage is present in the wall of the cyst. The cysts may be single or multiple and may be associated with cysts of the pancreas, liver, and kidney.

E. Bronchopulmonary dysplasia is visible in the lungs of neonates following respiratory failure. It occurs particularly in premature infants who have received oxygen and mechanical ventilation for hyaline membrane disease. It probably represents organization of diffuse alveolar damage, such as occurs in oxygen toxicity.
   1. Bronchopulmonary dysplasia causes chronic pulmonary disease in affected infants. Prominent clinicopathologic features include bronchospasm from smooth muscle hypertrophy in the airways and interstitial edema from endothelial cell damage.
   2. The nucleoprotein hyaline membrane lining the damaged alveolar surfaces resembles that seen in adult respiratory distress syndrome (ARDS).

III. VASCULAR DISORDERS OF THE LUNG

A. Pulmonary hypertension

1. **Pathology**
   a. **Morphologically,** pulmonary hypertension is represented by intimal proliferation, medial hypertrophy, and arterial sclerosis of the pulmonary vascular bed.
   b. **Macroscopically,** yellow linear intimal streaks are seen in the endothelial surfaces.

2. **Pathogenesis and clinical features.** The disorder is divided into primary and secondary forms.
   a. The **primary,** or **idiopathic, form** occurs in young women and is rapidly fatal. It develops in the absence of heart or lung disease.
   b. The **secondary form** arises as a sequela to disorders that alter the intraluminal pulmonary pressure, volume, or flow.
      (1) These disorders include congenital heart disease (e.g., pulmonic stenosis, interventricular septal defects, atrial septal defects), pulmonary arterial thromboemboli, left ventricular heart failure, aortic valve disease, chronic pulmonary diseases (e.g., chronic bronchitis, primary emphysema), pneumoconiosis, idiopathic interstitial fibrosis, sarcoidosis, tuberculosis, and vascular disorders (e.g., systemic polyarteritis nodosa, Wegener's granulomatosis).
      (2) All of these conditions produce a **vascular sclerosis of the pulmonary bed,** with increased pulmonary artery pressure (as measured by wedge pressure) and eventual development of **cor pulmonale**.
   c. Recurrent and multiple **small pulmonary emboli** also lead to pulmonary hypertension because silent emboli may lodge in small arteries and occlude them.

3. **Complications.** If long standing, pulmonary hypertension leads to right ventricular heart failure (cor pulmonale) and venous thromboses.

B. Pulmonary thromboembolism and infarction

1. **Pulmonary occlusion and infarction**
   a. Occlusion of pulmonary arteries may result from in situ thrombosis or, more commonly, from an embolus that arises in sites such as pelvic and lower extremity veins. In either case, the consequence may be **pulmonary parenchymal infarction.**
   b. This combination of occlusion and infarction occurs in most clinical conditions that compromise the venous system, such as congestive heart failure (CHF), states of vascular insufficiency (shock), septicemia, inanition related to malignancy, and confinement to bed.

2. **Pulmonary embolism** is a major cause of sudden death in hospitalized patients, especially if it involves the large pulmonary artery near its origin from the right ventricle (this type is known as a **saddle embolus**).
   a. Important causes of this condition include fractures of long bones, immobilization, and certain malignancies (e.g., pancreatic carcinoma).
   b. Advanced age and morbid obesity significantly increase the risk of saddle embolism occurring.

C. Pulmonary congestion and pulmonary edema

1. **Etiology and pathogenesis**
   a. A major cause of congestion and edema of proteinaceous fluid in the alveolar sacs is CHF with failure of the left ventricle, which results in increased pulmonary capillary pressure. This pressure buildup leads to accumulation of fluid from regurgitation into the pulmonary capillary interstitial bed.
   b. Other conditions leading to volume overload—such as **massive intravenous infusions of saline,** especially if accompanied by a low level of plasma protein—also can result in pulmonary edema. Intraalveolar edema fluid does not accumulate until the lymphatic drainage capacity is exceeded.
   c. **Chronic pulmonary congestion,** as occurs in mitral stenosis, is histologically reflected by numerous hemosiderin-laden macrophages filling the alveolar lumen.
   d. Pulmonary edema also may result from **any condition that increases alveolar capillary permeability,** such as pneumonia, chemical agents, and toxic gases and fumes.

2. **Clinical example.** A prime example of acute alveolar injury with pulmonary edema and respiratory failure is **acute adult respiratory distress syndrome (ARDS).**
   a. ARDS is recognized in many conditions that are characterized by **poor vascular perfusion of the lungs,** such as the postoperative state, septicemia, pancreatitis, severe thermal burns, severe pulmonary infections, oxygen toxicity, alveolar damage by inhalation of chemical irritants, drug overdose, anaphylactic and other hypersensitivity reactions, and major tissue trauma.
   b. Common to many of these conditions is the use of **high concentrations of oxygen as supportive therapy.** Oxygen-derived free radicals (superoxide and hydroxyl ions) may cause necrosis of alveolar epithelium by affecting the cell membrane lipids. Focal atelectasis and alveolar collapse occur because of altered surface tension. The ultimate cause of the syndrome, however, is unknown.
   c. Important in the **pathogenesis** is hypoperfusion of the distal pulmonary microvasculature.
      (1) **Direct pulmonary vascular endothelial damage** occurs, often accompanied by platelet microthrombi, sludging of capillary red blood cells, and sequestration of neutrophils.
      (2) The result is pulmonary microvascular constriction from platelet-derived serotonin, physiologic shunting of blood away from atelectatic areas, and local tissue acidosis.
   d. **Morphologic findings** include alveolar wall damage, pulmonary edema, hyaline membrane formation, and proliferation of type II pneumonocytes.

D. **Pulmonary veno-occlusive disease** occurs predominantly in children younger than age 15, but it can occur in adults as well. Thromboses develop in small veins, with or without recanalization.

   1. **Etiology.** The cause of this condition is unknown, but several conditions (chiefly infectious or immunologic disorders) have been proposed.

   2. **Clinical features**
      a. Clinical signs include severe pulmonary hypertension, accompanied by right ventricular hypertrophy and enlarged central pulmonary arteries.
      b. Patients develop congestion, edema, interstitial fibrosis, hemosiderosis, and arterial hypertensive changes with lymphatic dilation.

E. **Pulmonary vasculitis** exists in Wegener's granulomatosis, Churg-Strauss syndrome, and polyarteritis nodosa.

IV. INFLAMMATORY LUNG DISORDERS

A. **Acute laryngotracheitis,** which mainly affects young children, is caused by streptococci, *Haemophilus influenzae,* and certain viruses. It is characterized clinically by a hoarse, high-pitched cough and stridor. The mucosa is hyperemic and edematous and may be covered by a fibrinous membrane. *Haemophilus*-induced epiglottitis–tracheitis in the pediatric patient may have a fulminating course, with rapid death due to tracheal obstruction.

B. **Bronchitis**

   1. **Acute bronchitis** affects the larger bronchi and often is caused by common cold viruses. Influenza viruses, bacteria (e.g., staphylococci, *H. influenzae,* streptococci), and irritant dusts and gases also are known etiologic agents. The pathologic spectrum includes an exudative infiltrate of neutrophils and fibrin, vascular congestion, and occasionally severe ulceration of the bronchial mucosa.

   2. **Chronic bronchitis** is the consequence of prolonged exposure to bronchial irritants. Because the resulting obstruction of the airways is the major concern, chronic bronchitis is now classified with emphysema as a component of chronic obstructive pulmonary disease (COPD) [see V B].

C. **Bronchial asthma.** Asthma is characterized by a hyperirritability of the airways, causing bronchial constriction, edema, and inflammation in response to various substances.

   1. **Classification.** Asthma is divided into two **forms,** which coexist in some patients.
      a. **Extrinsic (allergic, atopic, reaginic) asthma** has an immunologic basis. Symptoms are precipitated by type I [immunoglobulin E (IgE)-mediated] hypersensitivity reactions to inhaled

allergens. The causative allergens vary widely—from bacterial proteins, to aspirin, to various organic and inorganic industrial and occupational materials. Serum levels of IgE usually are elevated.

  b. Intrinsic (nonallergic) asthma has an unknown basis. Symptoms are precipitated by nonallergenic factors, such as inhaled irritants or infection.

2. Clinical features. The manifestations may vary from occasional wheezing to paroxysms of dyspnea and respiratory distress; rarely, acute attacks fail to remit and become potentially lethal (a condition referred to as **status asthmaticus**).

3. Pathology. The pathologic findings are similar in both types.

  a. The bronchi have thickened walls with narrowed lumina and generally are filled with plugs of mucus in the acute attack. They undergo constrictive spasms, with edema of the bronchial wall and release of viscid mucus.

  b. The subepithelial basement membrane is markedly hyalinized, and goblet cells are accentuated. Bronchial smooth muscle is hypertrophic, and infiltration of eosinophils may occur. Charcot-Leyden crystals and Curschmann's spirals are present within the sputum and emanate from the eosinophils.

D. Infectious pneumonias

1. General considerations

  a. Etiology. Infectious pneumonia in adults is usually a bacterial pneumonia; in children and young adults, it is usually viral or mycoplasmal. In patients with altered host defense mechanisms (e.g., patients receiving antibiotics, cancer chemotherapy, or immunosuppressant drugs; patients with immunodeficiency diseases), pneumonia is apt to be caused by opportunistic organisms such as yeasts (*Histoplasma, Candida)* or *Pneumocystis carinii.*

  b. Pathogenesis. Bacteria tend to cause **pneumonia,** which is characterized by an intraalveolar exudate that leads to consolidation. Viruses and mycoplasmas tend to cause **pneumonitis,** which is chiefly an interstitial inflammation. However, in common usage, the term "pneumonia" is used for both types of inflammation.

  c. Pathology. If roentgenography shows that the inflammatory process is patchy or affects only a segment of a lobe, it is termed **segmental** or **lobular pneumonia;** if it affects an entire lobe, it is called **lobar pneumonia;** if it affects both alveoli and bronchi, it is **bronchopneumonia;** and if it affects chiefly interstitial tissues (i.e., if it is pneumonitis), it is termed **interstitial pneumonia**.

  d. Complications. The infection and inflammation may be complicated by CHF or by other conditions of the lungs, such as poor ventilation (as occurs in bedridden patients) or reduced vascular perfusion (as in ARDS).

2. Bacterial pneumonia

  a. Bacterial pneumonia often is caused by *Streptococcus pneumoniae;* and typically, one lobe is involved. It is characterized by early congestion, leukocyte infiltration, consolidation, and eventual resolution.

   (1) Pneumococcal pneumonia characteristically occurs in alcoholics or malnourished, debilitated persons.

   (2) In the acute phase, the alveolar sacs are filled with an exudate of red cells, neutrophils, and fibrin. The exudate eventually is removed by an ingress of macrophages and lymphocytes, with eventual resolution.

  b. Bacterial pneumonia may secondarily complicate pulmonary damage caused by trauma, hemorrhage, neoplastic obstruction of large bronchi, or pulmonary infarction. It also may follow pneumonitis resulting from aspiration of gastric contents or inhalation of chemicals or toxic fumes.

3. Bronchopneumonia produces changes similar to those of bacterial pneumonia, but it involves purulent bronchitis as well.

  a. Bronchopneumonia may be caused by *Staphylococcus, Pseudomonas, Proteus, Klebsiella,* and other gram-negative coliform bacteria. Some of the latter organisms may be acquired within the hospital setting (a **nosocomial infection**).

  b. Bronchopneumonia, especially when caused by coagulase-positive staphylococci, may be complicated by abscesses, empyema, pneumatocele, and pyopneumothorax.

4. Interstitial pneumonia usually is a viral pneumonia (e.g., the pneumonia of influenza). Cytomegalovirus (CMV), herpesvirus, measles virus, and respiratory syncytial virus are especially important in causing pneumonitis in immunosuppressed patients.

a. Atelectasis may be present in the inner lobule, whereas the septa become prominent and edematous. The predominant inflammatory infiltrate consists of lymphocytes, plasma cells, and histiocytes, and it extends into the interstitium and the septum.

b. Viruses directly attack the lower respiratory tract epithelium, which results in cell necrosis. Adenovirus may cause necrotizing bronchitis and terminal bronchiolitis.

c. Severe cases of all types may be associated with the formation of **hyaline membranes** lining the alveoli.

5. **Primary atypical pneumonia** can be caused by organisms such as mycoplasmas, chiefly *M. pneumoniae,* legionella and chlamydia. It is a common form of infectious pneumonia in children and young adults.

   a. Primary atypical pneumonia is an interstitial inflammation with bronchiolitis, erosion of the bronchial epithelium, and lymphoplasmacytic infiltration around the bronchial wall. It has been dubbed "atypical" because the typical exudates and consolidation of pneumococcal pneumonia are absent.

   b. This form of pneumonitis is associated with a rising titer of cold agglutinins (i.e., red blood cell–agglutinating antibodies that react at 4°C to 6°C). Very high titers (in excess of 1:10,000) often correlate with red cell clumping seen in microscopic examination of a blood smear.

E. Noninfectious pneumonias may be complicated by opportunistic, secondarily invading bacteria.

1. **Aspiration and chemical pneumonitis** are caused by aspiration of liquid vomitus or any chemical irritant.

   a. Bloody sputum may be visible, resulting from acute tracheobronchitis, with edema and hyperemia of the airways, and from eventual necrosis of the bronchial mucosa, with consequent peribronchiolar hemorrhages. Other pathologic changes include pulmonary edema, congestion, and acute infiltration of inflammatory cells, which become extensive.

   b. Complications include abscesses, bronchiectasis, and extensive necrosis.

2. **Lipid pneumonia** results from the aspiration of small oil droplets (e.g., from oily nose drops or mineral oil). It produces peribronchial consolidation. Lipid-laden macrophages and moderate inflammatory infiltrates are found within the alveolar spaces.

3. **Hemorrhagic pneumonitis** is associated with interstitial pneumonitis as well as glomerulonephritis (Goodpasture's syndrome). Pathologically, there is acute necrotizing alveolitis with marked hemorrhages.

4. **Eosinophilic pneumonia** is characterized by marked peripheral blood eosinophilia and infiltration of the lungs by eosinophils, in addition to bronchopneumonia and variable degrees of pulmonary edema. Eosinophilic pneumonia is a component of Löffler's syndrome, in which necrotizing arteritis, granuloma formation, and lymphoid interstitial inflammation also occur. Other causes of eosinophilic pneumonia are *Ascaris* infestations, hypersensitivity states, and polyarteritis nodosa.

5. **Hypersensitivity pneumonitis** is an immunologically mediated interstitial granulomatous pneumonitis. **Farmer's lung,** a prime example, is due to antigens of the mold *Micropolyspora faeni,* which grows on improperly stored hay, corn, tobacco, and barley. In the early stages, focal peribronchiolar granulomas are visible as well as an interstitial infiltrate of giant cells, lymphocytes, and macrophages. Eventual pulmonary fibrosis and emphysema may ensue.

F. Suppurative disorders

1. **Bronchiectasis** is a permanent bronchial dilatation associated with suppuration. The lower lobes are involved in many cases.

   a. Etiology and pathogenesis. Bronchiectasis occurs commonly with situs inversus viscerum **(Kartagener's syndrome)** and with cystic fibrosis.

   (1) The development of bronchiectasis appears to involve an interplay between peribronchial fibrosis and overdistention of the bronchi. Concurrent bronchial inflammation appears to weaken the bronchial walls, allowing further dilation.

   (2) There also is a component of bronchial obstruction, with distal accumulation of retained mucus and superimposed bacterial infection.

   b. Pathology. The bronchi are dilated and filled with mucus and numerous neutrophils. Chronic inflammation may occur in the surrounding parenchyma as well as alveolar fibrosis.

2. **Lung abscess** refers to a confined area of suppuration within the parenchyma. It can result from bronchiectasis; lobar pneumonia; bronchopneumonia; aspiration of gastric contents or foreign objects; a septic embolism arising from osteomyelitis, cavernous sinus thrombosis, or postpartum endometritis; and pulmonary embolism.

G. Infectious granulomatous disorders

1. **Primary pulmonary tuberculosis** continues to be an important cause of morbidity worldwide, although the death rate has improved since the last century. The causative organism is *Mycobacterium tuberculosis.*
   a. The initial tuberculous lesion (**Ghon's lesion**) is subpleural and occurs either in the inferior portion of the upper lobe or in the superior segments of the lower lobe. The **Ghon complex** consists of the initial primary lesion plus involved lymph nodes.
   b. The pulmonary granulomas characteristically show a **grossly** visible central necrosis and have a cheesy, crumbly (caseous) character. **Histologically,** multinucleate giant cells are present, surrounding areas of central necrosis.
   c. Most commonly, the apices of the lungs are involved in active disease, but the lower lobes or any other site may be affected. In active disease, caseous necrosis is followed by cavity formation and spread of infection to other sites.
   d. Tuberculosis may spread to distant organs via the lymphatics or, as in the case of miliary tuberculosis, via the bloodstream to involve all areas of the lungs as well as distant body sites. In immunosuppressed patients, widespread dissemination can occur.

2. **Histoplasmosis** has a natural history like that of tuberculosis.
   a. Histoplasmosis, which is caused by a small yeast, *H. capsulatum,* is endemic to the Ohio and Mississippi river valleys and the southern Appalachian mountain area.
   b. An asymptomatic primary lung infection is common, although it sometimes progresses to chronic cavitary disease. Occasionally, particularly in immunosuppressed persons, histoplasmosis disseminates hematogenously.
   c. The primary lesion is a mass of phagocytes containing the engulfed organisms; scarred calcified granulomas are the usual result in immunologically intact persons.

3. **Coccidioidomycosis,** endemic in the San Joaquin Valley and in arid desert regions of the southwestern United States, follows a similar pattern. It usually is an asymptomatic or mild infection in its primary form in the lungs but may progress to an active granulomatous pulmonary disease. In immunosuppressed persons, coccidioidomycosis may disseminate to become a widespread suppurative disorder.

4. **Aspergillosis** and **phycomycosis** occur less commonly than other suppurative disorders but are important in the presence of immunosuppression or malignancy. Branching hyphae are seen microscopically in cases of aspergillosis.

H. Pneumoconioses are lung disorders that result from inhalation of particulate material. They are often occupational diseases. Since pneumoconioses are caused primarily by pollutants, they are discussed in Chapter 4 VI C.

V. CHRONIC OBSTRUCTIVE PULMONARY DISEASE. Clinicians have combined **emphysema** and **chronic bronchitis** under the umbrella term of chronic obstructive pulmonary disease (COPD) because the two disorders are clinically similar and often occur concomitantly, particularly in cigarette smokers. However, pathologically they are quite distinct. Some authors include **asthma** in COPD, although its airflow obstruction is spasmodic and not usually chronic.

A. Emphysema

1. **Pathogenesis and pathology.** Emphysema is characterized pathologically by dilatation of the acinar airspaces due to destruction of the interalveolar septa. The septal destruction is thought to be due to the action of **proteolytic enzymes,** which are released from leukocytes during inflammation. Several facts support this theory.
   a. Emphysema shows a strong association with air pollution and cigarette smoking, both of which cause chronic, low-grade pulmonary inflammation.
   b. In α_1-antitrypsin deficiency, an autosomal dominant disorder, the normal antiproteolytic activity of serum globulins is lacking. Patients with this disorder are likely to develop early and severe emphysema.
   c. Cigarette smoke, because of its oxidants, also inhibits normal antiproteolytic activity.

2. **Clinical features.** The septal destruction has several **consequences**.
   a. Elasticity of lung tissue is reduced, restricting airflow to the respiratory portion of the lung and causing airways to collapse during expiration.
   b. The surface area available for gas exchange is reduced.
   c. Clinically, the consequence is progressive dyspnea and hypoxemia, with all their resultant ramifications. In advanced disease, increased pulmonary artery pressure eventually leads to cor pulmonale.

3. **Major subtypes.** The two major forms of emphysema seen in COPD are classified by the site of involvement.
   a. **Centrilobular emphysema** is the most common subtype. It primarily involves the respiratory bronchioles (i.e, the central acinus) and spares the alveoli, at least initially. Centrilobular emphysema begins in the upper lobes, occurs predominantly in men, and is associated with cigarette smoking.
   b. **Panlobular (panacinar) emphysema** begins distally in the alveolar ducts and sacs and advances proximally to involve the respiratory bronchioles. It tends to begin in the lower lobes in older persons and may occur in scoliosis, silicosis, and Marfan syndrome. This type is much less strongly associated with cigarette smoking, but it is the type seen in α_1-antitrypsin deficiency.

4. **Other subcategories** of emphysema also are defined.
   a. **Obstructive emphysema** is the term sometimes used when airway obstruction (e.g., from chronic bronchiolitis) appears to contribute to alveolar sac distention and rupture.
   b. **Focal,** or **irregular, emphysema** refers to the large bullae and subpleural cystic changes that are found adjacent to scars and areas of healed tuberculosis or anthracosis. Unless widespread, this form has little effect on respiratory function.
   c. In **senile emphysema,** the lungs become markedly increased in volume; the pleural cavities are filled, and the thorax becomes barrel-chested.

B. **Chronic bronchitis.** Although today's convention is to classify chronic bronchitis under COPD, strictly speaking it is small-airway disease—**chronic bronchiolitis**—that leads to COPD. However, chronic bronchiolitis rarely if ever occurs without chronic bronchitis. Both chronic bronchitis and chronic bronchiolitis are the result of long-standing irritation of the airways. Thus, there is a strong association with air pollution and cigarette smoking.

1. **Pathogenesis and pathology of chronic bronchitis**
   a. Hypersecretion of mucus, often leading to a chronic productive cough ("smoker's cough"), is typical. Pathologically, this condition is seen as hyperplasia of the glandular epithelium, accompanied by an increase in goblet cells and a loss of ciliated epithelial cells.
   b. Other changes include squamous metaplasia of the bronchial mucosa, submucosal edema, fibrosis, and varying amounts of lymphocytic infiltration. Some degree of intraalveolar fibrosis often accompanies chronic bronchitis.

2. **Pathogenesis and pathology of chronic bronchiolitis**
   a. Inflammatory narrowing and fibrosis of the bronchioles occur, markedly impeding the airflow into and out of the alveoli, even when the bronchiolar lumina are not totally obliterated.
   b. The bronchiolar epithelium may develop goblet cell metaplasia, with secretion of mucus that further restricts the flow of air.
   c. The loss of tissue elasticity and obstruction of the bronchioles can lead to alveolar sac distention and rupture (i.e., emphysema).

VI. **INTERSTITIAL LUNG DISEASE** (also called **restrictive,** or **infiltrative, lung disease**) includes a large category of disorders that produce a marked decrease in pulmonary compliance (**"stiff lung"**). Ventilation–perfusion disruption, with consequent hypoxemia, occurs in most patients. Also, the interstitium becomes generally thickened in most patients; and, thus, diffusing capacity decreases.

A. **Diffuse alveolar damage**

1. With diffuse injury to the alveoli, the lungs become remarkably heavy and stiff because of inflammation and edema, with hyaline membrane formation in the alveolar lining. Interstitial fibrosis and inflammation also are present.

2. A variety of agents can cause this disorder, including oxygen toxicity, prolonged treatment with mechanical respirators, both adult and neonatal respiratory distress syndromes, uremia, aspiration pneumonitis, fat embolism, toxic inhalants, drugs, thermal burns from smoke inhalation, radiation damage, and viral pneumonitis.

B. Chronic interstitial pneumonia

1. This disorder follows many of the acute forms of pneumonia, and its characterizing feature is organization of the interstitial infiltrate, which may proceed over a period of years and eventually results in pulmonary fibrosis. This fibrotic condition yields lungs with a honeycomb appearance, both microscopically and radiologically.

2. Causes include pneumoconiosis, chronic passive congestion, nitric oxide inhalation, systemic lupus erythematosus (SLE), rheumatoid arthritis, progressive systemic sclerosis (scleroderma), radiation, and viral pneumonia. Idiopathic cases are common.

3. Specific forms

   a. Usual interstitial pneumonitis [UIP; idiopathic pulmonary fibrosis (Hamman-Rich syndrome); fibrosing alveolitis] is the most common type of chronic interstitial pneumonia. Although causes are many, UIP is idiopathic in at least half of the cases. Many of the collagen vascular diseases are associated with it. **Microscopically,** the alveolar spaces are still intact, although the walls become markedly widened by fibrosis and mononuclear cell infiltration (Figure 11-1).

   b. Desquamative interstitial pneumonitis (DIP) is characterized by a marked proliferation and desquamation of the alveolar lining cells, which fill the alveolar spaces (Figure 11-2). The cells are alveolar macrophages admixed with type II pneumonocytes.

   c. Lymphoid interstitial pneumonitis (LIP) may occur in association with Sjögren's syndrome. It is characterized by interstitial aggregations of lymphoid cells, which may be marked enough to suggest lymphoma.

VII. MISCELLANEOUS PULMONARY DISORDERS

A. Pulmonary alveolar proteinosis is a chronic lung disease of unknown cause. It is characterized clinically by progressive dyspnea, expectoration of thick yellow sputum, chest pain, and marked fatigue. **Pathologically,** the alveolar spaces become filled with lipoproteinaceous material that is

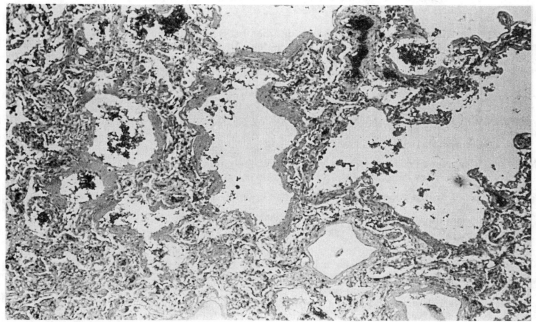

Figure 11-1. Usual interstitial pneumonitis (UIP). The interstitium is widened from fibrosis and infiltration of sparse mononuclear inflammatory cells, but the alveolar spaces remain patent.

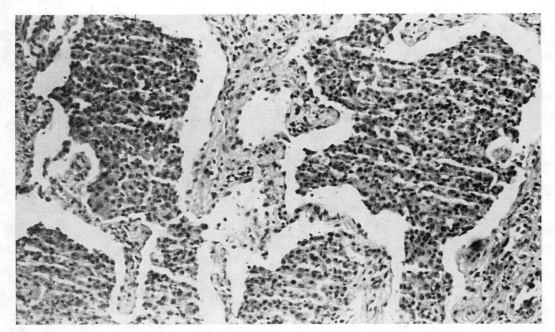

Figure 11-2. Desquamative interstitial pneumonitis (DIP). Mononuclear inflammatory cells, desquamated alveolar lining cells, and alveolar macrophages fill the alveolar spaces. This contrasts with the patent airspaces of UIP, shown in Figure 11-1.

markedly eosinophilic and granular, with needle-shaped, doubly refractile crystals and laminated bodies. Concomitant nocardiosis is found in some cases.

B. Sarcoidosis (Figure 11-3) is a multisystem granulomatous disorder of unknown cause. Pulmonary manifestations are common and occur characteristically as noncaseating, nonnecrotizing **epithelioid granulomas** in the subpleural lung, parenchyma, interstitium, and peribronchial (especially central hilar) lymph nodes.

C. Alveolar microlithiasis is a rare chronic disorder that is occasionally familial and may be due to an **abnormality of the carbonic anhydrase system.** An increase in pH causes calcium salts to precipitate within the alveolar spaces, thus forming laminated calcific concretions composed of calcium phosphate, calcium carbonate, and magnesium carbonate, throughout both lungs. Marked pulmonary fibrosis and cardiac hypertrophy result.

VIII. PULMONARY NEOPLASMS

A. Benign tumors occur infrequently in the lung.

1. **Hamartomas** consist of lobular masses of hyaline cartilage, with a component of myxoid connective tissue, adipose cells, smooth muscle cells, and clefts lined by respiratory epithelium.

2. **Other benign pulmonary tumors** include lipomas, leiomyomas, and rare neural tumors.

B. Malignant tumors

1. **General considerations**
   a. Most lung tumors are malignant, and many of these malignant tumors are **metastases** from primary tumors elsewhere in the body. Fully 95% of those originating in the lung are **bronchogenic carcinomas,** arising from the bronchial epithelium in or around the larger airways (first- and second-order bronchi).
   b. The **risk** of developing lung cancer is 20 times higher in heavy cigarette smokers. Benzopyrene in cigarette tar can initiate carcinoma; many other contaminants, such as radioactive substances and heavy metals, also are present. However, simply living in an urban industrial area can play a role.

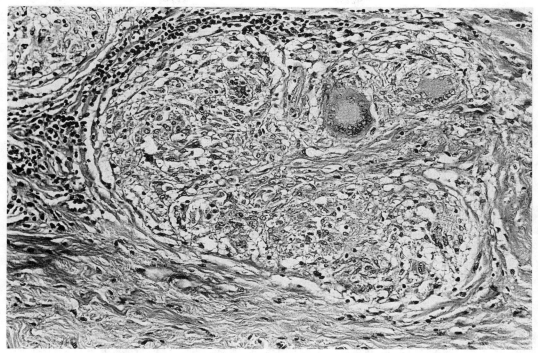

Figure 11-3. Nonnecrotizing epithelioid granuloma characteristic of sarcoidosis.

   c. Cancer deaths in men are predominantly due to lung cancer. Although breast carcinoma causes the most cancer deaths in women, the incidence of lung cancer in women is increasing rapidly.

   d. Paraneoplastic syndromes are relatively common accompaniments of bronchogenic carcinoma, especially the small cell and squamous cell types. Digital clubbing, pulmonary osteoarthropathy, and Horner's syndrome (ptosis and miosis) are also peripheral clinical signs found in all types of lung cancer.

2. Squamous cell carcinoma (SCC) is a tumor of the large, segmental, more central bronchi within the pulmonary parenchyma. It is the tumor most closely associated with cigarette smoking in men.

   a. Clinical course and features

      (1) The tumor is frequently silent until it causes narrowing of the bronchi, collapse of the parenchyma with obstruction, and consequent pneumonia distal to the obstruction.

      (2) Metastasis occurs via lymphatic and hematogenous routes.

      (3) A **paraneoplastic syndrome** may develop, usually manifested as hypercalcemia.

   b. Pathology. Depending on the degree of keratin and intercellular bridge formation, the tumors vary from well differentiated to poorly differentiated (Figure 11-4). Squamous dysplasia, metaplasia, or carcinoma in situ often is present in the vicinity of the tumor.

3. Adenocarcinoma also arises in first- and second-order bronchi but tends to occur more peripherally than SCCs and is found equally in both sexes. Its association with cigarette smoking is not as close as SCCs.

   a. Pathogenesis. Adenocarcinoma is said to occur in association with old trauma, tuberculosis, and infarctions and, hence, has been connected with the development of scars. This connection is controversial, however, because some tumors have the ability to form their own fibrous stroma.

   b. Clinical course and features. Adenocarcinoma grows more slowly than squamous cell or undifferentiated carcinomas and tends to have a better prognosis.

   c. Pathology. The tumor may vary from well differentiated to poorly differentiated. Most lesions contain epithelial mucin that stains positive with mucicarmine.

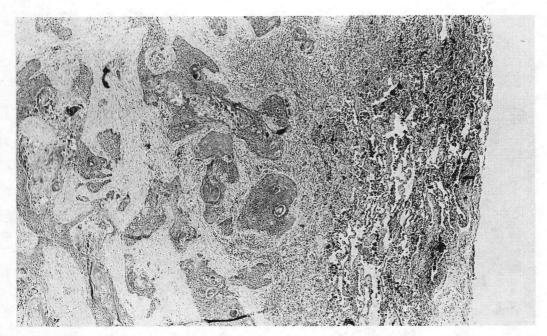

Figure 11-4. Well-differentiated squamous cell carcinoma (SCC). The nests of malignant squamous epithelium contain keratin pearls on the *left side* of the photomicrograph. Note the compressed (atelectatic) lung tissue on the *right side* of the photomicrograph.

4. **Bronchioalveolar carcinoma** is a variant form of adenocarcinoma. It has a pneumonia-like picture, both grossly and radiologically. Uniformly tall and columnar cells line the alveolar spaces, appear to reproduce terminal bronchial cell architecture, and grow in a diffuse pattern throughout the lung; but they maintain an airspace in the alveolar sacs. Mitoses are rarely seen.

5. **Undifferentiated (anaplastic) carcinomas** do not demonstrate distinguishing features that enable them to be characterized as SCC or adenocarcinoma. They are associated with a poor prognosis.
   a. **Small cell carcinoma** is divided into two types: **oat cell** (Figure 11-5), which resembles lymphocytes, and **intermediate cell,** which is fusiform in appearance. In both types, the tumor contains dense core granules similar to the argentaffin cell granules of the gastrointestinal tract and is active in the secretion of hormones and hormonelike products. The granules are thought to be identical to secretory granules of the amine precursor uptake and decarboxylation (APUD) system.
      (1) The hormonal substances produce a variety of **paraneoplastic syndromes,** including Cushing's syndrome from excess adrenocorticotropic hormone (ACTH), diabetes insipidus from insufficient antidiuretic hormone (ADH), and carcinoid syndrome from biogenic amines.
      (2) **Myasthenic (Eaton-Lambert) syndrome** may also occur; of unknown cause, it appears to be related to a lack of acetylcholine.
   b. **Large cell undifferentiated carcinoma** consists of sheets of large, round to polygonal malignant cells; some cases may represent a poorly differentiated adenocarcinoma. The prognosis is poor, especially in the giant cell carcinoma form.

6. **Bronchial gland neoplasms** are thought to arise from the subbronchial seromucous glands and were once erroneously classified as bronchial adenomas.
   a. **Mucoepidermoid carcinoma** consists of nests and cords of malignant squamous cells, with areas of mucopolysaccharides. Both low- and high-grade forms of the tumor exist.
   b. **Adenoid cystic carcinoma** is thought to arise from the larger bronchial seromucous glands and morphologically resembles the adenoid cystic carcinoma that is found within the salivary glands. It grows slowly initially but eventually metastasizes to regional lymph nodes and shows a propensity for perineural involvement.

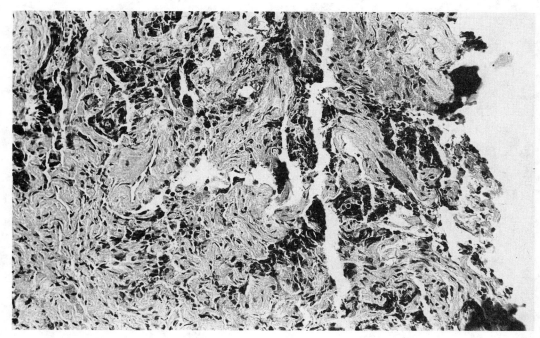

Figure 11-5. Small cell (oat cell) carcinoma. Note the crush artifact of the hyperchromatic undifferentiated malignant cells; this artifact is commonly seen in biopsies of this form of lung cancer. Close inspection reveals the lymphocytelike character of some of the tumor cells.

7. **Bronchial carcinoid tumors,** previously and erroneously called bronchial adenomas, comprise a group of malignant tumors demonstrating an endocrinoid microscopic pattern, with nests of uniform circular to polygonal cells, which abut blood vessels (Figure 11-6). The tumors occur primarily in patients under age 45.
   a. The tumor usually involves the large bronchi and has an endobronchial growth pattern that can fill the bronchial lumina. It can invade locally and is capable of metastasis.
   b. Carcinoid tumors belong to the APUD group of tumors by virtue of their ultrastructural dense core of argentaffin granules. The tumors secrete a variety of biogenic amines, especially serotonin. Nonetheless, the **carcinoid syndrome** (diarrhea, wheezing, and facial flushing and cyanosis) rarely occurs when lesions are confined to the lung.
   c. The prognosis is generally good, with an 80% 5-year survival rate.
   d. Several **variant forms** of bronchial carcinoid occur.
      (1) The **spindle-cell variant (atypical carcinoid)** histologically shows more mitoses and more spindle cells than the classic carcinoid tumor and has a more aggressive course, with a high incidence of metastasis.
      (2) The **tumorlet variant,** which consists of small round or spindle-shaped cells, is small in diameter and is present around the peribronchial arteries. Its malignant potential is very low.

IX. **DISORDERS OF THE PLEURA.** The visceral pleural surface of the lungs is the site of secondary involvement by various underlying conditions, such as pneumonia, collagen vascular disease, rheumatoid arthritis, CHF, and tumor metastases. The pleural mesothelial cells readily react, releasing a fluid effusion into the space between the visceral and parietal pleurae.

A. **Pleural effusions** may be **transudative** or **exudative.**

1. **Hydrothorax** is the accumulation of clear serous fluid **(transudate)** in the pleural cavity. Transudation is not due to pleuritic inflammation, but rather to an increase in extravascular fluid. Thus, hydrothorax commonly results from CHF, renal failure, and cirrhosis.

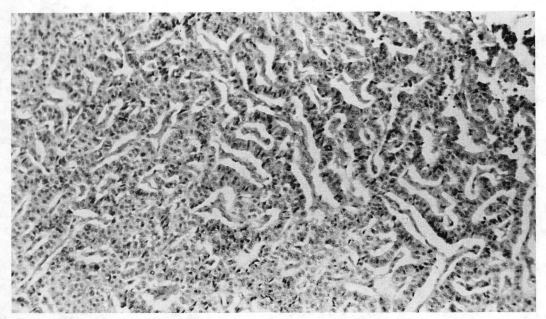

Figure 11-6. Bronchial carcinoid tumor. The tumor cells are arranged in tubular glands and ribbons. This pattern resembles that of carcinoids arising from the small intestine and appendix.

2. **Pleural exudates** are due to pleural inflammation or lymphatic obstruction. The exudate may be **serosanguineous** (e.g., in primary or metastatic lung cancer), grossly **bloody** (in pulmonary infarction), **fibrinous** (in pneumococcal pneumonia), or **suppurative** (in pneumococcal pneumonia); a suppurative exudate is known as **empyema**.

3. **Other pleural collections** also occur.
   a. **Chylothorax** is the accumulation of milky (chylous) lymph, usually in the left pleural cavity, as a result of lymphatic duct obstruction by tumors or trauma.
   b. **Hemothorax** is hemorrhage into the pleural space; it results from damage to any large vessel but especially occurs as a result of ruptured aortic aneurysms or trauma to the ascending aorta.
   c. **Pneumothorax** is the presence of air in the pleural cavity. The air may enter from the lung, as in emphysema or mechanical ventilation, or from the atmosphere, as in a stab wound or thoracentesis. A collapsed lung or infection may ensue.

B. **Inflammation of the pleura (pleurisy; pleuritis)** may be infectious or noninfectious.

1. **Infectious pleurisy** may be bacterial, viral, or fungal. Bronchopleural fistula and empyema result from staphylococcal and other infections of the lung.

2. **Noninfectious pleurisy** can result from pulmonary infarction, rheumatoid arthritis, SLE, or uremia.

C. **Pleural tumors** are mainly the result of metastasis from other sites (e.g., the breast); any visceral carcinoma may reach the pleural surfaces by lymphatic routes. Pleural effusion resulting from metastatic carcinoma can be easily demonstrated by cytologic study of the aspirated fluid.

1. **Benign pleural tumors** are uncommon and usually are local fibrous mesotheliomas.

2. **Malignant mesotheliomas** (Figure 11-7) are identified today with occupational exposure to asbestos. These tumors spread diffusely over the surfaces of both lungs, eventually completely encasing them in a thick **rind of fibrous stroma,** which contains the infiltrating nests and ducts of malignant mesothelial cells. The prognosis is very poor.

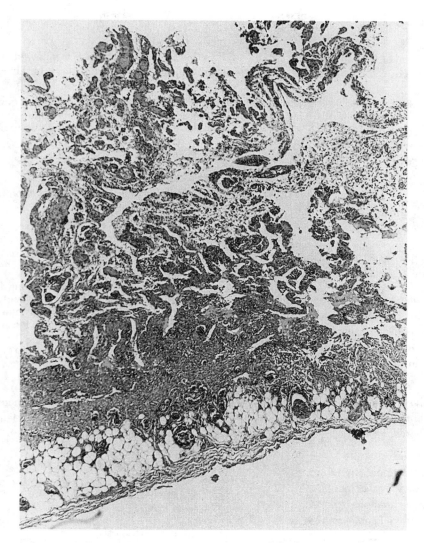

Figure 11-7. Malignant mesothelioma of the pleura. The papillary-like configuration of the small cords and glands is accompanied by a fibrous stromal reaction.

STUDY QUESTIONS

Directions: Each of the numbered items or incomplete statements in this section is followed by answers or by completions of the statement. Select the **one** lettered answer or completion that is **best** in each case.

1. Which infection is often the cause of interstitial pneumonia?

(A) Gram-positive bacterial
(B) Gram-negative bacterial
(C) Viral
(D) Fungal
(E) Parasitic

2. Which form of chronic interstitial pneumonia is characterized by marked proliferation and desquamation of alveolar lining cells?

(A) Usual interstitial pneumonitis (UIP)
(B) Idiopathic pulmonary fibrosis
(C) Desquamative interstitial pneumonitis (DIP)
(D) Lymphoid interstitial pneumonitis (LIP)
(E) Hamman-Rich syndrome

3. Of the lung tumors listed, which type belongs to the amine precursor uptake and decarboxylation (APUD) group of tumors?

(A) Hamartoma
(B) Mucoepidermoid carcinoma
(C) Adenoid cystic carcinoma
(D) Bronchial carcinoid
(E) Squamous cell carcinoma (SCC)

4. Which tumor is associated mainly with occupational exposure to asbestos?

(A) Bronchioalveolar carcinoma
(B) Oat cell carcinoma
(C) Mesothelioma
(D) Squamous cell carcinoma (SCC)
(E) Adenocarcinoma

5. A fire victim with massive thermal burns develops acute onset of respiratory failure, with diffuse pulmonary infiltrates seen on a chest radiograph. The predominant histologic finding of the most likely etiology is

(A) intraalveolar hemorrhage
(B) intraalveolar fibrin and polymorphonuclear leukocytes
(C) interstitial fibrosis
(D) granuloma formation
(E) type II pneumonocyte hyperplasia and hyaline membrane formation

6. A 65-year-old woman with a long history of smoking develops a hilar lung mass and mediastinal lymphadenopathy. From the histology of a biopsy of a mediastinal lymph node, it is impossible to distinguish between small cell cancer and malignant lymphoma. A logical next step to make the diagnosis would be

(A) lung resection
(B) electron microscopy of biopsy material
(C) a bone marrow biopsy to rule out leukemic involvement
(D) a medical workup for paraneoplastic conditions
(E) flow cytometry of peripheral blood

7. Which disorder is a common cause of chronic obstructive pulmonary disease (COPD) in the United States?

(A) Pneumoconiosis
(B) Pneumonia
(C) Interstitial lung diseases
(D) Emphysema
(E) Cystic fibrosis

8. Which carcinoma grows as well-differentiated cells that line the respiratory airspaces without invading the stroma of the lung?

(A) Squamous cell
(B) Anaplastic
(C) Large cell
(D) Small cell
(E) Bronchioalveolar

1-C	4-C	7-D
2-C	5-E	8-E
3-D	6-B	

ANSWERS AND EXPLANATIONS

1. The answer is C *[IV D 4]*.
Interstitial pneumonia usually is caused by a virus, including influenza virus, adenovirus, cytomegalovirus (CMV), herpesvirus, measles, and respiratory syncytial virus. These viruses produce alveolar cell necrosis and may be associated with formation of hyaline membranes along the alveoli.

2. The answer is C *[VI B 3 b]*.
Desquamative interstitial pneumonitis (DIP) is characterized by proliferation of desquamated alveolar lining cells within the alveolar spaces. These hyperplastic cells have the features of macrophages mixed with type II pneumonocytes. The causes of this disorder are thought to include viral, immunologic, and toxic injuries to the lungs, which induce the cellular proliferation and the pneumonia.

3. The answer is D *[VIII B 7]*.
Bronchial carcinoid tumor cells, in electron micrographs, have dense cores of argyrophilic granules and numerous mitochondria. The argentaffin granules are typical of amine precusor uptake and decarboxylation (APUD) cells, which produce a number of biogenic amines. Most bronchial carcinoids, however, do not produce the typical carcinoid syndrome. Although bronchial carcinoid is a relatively rare tumor, making up less than 5% of bronchial neoplasms, it is potentially curable by surgical resection in most cases.

4. The answer is C *[IX C 2]*.
It is now estimated that nearly two-thirds of all malignant mesotheliomas are associated with a history of industrial exposure to asbestos. However, asbestos is so widespread in the environment that nearly half of all individuals now autopsied in the United States have asbestos bodies in their lungs. The two histologic forms of malignant mesothelioma are fibrous and epithelial. The prognosis is poor for both; however, individuals with the fibrous type have a slightly better survival rate than do those with the epithelial type. Although bronchogenic carcinomas also occur more often in asbestos workers than in the general public, these cancers are far more strongly associated with cigarette smoking.

5. The answer is E *[III C 2]*.
The clinical history is typical of adult respiratory distress syndrome (ARDS), which is due to diffuse alveolar damage. Hemorrhage, acute pneumonia, and granulomatous inflammation are not part of this pathologic process. Although fibrosis may be seen as a late complication of diffuse alveolar damage, it is not a component of the acute process. Type II pneumonocytes predominate in ARDS.

6. The answer is B *[VIII B 5 a]*.
Occasionally it is impossible to distinguish between different types of poorly differentiated tumors by their light microscopic appearance, so adjuvant methods must be used to make a tissue diagnosis. Electron microscopy will reveal the neurosecretory dense core granules in small cell carcinoma. Since resection is not indicated for every type of lung tumor (including small cell carcinoma and malignant lymphoma), this procedure should not be carried out before a firm tissue diagnosis, which the other choices listed would not provide.

7. The answer is D *[V A]*.
Emphysema is one of the most common causes of chronic obstructive pulmonary disease (COPD) in the United States. It is characterized by distended lung alveoli, with variable amounts of alveolar septal wall destruction. Emphysema shows a strong association with cigarette smoking and with residence in an urban environment, with its attendant air pollution.

8. The answer is E *[VIII B 4]*.
Bronchioalveolar carcinoma is a special type of adenocarcinoma that consists of tall columnar or cuboidal epithelial malignant cells. The cells line respiratory spaces without invading the stroma of the lung. This tumor usually arises from bronchiolar epithelium, including that composed of the Clara cells, and then spreads to and intermixes with the alveolar epithelium. The tumor can present radiographically as a single peripheral nodule, as multiple nodules, or as a diffuse, pneumonia-like infiltrate.

12
Mediastinum

Maria J. Merino

I. NORMAL ANATOMY. The mediastinum lies between the pleural cavities of the thorax. Its boundaries are the thoracic inlet above and the diaphragm below, and it extends from the sternum anteriorly to the spine posteriorly. The mediastinum is divided into four **compartments**. Tumors can occur in any of these compartments (Table 12-1).

A. The superior mediastinum is located above the pericardium. It contains the aortic arch, thymus, great vessels, trachea, upper esophagus, and thoracic duct.

B. The anterior mediastinum is the space between the pericardium and the sternum. It contains lymph nodes, vessels, and fat.

C. The middle mediastinum contains the heart, pericardium, tracheal bifurcation, pulmonary arteries, and pulmonary veins.

D. The posterior mediastinum lies behind the trachea and pericardium and in front of the vertebral column. It contains the descending aorta, esophagus, thoracic duct, greater and lesser azygos veins, intercostal veins, vagal nerves, and greater splanchnic nerves.

II. CONGENITAL ABNORMALITIES. Mediastinal cysts are rare, but can occur in locations such as the pericardium and the lymphatic, tracheal, bronchial, and gastroenteric systems. The cysts probably form as defects during embryonic life and may reach different sizes. They are benign and largely asymptomatic. Surgical resection of the cysts is curative.

A. Bronchogenic cysts commonly arise in the middle mediastinum and in the tracheal area. They are filled with liquid; and when they communicate with the trachea or a bronchus, the liquid may empty into the air passages. Infection leads to abscess formation.

B. Enteric cysts occur along the esophagus, and their lining is intestinal or gastric epithelium. Abscesses may form; and if the cysts contain acid-secreting cells, the result can be perforation, ulceration, and hemorrhage.

C. Pericardial cysts are benign, and their usual location is the middle mediastinum near the right cardiophrenic angle. They are unilocular and filled with clear fluid.

III. INFLAMMATORY DISORDERS

A. Acute mediastinitis is a serious inflammation caused by descending infections, traumatic rupture and perforation of the esophagus, or infiltration of the esophagus and trachea by carcinoma. The resulting abscess formation usually requires surgical drainage.

B. Chronic mediastinitis frequently occurs in the anterior mediastinum in front of the tracheal bifurcation. It is generally a manifestation of granulomatous diseases such as tuberculosis or histoplasmosis. Cases of idiopathic fibrous mediastinitis have been reported, but they are uncommon.

1. **Histologically,** the diffuse fibrosis reveals caseating or noncaseating epithelioid granulomas. Culture and special stains may be helpful in identifying the causative organisms.

Table 12-1. Typical Lesions of Specific Mediastinal Compartments

Superior	**Posterior**
Thymoma	Neural tumors
	Enteric cyst
Anterior	
Germ cell tumors	**Any mediastinal compartment**
Middle	Malignant lymphoma and Hodgkin's
Pericardial cyst	disease
Bronchogenic cyst	Mesenchymal tumors

2. The major **complications** are due to constriction of the superior vena cava, but obstruction may appear in the tracheobronchial tree, pulmonary veins, and esophagus.

IV. TUMORS OF THE MEDIASTINUM

A. **Thymomas** are the most common neoplasms of the mediastinum. They arise in the superior mediastinum and occur in either sex and at any age, although the average age of patients is 49 years.

1. **General concepts.** Thymomas are tumors of the **thymus,** which is essentially an epithelial organ seeded by large numbers of developing T lymphocytes and other mesenchymal cells and covered by a thin fibrous capsule. Prominent during infancy and puberty, the thymus physiologically disappears or involutes in the adult.

2. **Clinical features**
   a. The majority of thymomas are slow-growing, well-encapsulated tumors with benign clinical behavior. One-third of the patients are asymptomatic, and the tumor is an incidental finding on routine chest x-ray.
   b. Other patients, however, present with an anterior mediastinal mass, cough, dysphagia, dyspnea, and retrosternal pain.
   c. Some thymomas are manifested through a systemic disorder (e.g., myasthenia gravis, red cell hypoplasia, or hypogammaglobulinemia).

3. **Pathology**
   a. **Grossly,** most thymomas are lobulated or multinodular and appear enclosed by a fibrous capsule of variable thickness, although some tumors are nonencapsulated and appear to extend by local invasion. Cut surface shows colors varying from pink to yellow. Cystic changes are encountered in up to 40% of the neoplasms.
   b. **Microscopic appearance**
      (1) **Histologically,** most thymomas are composed of an admixture of epithelial cells and lymphocytes.
         (a) The **epithelial cells,** believed to be the neoplastic cells, are characterized by eosinophilic cytoplasm and large vesicular nuclei. Ultrastructurally, they show branching tonofilaments, desmosomes, elongated cell processes, and basal laminae. Occasionally, the epithelial tumor cells are arranged in whorls, parallel bundles, or cartwheel patterns. Hassall's corpuscles may be present, but rarely are.
         (b) The **lymphocytes** are in close association with the epithelial cells and may look reactive.
      (2) Fibrous septa may divide the tumor into nodules.
   c. **Malignant thymomas** are characterized by extensive infiltration and invasion of the capsule and adjacent structures. They are also manifested by the presence of pleural implants or distant metastases. Nuclear pleomorphism, mitosis, and necrosis are not reliable signs of malignancy.

4. **Prognosis**
   a. The most important factor determining the prognosis of a patient with a thymoma is the **growth behavior and extent of the tumor**. The histologic type of a thymoma has no value in predicting prognosis. Moreover, various syndromes, especially myasthenia gravis and red cell hypoplasia, affect survival to a greater extent than do the direct effects of the tumor.
   b. **Well-encapsulated thymomas** rarely recur after surgical excision, and the 10-year survival rate for patients with these tumors approaches 100%.

     c. With **malignant thymomas,** surgical resection is difficult due to the extensive infiltration and invasion of the capsule and adjacent structures. The 10-year survival rate for patients with malignant thymomas is close to nil.

   5. Treatment. The primary form of therapy for these lesions is **surgical excision**. The role of postoperative radiation is debatable for tumors that are well encapsulated and completely resected.

B. Malignant lymphomas are one of the most common neoplasms of the mediastinum. They occur in all mediastinal compartments and may present as primary mediastinal disease or as a manifestation of a disseminated process.

   1. Most mediastinal malignant lymphomas originate in one or more of the lymph nodes that are normally present in this location. The most common type is **Hodgkin's disease** (60%); other types, such as **follicular center cell lymphomas** and **T-cell lymphoblastic lymphomas in children,** are also encountered.

   2. The tumors are histologically identical to those found in the hematopoietic system.

C. Germ cell tumors. The histogenesis of these tumors is unclear, but authorities think that they arise from misplaced germ cells during embryonic life.

   1. Teratomas can occur in both the anterior and middle mediastinum.
     a. Mature (benign cystic) teratomas are the most common of the benign germ cell neoplasms. They present during adult life as different-sized growths that may adhere to and perforate adjacent structures. **Histologically,** they are identical to benign cystic teratomas of the ovary. Surgical resection is curative.
     b. Malignant teratomas comprise fewer than 5% of mediastinal teratomas and predominantly affect men. These tumors are characterized by rapid growth.
       (1) Pathology. Grossly, the tumor appears as a solid mass with extensive areas of hemorrhage and necrosis. **Histologically,** the malignant components are usually squamous or undifferentiated carcinomas and rarely are sarcomas.
       (2) The **prognosis** for patients with these tumors is poor, the typical patient surviving less than 1 year.

   2. Seminomas are the most common malignant germ cell tumors of the mediastinum. They arise in the anterior mediastinum and are histologically identical to seminomas of the testis.

   3. Choriocarcinomas are highly malignant tumors that sometimes occur in the anterior mediastinum, predominantly in men, and present as friable, hemorrhagic, soft masses. They are histologically identical to choriocarcinomas of the uterus or testis. When a mediastinal choriocarcinoma is found, a primary testicular choriocarcinoma should always be sought.

   4. Other types of germ cell tumors, such as **endodermal sinus tumors** and **embryonal cell carcinomas,** do occur in the mediastinum, but are rare.

D. Tumors of neural origin found in the mediastinum are almost exclusively in the posterior compartment.

   1. Neurofibromas present as large, nonencapsulated, tan masses. Histologically, they show a myxoid background interspersed with wavy collagen bands and mast cells. Surgical resection of the lesion is curative.

   2. Neurilemmomas (schwannomas) also present as encapsulated tumor masses, but histologically the Antoni A and Antoni B patterns are characteristic [see Chapter 21 VIII B 6 and Chapter 25 III B 5 a (2)]. Surgical resection is curative.

E. Mesenchymal tumors, such as **lipomas, lymphangiomas,** and **hemangiomas,** can occur anywhere in the mediastinum. Histologically, these lesions are identical to those found in soft tissue elsewhere.

F. Metastatic tumors frequently involve the mediastinum and simulate primary tumors in this area.

   1. Bronchogenic carcinoma is the most common malignant neoplasm to involve the mediastinum secondarily, and it indicates extension of the tumor outside the lungs, worsening the prognosis of the patients.

   2. Other tumors known to metastasize to the mediastinum are **germ cell tumors** of the testis, **melanoma,** and **breast** and **kidney cancers.**

STUDY QUESTIONS

Directions: The numbered item or incomplete statement in this section is followed by answers or by completions of the statement. Select the **one** lettered answer or completion that is **best** in this case.

1. Which germ cell tumor is the most common malignant tumor of the anterior mediastinum?

(A) Cystic teratoma
(B) Embryonal cell carcinoma
(C) Choriocarcinoma
(D) Seminoma
(E) Endodermal sinus tumor

Directions: The group of items in this section consists of lettered options followed by a set of numbered items. For each item, select the **one** lettered option that is most closely associated with it. Each lettered option may be selected once, more than once, or not at all.

Questions 2–6

Match each statement with the mediastinal compartment that it describes.

(A) Superior mediastinum
(B) Anterior mediastinum
(C) Middle mediastinum
(D) Posterior mediastinum
(E) Entire mediastinum

2. This mediastinal compartment is the one most likely to contain a bronchogenic cyst

3. The heart lies within the pericardial sac in this mediastinal compartment

4. Rupture of the lower esophagus can cause an inflammation of this mediastinal compartment, resulting in acute mediastinitis

5. The great vessels originate from the aortic arch in this compartment of the mediastinum

6. Granulomatous disease such as tuberculosis or histoplasmosis can produce chronic mediastinitis of this compartment

1-D	4-D
2-C	5-A
3-C	6-B

ANSWERS AND EXPLANATIONS

1. The answer is D *[IV C 2].*
The most common malignant germ cell tumor occurring in the mediastinum is the seminoma. This tumor is thought to arise from germ cells that do not locate normally during embryonic development. Histologically, a seminoma that arises in the mediastinum is identical to a seminoma arising in the testes.

2–6. The answers are: 2-C *[I C; II A],* **3-C** *[I C],* **4-D** *[I D; III A],* **5-A** *[I A],* **6-B** *[I B; III B].*
The midsection of the thorax, which is the extrapleural space between the lungs, has been divided arbitrarily by anatomists and surgeons into subdivisions. The division of the mediastinum into superior, anterior, middle, and posterior compartments is the generally accepted breakdown; however, differences in terminology and referencing do exist.

   The mediastinal compartments contain specific organs and tissues. For example, the heart and pericardium are contained within the middle mediastinum, and the great vessels and aortic arch are contained within the superior mediastinum.

   Disease arising in the particular compartments of the mediastinum can be better diagnosed with an appreciation of the mediastinal anatomy. For example, although rare, bronchogenic cysts can produce serious infections in the middle mediastinum, with the possible formation of lung abscesses if an infected bronchogenic cyst should rupture into the airways. Similarly, acute mediastinitis can be a life-threatening condition requiring surgical attention when traumatic perforation of the esophagus leads to spilling of esophageal contents into the posterior mediastinum. Chronic mediastinitis is most likely to occur in the anterior mediastinum, in front of the tracheal bifurcation, as a result of granulomatous disease (e.g., tuberculosis).

13
Gastrointestinal Tract
Scott H. Saul

I. ESOPHAGUS

A. Normal anatomy and histology. The esophagus is a muscular tube about 25 cm long that extends from the pharynx to the gastroesophageal junction. It is lined with nonkeratinized squamous epithelium; some columnar epithelium may be found in the most distal 2 cm to 3 cm, in the region of the lower esophageal sphincter.

B. Congenital anomalies

1. **Esophageal atresia and tracheoesophageal fistula.** Esophageal atresia (EA) and congenital tracheoesophageal fistula (TEF) occur once in every 2000 to 4000 live births. These congenital defects usually occur together; only rarely does one exist without the other, reflecting the common embryologic development of the trachea and esophagus. In 50% of cases, other malformations also are present.
   a. EA with a fistula connecting the blind lower esophageal pouch to the trachea is seen in 90% of cases.
   b. Infants usually present with respiratory distress, excessive salivation, and regurgitation within 24 hours of birth. About 35% of the infants are premature, and maternal hydramnios occurs in 85% of cases.
   c. Although these defects previously were fatal, early recognition and surgical intervention have raised the survival rate to almost 90%.

2. **Heterotopia.** Occasionally, **ectopic rests** containing gastric epithelium, with parietal cells, may be found in the esophagus, particularly in the cervical region.
   a. Rarely, adenocarcinomas arise in these foci.
   b. Ectopic rests must be distinguished from the parietal cells found in Barrett's esophagus [see I D 2 a (3)], which is a metaplastic phenomenon.

3. **Rings and webs.** These concentric constrictions of the esophagus consist of folds of mucosa, usually containing little smooth muscle. Patients may present with dysphagia, or these structures may be incidental findings. Their pathogenesis is obscure. Although often considered to be congenital abnormalities, some of these structures are clearly postinflammatory adhesions.
   a. **Upper esophageal webs** may be found in middle-aged women in association with iron deficiency anemia, atrophic glossopathy, and dysphagia (the **Plummer-Vinson** or **Paterson-Kelly syndrome**) or may be an isolated finding.
   b. **Lower esophageal (Schatzki's) rings** occur close to the gastroesophageal junction. They show no association with iron deficiency anemia and no female predominance.

C. Hiatal hernia. Upward herniation of the stomach through the esophageal hiatus can occur in two forms.

1. The **sliding type** represents about 90% of all hiatal hernias. The esophagogastric junction and a bell-shaped portion of the stomach lie above the diaphragm. This type is present in 10% of the general population and in 50% or more of patients with reflux esophagitis (see I D 2 a).

2. The **rolling type** represents only 10% of hiatal hernias. A portion of the gastric fundus "rolls" alongside the distal esophagus; the esophagogastric junction remains in its normal location.

D. Esophagitis

1. **General description.** A variety of insults can cause inflammatory disease of the esophagus (i.e., esophagitis). Regardless of etiology, there are similar **symptoms**—retrosternal pain ("heartburn") and dysphagia—and similar **pathologic findings**—chronic and acute inflammation, epithelial hyperplasia, hyperemia, and ulcers, sometimes with formation of fibrous strictures.

2. **Classification.** The more common forms of esophagitis and their causes are as follows.

   a. **Reflux esophagitis,** the most common form of esophagitis, is also the most common motor disorder of the esophagus. Reflux esophagitis is a chronic condition, whereas most other forms of esophagitis are acute.

      (1) **Reduced lower esophageal sphincter pressure** allows gastroesophageal reflux. The degree of mucosal damage depends on the nature of the refluxing fluid (acid, pepsin, bile), the duration of exposure to the reflux, and the efficiency of the clearing mechanism.

      (2) The motor disorder is usually idiopathic, but it may be secondary to a variety of conditions (e.g., pregnancy, diabetes mellitus, ethanol abuse, prolonged intubation, prior surgery).

      (3) **Barrett's (columnar lined) esophagus** complicates reflux esophagitis in about 10% of cases.

         (a) The types of epithelia seen in this metaplastic disorder include the following.

            (i) **Columnar epithelium** (similar to **gastric cardiac** and **gastric fundic** epithelium) may be found at least 2 cm to 3 cm above the gastroesophageal junction.

            (ii) More importantly, **intestinal ("specialized" columnar) epithelium** (showing villous architecture, goblet cells, and occasionally, Paneth's cells), occurring anywhere in the distal esophagus, is considered diagnostic of Barrett's esophagus.

         (b) Endoscopically, this epithelium has a red, velvety appearance, contrasting with the grayish-white squamous mucosa. **Ulcers,** sometimes deep and resembling peptic ulcers, may occur in this setting.

         (c) Although **strictures** in the distal esophagus may occur with reflux alone, more proximal strictures are nearly always associated with Barrett's metaplasia.

         (d) **Progressive dysplastic epithelial abnormalities** may be noted in the columnar epithelium, particularly the specialized type. Of major importance, 3%–10% of patients with Barrett's esophagus present with or develop **esophageal adenocarcinoma**.

         (e) **Surveillance biopsies** are typically performed annually to look for prominent (high-grade) dysplasia [see IV E 4 a (4)]. When it is found, esophagogastrectomy is often performed in suitable candidates for surgery, because up to 50% of these patients harbor an invasive adenocarcinoma. Some reserve esophagogastrectomy for those who demonstrate invasive adenocarcinoma on biopsy.

   b. **Infectious esophagitis.** The esophagus is remarkably resistant to infection; infectious esophagitis usually is seen only in debilitated or immunosuppressed patients (i.e., as an opportunistic infection).

      (1) **Candidal esophagitis** causes ulcers, which often are linear with white elevated plaques. Typical yeasts and pseudohyphae also are found.

      (2) **Herpetic esophagitis** causes discrete punched-out ulcers with raised margins. Typical herpetic viral inclusions (multinucleate epithelial cells with nuclear molding and intranuclear inclusions) are present at the ulcer margin.

      (3) Rarely, other organisms [e.g., cytomegalovirus (CMV) or various bacteria] may cause esophagitis. *Mycobacterium tuberculosis* causes the formation of caseating granulomas.

   c. **Iatrogenic esophagitis.** Drugs (particularly chemotherapeutic agents), irradiation, and instrumentation may cause esophagitis.

   d. **Esophagitis from corrosive chemicals,** either acid or alkaline, may follow accidental ingestion (generally in children) or an attempted suicide (generally in adults or adolescents). Coagulative necrosis occurs and may result in perforation and death. Healing usually results in stricture formation (**"lye stricture"**).

   e. **Other disorders,** such as pemphigus vulgaris, Crohn's disease (CD), or Behçet's syndrome, also may cause esophagitis.

E. Motor disorders. The **swallowing mechanism** requires a series of coordinated motions: Relaxation of the upper esophageal sphincter (normally constricted at rest) allows the food bolus to enter the esophagus, where peristaltic contractions propel it downward until it passes through the lower esophageal sphincter, which also has relaxed. Abnormalities anywhere along this pathway may lead to esophageal dysfunction.

1. **Reflux esophagitis** (see I D 2 a)

2. **Achalasia** is a disorder characterized by incomplete relaxation of the lower esophageal sphincter, typically with elevated resting lower esophageal sphincter pressure and lack of propulsive esophageal peristalsis. This combination produces functional obstruction of the distal esophagus.
    a. **Etiology.** It is unknown in virtually all cases, although various neurogenic defects have been postulated. Destruction of the myenteric plexus by *Trypanosoma cruzi* in Chagas' disease causes an identical clinicopathologic picture, supporting the hypothesis of primary neural dysfunction. Achalasia may be caused by tumors in close proximity to the esophagus; therefore, a neoplastic disorder must be ruled out.
    b. **Clinical features and diagnosis**
        (1) Achalasia may affect both sexes at any age but usually starts in the third or fourth decade. Patients present with dysphagia for both solids and liquids. Regurgitation and aspiration are common.
        (2) A barium esophagogram reveals a characteristic beaklike fusiform tapering. This feature, along with demonstration of failure of the lower esophageal sphincter to relax on swallowing, complete absence of peristalsis, frequently elevated resting lower esophageal sphincter pressure, and increased esophageal contraction in response to methacholine, establishes the diagnosis.
        (3) Long-standing achalasia is associated with an increased risk of esophageal squamous carcinoma.
    c. **Pathology.** A dilated proximal esophagus (**megaesophagus**) with distal tapering is found. Myenteric ganglion cells are absent or markedly decreased in the dilated esophageal body but may or may not be decreased in the distal tapered region. Chronic inflammation of the myenteric plexus (**ganglionitis**) may be present. Vagal fibers leading to the esophagus may show degenerative changes.

3. **Progressive systemic sclerosis (scleroderma)** is a systemic disease characterized by fibrosis, smooth muscle atrophy, and a variable inflammatory infiltrate. The skin, gastrointestinal tract, kidney, heart, lungs, and musculoskeletal system frequently are involved.
    a. **Clinical features.** Overall, about 80% of patients have esophageal dysfunction, with symptoms of obstruction, reflux, or both. Patients with the **CREST syndrome** (**c**alcinosis, **R**aynaud's phenomenon, **e**sophageal dysmotility, **s**clerodactyly, and **t**elangiectasia) have a better prognosis than do patients with other forms of the disease.
    b. **Pathology.** Smooth muscle atrophy, affecting the distal two-thirds of the esophagus, and fibrosis are typical findings, often associated with hyaline thickening of small arterioles. The esophagus often is thickened and stenotic (fibrotic) distally and dilated proximally. Damage to the lower esophageal sphincter causes associated reflux esophagitis and Barrett's esophagus, with the related risk of developing adenocarcinoma.

4. **Diffuse esophageal spasm** is characterized by simultaneous painful, nonrepetitive, nonperistaltic contractions of high amplitude in the distal two-thirds of the esophagus, associated with thickening of the tunica muscularis (muscularis propria) in this region (**idiopathic muscular hypertrophy**). Ganglion cells are present but may be inflamed (ganglionitis).

F. **Esophageal diverticula**

1. These **congenital or acquired outpouchings,** which may occur at any level of the esophageal wall, are commonly associated with a motility disorder. They often are asymptomatic but may cause dysphagia and regurgitation.

2. **Pharyngoesophageal (Zenker's) diverticulum** is probably the most common. It is located just behind the cricoid cartilage in the region of the upper esophageal sphincter and often contains all layers of the esophageal wall.
    a. The prolonged stasis of trapped food associated with the diverticulum appears to increase the risk of developing **squamous cell carcinoma (SCC)**.
    b. This disorder is presumably related to increased contact of the epithelium with carcinogens or increased epithelial turnover secondary to stasis-induced inflammation.

G. Esophageal lacerations and rupture

1. **Mallory-Weiss syndrome** is characterized by increased intraabdominal pressure, usually from strenuous vomiting (often in alcoholics) and failure of the lower esophageal sphincter to relax. This pressure causes one or more **partial-thickness lacerations** parallel to the long axis of the esophagus, in the region of the gastroesophageal junction and gastric cardia. These lacerations may be responsible for up to 15% of cases of massive upper gastrointestinal bleeding. Most patients respond to conservative therapy.

2. **Boerhaave's syndrome** is characterized by **complete rupture** of the esophagus. In 90% of cases, this break occurs in a weak spot located in the left posterior distal esophagus. The rupture results from the sudden propulsion of gastric contents into a fully relaxed esophagus, possibly with a delay in opening of the upper esophageal sphincter. Pneumothorax and subcutaneous emphysema, but not massive bleeding, usually result. The mortality rate is quite high.

H. Esophageal varices. Esophageal submucosal veins become dilated as a result of portal hypertension and shunting within the portal venous system (left coronary vein to esophageal veins). About two-thirds of patients with cirrhosis develop varices. Esophageal varices appear endoscopically as bluish linear streaks in the distal esophagus. They often bleed (secondary to mucosal ulceration) and are associated with significant morbidity and mortality rates.

I. Esophageal carcinoma

1. **Frequency and classification.** Esophageal carcinoma represents about 10% of all gastrointestinal cancers and accounts for 2%–5% of all cancer deaths in the United States. About 70%–80% of the tumors are **SCC;** however, **adenocarcinoma,** almost always arising in Barrett's esophagus, forms another important group, comprising nearly all of the remaining 20%–30%.

2. **Epidemiology and risk factors.** The incidence of esophageal SCC in the United States is 2–8 per 100,000 population per year; the rates are more than 10 times higher in areas of China, Iran, and Russia. Esophageal carcinoma is a tumor occurring in adult life, reaching peak incidence between age 50 and 70, and affecting three times more men than women in the United States.

   a. **Alcohol** and **tobacco** abuse are important **associated factors** in areas of low risk; other environmental or genetic factors may be operative in high-risk regions. A role for human papillomavirus (HPV) is under investigation.

   b. SCC may be associated with various conditions characterized by **stasis,** such as diverticula, achalasia, lye or peptic strictures, and the Plummer-Vinson syndrome.

   c. **Barrett's esophagus** and **adenocarcinoma** may develop in conditions associated with reflux esophagitis.

3. **Clinical features and diagnosis**

   a. Symptoms occur late, with progressive dysphagia, weight loss, and pain being the most common. Symptoms of reflux esophagitis may be absent in one-third of patients with adenocarcinoma.

   b. The tumors spread locally to regional lymph nodes before metastasizing to distant sites, such as the liver and lung. TEF may occur.

   c. Diagnosis is confirmed by biopsy and cytology. In high-risk areas or in patients with known risk factors, endoscopic screening to detect early lesions may be advisable.

4. **Pathology**

   a. **Macroscopic appearance.** In the overwhelming majority of cases, lesions of SCC and adenocarcinoma are located in the distal or middle third of the esophagus. Tumors most commonly are fungating, polypoid, or nodular; less often, they are ulcerating (Figure 13-1) or diffusely infiltrating. Early lesions may appear as small, flat, or slightly elevated zones.

   b. **Microscopic appearance.** In both SCC and adenocarcinoma, the degree of differentiation is quite variable. Both well and poorly differentiated foci often occur in the same tumor. Differentiation has little relationship to survival.

5. **Prognosis and treatment**

   a. **Prognosis.** Overall, the 5-year survival rate for esophageal carcinoma of either type is about 10%. There is a strong correlation between the degree of mural invasion and survival: The fact that most patients have tumors that extend into the adventitia at the time of diagnosis explains the poor prognosis. If the carcinoma is confined to the submucosa, with negative

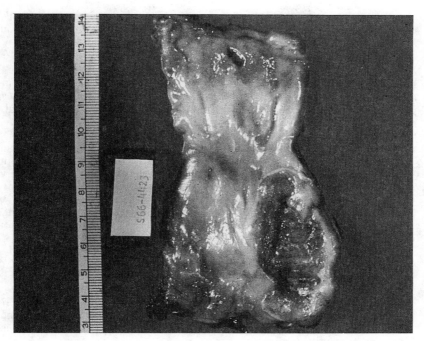

Figure 13-1. Gross view of an ulcerating carcinoma involving the distal segment of the esophagus.

lymph nodes (**early esophageal cancer**), the 5-year survival rate may reach 90%. Clearly, early detection of carcinoma or its precursor lesion (**dysplasia**) is the only way to improve survival.

    b. Treatment is basically surgical, although radiation may be used for palliation.

J. Other tumors, both **malignant** (small cell carcinoma, leiomyosarcoma) and **benign** (leiomyoma, granular cell tumor), may occur but are rare or clinically unimportant.

II. STOMACH

A. Normal anatomy and histology

    1. The stomach is divided into four anatomic **regions,** all of which have a surface lining of tall columnar mucin-secreting cells.

        a. The **cardia** is located directly adjacent to the gastroesophageal junction. It contains mucin-secreting glands.

        b. The **fundus** is located to the left of the esophagus cephalad to the gastroesophageal junction. Its lining is similar to that of the body.

        c. The **body** is the largest anatomic compartment. It contains the acid-secreting gastric glands, which are characterized by numerous **parietal cells** (producing hydrochloric acid and intrinsic factor) and **chief cells** (producing pepsinogen).

        d. The **antrum** comprises the distal third of the stomach, including the region of the pyloric sphincter (pyloric antrum), and ends at the pyloroduodenal junction. Mucin-secreting glands are found, as are the gastrin-secreting **G cells.**

    2. The **gastric mucosal barrier,** which prevents autodigestion by intraluminal gastric acid, appears to consist of the tight junctions between the epithelial cells, the layer of mucus attached to the epithelial surface, and the buffers secreted by the surface cells.

B. Congenital anomalies

    1. Pyloric stenosis occurs in approximately 0.4% of all live births. It is familial and is three times more common in males, particularly firstborn males. Infants usually present at 3 to 4 weeks of age with vomiting. Marked thickening of the pyloric musculature is a characteristic finding. Myotomy usually is curative.

2. Heterotopic pancreatic tissue may be present in the distal stomach, predominantly in the submucosa. These foci are usually less than 1 cm in diameter. Normal pancreatic acini and ducts are noted, but islets are rare. Clinically, pyloric obstruction and epigastric pain may be present.

C. Gastritis

1. Acute (erosive or hemorrhagic) gastritis. This condition usually is sudden in onset and, although often transient, may cause extensive, life-threatening gastric bleeding. The clinical and pathologic findings form a continuum from more mild forms (acute superficial gastritis) to more severe forms (acute hemorrhagic gastritis, stress erosions, ulcers). The term "acute" refers to the rapidity of onset rather than the type of inflammatory infiltrate.

    a. Etiology. Well-documented associations include use of nonsteroidal anti-inflammatory drugs (NSAIDs), such as aspirin; chronic ethanol abuse; heavy smoking; antineoplastic agents; severe stress, as from extensive burns (**Curling's ulcer**), or central nervous system (CNS) trauma (**Cushing's ulcer**); and mucosal hypoperfusion. A few cases of acute gastritis associated with *Helicobacter pylori* have been reported.

    b. Clinical features. Patients may complain of abdominal pain, nausea, vomiting, hematemesis, or melena or may be entirely asymptomatic, depending on the severity of the lesion.

    c. Pathology
        (1) Macroscopic appearance. Changes range from thickening (edema) and erythema of the mucosal folds to a number of randomly distributed **erosions** (limited to the mucosa) and **ulcers** (extending below the mucosa) with adherent blood clots.
        (2) Microscopic appearance. In milder forms, the surface epithelium may be intact, with edema, focal hemorrhage, and occasional leukocytes in the lamina propria. Conspicuous in more severe cases is necrosis of the mucosa (and perhaps of deeper layers of the gastric wall), with an associated acute (neutrophilic) inflammatory infiltrate and prominent hemorrhage.

    d. Treatment and prognosis. Conventional peptic ulcer regimens are usually tried first. Lesions may wax and wane over months to years. No treatment is consistently effective.

2. Specific forms of chronic gastritis. Several unusual forms of chronic gastritis have specific distinguishing histologic features.

    a. Granulomatous gastritis may be idiopathic or associated with CD, tuberculosis, or, very rarely, sarcoidosis.

    b. Eosinophilic gastritis, characterized by numerous eosinophils within the gastric wall, often is associated with peripheral blood eosinophilia and other evidence of allergy. Other portions of the gastrointestinal tract may be involved.

    c. Lymphocytic gastritis is characterized by the presence of numerous intraepithelial lymphocytes. It has been described as an isolated phenomenon or in association with celiac disease, *H. pylori* infection, or protein-losing enteropathy or occasionally with several other unrelated disorders.

3. Chronic nonspecific gastritis. Chronic nonspecific gastritis is characterized by progressive inflammatory changes, which may result in glandular atrophy and intestinal metaplasia. Although chronic gastritis may be diffuse, it often preferentially involves the body or antrum.

    a. Etiology and classification
        (1) Fundic gastritis (type A) may be associated with pernicious anemia. In pernicious anemia, antibodies to parietal cells and to intrinsic factor often are found in the serum.
        (2) Antral gastritis (type B) has been ascribed to chronic ethanol or NSAID use, postgastrectomy states, peptic ulcer disease, and bile reflux.
        (3) Recently gastric *H. pylori* has been found in the majority of cases which were previously classified as type B.
            (a) This gram-negative bacterium can survive in the mucous layer of the stomach despite the low intragastric pH because it possesses a urease enzyme that breaks down urea, thereby creating a locally more alkaline environment.
            (b) Current data suggest that *H. pylori* has an important role in the pathogenesis of chronic gastritis and peptic ulcer disease (see II D 2 b).

    b. Clinical features. Patients often are asymptomatic, although they may have nonspecific abdominal complaints.

    c. Pathology
        (1) Macroscopic appearance. The mucosa may appear relatively normal, may be slightly nodular, or, in late stages, may be quite thin and shiny, with visible submucosal vasculature.

(2) **Microscopic appearance**

    (a) Chronic nonspecific gastritis may be divided into **superficial** and **atrophic (deep)** forms, depending on the depth of lymphocyte and plasma cell infiltration.

    (b) Active disease is manifested by a **neutrophilic infiltrate** that may progressively destroy the glands, causing them to become shortened and dilated and to develop intestinal metaplasia (with goblet cells, Paneth's cells, absorptive cells, and a villous architecture). Parietal and chief cells also may be replaced by pyloric-type glands representing so-called pyloric metaplasia.

    (c) The end stage, **gastric atrophy,** shows nearly complete glandular atrophy, with a loss of parietal cells in the fundic type of gastritis.

  d. Prognosis. Metaplastic epithelium may become dysplastic, and the risk of adenocarcinoma increases, particularly in patients with marked atrophic gastritis and pernicious anemia. Carcinoids also may develop in patients with chronic type A gastritis.

  e. Treatment [see I D 2 a (3) (e)]

D. Chronic peptic ulcer disease. In 80% of cases, chronic ulcers are solitary excavations. They extend at least into the submucosa and frequently more deeply. Gastric acid and pepsin are necessary for their production. Peptic ulcers may occur at any age but are most common in middle age. Men are more often affected than women.

  1. Location. Although ulcers may occur anywhere within the gastrointestinal tract, 98% are located in the proximal duodenum or in the stomach (usually in the antrum on the lesser curvature). Peptic ulcers also occur in the distal small bowel in Zollinger-Ellison syndrome; in Barrett's esophagus; adjacent to heterotopic gastric mucosa in Meckel's diverticulum; or at the margin of a gastroenterostomy.

  2. Pathogenesis. The integrity of the gastric and duodenal mucosa is determined by the balance between the protective and the damaging factors (Table 13-1). Infection with *H. pylori* and use of NSAIDs are the most important damaging factors in the presence of acid and pepsin.

    a. Lowering of mucosal resistance by various irritants in a person with normal or low acid–pepsin secretion is typical for a gastric ulcer. Associated chronic gastritis invariably is present.

    b. Gastric infection with *H. pylori* appears to be an important factor, since it is found in nearly all patients with duodenal ulcer and in the majority of those with gastric ulcer. Complete eradication of *H. pylori* generally results in ulcer healing.

    c. Increased acid–pepsin secretion appears to be very important in the genesis of duodenal ulcers. Patients who are blood group O and are nonsecretors (of ABO blood group antigens in body fluids, such as saliva) appear to be at increased risk.

  3. Pathology

    a. Macroscopically, a sharply punched-out hole, 2 cm to 4 cm in diameter, penetrates into the tunica muscularis (muscularis propria). The ulcer base is clean and lacks the heaped-up margins often seen in ulcerating cancer.

Table 13-1. Protective and Damaging Factors Affecting Peptic Ulcer Disease and Gastroduodenal Mucosal Integrity

Protective Factors	Damaging Factors
Bicarbonate	Acid*
Mucus	Pepsin*
Cell renewal	*H. pylori*[†]
Prostaglandins	NSAIDs[†]
Good blood flow	Ischemia
	Ethanol
	Bile salts
	Cigarette smoking

NSAIDs = nonsteroidal anti-inflammatory drugs.
*Acid and pepsin are required to produce peptic ulcers.
[†]*H. pylori* and NSAIDs, alone or in combination, are found in association with almost all peptic ulcers.

   b. Microscopically, the appearance varies with activity and degree of ulcer healing. Active lesions have four layers: surface fibrin, an inflammatory layer rich in neutrophils, a zone of granulation tissue, and, deepest, a fibrous scar with thick-walled blood vessels. Progressive healing may lead to reepithelialization.

   c. Biopsy and cytologic examination are important to rule out malignancy [see II G 1 c (2)].

4. Complications
   a. Hemorrhage, the most common complication, occurs in 25% to 33% of cases and is due to damage of vessels at the ulcer base. Sometimes massive, it is responsible for 25% of ulcer deaths.

   b. Perforation (Figure 13-2) and **penetration** into an adjacent organ, such as the pancreas, are rare, but often fatal complications.

   c. Obstruction of the duodenum or pylorus can result from scarring.

   d. Malignant transformation is rare, occurring in fewer than 1% of cases. Nearly all ulcerating carcinomas were neoplasms at their inception.

5. Prognosis and treatment. Peptic ulcer is a relapsing condition marked by recurrent gastric pain. Treatment modalities include medication to reduce gastric acidity, antibiotics and bismuth-containing compounds to eradicate *H. pylori,* and, sometimes, surgery.

E. Hyperplastic gastropathy. Although often designated as "hypertrophic gastritis," this group of disorders is not characterized by hypertrophy or gastritis, but by marked thickening of the gastric rugae owing to hyperplasia of various mucosal epithelial cell types. The prominent gastric folds may be misinterpreted radiographically or endoscopically as diffusely infiltrating carcinoma or lymphoma. Two characteristic disorders are described.

1. Ménétrier's disease is characterized by hyperplasia of gastric mucous cells and by protein-losing enteropathy, hypoalbuminemia, and, often, hypo- or achlorhydria. Patients may be asymptomatic or may present with nausea, vomiting, or intense gastric pain. Rare cases of associated gastric carcinoma have been reported. Gastrectomy may be necessary.

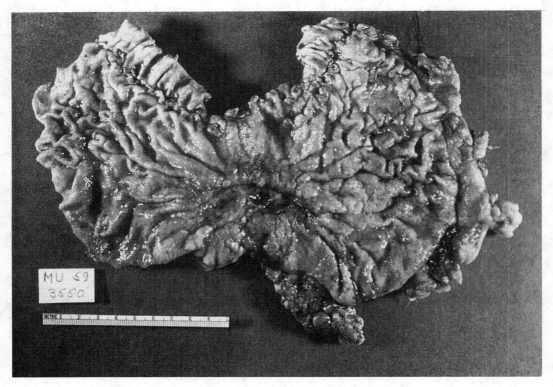

Figure 13-2. Chronic peptic ulcer of the stomach, with acute perforation.

2. Zollinger-Ellison syndrome is characterized by hyperplasia of parietal and chief cells secondary to the excessive secretion of gastrin by a **gastrinoma** (see Chapter 20 V C 2 c). This secretion of gastrin leads to gastric acid hypersecretion and one or more peptic ulcers. Occasionally, these ulcers may be in unusual locations, such as the distal small bowel. The gastrinomas usually arise in the pancreas or duodenum, and two-thirds are malignant. The acid hypersecretion usually can be controlled medically. If possible, the gastrinoma is resected. Primary antral G-cell hyperplasia also may result in parietal and chief cell hyperplasia.

F. Benign tumors. Although not infrequent incidental findings at autopsy, on endoscopy, or from radiographs, benign gastric tumors are only occasionally the cause of clinical symptoms.

  1. Epithelial growths. Although the term "gastric polyp" usually applies to an epithelial lesion, strictly speaking, any protrusion into the lumen can be considered a polyp.

   a. Hyperplastic polyps constitute 80% to 90% of benign gastric epithelial tumors. They may be single or multiple and commonly have a diameter of 1 cm or less. Microscopically, they are characterized by a proliferation of elongated and often cystically dilated glands lined by surface mucus-type cells. Their neoplastic potential is negligible.

   b. Fundic gland polyps (found in 1% of all gastroscopies) are characterized by a nonneoplastic proliferation of cystically dilated acid-secreting glands. They occur as single or, more commonly, multiple small (diameter of a few millimeters) polyps in the gastric fundus or body. They have no precancerous potential. They are, most commonly, incidental findings in normal middle-aged women, although patients with familial adenomatous polyposis (FAP) more frequently have such polyps.

   c. Adenomas (constituting 10% to 20%) usually are solitary and sessile, although occasionally they may be pedunculated. They are usually greater than 2 cm in diameter.

     (1) Microscopically, gastric adenomas consist of a tubular, tubulovillous, or villous proliferation of dysplastic columnar epithelial cells with varying degrees of nuclear hyperchromatism, an increased nucleus:cytoplasm ratio, and glandular crowding. The histologic appearance is quite similar to that of colonic adenomas (see IV E 4).

     (2) Gastric adenomas are, by definition, neoplastic polyps, and roughly 50% (almost always larger than 2 cm in diameter) are associated with invasive adenocarcinoma.

   d. Polyps characteristic of various gastrointestinal **polyposis syndromes** such as Peutz-Jeghers syndrome, juvenile polyposis, and FAP (see IV E 3 a, b, 4 c), may be found in the stomach.

  2. Mesenchymal tumors. The most common benign mesenchymal tumors of the stomach are **leiomyomas.** The term **benign stromal tumor** sometimes is used instead of leiomyoma because ultrastructural and immunohistochemical evidence of smooth muscle differentiation often is difficult to identify, and there is some controversy regarding the cell of origin of these spindle cell and epithelioid cell tumors.

   a. Leiomyomas may be found at any age, but patients are typically ages 30 to 70. Although leiomyomas may be incidental findings, patients with tumors greater than 3 cm in diameter often present with bleeding, pain, or other symptoms.

   b. Size varies from 1 cm to 20 cm, although leiomyosarcoma must be considered when lesions are greater than 6 cm in diameter. The tumors are usually intramural, causing slight elevation of the mucosa; occasionally, they are attached to the muscularis propria by a thin pedicle and thus project into the omentum. Microscopically, leiomyomas are similar to benign smooth muscle neoplasms found elsewhere.

  3. Other benign tumors, such as schwannomas or lipomas, occasionally arise in the stomach.

G. Malignant tumors. Over 95% of primary gastric malignancies are adenocarcinomas; however, lymphoma, leiomyosarcoma, and carcinoid tumors also occur.

  1. Adenocarcinoma

   a. Epidemiology. Adenocarcinoma of the stomach is a common neoplasm in certain regions, such as Japan (where it is the leading cause of cancer death in men), the Scandinavian countries, and Iceland. In the United States, although still ranking in the top 10 causes of death (causing 5% of all cancer deaths), its incidence has declined since 1930, from 33 cases to 6 cases per 100,000 population per year. This decline is related to a prominent decrease in the number of distal tumors, whereas the number of cardiac adenocarcinomas has actually increased. Currently, men are affected slightly more often than women; in the past, the difference was more striking.

b. Pathogenesis
  (1) Environmental factors appear to be important in the pathogenesis of gastric carcinoma. Among persons moving from a high-risk to a low-risk region, there is a progressive decline in incidence. Diet, particularly the presence of nitrites (used as food preservatives), has received much attention as an important factor in the pathogenesis of gastric cancer.
  (2) Genetic factors appear to play only a small role; only 4% of patients have a family history of gastric cancer.
  (3) Predisposing conditions include the following.
    (a) Chronic atrophic gastritis with intestinal metaplasia, often occurring in patients with pernicious anemia, is associated with an increased risk for developing gastric adenocarcinoma.
    (b) Postgastrectomy states. Roughly 3% of postgastrectomy patients develop adenocarcinoma, usually 20 years or more after the surgery. The risk probability is related to the occurrence of gastritis in the gastric stump.
c. Clinical features and diagnosis
  (1) Patients may be asymptomatic or may have symptoms indistinguishable from peptic ulcer disease, (e.g., pain, anorexia, weight loss, melena, and anemia). An epigastric mass and evidence of metastases are characteristic of later stages.
  (2) Gastric cancer may mimic peptic ulcers endoscopically and radiographically. Biopsy and cytologic examination of every ulcer to confirm its benign or malignant nature, therefore, are of utmost importance.
d. Pathology
  (1) Early versus advanced gastric cancer
    (a) Early gastric cancer (EGC) is carcinoma that is limited to the mucosa and submucosa and has not invaded the muscularis propria. However, lymph node metastases may be present. Because endoscopic surveillance is common in high-risk countries, EGC accounts for one-third of all gastric cancers in Japan, but only 10% to 20% in the United States.
    (b) Advanced gastric cancer (AGC) indicates extension into or beyond the muscularis propria. AGC accounts for about 70% of cases in high-risk regions and 80% to 90% in low-risk regions.
  (2) Macroscopic appearance
    (a) EGC lesions may be found anywhere in the stomach and appear elevated, flat, or, most commonly (in 70%), depressed. Size is variable (up to 8 cm); lesions often are quite small.
    (b) AGC involves the antrum in 50% of cases and the body in 25% of cases; the remainder of advanced lesions are localized to the cardia or involve the entire stomach. AGC may be fungating, polypoid, flat (superficial), ulcerated, or diffusely infiltrating (linitis plastica, or "leather-bottle stomach").
      (i) Ulcerating carcinomas must be distinguished from benign ulcers. The former usually are larger, with heaped-up rather than punched-out borders and a shaggy rather than clean base. The ulcerating and fungating forms account for 60% to 70% of all gastric carcinomas.
      (ii) The **linitis plastica** variant has no luminal mass, but nearly the entire gastric wall is markedly thickened by tumor. This type accounts for 10% to 20% of cases.
  (3) Microscopic appearance. Both EGC and AGC may be divided into two basic patterns.
    (a) Intestinal (expanding) type. Cohesive masses of fairly well-differentiated glands or cords of tumor cells tend to push as a broad front into the gastric wall. This type often is associated with adjacent intestinal metaplasia of the gastric mucosa. This histologic pattern appears to be decreasing in frequency.
    (b) Diffuse (infiltrative) type. Individual tumor cells permeate the gastric wall diffusely. Frequently, cytoplasmic mucin pushes the nucleus to the side, forming the so-called **signet-ring cell** (Figure 13-3). This histologic type of gastric cancer is relatively more common in women and has not changed in frequency.
e. Prognosis and treatment
  (1) Patients with EGC have a 5-year survival rate of about 70% to 90%, whereas those with AGC have a poor prognosis, with attempts at curative surgical resection in only about 40% of cases and an overall 5-year survival rate of 5% to 15%. Thus, early diagnosis is critical.

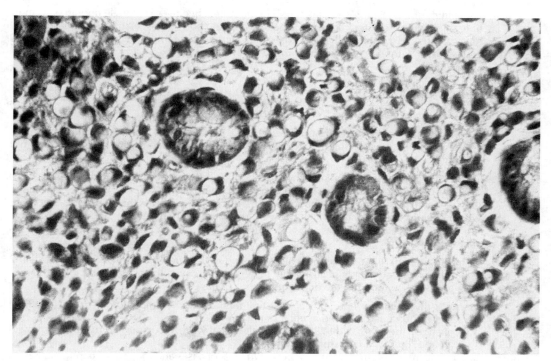

Figure 13-3. Numerous signet-ring cells, characteristic of the diffuse or infiltrative microscopic pattern of gastric cancer. This cell type typically is associated with the linitis plastica macroscopic appearance [hematoxylin and eosin (H and E) stain; × 400].

    (2) Regional lymph nodes and the liver often are sites of metastases, although spread to the ovaries, supraclavicular (Virchow's) nodes, or peritoneal cul-de-sac may be the first sign of disease. Ovarian tumors that contain signet-ring cells are termed **Krukenberg's tumors**.

        (a) Krukenberg's tumors typically are bilateral. They are most frequently metastatic from the stomach but occasionally originate in the colon, appendix, or another site.

        (b) The great majority of gastric tumors that metastasize to the ovary are Krukenberg's tumors. Primary ovarian Krukenberg's tumors rarely, if ever, occur.

2. Gastrointestinal lymphomas

    a. Almost always of the **non-Hodgkin's type,** lymphomas in the gastrointestinal tract usually are secondary foci of widely disseminated lymphoma. Primary gastrointestinal lymphoma is most commonly gastric and comprises only 3% to 5% of all gastric malignancies. Less commonly involved are (in decreasing order) the ileum, large bowel, and other gastrointestinal sites.

    b. **Macroscopically,** these tumors may be polypoid, ulcerative, infiltrative, or even resemble gastritis. Most of the primary lymphomas are derived from B cells, which are part of the mucosa-associated lymphoid tumor (MALT); **histologically** they may be divided into low-grade (small lymphoid cells) and high-grade (large lymphoid cells) types.

    c. **Prognosis** for gastrointestinal lymphomas is related to stage and histologic type of disease; overall, it is better than the prognosis for patients with carcinoma.

3. Leiomyosarcoma represents about 1% of gastric malignancies. Distinction from leiomyoma can be difficult since symptoms are similar.

    a. As with gastric leiomyoma, the histogenesis of this malignant tumor is controversial; thus, it sometimes is termed **malignant gastric stromal tumor**.

    b. **Histologically,** the gastric lesions are similar to leiomyosarcomas found at other sites (see Chapter 25 III D 3 b). Mitotic rate and size (usually greater than 6 cm) are the best predictors of metastatic potential.

    c. Hematogenous dissemination to the liver and lung occurs frequently. Complete surgical resection is the treatment of choice.

4. Carcinoid tumors occasionally are found in the stomach, either as a single nodule or as multiple small foci. The latter frequently arise in the gastric body in association with chronic atrophic gastritis and secondary hypergastrinemia. Overall, long-term survival is the rule, although metastases to lymph nodes and liver may occur.

III. SMALL BOWEL

A. Normal anatomy and histology

1. The adult small bowel ranges from 12 feet to 20 feet in length. It is divided into the duodenum, jejunum, and ileum. The small bowel is specialized to facilitate the absorption of required nutrients.

2. The **histologic hallmark** of the small bowel mucosa is the presence of **villi,** fingerlike structures lined by absorptive cells with an extensive microvillous brush border. Interspersed among these cells are goblet and neuroendocrine cells. Between the villi are the **crypts of Lieberkühn,** which contain undifferentiated cells as well as goblet, neuroendocrine, and Paneth's cells.

B. Congenital anomalies

1. **Heterotopic pancreatic tissue** most often is found in the duodenum; it is rarely more than 2 cm in diameter and is only occasionally responsible for symptoms. Heterotopic gastric mucosa also may be found in the duodenum.

2. **Meckel's diverticulum** represents a persistent remnant of the omphalomesenteric (vitelline) duct and is found in 2% of the general population.
   a. It occurs in the ileum within 90 cm of the ileocecal valve. It contains all layers of the bowel wall and, thus, is a **true diverticulum**.
   b. Acid-secreting gastric mucosa is present in 50% of cases and may cause peptic ulceration and bleeding. Perforation rarely results. Occasionally, other heterotopic tissue (e.g., pancreas) is present.

C. Malabsorption. Numerous disorders can impair the transport of foodstuffs from the intestinal lumen into the portal and lymphatic circulations. The consequence is abnormal fecal excretion of fat, protein, or carbohydrates.

1. **Etiology.** Malabsorption may result from one or more of the following conditions.
   a. **Maldigestion** (due to diseases of the pancreas, biliary tree, or stomach, or to intestinal overgrowth of bacteria); the term connotes an inability to break down foodstuffs into small molecules suitable for transport across the intestinal mucosa.
   b. **Reduced absorptive capacity** (due to intrinsic disease of the small bowel)
   c. **Transport abnormalities** (due to lymphatic obstruction)

2. **Clinical features.** Patients often present with diarrhea, bulky stools, weight loss, fatigue, and evidence of vitamin deficiencies.

3. **Selected malabsorptive disorders** of the small bowel are summarized next.
   a. **Celiac disease (gluten-sensitive enteropathy, nontropical sprue)** is a malabsorptive disorder characterized by a flat small-bowel mucosa and by prompt clinical improvement following withdrawal of foods that contain gluten (wheat, barley, rye). Antigliadin, antireticulin, and antiendomysial antibodies are frequently detectable in the serum of patients with celiac disease and have diagnostic utility.
      (1) **Pathogenesis**
         (a) Celiac sprue appears to represent an immunologic disorder in which reactivity to **gliadin** (a glycoprotein in gluten) results in damage to the epithelial cells lining the villus. Whether the immune injury is cell-mediated or humoral is unknown Previous exposure to **adenovirus type 12,** which contains a protein that shares homology with α-gliadin, may "prime" patients to develop celiac disease.
         (b) About 80% of patients are positive for the human leukocyte antigens HLA-B8 and HLA-Dw3, which are found in only 20% to 25% of the general population.
      (2) **Pathology.** Changes are most severe in the proximal small bowel. **Microscopically,** the villi are often absent (**"flat biopsy"**), but in less severe cases they may demonstrate more subtle abnormalities. Surface lining cells become more cuboidal, and intraepithelial lymphocytes are prominent. The lamina propria is expanded by a

chronic inflammatory infiltrate. In **collagenous sprue,** a thick layer of collagen is deposited just under the surface epithelium. Celiac disease is the most common cause of a flat small bowel biopsy in the United States.

    (3) Prognosis and treatment. Prompt clinical response to gluten withdrawal is typical, but histologic improvement often is delayed.

    (4) Complications. Three major complications may develop, causing the patient to stop responding to a gluten-free diet (**refractory sprue**).

        (a) Ulcerative jejunoileitis is characterized by multiple ulcers, which may result in the formation of strictures. There is a high mortality rate. Some of these patients actually may have undiagnosed T-cell lymphomas.

        (b) Malignant small bowel tumors are chiefly T-cell lymphomas and less frequently adenocarcinomas.

        (c) Mesenteric lymph node cavitation is characterized by massive enlargement and replacement of the mesenteric nodes by inspissated hyaline and lipid material that appears to represent chylomicrons.

b. Tropical sprue, found chiefly in tropical regions, is a malabsorptive disorder that usually begins as an acute intestinal illness and is most likely secondary to a bacterial infection. **Microscopically,** a more variable degree of villous atrophy is found than in celiac disease. Patients respond dramatically to broad-spectrum antibiotics plus folic acid.

c. Disaccharidase deficiency is a collective term for several malabsorptive states in which a disaccharide cannot be digested because one or more enzymes are lacking. **Lactase deficiency** is the most common.

    (1) Disaccharidases are localized to the small intestinal brush border, where they split sugars into the monosaccharides required for intracellular transport. Without its appropriate enzyme, a sugar ferments in the intestinal lumen, which causes an osmotic diarrhea.

    (2) The small bowel mucosa is **histologically unremarkable,** but the enzymatic defect can be detected by specific enzymatic assays.

    (3) Treatment is to avoid the indigestible sugar or to add the missing enzyme to the diet.

d. Whipple's disease (intestinal lipodystrophy) is a multisystem disorder that usually occurs in adult males.

    (1) Clinical features. Patients characteristically present with malabsorption, although polyarthritis and CNS symptoms may first bring the patient to a physician. Also common are anemia, abnormal pigmentation, lymphadenopathy, and cardiac, hepatic, or pulmonary symptoms.

    (2) Etiology. Whipple's disease is a **bacterial disease,** although the particular responsible bacterium has remained elusive. Recent studies utilizing molecular biologic techniques suggest that the bacillus is a previously uncharacterized actinomycete, provisionally named *Tropheryma whippelii.* The patient's macrophages appear to have a lysosomal defect that prevents the ingested bacteria from being killed in the usual fashion.

    (3) Pathology

        (a) On **light microscopy,** the small bowel villi are seen to be distended by numerous foamy histiocytes (Figure 13-4), which contain granules that can be stained with periodic acid–Schiff (PAS) stain. They are gram-positive but **not** acid-fast. Lymphangiectasia and extracellular lipid droplets also may be present. Identical macrophages may be found at other sites, including lymph nodes, spleen, heart, kidney, liver, synovium, and CNS.

        (b) By **electron microscopy,** bacillary structures are found both within the histiocytes and in the extracellular space. The PAS-positive granules are seen to represent lysosomes containing products of bacterial degradation.

    (4) Diagnosis and treatment. Diagnosis depends on finding the characteristic histiocytes. Treatment with antibiotics often results in cure, although relapse, particularly in the CNS, is not uncommon.

e. Microvillous inclusion disease, an autosomally inherited recessive condition in newborns, is characterized by intractable diarrhea and steatorrhea. Villi are absent by light microscopy. Microvillous inclusions found just below the cell surface by electron microscopy or special histochemical techniques are the pathognomonic finding of this disease. Death typically occurs prior to 2 years of age.

f. Other causes of malabsorption include infectious agents, short bowel syndrome, bacterial overgrowth, CD, and various extraintestinal conditions.

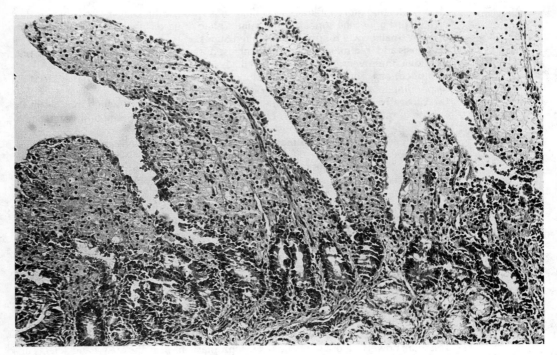

Figure 13-4. Whipple's disease of the small bowel. The lamina propria of the intestinal villi are filled with aggregates of macrophages. These macrophages typically demonstrate numerous granules when stained with periodic acid–Schiff (PAS) stain (H and E stain; × 100).

D. Tumors. Only 5% of all gastrointestinal tumors occur in the small bowel, where about half are benign and half are malignant.

1. **Benign tumors.** Most benign tumors of the small bowel (lipomas, leiomyomas, adenomas, hemangiomas) are incidental findings at autopsy. Small bowel **adenomas** occur most commonly in the duodenum. Of adenomas requiring surgical excision, the majority disclose foci of invasive adenocarcinoma. Polyps in patients with Peutz-Jeghers syndrome or FAP are discussed in IV E 3 a, 4 c.

2. **Malignant tumors.** The most important malignant tumors of the small bowel are adenocarcinoma (most commonly duodenal), lymphoma, carcinoids, and leiomyosarcoma. Pathologically, these tumors are identical to their counterparts at other sites. Only **carcinoid tumors** are discussed here. These neoplasms (also referred to as endocrine cell tumors, neuroendocrine neoplasms, argentaffinomas, or APUDomas) are derived from neuroendocrine cells or their precursors, which normally are dispersed throughout the gut mucosa.

   a. **Neuroendocrine cell origin.** Gut neuroendocrine cells currently are believed to have arisen from undifferentiated cells at the crypt base and not to have migrated from the neural crest, as do neuroendocrine cells located in some other organs. Although neuroendocrine cells may develop by different mechanisms, all have the ability to synthesize biogenic amines or peptide hormones and, thus, possess similar biochemical pathways. Those cells producing biogenic amines are sometimes termed **APUD cells,** an acronym for amine precursor uptake and decarboxylase. Carcinoid tumors are, therefore, sometimes called **APUDomas.**

   b. **Location.** Carcinoids of the gastrointestinal tract are most commonly found in the appendix, followed (in order of decreasing frequency) by the small bowel (usually the ileum), the rectosigmoid region, and finally the remainder of the colon. Tumors may be multiple.

   c. **Clinical features**
      (1) The majority of gastrointestinal carcinoids are incidental findings at surgery or autopsy, although they may cause bleeding or obstruction.
      (2) About 5% to 10% are associated with the **carcinoid syndrome** (cutaneous flushing, cyanosis, diarrhea, abdominal pain, wheezing, pulmonic valvular lesions), which is

caused by the tumor's production of vasoactive amines (e.g., serotonin, histamine, bradykinin). Patients almost always have extensive liver metastases. The carcinoid syndrome rarely is due to tumors arising in other organs (bronchi, pancreas, gonads).

  d. Pathology

  (1) Macroscopically, the tumors appear as gray, white, or yellow mucosal plaques, usually 1 to 2 cm in diameter, with an intact overlying epithelium. Some tumors may penetrate the muscularis propria and extend into the mesentery, inciting a desmoplastic reaction with fibrous adhesions that lead to kinking of adjacent bowel loops.

  (2) On **light microscopy,** carcinoids are characterized by a uniform proliferation of round or cuboidal cells with bland, round central nuclei, abundant eosinophilic cytoplasm, and usually only rare mitoses. The cells often are arranged in solid islands, trabeculae, or rosettes.

  (3) Special studies. Electron microscopy reveals electron-dense, membrane-bound neurosecretory granules that often prove to have an affinity for silver salts, either with (**argyrophil**) or without (**argentaffin**) the need for an added reducing agent. **Immunohistochemical stains** utilizing antibodies to several "neuroendocrine" markers (chromogranin, synaptophysin, neuron-specific enolase) often are positive.

  e. Prognosis. Any carcinoid may metastasize, but extraappendiceal carcinoids, those larger than 2 cm, and those showing extensive mural invasion are most likely to do so. However, even with liver metastases, the 5-year survival rate may approach 40%.

  f. Treatment. Resection of the lesion is curative if distant metastases have not developed and there is no evidence of the carcinoid syndrome. Because 10% to 30% of patients may have another malignant neoplasm, either within the gastrointestinal tract or at another location, careful surgical exploration must accompany surgical excision.

IV. LARGE BOWEL

A. Normal anatomy and histology

  1. The large bowel, measuring about 150 cm, includes the cecum, ascending colon, transverse colon, descending colon, and rectum. It joins distally to the anal canal, which extends another 3 to 5 cm. The colon and proximal rectum are intraperitoneal, whereas the distal rectum is extraperitoneal. The large bowel is important for fluid absorption, fecal storage, and defecation.

  2. Microscopically, the bowel mucosa consists of an orderly arrangement of straight tubular **crypts** containing many goblet cells and occasional neuroendocrine cells. Villi are absent. Cell proliferation normally takes place in the lower half of the crypt.

B. Congenital anomalies. Hirschsprung's disease (aganglionic megacolon) is caused by a congenital failure of ganglionic development in the colonic submucosal (Meissner's) and myenteric (Auerbach's) plexuses. This lack of development leads to a failure of muscular relaxation and, thus, to functional colonic obstruction. An absence of intramural ganglion cells at the anorectal junction usually involves the rectosigmoid region and sometimes extends more proximally.

  1. Epidemiology. Hirschsprung's disease occurs in 1 in 5000 live births. Siblings are affected in approximately 4% of cases, and men predominate (4:1), except with long-segment involvement and in familial cases. There is an association with other congenital disorders, particularly Down syndrome.

  2. Clinical features

  a. The disorder usually becomes apparent shortly after birth when the infant passes little meconium and the abdomen becomes distended. Severe constipation and vomiting follow. Abdominal radiographs reveal dilation of the proximal large bowel above the narrow distal aganglionic segment.

  b. Occasionally the disease appears later in life, when the patient may present with chronic constipation. It must then be differentiated from other causes of megacolon, such as ganglion cell and neuronal proliferation (ganglioneuromatosis or neuronal dysplasia) and organic obstruction.

  3. Diagnosis. Rectal suction biopsy (including both mucosa and submucosa) or full thickness biopsy will document the absence of ganglion cells. Immunohistochemical staining for neuron-specific enolase aids in the detection of ganglion cells, which, if found, exclude the diagnosis of Hirschsprung's disease. Immunohistochemical staining for S100 protein or enzyme histochemistry studies to detect cholinesterase activity can be used to demonstrate the hypertrophied nerve twigs frequently found in the lamina propria and throughout the bowel wall in this disorder.

4. **Treatment.** Surgical resection of the aganglionic segment is curative and avoids the major complications, namely, enterocolitis and perforation.

C. **Diverticular disease**

1. **General description.** Colonic diverticula are actually **pseudodiverticula,** as they represent **herniations** of the mucosa, submucosa, and occasionally a portion of the outer longitudinal muscle layer into the pericolonic fat. Striking hypertrophy of the sigmoid muscularis propria is found in 75% of cases and occasionally may be seen without diverticula. The term "diverticular disease" is clinically appropriate since symptoms often do not distinguish uninflamed diverticula (**diverticulosis**) from acutely inflamed ones (**diverticulitis**).

2. **Location.** Fully 95% of colonic diverticula are found in the sigmoid colon. The outpouchings occur between the mesenteric and antimesenteric taeniae, since the penetration of blood vessels in this region causes weak spots.

3. **Clinical and epidemiologic features.** Diverticular disease is a disorder of Western civilization, where the prevalence has markedly increased since the beginning of this century. It is a disease of the elderly, rarely seen before age 40 and found at autopsy in 30% to 50% of persons over age 60. Roughly 10% to 20% of patients are symptomatic and may complain of left lower quadrant pain, rectal bleeding, and constipation or diarrhea.

4. **Pathogenesis.** Dysmotility and relative weakness of the colon wall both appear to be important factors. Decreased dietary fiber is associated with increased risk for developing diverticula.

5. **Treatment, prognosis, and complications.** In many cases, symptoms resolve with conservative therapy. A high-fiber diet, by increasing stool bulk, may decrease the frequency and severity of symptoms. Complications include pericolic abscess, perforation, fistulas, and hemorrhage.

D. **Vascular disorders**

1. **Angiodysplasia (vascular ectasia, arteriovenous malformation),** consisting of single or multiple small (often less than 5 mm) areas of vascular dilation, are usually (in 80% to 90%) found in the cecum and ascending colon.
   a. **Pathogenesis.** The leading hypothesis states that obstruction of submucosal veins impedes venous return and, thereby, causes venous ectasia and arteriovenous fistulas. The usual occurrence of these lesions in the cecum probably reflects the increased wall tension in this region.
   b. **Clinical features.** This condition is a major cause of **lower gastrointestinal bleeding,** particularly in patients over age 60. However, the lesions are often incidental findings. Vascular ectasia may be seen during colonoscopy or may be demonstrated by angiography.
   c. **Pathology.** Dilated veins and capillaries are present in the submucosa and, with advanced lesions, in the lamina propria. The pathologist usually needs special techniques, such as latex or silicon injection, to visualize these lesions in gross specimens.
   d. **Treatment.** Surgical resection often is performed once a bleeding angiodysplasia is detected.

2. **Hemorrhoids** are variceal dilations of the anorectal submucosal venous plexus. They occur in 50% of persons over age 50. Their frequency increases in the elderly and during pregnancy.
   a. Important **pathogenetic factors** include constipation and straining, which cause a downward displacement of specialized cushions of submucosal tissue. These cushions contain a plexus of veins and a rich accompanying arterial supply. Internal hemorrhoids arise above the pectinate line (see VII A), and external hemorrhoids arise below it. Hemorrhoids only rarely result from portal hypertension.
   b. Bleeding, ulceration, thrombosis, and prolapse are potential **complications**.

E. **Polyps (Table 13-2).** By definition, any circumscribed protuberance into the bowel lumen is a polyp; thus, the term lacks specificity. A polyp should be classified according to its **specific type**.

1. **Reactive polyps.** Included are both the **inflammatory polyp** (often called a **"pseudopolyp"**), which typically is seen in UC and CD, and the **lymphoid polyp,** which represents a localized lymphoid hyperplasia.

Table 13-2. Common Polyps: Summary of Important Clinicopathologic Features

Polyp Type	Frequency of Polyps in Adults	Usual Size	Histologic Characteristics	Presence of Invasive Carcinoma	Polyposis Syndrome
Neoplastic					
Adenoma	40%–70%	< 1–3 cm	Dysplastic glands; T, TV, V	5%	FAP; Gardner's syndrome
Hyperplastic	30%–60%	< 1 cm	Serrated glands	Rare	Hyperplastic polyposis
Hamartomatous					
Juvenile	Uncommon (most common polyp in children)	1–3 cm	Cystically dilated glands	Rare*	Juvenile polyposis
Peutz-Jeghers	Uncommon	1–3 cm	Normal or cystically dilated glands; arborized muscularis mucosae	Rare*	Peutz-Jeghers syndrome
Reactive					
Inflammatory	Uncommon	Variable	Inflamed mucosa	No	Inflammatory polyposis (associated with IBD)
Lymphoid	Common	< 1 cm	Benign lymphoid aggregates	No	Nodular lymphoid hyperplasia

FAP = familial adenomatous polyposis; IBD = inflammatory bowel disease; T = tubular; TV = tubulovillous; V = villous.

*While single juvenile or Peutz-Jeghers polyps have minimal risk of malignant change, the risk is significantly greater in patients with juvenile polyposis or Peutz-Jeghers syndrome. Patients with FAP have virtually a 100% chance of developing colon cancer if colectomy is not performed. Colorectal carcinomas occurring in polyposis syndromes often occur before age 40.

2. Hyperplastic (metaplastic) polyps

a. These polyps account for 30%–60% of all colorectal polyps. They are found primarily in the rectosigmoid region and are seen in 75% of all persons over age 40. Hyperplastic polyps are always asymptomatic and, thus, are incidental findings.

b. Pathogenesis. Hyperplastic polyps result from an imbalance in cell renewal, with epithelial cell proliferation exceeding desquamation.

c. Pathology

    (1) Macroscopically, the polyps are sessile, usually small (1 to 5 mm), pink or gray teardrop-shaped protrusions of mucosa.

    (2) Microscopically, they consist of elongated crypts, with a serrated epithelial lining composed of absorptive cells and goblet cells (Figure 13-5). Only occasionally is a mixed hyperplastic–adenomatous polyp found.

d. Prognosis. Hyperplastic polyps have virtually no premalignant potential.

3. Hamartomatous polyps

a. Peutz-Jeghers polyps. These polyps usually, but not always, are associated with **Peutz-Jeghers syndrome,** an autosomal dominant disorder characterized by mucocutaneous pigmentation and multiple gastrointestinal hamartomatous polyps. As many as 50 to 100 polyps may be found. They occur most often in the small bowel but may be seen in any portion of the gastrointestinal tract.

    (1) Clinical features. Patients with the Peutz-Jeghers syndrome typically have mucocutaneous melanin pigmentation (found chiefly on the perioral skin, lips, buccal mucosa, hands, and feet) and often present with small bowel intussusception before age 10.

    (2) Pathology

        (a) Macroscopically, Peutz-Jeghers polyps appear firm and lobulated and usually are 2 to 3 cm in diameter. They may be pedunculated or sessile.

        (b) Microscopically, an arborization of the muscularis mucosae is seen separating an increased number of relatively normal or cystically dilated crypts.

    (3) Prognosis and treatment. An increased but uncertain number (probably 10% to 20%) of patients with Peutz-Jeghers syndrome develop gastrointestinal carcinomas, usually before age 40. There also appears to be an increased risk for developing extraintestinal carcinomas, particularly bilateral breast carcinomas and well-differentiated

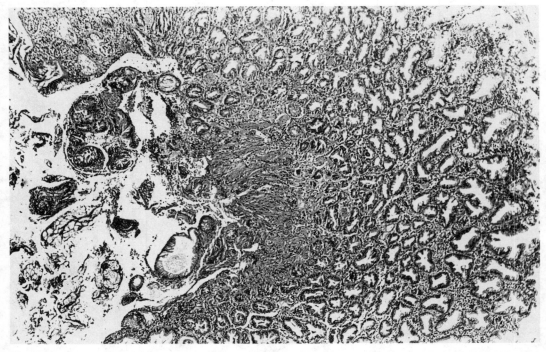

Figure 13-5. Low-power view of a hyperplastic polyp, showing elongated crypts with a serrated epithelial lining (H and E stain; × 100).

adenocarcinoma of the uterine cervix. A rare ovarian tumor [sex cord tumor with annular tubules (**SCTAT**)] can be identified in almost all women patients if the ovaries are carefully sampled. Currently, Peutz-Jeghers polyps are removed when they cause symptoms or are under surveillance.

   b. Juvenile (retention) polyps. These hamartomas may occur as one or a few polyps or as a polyposis syndrome.

      (1) Most commonly, a **single polyp** is found in the rectosigmoid region in a child under age 10. However, this type of polyp may also be found in adult life.

         (a) Macroscopically, juvenile polyps usually appear pedunculated, deep red, and smooth and usually are no more than a few centimeters in diameter.

         (b) Microscopically, cystically dilated glands containing inspissated mucin (hence, the term "retention polyp") are seen embedded in an inflamed and edematous lamina propria.

         (c) A juvenile polyp may be impossible to distinguish from an inflammatory polyp.

      (2) Juvenile polyposis may occur sporadically or be inherited as an autosomal dominant trait. Associated congenital defects occur in 25% of patients.

         (a) Patients usually present before age 10 with intussusception, gastrointestinal hemorrhage resulting in anemia, or protein-losing enteropathy. These complications often require bowel resection. From 10 to 100 polyps often are found most commonly in the colorectum, but the stomach and small bowel may also be involved.

         (b) In 20% of patients with juvenile polyps, one or more of the polyps may display dysplastic (adenomatous) change. This alteration is probably responsible for the 15%–20% prevalence of colon carcinoma, which occurs at a mean age of 34 years in this patient population. Family members without polyps also have an increased risk of both gastrointestinal and extraintestinal malignancies.

4. Neoplastic polyps (adenomas, adenomatous polyps)

   a. General concepts

      (1) Incidence. Adenomatous polyps account for about 40% to 70% of all colorectal polyps. Adenomas are found in 10% to 15% of the adult population and in 66% of persons over age 65. If found prior to age 30, a polyposis syndrome or a heritable nonpolyposis syndrome must be ruled out.

      (2) Appearance. In 50% of cases, the adenomas are multiple. The polyps may be pedunculated, sessile, or flat. While often greater than 1 cm in diameter, adenomas also account for roughly 50%–60% of all diminutive (less than 5 mm in diameter) polyps. Cell division is unrestricted and is observed at all levels of the crypt. Cell differentiation is incomplete or absent.

      (3) Clinical features. Most adenomas are asymptomatic. When symptoms occur, they most frequently result from bleeding (either melena or hematochezia). Rarely, villous adenomas cause watery diarrhea and consequent hypokalemia.

      (4) Cytologic features

         (a) The typical adenoma, regardless of histologic type, has classic cytologic features (i.e., a "picket-fence" arrangement of cells having elongated, hyperchromatic nuclei). These epithelial abnormalities often are termed **"dysplasia."** Therefore, a circumscribed proliferation of dysplastic epithelium is an adenoma.

         (b) More marked degrees of dysplasia demonstrate nuclear stratification, prominent nucleoli, an increased nuclear:cytoplasmic ratio, and a cribriform pattern. These features are seen in some adenomas.

         (c) About 5% of adenomas harbor invasive adenocarcinoma (defined as invasion through the muscularis mucosae).

      (5) Treatment. Polypectomy is curative for those adenomas without invasive adenocarcinoma. Treatment for those with invasion is discussed in IV E 4 e.

   b. Histologic classification

      (1) Tubular adenomas represent 75% of the total. They often are round, smooth, pedunculated, and less than 1 cm in diameter. Microscopically, there is a proliferation of tubules, which often are branched and possess the cytologic features mentioned previously. Less than 20% of the lesion has a villous architecture.

      (2) Villous adenomas represent 10% of the total. The majority are greater than 2 cm in diameter. They typically have a shaggy, cauliflower-like appearance, and 90% are sessile. The **histologic hallmark** is the presence of villi (i.e., fingerlike projections with a lining of epithelium and a fibrovascular core), which comprise more than 50% of the lesion.

(3) Tubulovillous adenomas, representing 15% of the total, possess pathologic features intermediate between tubular and villous adenomas; 20% to 50% of the lesion has a villous architecture.

c. **Familial adenomatous polyposis and Gardner's syndrome**

(1) By definition, patients with **FAP** have 100 to more than 1000 adenomas, which carpet the colon. Less frequently, adenomas also are found in the stomach and small bowel, particularly the duodenum. The lesions usually are less than 1 cm in diameter and have a tubular histology.

(a) The disorder has a prevalence of 1 in 7000 to 1 in 24,000 of the population, and it is most commonly inherited in an autosomal dominant fashion, although one-third of cases are sporadic. The adenomatous polyposis coli (APC) gene, located on the long arm of chromosome 5, has recently been cloned.

(b) Adenomas usually appear in the second and third decades, with symptoms occurring one decade later. If colectomy is not performed, all patients will develop adenocarcinoma, usually by age 40; and in 40%–50% of cases, these malignancies are multiple. By the time symptoms occur, two-thirds of patients already have developed carcinoma. Carcinomas may also develop at other gastrointestinal sites.

(2) **Relationship of FAP and Gardner's syndrome.** The colonic adenomas are identical in these two entities. Although the presence of duodenal adenomas, soft-tissue lesions (epidermoid cysts, lipomas, fibromatosis), and congenital hypertrophy of the retinal pigment epithelium were considered to be characteristic of Gardner's syndrome, identical lesions have been found in FAP patients, although they are often subclinical. Recently, genetic linkage to the long arm of chromosome 5 has also been found in Gardner's syndrome. While the exact relationship between these two entities still remains controversial, most investigators consider Gardner's syndrome a variant of FAP.

d. **Turcot's syndrome.** The inheritance is controversial. Patients have multiple adenomas (fewer than in FAP) plus malignant tumors of the CNS. These patients have an increased risk for developing colorectal cancer.

e. The **adenoma–carcinoma sequence.** It appears that **virtually all colon carcinomas arise in adenomas,** and that this sequence takes 10 to 15 years.

(1) **Evidence for this relationship** is substantial.

(a) Adenomas and carcinomas are similar in location and epidemiologic characteristics.

(b) Minute carcinomas rarely if ever arise de novo, independent of adenomatous foci.

(c) Adenomas can display a continuum of dysplastic changes, including carcinoma in situ and invasive carcinoma.

(d) Both adenomas and carcinomas frequently are associated with mutational activation of oncogenes and with allelic deletions of one or more chromosomes.

(e) The more adenomas a patient has, the greater the risk of carcinoma.

(f) Carcinomas, particularly if they are only superficially invasive, often contain residual adenoma.

(g) Systematic removal of adenomas drastically reduces the incidence of carcinoma.

(2) **Risk factors for the presence of invasive adenocarcinoma in adenomas** include the following.

(a) **Size.** For adenomas smaller than 1 cm in diameter, the risk is 1%; for those larger than 2 cm, the risk is 10% to 50%.

(b) **Degree of epithelial dysplasia.** Increasing degrees of dysplasia correlate with the risk of finding a focus of invasive carcinoma.

(c) **Histologic type.** Villous adenomas have the greatest risk, followed by tubulovillous and tubular types.

(d) **Number of adenomas.** The greater the number of adenomas, the greater the risk of carcinoma.

(3) **Treatment of resected adenomas harboring carcinoma.** The clinical potential for metastasis exists only when invasion proceeds beyond the muscularis mucosae.

(a) However, for a **pedunculated lesion,** even when such invasion is present but the stalk margin is free of tumor, lymphatic invasion is absent, and the tumor is not poorly differentiated. Then polypectomy alone, without bowel resection, is almost always curative.

(b) If the adenoma is **sessile** rather than pedunculated, then invasion implies extension into the bowel wall itself, and standard cancer surgery usually is performed.

F. Malignant tumors

1. **Carcinoma.** Representing 95% of all primary colorectal malignancies, colorectal carcinoma is the second most common cause of all cancer deaths (about 60,000 deaths annually).
   a. **Epidemiology and risk factors**
      (1) The peak incidence is in the seventh decade, with only 20% of cases occurring prior to age 50. It is rare before age 40 without associated polyposis or hereditary nonpolyposis syndromes, or IBD. Women with a history of genital or breast cancer also are considered to be at increased risk. Rectal cancers are more frequent in men, whereas colon carcinomas are slightly more common in women.
      (2) Colorectal carcinoma is most common in industrialized nations and urban regions, where diets are higher in animal fat, protein, and refined carbohydrate and lower in fiber. This so-called "Western diet" may increase the anaerobic gut flora, leading to the formation of secondary bile acids, which may be carcinogens or cocarcinogens. The decreased fiber content causes a decreased colonic transit time, thereby increasing the time that potential carcinogens are in contact with the epithelium.
      (3) **Genetic influences** also appear to be important.
         (a) **Hereditary nonpolyposis colorectal carcinoma (HNPCC)** accounts for 5%–13% of all colorectal carcinomas. The disorder has been recently linked to chromosome 2; inheritance is autosomal dominant. Patients with HNPCC have families in which three or more members have been affected before age 50 over the course of two successive generations. Patients are often 30–50 years old. Their cancers are often right-sided (50%) and multiple (20%); a few adenomas may also be present. Two syndromes have been described, although their distinction is controversial.
            (i) In **site-specific colon cancer,** cancer is found only in the colon or rectum.
            (ii) In the **cancer family syndrome,** cancers are found at multiple sites, including the colon or rectum, other gastrointestinal sites, and the female sex organs.
         (b) Colorectal cancer in the general population is also believed to be inherited in an autosomal dominant fashion but with a low penetrance. First-degree relatives of patients with these tumors have a threefold increased risk of colorectal cancers. It appears that environmental influences and genetic susceptibility interact to determine a person's risk for developing colorectal carcinoma.
         (c) Genetic studies of colon carcinoma cells demonstrate frequent mutation or deletion of tumor suppressor genes located on chromosomal segments 5q, 17p, and 18q as well as oncogene activation (particularly *ras*).
   b. **Location**
      (1) From 60% to 75% of tumors are located in the rectum and the rectosigmoid and sigmoid regions, with the remainder being distributed throughout the bowel. Over the last several decades, a shift in the location of colorectal cancer has been noted, with a decrease in the number of rectal tumors and an increase in the number of those located more proximally.
      (2) In the general population, only 2% to 5% of large bowel carcinomas are multiple, whereas 20% to 50% of the carcinomas which develop in patients with ulcerative colitis or FAP are multiple.
   c. **Clinical features and diagnosis**
      (1) Patients often have had **symptoms** for months or years prior to diagnosis. Rectosigmoid lesions more frequently present as overt rectal bleeding or obstruction, whereas cecal and right colonic tumors often present as anemia and occult gastrointestinal blood loss.
      (2) The **diagnosis** usually can be made by barium enema and is confirmed by sigmoidoscopy or colonoscopy with biopsy. Testing of the stool for occult blood is an important screening procedure.
   d. **Pathology**
      (1) **Macroscopically,** right-sided lesions often form a polypoid fungating mass; left-sided lesions, an ulcerated annular plaque ("napkin-ring" lesion; Figure 13-6). Rarely, colon cancer may cause rigid thickening of the wall (**linitis plastica** type) with little mucosal abnormality.
      (2) **Microscopically,** 95% of these tumors are **adenocarcinomas** that usually are well differentiated or moderately differentiated (Figure 13-7). Occasionally, variants produce large amounts of extracellular mucin (**colloid or mucinous adenocarcinoma**) or, in the

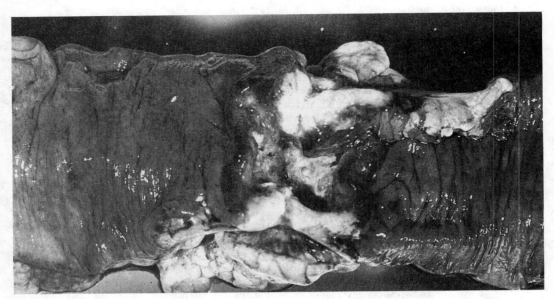

Figure 13-6. A carcinoma of the rectosigmoid, showing the characteristic "napkin-ring" configuration.

rare linitis plastica variant, they contain numerous signet cells. Squamous, adeno-squamous, and small cell carcinomas are quite rare.

e. Staging and prognosis (Table 13-3). Dukes described the original staging system for rectal carcinoma. Among the numerous modifications now used for colorectal carcinoma, two that are frequently employed are the Astler-Coller modification and the system of the American Joint Committee on Cancer (AJCC). All of these staging systems emphasize that prognosis is related to the depth of mural invasion by the tumor and the status of the

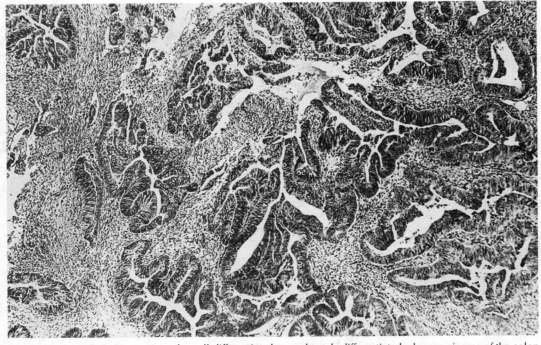

Figure 13-7. Medium-power view of a well-differentiated to moderately differentiated adenocarcinoma of the colon (H and E stain; × 200).

pericolorectal lymph nodes. Tumors with an abnormal chromosome number (aneuploidy), an increased growth fraction, or specific chromosomal deletions may behave in a more aggressive fashion. These prognostic factors are currently under evaluation.

   f. Treatment and surveillance. The cornerstone of treatment is **surgical resection.** Adjunctive radiotherapy and chemotherapy have been used for the treatment of rectal carcinoma, and recently a survival advantage has been found for patients with stage C colon carcinoma treated with 5-fluorouracil and levamisole. Patients may be followed after treatment by monitoring serum carcinoembryonic antigen (CEA) levels.

  2. Other primary tumors may occur in the large bowel, such as carcinoid (III D 2), leiomyosarcoma (see II G 3), and lymphoma (see II G 2), as may metastatic neoplasms, particularly melanoma, carcinomas from the lung and breast, and lymphoma or leukemia.

V. INFLAMMATORY BOWEL DISEASES.

The term "inflammatory bowel disease" (IBD) includes a number of disorders of the small and large bowel in which inflammation plays an important role and diarrhea usually results, although the term sometimes is used to designate only the idiopathic cases.

  A. General considerations

    1. Pathology. Mucosal biopsies of the colon often disclose an inflammatory infiltrate in the lamina propria with crypt abscesses (neutrophils in the lumen of a crypt).

     a. A prominence of **neutrophils in the lamina propria** in the absence of architectural distortion, atrophy, or metaplastic changes in the crypt favors a diagnosis of infectious colitis over idiopathic IBD.

     b. The presence of **leukocytes in the stool** indicates a destructive inflammatory process; however, it does not indicate a specific diagnosis, as fecal leukocytes may be found in association with invasive bacteria or parasites, the effects of a toxin such as that of *Clostridium difficile,* ischemic bowel disease, or idiopathic IBD.

    2. Differential diagnosis. The diagnosis of idiopathic IBD (i.e., UC and CD) requires exclusion of a broad range of conditions of known etiology, either noninfectious (e.g., ischemia, radiation injury, uremia, cytotoxic drug injury) or infectious. Infectious disorders may be diagnosed by morphologic, serologic, or cultural evidence of a particular organism. Infectious etiologies are summarized in Table 13-4.

  B. Idiopathic inflammatory bowel disease

    1. General considerations

     a. Epidemiology. Data apply to either UC or CD, although UC is somewhat more common. The prevalence of idiopathic IBD is 5 to 60 per 100,000 population. The ratio of white to

Table 13-3. Colorectal Carcinoma: Prognosis*

	Modified Dukes' / AJCC Stage				
Diagnostic Feature	**A / ST 0**	**B1 / ST I**	**B2 / ST II**	**C1 / ST III**	**C2 / ST III**
Depth of mural invasion	Limited to mucosa	Limited to muscularis propria	Beyond muscularis propria	Limited to muscularis propria	Beyond muscularis propria
Positive lymph nodes	No	No	No	Yes	Yes
5-Year survival rate	100%	80%–90%	75%–80%	65%–75%	30%–45%

*According to the Astler-Coller modification of Dukes' staging system and the American Joint Committee on Cancer (AJCC) staging system. The complete AJCC staging system is as follows:

    Stage 0   Tis (carcinoma in situ); N0 (negative lymph nodes); M0 (no distant metastases).
    Stage I   T1 or T2 (tumor invades submucosa or muscularis propria, respectively); N0; M0.
    Stage II   T3 or T4 (tumor invades through the muscularis propria without or with invasion of the adjacent viscera, respectively); N0; M0.
    Stage III Any T; N1, N2, or N3 (positive lymph nodes); M0.
    Stage IV Distant metastases with any T or N.

Some investigators use Dukes' stage "D" to indicate the presence of distant metastases. The 5-year survival rate of patients with stage D (AJCC Stage IV) disease is only 5%.

Table 13-4. Infectious Forms of Inflammatory Bowel Disease

Infectious Agent	Clinical Features	Pathologic Features
Bacteria		
Preformed enterotoxin		
C. perfringens, S. aureus, B. cereus	Food poisoning	None
C. botulinum	Botulism	None
Enterotoxin after colonization		
V. cholerae, E. coli	Marked fluid loss	None
Shigella, E. coli	Enterocolitis (dysentery)	Acute mucosal inflammation, ulcers
C. difficile	Enterocolitis diarrhea; usually antibiotic-associated	As above, with pseudomembranes (pseudomembranous enterocolitis)
E. coli (verotoxin-producing*)	Bloody diarrhea; hemolytic-uremic syndrome; TTP	Hemorrhagic enterocolitis
Bacterial invasion of mucosa		
Shigella, Salmonella, Campylobacter, Yersinia, E. coli†	Enterocolitis: Yersinia may mimic appendicitis or Crohn's disease	Acute mucosal inflammation, ulcers; microabscesses in lymphoid aggregates with Yersinia; granulomas with Y. pseudotuberculosis
Mycobacteria		
M. tuberculosis	Now rarely involves GI tract (usually ileocecal region)	Caseating granulomas; AFB
M. avium–intracellulare (MAI)	Typically found in AIDS patients; small bowel predominately affected	Poorly formed histiocytic aggregates which are PAS-positive; numerous AFB ("pseudo-Whipple's disease")
Chlamydia trachomatis‡	Proctitis; occasionally more proximal disease	Inflammation; occasionally strictures and fistulae
Viruses		
Rotavirus	Most common cause of early childhood diarrhea (often severe)	Mild enteritis
Norwalk virus group	Most common cause of diarrhea (often mild) in older childhood and adults	Mild enteritis
Caliciviruses, astroviruses, coronaviruses, enteric adenoviruses	Diarrhea	Mild enteritis
CMV	Diarrhea in immunocompromised host	Nuclear and cytoplasmic inclusions in mesenchymal or epithelial cells; ulcers

Fungi

Candida, Aspergillus	Immunocompromised host	Ulcers; yeasts and pseudohyphae (*Candida*); septate hyphae (*Aspergillus*)
Other fungi	Rare; manifestation of disseminated disease	Fungal forms characteristic of specific genus

Parasites
Protozoa

Giardia lamblia	Diarrhea; patients with hypogammaglobulinemia (especially IgA deficiency) at increased risk	Trophozoites with pear-shaped binucleate morphology found adjacent to duodenal villi; villi usually normal
Amebiasis	Amebic dysentery; hepatic amebic abscesses in 40% of cases	Flask-shaped colonic ulcers; sometimes masses (ameboma); characteristic trophozoites with erythrophagocytosis or cysts (diagnostic feature)
Cryptosporidium	Diarrhea, most severe in immunocompromised (AIDS) patients	Tiny round extracellular organisms found adjacent to epithelial cells, most commonly in small bowel; little inflammation
Isospora belli, Microsporidium	Diarrhea in immunocompromised (AIDS) patients	Intracellular; found in surface epithelium most commonly in small bowel; Little inflammation

Helminths

Schistosomiasis	Common worldwide, causing chronic diarrhea and portal hypertension (*S. mansoni, S. japonicum*) or cystitis (*S. hematobium*)	Ulcers, strictures, inflammatory polyposis; granulomatous response to ova; sometimes eosinophils
Strongyloides stercoralis	Chronic diarrhea; vomiting; malabsorption; may be rapidly fatal in immunocompromised (AIDS) patients	Larvae, eggs, or adult worms may be seen in the crypts; villus atrophy, inflammation, and granulomas may be found

AFB = acid-fast bacilli; AIDS = acquired immunodeficiency syndrome; CMV = cytomegalovirus; GI = gastrointestinal tract; IgA = immunoglobulin A; LGV = lymphogranuloma venereum; MAI = *M. avium–intracellulare*; PAS = periodic acid–Schiff; TTP = thrombotic thrombocytopenic purpura.

*Especially the 0157:H7 serotype.

†Some *E. coli* serotypes may cause bowel damage merely by adhering to the surface epithelium (enteroadhesion).

‡LGV and non-LGV serotypes.

black patients is 20:1, and Jewish persons are affected 2 to 4 times as often as non-Jews. Age of onset shows two peaks, in the second to third decade and the sixth to seventh decade; men and women are affected equally. From 15% to 40% of patients have a family history of idiopathic IBD.

  b. **Pathogenesis.** Currently, the pathogenesis of idiopathic IBD is unknown; transmissible agents, environmental factors, genetic predisposition, and various immunologic mechanisms have been postulated.

  c. **Differential diagnosis.** Idiopathic IBD includes two disorders, **UC** and **CD**.

  (1) Although these two disorders often can be distinguished by clinical criteria, overlapping features are common, thus requiring pathologic examination of tissue specimens for a definitive diagnosis (Table 13-5).

  (2) About 5% to 10% of cases involving the colon cannot be classified as either UC or CD, even after histologic study; the term **indeterminant colitis** is used for these cases, which typically demonstrate severe colitis.

  (3) Before a diagnosis of either UC or CD can be assigned, all specific etiologic agents of IBD must be excluded (see V A 2).

2. **Ulcerative colitis.** UC is a chronic recurrent inflammatory and ulcerative disease of the colon and rectum characterized by **continuous** mucosal ulceration that begins in the **rectum** and by relatively **superficial inflammation.**

  a. **Clinical features**

  (1) During the recurrent bouts of active disease, rectal bleeding and tenesmus are the most common complaints. Crampy abdominal pain, malnutrition, and perianal disease are less common. Fistulas occur rarely.

  (2) Severe (fulminant) colitis occurs in 10% to 15% of patients. **Toxic megacolon,** defined as colonic dilation to at least 6 cm in diameter, with systemic toxicity, occurs in 10% to 15% of patients with fulminant colitis (overall, in 2% to 8% of all UC patients).

Table 13-5. Ulcerative Colitis and Crohn's Disease—Differential Diagnosis

Findings	Ulcerative Colitis	Crohn's Disease
Clinical features		
Rectal bleeding	In 85%	In 40%
Weight loss, malnutrition	Unusual	Common in small bowel disease
Anal or perianal disease	In < 20%	In 20% to 80%
Internal fistulas	Rare	In 20% to 40%
Risk of carcinoma	Increases progressively after 7 to 10 years of disease; more common than in Crohn's disease	Increases progressively after 25 years of disease; less common than in ulcerative colitis
Macroscopic features		
Continuity of lesions	Continuous	Discontinuous (segmental)
Ileal involvement	Rare	In 70% to 80%
Mucosal appearance	Granular, deep, broad ulcers	Discrete ulcers, fissures, cobblestone appearance
Serosa	Normal	Often shows "creeping fat"
Bowel length	Shortened	Usually normal
Benign fibrous stricture	Very rare	Very common
Microscopic features		
Location of inflammation	Mucosa, upper submucosa	Transmural
Ulcers	Broad and deep	Superficial, aphthous
Knifelike fissures	Rare	Common
Granulomas	Absent	In 60% to 70%
Submucosal fibrosis, lymphoid hyperplasia, edema, lymphangiectasia, neuromatous hyperplasia	Rare	Common

b. Pathology
  (1) Macroscopic appearance
  - **(a)** UC affects the bowel **continuously** and always begins in the rectum, with only 10% of cases showing mild involvement of the terminal ileum (**"backwash" ileitis**).
    - **(i)** Initially, about 25% of patients have disease confined to the rectum (**ulcerative proctitis**), with only 15% of patients having disease that extends into the right colon (**pancolitis,** or **universal colitis**).
    - **(ii)** After 10 years of disease, about one-third of patients have pancolitis.
  - **(b)** With active disease, the mucosa is friable and hemorrhagic with broad areas of ulceration. Residual areas of mucosa protrude as "mucosal islands," or "pseudopolyps." Often these mucosal islands are inflamed; thus, the term **"inflammatory polyp"** is used. Fibrotic strictures are rare unless there is associated carcinoma. Benign strictures may result from hypertrophy of the muscularis mucosae.
  - **(c)** The colon typically is shortened; this is due to muscular spasm, not fibrosis.

  (2) Microscopic appearance. UC is basically a **mucosal disease** with superficial submucosal involvement. The crypt architecture is distorted, with an infiltrate of chronic inflammatory cells (particularly plasma cells) in the lamina propria. Paneth's cells and gastric pyloric metaplasia may be seen. With active disease, neutrophils invade the crypt epithelium (**cryptitis**) and cluster in the crypt lumen (**crypt abscess**) in association with the mucosal ulceration (Figure 13-8). Goblet cell mucin typically is decreased.

c. Treatment and prognosis
  (1) Patients often respond to symptomatic medical treatment with corticosteroids and sulfasalazine or other related compounds. However, about 25% of patients require colectomy within 5 to 10 years after onset of the disease, usually for intractable disease, a severe episode, toxic megacolon, or colon perforation.

  (2) Because of the great variation in the frequency and severity of individual attacks and the extent of colonic disease, it is difficult to estimate the long-term prognosis in a given patient. About 5% of patients die within 1 year after their first attack.

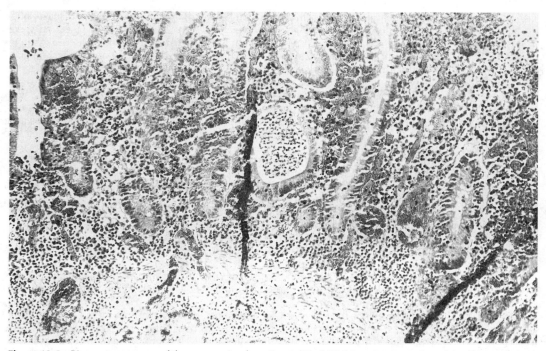

Figure 13-8. Biopsy appearance of the mucosa in ulcerative colitis (UC). Note the expansion of the lamina propria by chronic inflammatory cells and the presence of crypt abscesses (H and E stain; × 250).

3. **Crohn's disease.** CD is a chronic recurrent inflammatory and ulcerative disease of the digestive tract extending **discontinuously** from mouth to anus, although clinically apparent disease most commonly involves the distal ileum (**regional** or **terminal ileitis**), the colon (**granulomatous colitis**), and the anal region, perianal region, or both. The inflammation is characteristically **transmural,** and **granulomas** often are present.
   a. **Clinical features.** Common symptoms include fever, crampy abdominal pain, and, with small bowel disease, weight loss and malnutrition. Rectal bleeding is less common than in patients with UC, and anal or perianal disease is more common. Enterocutaneous and enteroenteric **fistulas** are each found in 15% to 20% of patients. Toxic megacolon occurs in about 5% of all patients, as with UC. However, intraabdominal abscesses are much more frequent in patients with CD.
   b. **Pathology**
      (1) **Location.** Both the small and the large bowel (ileum and proximal colon) are affected in 55% of patients; only the small bowel in 30%, and only the large bowel in 15%. The right colon often is involved, and the rectum frequently is spared.
      (2) **Macroscopic appearance.** CD is a **segmental (discontinuous)** disease, with intervening **"skip" areas** of normal mucosa.
         (a) Small **aphthous ulcers** resembling oral canker sores may be the earliest lesions; later in the course, long, longitudinally oriented ulcers often impart a "tram-track" or rakelike appearance to the colon mucosa. The aphthous ulcers often give rise to narrow knifelike fissures that subsequently may develop into fistulas. The spared mucosa between the ulcers typically has a cobblestone appearance because of marked submucosal edema.
         (b) **Inflammatory polyps ("pseudopolyps")** also may be a prominent feature. The bowel wall may be markedly thickened, and mesenteric fat may extend over the serosal surface ("creeping fat").
         (c) **Fibrous strictures** most frequently occur in the ileum. The thickened fibrotic wall reduces the fecal stream to a thin column causing the "string sign" radiographically and the "hosepipe" appearance macroscopically. The colon is only occasionally shortened.
      (3) **Microscopic appearance**
         (a) **Transmural chronic inflammation,** the **histologic hallmark** of this disease, often is accompanied by epithelioid **granulomas** (in 60% to 75% of resection specimens). Granulomas also may be noted in regional lymph nodes. Mucosal changes similar to those of UC may be found, such as cryptitis, crypt abscesses, and glandular metaplasia, but crypt distortion and goblet-cell depletion often are less severe and mucosal inflammation more patchy.
         (b) In the absence of granulomas, colonic CD can be distinguished from UC by its segmental nature, transmural chronic inflammation, aphthous ulcers, fissures, prominent submucosal fibrosis, lymphoid hyperplasia, edema, lymphangiectasia, and neuromatous hyperplasia of both Meissner's and Auerbach's plexuses (see Table 13-5).
   c. **Treatment.** Although patients often respond to medical therapy, about 40% to 50% still require surgery for bowel obstruction or complications of fistulas. Surgical resection attempts to save as much macroscopically disease-free bowel as possible. From 10% to 20% of patients ultimately die of CD or its complications.

4. **Complications of idiopathic IBD**
   a. **Systemic complications.** More than 100 systemic complications have been identified, including ankylosing spondylitis, erythema nodosum, arthritis, uveitis, pyoderma gangrenosum, sclerosing cholangitis, and intestinal carcinoma.
   b. **Intestinal carcinoma as a complication.** Patients with UC and, to a lesser extent, CD are at increased risk for developing adenocarcinoma of the bowel, although the magnitude of this risk is somewhat controversial.
      (1) For **UC patients,** the risk of developing colon adenocarcinomas increases after 7 to 10 years of disease, particularly for patients with pancolitis. The exact risk is unknown. It has varied from less than 10% to greater than 30% after 25 years of disease, in several series. Colon carcinoma in the UC patient population occurs earlier (mean is 40 years) and is more often multiple (in 25%) than in the general population. Monitoring UC patients by multiple colorectal biopsy to look for epithelial dysplasia appears to be a

more rational approach than performing indiscriminate proctocolectomy after 10 years of disease; however, the problem of cost-effectiveness must be addressed.

    (a) Finding high-grade dysplasia similar to that seen in some colonic adenomas [see IV E 4] indicates a significant (30% to 50%) risk for invasive carcinoma, and, thus, colectomy usually is performed.

    (b) Finding any degree of dysplasia in a macroscopically visible lesion also suggests that foci of carcinoma are present deeper in the bowel wall. Colectomy may also be performed in this situation.

  (2) **CD patients** may develop gastrointestinal adenocarcinoma at colonic or extracolonic sites, usually after 25 years of disease. As the bowel is often strictured, endoscopic surveillance is quite difficult.

C. Collagenous and lymphocytic (microscopic) colitis are recently described forms of colitis that appear to be distinct from UC or CD.

  1. Clinical features. Patients typically are middle-aged women who present with watery diarrhea. In the past, these patients were often thought to have idiopathic IBD or irritable bowel syndrome, a disorder of bowel motility without a demonstrable organic cause.

  2. Pathology. Colonoscopic examination usually is **normal,** and thus quite dissimilar from other forms of IBD. Microscopically, the presence of a thick collagenous band under the surface epithelium distinguishes collagenous colitis from lymphocytic (microscopic) colitis. In both disorders one sees chronic inflammation in the lamina propria, preserved crypt architecture, and generally an increased number of intraepithelial lymphocytes. The relationship of these two entities is controversial.

  3. Treatment. Although patients often appear to respond to medical therapy, spontaneous remissions also occur.

VI. ISCHEMIC BOWEL DISEASE. Many terms have been used when describing ischemic bowel disease: ischemic enteritis, colitis, or enterocolitis; hemorrhagic necrosis or infarction; and gangrene of the gastrointestinal tract. Although pseudomembranous colitis typically is associated with *C. difficile* enterotoxin, occasional cases appear to be secondary to bowel ischemia.

A. Normal anatomy of the intestinal arterial supply. The intestines are supplied nearly entirely by three major arterial trunks. The anatomy of these vessels and their ability to form collaterals determine the consequences of a particular vascular occlusion.

  1. The **celiac trunk** supplies the first portion of the duodenum.

  2. The **superior mesenteric artery (SMA),** via a series of vascular arcades, supplies the remainder of the small bowel and the colon to the level of the midtransverse region or splenic flexure.

  3. The **inferior mesenteric artery (IMA)** supplies the distal colon and most of the rectum. The distal rectum is supplied via branches of the **internal iliac artery,** which is part of the systemic circulation.

  4. The **marginal artery of Drummond** often connects the SMA and IMA; the IMA also receives collaterals distally from branches of the internal iliac artery.

B. Pathophysiology. In the resting state, the intraabdominal digestive organs (the splanchnic bed) receive 25% to 30% of the cardiac output.

  1. Hypotension causes mesenteric arterial vasoconstriction, with shunting of blood to the heart and brain. Often the bowel can tolerate marked decreases in blood flow (to 30% of normal) without suffering tissue damage. The mucosa is the tissue most sensitive to ischemic damage; the muscularis propria is least sensitive.

  2. An **inadequate blood supply (ischemia)** leads to tissue hypoxia and the buildup of metabolic waste products, which may cause tissue necrosis (**infarction**). The degree of bowel damage can vary from focal forms to massive infarction involving both the small and large bowel, depending on the following factors.

    a. The rapidity of onset and the type, severity, and duration of the insult

    b. The extent of collateral circulation

    c. The metabolic requirements of the affected segment of bowel

   d. The nature of the bowel flora; for example, anaerobes such as several *Clostridium* species may produce toxins that result in extensive tissue damage

   3. Acute mesenteric ischemia involves at least the SMA distribution and often that of the IMA. When the colon is involved, often the region of the splenic flexure is damaged, as it is the watershed area between the SMA and the IMA.

C. Pathogenesis

   1. SMA occlusion (comprising 30% to 50% of cases) can be thrombotic or embolic in origin.
      a. A **thrombus** almost always lodges in the proximal 2 cm of the SMA, overlying an ulcerated atheromatous plaque.
      b. Emboli typically arise from the heart, either from intraatrial thrombi, which have formed as a complication of atrial fibrillation, or from a dislodged mural thrombus overlying a myocardial infarct. The embolus may lodge in proximal or more distal branches of the SMA.

   2. Nonocclusive ischemia (occurring in 30% to 50% of cases) represents hypoperfusion of the bowel due to splanchnic vasoconstriction, which can occur in various conditions (e.g., myocardial infarction, shock, congestive heart failure).

   3. Mesenteric venous thrombosis (occurring in 10% to 15% of cases) may be idiopathic or secondary. Causes include portal vein thrombosis, intraabdominal sepsis, oral contraceptives, and hypercoagulable states such as polycythemia vera.

   4. IMA occlusion (occurring in fewer than 10% of cases) has the same causes as SMA occlusion. The artery also may be inadvertently ligated at the time of cardiac bypass surgery or aortoiliac reconstruction.

   5. Systemic vasculitis (e.g., polyarteritis nodosa) and extension of a dissecting aortic aneurysm are rare causes of acute mesenteric ischemia. They may cause segmental areas of infarction that do not conform to the distribution of major arteries.

   6. Ischemia secondary to intestinal obstruction can result from mechanical causes.
      a. Intraabdominal hernias represent portions of bowel (usually small intestine) that become trapped in a narrow orifice, such as the inguinal or femoral canal, a surgical scar, or the umbilicus.
      b. Intestinal adhesions, which are fibrotic bridges of inflamed peritoneum, usually are sequelae of prior surgery or infection. They may trap and kink bowel segments.
      c. Intussusception is the telescoping of a proximal portion of the bowel into an immediately distal segment. Peristalsis then propels the telescoped segment further into the distal segment. Intussusception is most common in children, often occurring spontaneously. In adults, a malignancy often is present at the leading edge of the entrapped segment.
      d. Volvulus, the twisting of a loop of bowel about its mesenteric base, is most commonly found in the small bowel or sigmoid colon.

D. Clinical features

   1. Acute mesenteric ischemia. Patients usually are over age 50 and appear seriously ill. They classically present with acute onset of severe abdominal pain that seems out of proportion to the minimal physical findings. Patients often demonstrate occult gastrointestinal bleeding. Abdominal pain beginning soon after eating is known as **intestinal angina**.

   2. Ischemic colitis usually is a chronic segmental process in elderly patients, typically affecting the watershed areas of the splenic flexure and rectosigmoid region. Although patients may present with acute onset of abdominal pain and rectal bleeding, these symptoms may occur intermittently for weeks or months prior to presentation. Clinical distinction from idiopathic IBD, infectious colitis, diverticulitis, and carcinoma may be quite difficult.

E. Pathology. Findings depend on the severity of the injury.

   1. Macroscopic appearance. Typically, a red or purple, moist, dilated bowel segment appears with a friable and often hemorrhagic mucosa. The wall may tear easily and perforation may occur.

   2. Microscopic appearance
      a. The least severe lesions consist only of mucosal necrosis. Occasionally, there are yellow mucosal plaques composed of mucin, necrotic debris, and inflammatory cells, with pseudomembrane formation. At this stage the changes are reversible, and the mucosa will regenerate if normal blood flow can be restored.

   b. With more severe injury, deeper layers of the bowel wall become necrotic (infarcted), and often many neutrophils are seen. If healing does occur, a fibrous stricture usually results.

F. Treatment and prognosis

1. Acute mesenteric ischemia in the past has been associated with a poor prognosis, that is, a 70% to 100% mortality rate. Recently, early recognition and prompt treatment have yielded better results. Necrotic bowel must be removed.

2. In some patients with ischemic colitis, the clinical symptoms resolve completely. In others, a stricture develops and may require surgical resection.

VII. ANAL CANAL

A. Normal anatomy and histology

1. The anal canal is 3 to 4 cm long. It is bounded by the anal opening (**anal verge** or **anal margin**) distally and by the upper border of the internal sphincter proximally.

2. About 2 cm above the anal verge, at the base of the anal valves, the **pectinate (dentate) line** marks the boundary between squamous and nonsquamous mucosa.

3. A region approximately 1 cm in diameter, known as the **transitional** or **cloacogenic zone,** extends proximally from the pectinate line to blend with the columnar mucosa of the rectum. This zone is characterized histologically by one or more epithelial types, including stratified sqamous epithelium, simple or stratified columnar epithelium, and transitional epithelium like that of the bladder. Anal glands arise in this region and normally may extend into and through the internal sphincter.

B. Imperforate anus.
Maldevelopment of the junction of the hindgut and the ectodermal anal dimple may result in an intact membranous septum or a more severe defect, such as agenesis, atresia, or stenosis of this region. Fistulas to the genitourinary tract may occur.

C. Inflammatory disorders

1. **Fissures** represent ulcers of the squamous mucosa. More than 90% of fissures are found in the midline posteriorly, probably because of impingement on this region by the fecal mass and the relative lack of muscular support. When fissures are found in other locations, CD and carcinoma must be considered. Nonspecific inflammation is seen microscopically.

2. **Fistulas** are characterized by an internal opening at the level of the dentate line and one or more openings in the perianal skin. The fistula tract is lined by nonspecific inflammation, granulation tissue, and at times, foci of epithelium. A foreign-body giant-cell reaction to fecal material commonly is seen. The pathogenesis is currently considered to be infection of an anal gland followed by rupture, formation of a perirectal abscess, and finally formation of the fistula tract.

3. **CD** and much less frequently **UC** (see V B) can involve the anal region. The noncaseating granulomas of CD must be distinguished from the foreign-body granulomas of nonspecific fistulas.

4. **Infections** such as syphilis, gonorrhea, chlamydial infection with LGV and non-LGV serotypes, herpes simplex, and HPV infection (e.g., condylomas, venereal warts) are STDs that may involve the anal region. They have been described with increasing frequency in the homosexual population.

D. Hemorrhoids (see IV D 2)

E. Neoplasms

1. **Squamous cell carcinoma**
   a. **Types and clinical features**
      (1) SCC (including its histologic variants) is the most common form of malignancy of the anal canal, accounting for 2% of all large bowel cancers. Most commonly, lesions arise in the region of the dentate line and, thus, are sometimes called **cloacogenic carcinomas**. Women are more frequently affected than men; however, an increase has recently been noted in the homosexual male population. Bleeding, pain, and a mass are the most common symptoms.

(2) **Squamous dysplasia,** including **carcinoma in situ (Bowen's disease),** is a precursor lesion. As in the cervix, HPV may play an important role in the pathogenesis of these tumors. Squamous carcinomas may arise in condylomas.

b. **Pathology.** Microscopically, nonkeratinizing (rarely, keratinizing) squamous, basaloid, and mucoepidermoid patterns of invasive carcinoma can be seen.

c. **Treatment and prognosis.** Combined radiation and chemotherapy have come to play a major role in treatment of these tumors, potentially eliminating the need for abdomino-perineal resection. The overall 5-year survival rate is about 60%, with the stage of disease being the most important prognostic factor. Metastases to inguinal lymph nodes occur in 40% of cases.

2. **Verrucous carcinoma.** This extremely well-differentiated, warty squamous growth demonstrates extensive local invasion but does not metastasize. It is probably identical to the lesion known as **giant condyloma** or (**Buschke-Löwenstein tumor**).

3. Other **malignant neoplasms** that arise less commonly at this site include malignant melanoma, small cell carcinoma, extramammary Paget's disease, and adenocarcinoma arising in the anal glands.

VIII. VERMIFORM APPENDIX

A. Normal anatomy and histology

1. The vermiform appendix, a worm-like structure, is a derivative of the cecum and is about 7 cm in length by 0.5 to 1 cm in diameter. It usually lies adjacent to the anterior taenia of the cecum, but its position is variable, leading to potential difficulties in the diagnosis of appendicitis.

2. The histologic structure is similar to that of the colon, except that the lamina propria and submucosa of the appendix contain numerous lymphoid follicles that encircle the lumen. With age, lymphoid atrophy and progressive fibrosis cause the lumen to become obliterated (fibrous obliteration).

B. Appendicitis

1. **Acute nonspecific appendicitis.** This common disorder predominantly affects young adults but may occur at any age.

a. **Pathogenesis.** Luminal obstruction leads to mural ischemia and secondary bacterial infection in the overwhelming majority of cases. The obstruction is caused by fecaliths in 67% of cases; other causes include hyperplasia of lymphoid tissue or adhesions.

b. **Clinical features.** Patients usually present with right lower quadrant or periumbilical pain, anorexia, vomiting, and fever. Leukocytosis often is present.

c. **Pathology.** The findings vary with the severity of the disorder.

(1) **Macroscopically,** mild cases show only minimal swelling of the appendix, with serosal congestion. More severe cases show extensive serosal exudate and mural necrosis (referred to as **gangrenous appendicitis**). With perforation, a periappendiceal abscess may result.

(2) **Microscopically,** mild cases show focal mucosal ulceration, with neutrophils extending into the submucosa. Severe cases show transmural necrosis, with numerous neutrophils and secondary vascular thrombosis.

d. **Treatment** is surgical removal of the appendix.

2. **Chronic nonspecific appendicitis** is a controversial disorder. Although bouts of acute appendicitis may occur and spontaneously subside, truly persistent chronic nonspecific inflammation of the appendix rarely, if ever, occurs.

3. **Specific types of appendicitis.** Enterobiasis, or oxyuriasis (caused by *Enterobius vermicularis,* or pinworms), is found in about 3% of appendixes and is believed to be a rare cause of appendicitis. Other rare causes include yersiniosis, actinomycosis, schistosomiasis, measles, adenovirus infection, and idiopathic IBD.

C. Tumors and other appendiceal masses

1. **Carcinoid tumors** of the appendix constitute 70% to 80% of all gastrointestinal carcinoids and are the most common appendiceal tumor. They usually are incidental findings at the

appendiceal tip. Pathologic features are identical to those of carcinoids at other sites (see III D 2). Metastatic spread and development of the carcinoid syndrome are exceedingly rare with appendiceal carcinoid tumors.

2. **Mucocele.** A dilated, saclike appendix filled with tenacious mucin can result from several causes.

   a. **Retention cysts** are nonneoplastic mucoceles. They cause only slight appendiceal dilation and usually are secondary to obstruction.

   b. **Neoplastic forms of mucocele** often dilate the appendix to more than 6 cm in diameter. With a benign **cystadenoma,** the epithelium is similar microscopically to that of colorectal adenomas. When the tumor invades the appendiceal wall, it is a **cystadenocarcinoma**.

   c. **Pseudomyxoma peritonei** is characterized by the presence of mucinous masses in the peritoneal cavity and is almost always due to rupture of an appendiceal cystadenoma, a cystadenocarcinoma, or an ovarian mucinous tumor. With rupture of an appendiceal cystadenoma, the mucinous material is nearly always confined to the right iliac fossa and resolves after appendectomy. Rupture of a cystadenocarcinoma may lead to generalized peritoneal seeding of mucinous adenocarcinoma. In these cases, the result is often death from bowel obstruction.

3. **Solid adenocarcinomas** similar to those seen in the colorectum can occur in the appendix, but are rare.

STUDY QUESTIONS

Directions: Each of the numbered items or incomplete statements in this section is followed by answers or by completions of the statement. Select the **one** lettered answer or completion that is **best** in each case.

1. Which type of esophagitis is the most common?

(A) Reflux
(B) Viral
(C) Fungal
(D) Acute corrosive
(E) Chronic granulomatous

2. An organism that is discovered (and appears to play a causative role) in many cases of chronic nonspecific gastritis and chronic peptic ulcer disease is

(A) *Enterobacter cloacae*
(B) *Escherichia coli*
(C) *Helicobacter pylori*
(D) *Klebsiella pneumoniae*
(E) *Citrobacter freundii*

3. Hirschsprung's disease usually is caused by the congenital absence of ganglion cells in which segment of the large intestine?

(A) Cecum
(B) Ascending colon
(C) Transverse colon
(D) Descending colon
(E) Rectum

4. Which inflammatory condition of the intestine is characterized by segmental involvement of the small or large bowel, or both, transmural inflammation, and the development of epithelioid granulomas?

(A) Crohn's disease (CD)
(B) Ulcerative colitis (UC)
(C) Cryptosporidiosis
(D) Diverticulitis
(E) Colitis cystica profunda

5. Which statement about disorders of the anal canal is true?

(A) Anal fistulas most often occur in association with Crohn's disease (CD)
(B) Adenocarcinoma is the most common primary malignancy of the anal canal
(C) The risk for squamous cell carcinoma (SCC) of the anal canal is equivalent for heterosexual and homosexual men
(D) Perirectal abscesses are believed to stem from infection of an anal gland
(E) External hemorrhoids originate above the pectinate line

6. The most common site of gastrointestinal carcinoid tumors is

(A) small bowel
(B) colon
(C) appendix
(D) esophagus
(E) stomach

7. Which statement about esophageal atresia (EA) is true?

(A) Other malformations typically are absent
(B) Symptoms develop after the first year of life
(C) Surgical correction is required for survival
(D) Patients with this disorder cannot regurgitate
(E) A fistula connecting the blind lower pouch to the trachea is rarely seen

8. Reflux esophagitis is an esophageal motor disorder characterized by

(A) inappropriately increased lower esophageal sphincter pressure
(B) the development of Barrett's epithelium in some chronic cases
(C) more frequent development of squamous cell carcinoma (SCC) rather than adenocarcinoma
(D) the lack of potential for stricture development
(E) a high frequency of associated *Candida* esophagitis

1-A	4-A	7-C
2-C	5-D	8-B
3-E	6-C	

9. Ménétrier's disease is characterized by

(A) thickened gastric folds, mucous cell hyperplasia, hypoproteinemia and protein-losing enteropathy
(B) thickened gastric folds related to infiltration by lymphoma
(C) the presence of numerous *Helicobacter pylori* organisms
(D) thickened gastric folds related to signet-ring cell adenocarcinoma
(E) loss of gastric folds related to chronic atrophic gastritis

10. Which colorectal polyp is considered to be nonneoplastic?

(A) Tubulovillous adenoma
(B) Villous adenoma
(C) The polyps of familial adenomatous polyposis (FAP)
(D) Hyperplastic polyp
(E) Leiomyoma

11. Which statement about pseudomembranous enterocolitis is true? It

(A) is caused by the enterotoxin of *Clostridium perfringens*
(B) causes constipation
(C) is usually associated with a recent history of antibiotic use
(D) is characterized histologically by transmural chronic inflammation
(E) is an uncommon but well-documented variant of ulcerative colitis (UC)

12. Acute bowel (mesenteric) ischemia is often characterized by

(A) an overall good prognosis
(B) celiac artery thrombosis
(C) the presence of splanchnic vasoconstriction
(D) a proclivity to affect young patients
(E) no relationship between degree of mural damage and the rapidity of onset or the severity or duration of the insult

13. The definition of early gastric cancer (EGC) requires

(A) a tumor smaller than 2 cm in diameter
(B) a patient with symptoms for less than 2 years
(C) no lymph node involvement
(D) tumor invasion no further than the submucosa
(E) a tumor with a raised macroscopic appearance

14. Which feature characterizes celiac disease, a malabsorptive disorder of the small bowel?

(A) Deranged immunologic reactivity to milk protein
(B) Marked villous atrophy on biopsy
(C) Primarily distal involvement
(D) Increased risk of colon carcinoma
(E) Numerous intraepithelial eosinophils on biopsy

15. A biopsy performed on a gastric ulcer reveals adenocarcinoma. When a partial gastrectomy is performed, it reveals invasive, moderately differentiated adenocarcinoma extending into, but not beyond, the submucosa. One of five regional lymph nodes is positive for metastatic adenocarcinoma. Which statement about adenocarcinoma is true?

(A) This case is unusual because squamous cell carcinoma (SCC) is the most common histologic type of gastric carcinoma
(B) This patient will most likely die of her disease within 5 years
(C) By definition, this patient has advanced gastric carcinoma (AGC)
(D) The size of the gastric carcinoma, rather than the degree of mural invasion, is the most important factor pertaining to patient prognosis
(E) Early gastric carcinoma (EGC) represents about 10% to 20% of all gastric carcinomas in this country

16. Achalasia is characterized by all of the following features EXCEPT

(A) regurgitation and aspiration
(B) incomplete relaxation of the lower esophageal sphincter on swallowing
(C) absence of esophageal peristalsis
(D) increased risk for esophageal squamous cell carcinoma (SCC)
(E) an esophagus that is narrowed proximally and widened distally

9-A	12-C	15-E
10-D	13-D	16-E
11-C	14-B	

17. Features of colonic adenomas that are associated with an increased risk for carcinoma include all of the following EXCEPT

(A) severe dysplasia
(B) villous architecture
(C) size exceeding 2 cm
(D) marked inflammation
(E) multiple adenomas

18. Diverticular disease of the colon is typically characterized by all of the following EXCEPT

(A) involvement of all layers of the bowel wall
(B) frequent occurrence in the sigmoid colon
(C) muscular hypertrophy of the bowel wall
(D) frequent occurrence in the elderly
(E) complications (e.g., pericolic abscess)

19. All of the following statements about colorectal carcinoma are true EXCEPT

(A) it is the second most common cause of cancer deaths in the United States
(B) the peak incidence is in the seventh decade
(C) adenocarcinoma is more common than squamous cell carcinoma (SCC)
(D) only a minority of colorectal carcinomas arise in the setting of inflammatory bowel disease (IBD)
(E) chromosomal abnormalities are rarely encountered in colorectal carcinoma

20. All of the following features are typical of Crohn's disease (CD) EXCEPT

(A) the presence of granulomas
(B) minimal submucosal involvement
(C) predominant involvement of the cecum and small bowel
(D) frequent fibrotic strictures and fistulas
(E) discontinuous inflammation

21. All of the following factors appear to predispose to chronic peptic ulcers EXCEPT

(A) colonic diverticula
(B) blood group O
(C) *Helicobacter pylori* infection
(D) excessive gastrin secretion in the Zollinger-Ellison syndrome
(E) nonsteroidal antiinflammatory drugs (NSAIDs)

22. All of the following statements about gastric ulcers are true EXCEPT

(A) *Helicobacter pylori* is found in association with chronic peptic ulcers of the stomach in the majority of patients
(B) nonsteroidal antiinflammatory drugs (NSAIDs) appear to be important in the pathogenesis of many gastric ulcers
(C) chronic gastritis is often found in association with chronic peptic ulcers
(D) carcinoma is easily distinguished from benign peptic ulcers on macroscopic (endoscopic) inspection
(E) bleeding, perforation, and penetration into adjacent viscera are all potential complications of peptic ulcer disease

17-D   20-B
18-A   21-A
19-E   22-D

ANSWERS AND EXPLANATIONS

1. The answer is A *[I D 2 a].*
Inflammation of the esophagus most often is the result of an incompetent lower esophageal sphincter, which permits reflux of gastric contents into the lower esophagus. Viral and fungal esophagitis occur primarily in patients with diminished immune responses. Corrosive esophagitis results from ingestion of corrosive chemicals, usually cleaning agents. Granulomatous esophagitis is an uncommon condition, occurring chiefly in patients with tuberculosis or Crohn's disease (CD).

2. The answer is C *[II C 3 a (3), D 2 b].*
Helicobacter pylori is a curved gram-negative rod that frequently has been found in gastric biopsies from patients with chronic nonspecific gastritis, gastric ulcer, and particularly duodenal ulcer. It is found in areas of gastric metaplasia adjacent to ulcers in the duodenum and only occasionally is found in histologically normal stomachs. *H. pylori* produces a urease that converts urea to carbon dioxide, ammonia, and water; thus, the bacterium can survive in spite of the low gastric pH by creating a more alkaline microenvironment in the gastric mucous layer where it resides. Patients seem to respond to combined therapy with a bismuth-containing compound and antibiotics. *Enterobacter cloacae, Escherichia coli, Klebsiella pneumoniae,* and *Citrobacter freundii* are not significant in the pathogenesis of chronic nonspecific gastritis and chronic peptic ulcer disease.

3. The answer is E *[IV B].*
In all cases of Hirschsprung's disease the internal anal sphincter is aganglionic, and in most cases the rectum and part of the sigmoid colon also are affected. Occasionally, the more proximal colonic segments also are aganglionic. Hirschsprung's disease, or aganglionic megacolon, results from a failure in the development of ganglion cells in Meissner's (submucosal) and Auerbach's (myenteric) plexuses in the colon. Innervation of the colon during embryogenesis proceeds from the cecum to the anus. Interruption of this sequential development leaves the more distal segments of the colon aganglionic.

4. The answer is A *[V B 3].*
Crohn's disease (CD) is a chronic inflammatory disorder of the gastrointestinal tract that most commonly involves the distal ileum, colon, and anorectal region. It typically has a segmental pattern of involvement. Transmural chronic inflammation, often with epithelioid granulomas, is the histologic hallmark of CD. Granulomas are seen in 60% to 75% of resection specimens and also may occur in regional lymph nodes. Ulcerative colitis (UC) is a chronic inflammatory disorder of the bowel that begins in the rectum and often extends continuously to involve more proximal segments of the colon. Chronic inflammation generally is confined to the mucosa and superficial submucosa, and epithelioid granulomas are absent.

5. The answer is D *[VII C 2].*
It currently is believed that a perirectal abscess stems from infection of an anal gland, which subsequently ruptures. A fistula, with an internal opening near the dentate line and one or more secondary openings in the perianal skin, may result if the perirectal abscess fails to resolve. Although anal fistulas are seen in Crohn's disease (CD), they most frequently occur in the absence of this disease. All hemorrhoids develop in the submucosal venous plexus. Internal hemorrhoids arise above the pectinate line; external hemorrhoids arise distal to the pectinate line. Squamous cell carcinoma (SCC), and its basaloid and mucoepidermoid variants, is the most common primary carcinoma of the anal canal. Adenocarcinoma occasionally may arise from the upper anal canal. The homosexual male population appears to be at an increased risk for the development of SCC of the anal canal, possibly related to human papillomavirus (HPV).

6. The answer is C *[VIII C 1].*
The appendix is the most common site of gastrointestinal carcinoid tumors, accounting for 70% to 80% of the total. At this site, the tumors usually are incidental findings, rarely giving rise to metastases or the carcinoid syndrome. Second in frequency is the ileum, which is the most common site of gastrointestinal carcinoid tumors that give rise to the carcinoid syndrome. Carcinoid tumors also are somewhat common in the rectosigmoid region and, to a lesser degree, occur in the remainder of the colon.

7. The answer is C *[I B 1].*
Although in the past esophageal atresia (EA) and tracheoesophageal fistula (TEF) were fatal in most cases, survival currently approaches 90% with early recognition and prompt surgical intervention. EA (i.e., discontinuity of the esophagus) and TEF occur once in every 2000 to 4000 live births. These congenital defects usually occur together and in 50% of cases are associated with other congenital malformations. In

90% of cases a fistula connects the blind lower esophageal pouch to the trachea. Affected infants usually present with excessive salivation, respiratory distress, and regurgitation within 24 hours after birth.

8. The answer is B *[I D 2 a].*
Reflux esophagitis is the most common form of esophagitis. Reduced lower esophageal sphincter pressure allows gastroesophageal reflux, with the degree of mucosal injury being a function of the nature of the refluxing fluid, the duration of exposure, and the efficiency of the clearing mechanism. Strictures are a common complication, and high strictures almost always are associated with Barrett's epithelium. Barrett's epithelium, the replacement of normal esophageal squamous mucosa by columnar (gastric) or intestinal epithelium, occurs in about 10% of cases of symptomatic reflux esophagitis. Barrett's epithelium is complicated by adenocarcinoma in about 3% to 10% of cases. *Candida* esophagitis has no direct relationship to reflux esophagitis.

9. The answer is A *[II E 1].*
Ménétrier's disease is characterized by marked enlargement of the gastric mucosal folds, well beyond the normal thickness of 1 mm. These thickened folds produce radiographic signs that can mimic those of gastric lymphomas and some carcinomas. Ménétrier's disease can lead to excessive leakage of plasma proteins, with resultant hypoalbuminemia. Replacement of acid-secreting mucosa by mucus-secreting cells may lead to hypo- or achlorhydria.

10. The answer is D *[II F 1 a; IV E 2, 4; Figure 13-5].*
Hyperplastic polyps are considered not to be neoplastic, with virtually no premalignant potential. They account for approximately 50% of all colorectal polyps, and they result from an imbalance of cell renewal. Adenomatous (neoplastic) polyps occur in three main histologic forms: tubular, tubulovillous, and villous. Virtually all colorectal carcinomas arise from adenomas. In the familial adenomatous polyposis (FAP) syndrome, it is very likely that the patient will develop one or more carcinomas of the colon unless a total colectomy is performed. Leiomyomas are benign neoplasms of smooth muscle.

11. The answer is C *[Table 13-4].*
Pseudomembranous enterocolitis nearly always is caused by the enterotoxin of *Clostridium difficile*. Intestinal overgrowth by this organism most commonly is due to treatment with antibiotics. Symptoms can range from mild diarrhea to severe colitis. Macroscopically, grayish-white mucosal plaques (pseudomembranes) are seen; microscopically, there are foci of relatively superficial mucosal necrosis associated with an outpouring of mucus and neutrophils ("volcano lesion"). Rarely, intestinal ischemia in the absence of *C. difficile* enterotoxin may be responsible for identical morphologic findings. While pseudomembranous colitis may complicate ulcerative colitis (UC), each is a distinct disorder.

12. The answer is C *[VI A–D 1].*
Nonocclusive ischemia, representing hypoperfusion of the bowel due to splanchnic vasoconstriction, accounts for 30% to 50% of all cases of acute mesenteric ischemia. Although earlier detection of this disorder has improved survival, the mortality rate remains high. In bowel ischemia, the degree of mural damage is directly related to the rapidity of onset and the type, severity, and duration of the insult. The extent of the collateral circulation, the metabolic requirements of the affected bowel segment, and the nature of the bowel flora are other important factors. Most cases of acute mesenteric ischemia involve the distribution of the superior mesenteric artery (SMA) and occur in patients who are over age 50. Involvement of the bowel supplied by the celiac artery is rare. Microscopically, the least severe lesions may demonstrate only foci of mucosal necrosis; with more severe injury, the entire bowel wall may become necrotic (infarcted), and perforation may result.

13. The answer is D *[II G 1 d–e].*
The definition of early gastric cancer (EGC) requires that the tumor invade no further than the submucosa, with or without the presence of lymph node metastases. The duration of symptoms and the size of the lesions are quite variable. EGC also varies considerably in appearance; lesions may be elevated, flat, or (in most cases) depressed.

14. The answer is B *[III C 3 a].*
Celiac disease is caused by a deranged immunologic reaction to gliadin, a component of gluten found in wheat, barley, and rye. The characteristic small-bowel biopsy findings are marked villous atrophy (a flat biopsy) with crypt hyperplasia, lamina propria chronic inflammation, and a prominent number of intraepithelial lymphocytes. The proximal small bowel demonstrates the most extensive and severe injury. Complications of celiac disease include ulceration and strictures of the small bowel, lack of responsiveness to a gluten-free diet (refractory sprue), formation of large mesenteric lymph nodes containing

inspissated chylomicrons (cavitated mesenteric lymph nodes), and development of malignant small bowel tumors (primarily T-cell lymphoma and, more rarely, adenocarcinoma).

15. The answer is E *[II G 1].*
Even in the presence of lymph node metastases, this patient's tumor is classified as an early gastric carcinoma (EGC) since it does not invade the gastric wall beyond the submucosa. The depth of mural penetration—not the size of the carcinoma—has prognostic importance. Overall, patients with EGC have a 5-year survival rate of 70% to 90% versus a 5-year survival rate of 5% to 15% for advanced gastric cancer (AGC). Over 95% of gastric malignancies are adenocarcinomas; squamous cell carcinoma (SCC) is quite rare.

16. The answer is E *[I E 2].*
In achalasia, the esophagus typically demonstrates a *dilated* proximal portion with distal *tapering*. Myenteric ganglion cells are absent or markedly decreased in the dilated portion but may be present in the distal tapered region. The diagnosis of achalasia is established by a barium enema that reveals the characteristic tapering combined with demonstration of incomplete relaxation of the lower esophageal sphincter during swallowing, absence of esophageal peristalsis, and increased esophageal contraction in response to methacholine. Patients with achalasia experience dysphagia for solids and liquids, and regurgitation and aspiration are common. Patients with long-standing achalasia are at an increased risk for squamous cell carcinoma (SCC) of the esophagus.

17. The answer is D *[IV E 4 e (2)].*
The degree of inflammation in the adenoma has no relationship to its propensity to develop carcinoma. Significant risk factors for the presence of adenocarcinoma in an adenoma of the colon include size (if larger than 2 cm, the risk is 10% to 50%), histologic type (villous, tubulovillous, tubular), degree of epithelial dysplasia, and the number of adenomas.

18. The answer is A *[III B 2 a, IV C].*
Colonic diverticula are actually pseudodiverticula, as they represent herniations of the mucosa, submucosa, and perhaps a portion of the outer longitudinal muscle layer. This separates them from "true" diverticula, such as Meckel's diverticulum, which contains all layers of the bowel wall. About 95% of colonic diverticula are found in the sigmoid colon, often in association with prominent muscular hypertrophy. Diverticula are rarely encountered before age 40. Pericolonic abscess, perforation, fistulas, and hemorrhage are important complications.

19. The answer is E *[IV F 1].*
Chromosomal deletions or mutations are frequently found, particularly involving tumor suppressor genes on chromosomal segments 5q, 17q, and 18q. Colorectal cancer is second only to lung cancer as the most common cause of cancer-related deaths in the United States. In about 95% of cases, the tumors are adenocarcinomas; squamous cell carcinomas (SCCs) are quite rare. Except in cases associated with polyposis or hereditary nonpolyposis syndromes or with inflammatory bowel disease (IBD), colorectal cancers are rare before age 40, having a peak incidence in the seventh decade. Several risk factors have been identified, most notably a diet that is high in animal fat and protein and low in fiber. A genetic predisposition also has been noted. Patients with so-called hereditary nonpolyposis syndromes inherit colorectal cancer as an autosomal dominant trait. Only about 1% of colorectal carcinomas are found in patients with idiopathic IBD.

20. The answer is B *[V B 2, 3; Table 13-5].*
Both Crohn's disease (CD) and ulcerative colitis (UC) are considered to be forms of chronic idiopathic inflammatory bowel disease (IBD); although the two disorders show many similarities, certain diagnostic differences exist. CD causes formation of granulomas in about 75% of affected persons, whereas granulomas are not found in patients with UC. The ulcers and inflammation of UC are predominantly mucosal, in contrast to the more typical transmural inflammation of CD. UC is a continuous disease that begins in the rectum; it may extend to involve the entire colon. CD is discontinuous and frequently involves the small bowel; the colonic involvement often is right-sided, with sparing of the rectum. Fibrotic strictures and fistulas are typical of CD and are quite rare in UC.

21. The answer is A *[II D 2, E 2].*
Chronic peptic ulcers of the gastrointestinal mucosa may occur at any site that is exposed to acid–pepsin secretion; however, nearly all peptic ulcers occur in the duodenum or stomach. Peptic ulcers may develop in a Meckel's diverticulum related to the presence of heterotropic gastric acid-secreting mucosa.

These ulcers do not occur in colonic diverticula. The balance between the integrity of the mucosal barrier and the degree of acid–pepsin secretion is quite important. *Helicobacter pylori* appears to be one of the most important factors in the pathogenesis of peptic ulcer disease. *H. pylori* has been found in the stomach in nearly all patients with duodenal ulcer and in the majority of those with gastric ulcers. The use of nonsteroidal antiinflammatory drugs (NSAIDs) is another very important predisposing factor. Persons with duodenal ulcers often have higher acid secretion levels than normal persons. In addition, an increased incidence of duodenal ulcers has been documented in persons with blood group O and in those who are nonsecretors of ABO blood group antigens. Increased gastrin secretion, as in patients with gastrin-secreting tumors, leads to hyperacidity, with the consequent development of peptic ulcers (Zollinger-Ellison syndrome).

22. The answer is D *[II D]*.
Gastric carcinomas, especially when they are small and minimally invasive [early gastric cancers (EGC)], can be indistinguishable from benign peptic ulcers. Therefore, endoscopic biopsies, often coupled with cytologic examination of the ulcer, are necessary to exclude malignancy. Healing of the ulcer surface with medical therapy does not ensure that the ulcer is benign.

14

Biliary Tract and Exocrine Pancreas

Scott H. Saul

I. GALLBLADDER

A. Normal anatomy and histology

1. The normal gallbladder is a thin-walled sac with a 50-ml capacity. Located under the right lobe of the liver in the gallbladder fossa, it consists of a fundus, body, and neck. The gallbladder is connected (via the cystic duct) to the common hepatic duct to form the common bile duct.

2. Histologically, the gallbladder has four layers:
   a. An inner mucosa, composed of a columnar epithelial lining and lamina propria
   b. A muscular layer
   c. A perimuscular layer of loose connective tissue
   d. A covering of peritoneum (serosa), except in the hepatic bed

B. Congenital abnormalities

1. **Abnormal shape** may occur [e.g., bilobate ("hourglass") gallbladder].

2. **Abnormal position,** such as lying within the liver or floating on a pendulous mesentery, may lead to problems at surgery.

3. **Variations in the length and course of the cystic duct** also can lead to surgical difficulties, especially when the area is inflamed.

4. **Folded fundus,** caused by angulation between the fundus and body (**phrygian cap**), may be noted on radiologic examination but has no clinical significance.

C. Gallstones (cholelithiasis)

1. **Frequency and diagnosis.** Gallstones affect approximately 20 million Americans (about 20% of all women and 8% of all men) and account for about $1 billion in medical expenses annually. They are common in those living in affluent countries, and frequency of occurrence increases with age. From 10% to 20% of gallstones are radiopaque. Ultrasonography is the diagnostic modality of choice, since it detects virtually all stones greater than 3 mm in diameter.

2. **Risk factors**
   a. Table 14-1 lists conditions associated with an increased risk of gallstones. The mnemonic known as the **five Fs** (fair, fat, fertile, female, forty) describes the typical patient with an increased risk for cholelithiasis, but also oversimplifies the situation.
   b. Two risk factors—obesity and a high-calorie diet—appear to increase the hepatic secretion of cholesterol. A diet rich in unrefined sugars may decrease the bile acid pool.

3. **Classification and pathogenesis**
   a. **Cholesterol stones** comprise about 85% of all stones.
      (1) **Pathogenesis**
         (a) Cholesterol-rich stones result from failure of the liver to provide enough bile salts and lecithin, from increased hepatic synthesis of cholesterol, or from both. **Supersaturation of bile with cholesterol** is the result.
         (b) Stone formation also requires an initial **nucleation step** that must involve a **nidus** (e.g., precipitated cholesterol, glycoproteins, calcium salts, cell debris). Once formed, the stone enlarges by continuous precipitation of cholesterol. Gallbladder

Table 14-1. Conditions Associated with Increased Risk of Gallstones

---

Cholesterol stones
   Racial background: Native American, Mexican American > white > black
   Demographic location: Europe > North America > Asia
   Obesity, high-calorie diet
   Old age
   Certain drugs: oral contraceptives, estrogen compounds
   Intestinal resection or bypass surgery
   Crohn's disease
   Pregnancy (?), multiparity (?)
   Diabetes mellitus (?)
   Hyperparathyroidism (?)

Pigment stones
   Black stones
      Old age
      Chronic hemolytic anemia (usually hereditary, such as hereditary
         spherocytosis, sickle cell anemia)
      Cirrhosis

   Brown stones
      Racial background: Asian > western
      Biliary tract infection

---

stasis favors gallstone growth. **Biliary sludge** represents highly viscous bile, which may be important in gallstone pathogenesis.

   (2) Types of cholesterol stones
      (a) Mixed cholesterol stones comprise about 75% of all gallstones. They usually are multiple, multifaceted, and laminated; have a crystalline appearance on cut surface; and measure up to 3 cm in diameter. Varying combinations of cholesterol (at least 60% of stone content, by definition), calcium carbonate, and calcium bilirubinate comprise the stones; the specific composition determines the color, which ranges from yellow to brown, and sometimes green.
      (b) Pure cholesterol stones (at least 90% cholesterol, by definition) comprise about 10% of the stones. They occur singly, are oval and crystalline, measure about 1 to 6 cm in diameter, and are white to pale yellow.

   b. Pigment stones comprise about 15% of the stones. They usually are multiple, measure a few millimeters in diameter, and contain a variety of insoluble calcium salts, including calcium bilirubinate, and cholesterol (usually less than 20% by weight). The two **types** are black and brown.
      (1) Black stones are deep brown to black and have an irregular surface. On fracturing, the stone is glass-like and featureless.
         (a) An insoluble calcium bilirubinate polymer is the major form of bile pigment in these stones. Although originally described only in patients with sickle cell anemia or other chronic hemolytic anemias or cirrhosis, black stones are most commonly found in elderly patients without predisposing disease.
         (b) The bile is **sterile,** and the degree of associated gallbladder inflammation is minimal. Approximately 50% of these stones are radiopaque.
      (2) Brown stones are soft and look rough and flaky. On cross section, they demonstrate alternating brown and tan layers of monomeric calcium bilirubinate and calcium salts of fatty acids.
         (a) The hydrolysis of bilirubin glucuronide by β-glucuronidases seems important in the pathogenesis of brown stones.
         (b) Brown stones are associated with **biliary stasis** and with the presence of **bacteria** (particularly *Escherichia coli* and anaerobes) and **parasites** in the bile. These stones are most common in Asians and are frequently associated with choledocholithiasis. They are rare in Americans.
   c. Calcium carbonate stones are rare. They are gray-white and amorphous.

4. Treatment options for gallstones have previously included only laparotomy with cholecystectomy and clinical observation. Recently, **laparoscopic cholecystectomy** has become the favored method of removing the gallbladder. Other nonsurgical methods used to dissolve or fragment gallstones include cholelitholytic (stone-dissolving) bile acids, transhepatic puncture of the gallbladder with instillation of methyl-tert-butyl ether, and, most recently, extracorporeal shock waves (lithotripsy).

5. **Complications** include acute and chronic cholecystitis, obstructive jaundice, ascending cholangitis, acute pancreatitis, and carcinoma of the gallbladder. An uncommon complication is **gallstone ileus,** a mechanical bowel obstruction resulting from a gallstone impacted in the intestinal lumen. The gallstone is more than 2.5 cm in diameter, nearly always enters via a cholecystoduodenal fistula, and typically becomes impacted in the ileum.

D. Cholecystitis

1. **Acute cholecystitis** almost always is a consequence of cholelithiasis. In the few remaining cases, it occurs as a complication of other serious illness or trauma.
   a. **Pathogenesis.** Although this topic is controversial, two mechanisms are cited.
      (1) **Acute calculous cholecystitis.** In 90% to 95% of patients, acute cholecystitis is initiated by gallstone impaction in the gallbladder neck or the cystic duct. The bile becomes increasingly concentrated and may act as a chemical irritant. The obstruction leads to increased intraluminal pressure, vascular compromise, necrosis, and, often, secondary bacterial invasion (*E. coli, Klebsiella,* enterococci, anaerobes, or other organisms in 40% to 65% of patients).
      (2) **Acute acalculous cholecystitis.** The remaining 5% to 10% of patients demonstrate a variety of conditions, including diabetes mellitus, shock, arteritis, sepsis, trauma, and burns. Probably one or more different mechanisms (e.g., ischemia, bacterial infection) are operative in a given case. In patients with AIDS, cytomegalovirus (CMV) and *Cryptosporidium* may cause acalculous cholecystitis.
   b. **Clinical features.** Women are 1.5 times more likely to be affected than men. The mean age of patients is 60 years. Common symptoms are right upper quadrant pain, particularly when the patient takes a deep breath (Murphy's sign); nausea; vomiting; fever; and slight jaundice. Prominent elevation of the serum bilirubin level may indicate the presence of stones in the common bile duct as well as in the gallbladder.
   c. **Pathology**
      (1) **Macroscopic examination** usually reveals an enlarged, discolored gallbladder, often with surface exudate. Pus may fill the lumen (**empyema**). Occasionally, gas may be found in the lumen or gallbladder wall (**emphysematous cholecystitis**) as a manifestation of gas-forming bacteria, particularly *Clostridium perfringens.*
      (2) **Microscopically,** acute inflammation accompanies vascular congestion and edema of the mucosa and often of the entire gallbladder wall. Mucosal erosion, deeper ulceration, and foci of necrosis may occur.
   d. **Clinical course.** Acute cholecystitis usually resolves but may become chronic. Resolution seems to result from relief of the cystic duct obstruction, either when a stone falls back into the gallbladder or when pressure within the gallbladder forces the stone past the obstruction in the duct. Cholecystectomy generally is considered the optimal treatment for acute cholecystitis. Patients who are poor operative risks may be managed medically.
   e. **Complications.** If the acute inflammation progresses, the mural blood vessels may become thrombosed secondarily, leading to gangrene (**gangrenous cholecystitis**) and perforation of the gallbladder, with consequent peritonitis. Perforation, the most serious complication, is seen in about 10% of patients and is much more common in acalculous patients. Mortality rates with free perforation approach 30%.

2. **Chronic cholecystitis** almost always develops in association with gallstones. Women are three times more likely to be affected than men.
   a. **Clinical features.** Chronic cholecystitis usually comes to clinical attention because of repeated bouts of acute cholecystitis or biliary colic. Sometimes the complications of gallstones, rather than the stones themselves, are responsible for the initial symptoms. Symptomatic chronic cholecystitis usually is treated by cholecystectomy, particularly when complicated by gallstones.
   b. **Pathology**
      (1) **Macroscopic findings** (Figure 14-1) are quite variable. One or more stones are present in the lumen of the gallbladder; multiple stones usually are faceted. When two or three "generations" of stones are present, they are recognizable by their different sizes. The

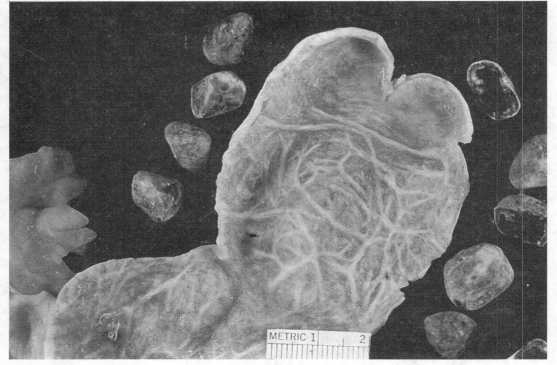

Figure 14-1. Opened gallbladder showing thickened walls with fibrous bands crisscrossing the mucosa. Numerous gallstones that originally were in the gallbladder lumen have been removed.

wall of the gallbladder becomes thickened, and the gallbladder itself may become so grossly shrunken by repeated bouts of inflammation that it is difficult to find at operation.

(2) Microscopic findings

(a) The degree of inflammation ranges from small scattered foci of chronic inflammatory cells to an extensive inflammatory infiltrate with prominent fibrosis, which causes the mural thickening. In addition, areas of mucosal ulceration may result from trauma by the stones.

(b) Rokitansky-Aschoff sinuses (outpouchings of mucosa that often extend into and beyond the muscular layer) are found in 90% of cases.

(c) Dystrophic calcification within the wall leads to **porcelain gallbladder**—a condition that may be detected radiographically.

E. Hydrops (mucocele). Impaction of a stone, usually in the cystic duct, may cause the gallbladder to be distended with a cloudy or mucoid fluid. Rarely, obstruction by a tumor may also cause hydrops.

F. Tumors of the gallbladder

1. Benign tumors are not unusual; most are nonneoplastic.

a. Nonneoplastic tumors. In addition to the types described next, inflammatory, lymphoid, and hyperplastic polyps also occur.

(1) Cholesterol polyps are the most common benign tumors of the gallbladder and have no association with serum cholesterol levels.

(a) Macroscopic appearance

(i) Macroscopically, cholesterol polyps appear as small yellow excrescences arising on a small pedicle from a mucosa that is usually otherwise normal. Rarely, diffuse cholesterolosis also is present; when striking, it is termed **strawberry gallbladder**.

(ii) Cholesterol polyps may become detached from their site of origin and float freely in bile. Conceivably, such free-floating polyps can provide a nucleus for the formation of gallstones.

      (b) Microscopically, the polyps consist of collections of foamy, cholesterol-rich macrophages in the lamina propria and a covering layer of surface columnar epithelium.

    (2) Adenomyoma and adenomyomatosis are characterized by hyperplasia of the mucosal epithelium and muscular layer of the gallbladder wall.

      (a) Macroscopically, the localized form (**adenomyoma**), which is usually found in the fundus, consists of a nodular protuberance, commonly with an umbilicated center. The cut surface is gray and cystic. The more diffuse form (**adenomyomatosis**) may cause marked thickening of the entire gallbladder wall.

      (b) Microscopically, there is hyperplasia of the muscle layer and the epithelium. The epithelium forms branched glandlike structures, an exaggeration of the Rokitansky-Aschoff sinuses seen in chronic cholecystitis. The projection of these structures into the surrounding hyperplastic muscle layer may lead to a misdiagnosis of adenocarcinoma. In fact, this process is not neoplastic at all, but is somewhat similar to diverticular disease of the colon.

  b. True benign epithelial neoplasms (i.e., **adenomas**) are uncommon in the gallbladder. Almost always less than 2 cm in diameter, they may be noted as isolated growths or may be found at the edge of a carcinoma. They have a tubular, tubulovillous, or villous architecture similar to that of colonic adenomas.

2. Malignant tumors. Carcinoma of the gallbladder accounts for 1% to 3% of all gastrointestinal malignancies.

  a. Pathogenesis

    (1) Gallstones are found in 75% of gallbladders containing carcinoma (Figure 14-2). However, whether they are the cause of the carcinoma or the effect of unknown carcinogenic influences is unknown. It is important to remember that only about 1% of patients with gallstones ever develops gallbladder carcinoma.

    (2) Some investigators have postulated that the mechanical irritation caused by gallstones and infection leads to neoplastic change.

    (3) From 10% to 15% of patients with gallbladder carcinoma have an **anomalous pancreaticobiliary junction** (see II A 1). Reflux of pancreatic enzymes into the common bile duct leads to increased lysophosphatidylcholine, which may initiate cellular damage, leading to carcinoma.

  b. Clinical features

    (1) Carcinoma of the gallbladder occurs most frequently in women; they are three to four times more likely to be affected than men. It is seen most often in Native Americans, Mexican–American women, and the Japanese.

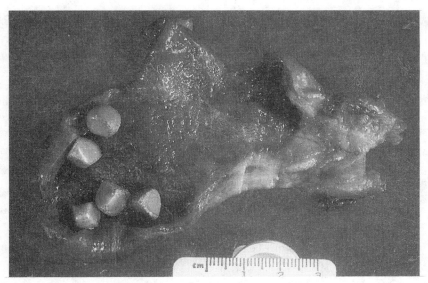

Figure 14-2. Gallbladder, surgically removed for chronic cholecystitis and cholelithiasis. An adenocarcinoma in the neck region (*right*) that caused marked mural thickening was also found. Metastatic tumor was found in the liver at the time of operation.

(2) The carcinoma usually occurs after age 50; the peak incidence is in the seventh decade of life. The rare patient who develops gallbladder carcinoma before age 40 is also likely to have ulcerative colitis or (much less commonly) Crohn's disease or familial adenomatous polyposis. Patients with a **porcelain gallbladder** are at increased risk.

(3) The most common symptoms are abdominal pain, jaundice, and weight loss. Most patients give a history of right upper quadrant pain.

c. Pathology

(1) **Macroscopically,** the tumor may form a bulky or papillary mass or may cause diffuse mural thickening (see Figure 14-2) that occasionally is indistinguishable from the mural thickening seen in chronic cholecystitis. The entire organ is involved in 80% of cases, and the fundus is the most common site of origin. If the cystic duct becomes obstructed, hydrops of the gallbladder may result.

(2) **Microscopically,** about 90% of the carcinomas are **adenocarcinomas** of variable differentiation. Rarely, squamous or adenosquamous carcinomas are found. Dysplastic gallbladder epithelium nearly always is found at the margins of the tumor and represents the **precursor lesion**. Microscopic signs of coexistent chronic cholecystitis are virtually always present.

d. Diagnosis is typically late, probably because early symptoms resemble those of chronic cholecystitis and cholelithiasis, which patients may have had for years. By the time a distinctive new symptom develops (e.g., jaundice or severe pain) and the disease is diagnosed, it usually has spread into the adjacent liver and perihilar lymph nodes.

e. Treatment depends on the extent of disease.

(1) For invasive disease confined to the gallbladder wall, cholecystectomy, possibly with excision of a wedge of surrounding liver and the adjacent lymph nodes, is the procedure of choice.

(2) Unfortunately, in most cases the tumor extends beyond the gallbladder wall and causes biliary obstruction. Palliation by placement of a bile duct stent is the treatment of choice.

f. Prognosis. The prognosis is poor; that is, the overall 5-year survival rate is less than 5%. Survival directly relates to the stage of mural invasion. The few survivors have small tumors that have not yet invaded the muscular layer and that are found incidentally in specimens surgically removed for chronic cholecystitis and cholelithiasis.

II. EXTRAHEPATIC BILE DUCTS

A. Normal anatomy and histology

1. The right and left hepatic ducts usually join to form the common hepatic duct within the porta hepatis. The cystic duct joins the common hepatic duct to form the common bile duct. The bile duct continues for 7 to 9 cm, passing through the pancreas into the duodenal wall, where it usually joins the pancreatic duct to form a common channel before emptying into the duodenum at the ampulla of Vater. An anomalous pancreaticobiliary junction is characterized by the ductal union occurring **outside** the duodenal wall.

2. Histologically, the bile duct mucosa consists of a single layer of tall columnar epithelium similar to that of the gallbladder; this epithelial layer connects with subepithelial mucous glands. The bile ducts have a supportive framework of connective tissue with rare smooth muscle fibers.

B. Congenital abnormalities

1. **Extrahepatic biliary atresia** is characterized by complete or incomplete discontinuity between the major hepatic or common bile ducts and the duodenum, resulting in persistent conjugated (direct) hyperbilirubinemia.

a. Pathogenesis. Extrahepatic biliary atresia, along with neonatal hepatitis and choledochal cyst, form part of the spectrum of infantile obstructive cholangiopathy.

(1) The disorder, once thought to be a developmental anomaly, is now recognized as an acquired condition that begins prenatally and continues after birth.

(2) An etiologic agent has not been identified. Viruses and maternal alcohol use both have been suggested as causes.

b. Clinical features

(1) Extrahepatic biliary atresia occurs once in every 10,000 live births. Females are two to three times more likely to be affected than males. Most patients are neonates who are born following an uncomplicated pregnancy and who have a normal birth weight, although various congenital defects may be found.

(2) The neonate, only a few weeks after birth, exhibits persistent conjugated (direct) hyperbilirubinemia.

(3) In most cases, a definitive diagnosis of extrahepatic biliary atresia is reached by 7 to 8 weeks of life.

c. **Pathology.** The extrahepatic biliary duct is transformed into a small threadlike cord embedded in fibrous tissue in the porta hepatis. The liver demonstrates features of mechanical obstruction, including bile duct proliferation and portal fibrosis.

d. **Treatment**
(1) Surgery, usually the **Kasai procedure** (portoenterostomy), should be performed by 10 to 12 weeks of life. Without successful surgical intervention, fatal biliary cirrhosis ensues, and average survival time is then only 10 to 12 months.

(2) Hepatic transplantation is an important treatment option, since the 5-year survival rate is as high as 75%.

2. Choledochal (bile duct) cysts are found in 1 in 13,000 live births; 80% occur in females. The cysts often are classified according to the portion of the biliary tree that is dilated. An anomalous pancreaticobiliary junction has been found in up to 90% of cases.

a. **Clinical features.** The majority of patients exhibit clinical manifestations within the first year of life, although presentation in adulthood may occur. Typical clinical findings include abdominal pain, jaundice, and an abdominal mass.

b. **Pathology.** The cysts are either spherical or fusiform. They can contain up to 1500 ml of bile and can attain a maximum diameter of 15 cm. The cyst wall is composed of fibrous tissue with a variable chronic inflammatory infiltrate. Remnants of biliary epithelium are seen in 20% to 60% of cases.

c. **Treatment** is cyst excision with a biliary drainage procedure.

d. **Complications.** Biliary tract carcinoma [i.e., adenocarcinoma or, rarely, squamous cell carcinoma (SCC)] may arise in association with a choledochal cyst in 2% to 8% of cases.

C. Choledocholithiasis (common bile duct stones)

1. Pathogenesis. Stones occasionally originate in the extrahepatic bile ducts (or in the intrahepatic ducts) but most often are the result of gallbladder calculi that have entered the common duct through the cystic duct. Patients with cholelithiasis have associated choledocholithiasis in 15% of cases. Duct stones are thought to be left behind in 3% to 4% of cholecystectomies. Primary duct stones are often brown stones.

2. Clinical features. The common bile duct is narrowest just proximal to the ampulla of Vater, so stones collect at that location, not at the actual opening. Pain, jaundice, and fever follow in 90%, 50%, and 33% of patients, respectively.

3. Course and complications. If stones cause obstruction, the patient risks infection and liver abscess. Unrelieved obstruction leads to secondary biliary cirrhosis. With recurrent attacks of obstruction, fibrosis, stricture, and stenosis may occur in the area of the sphincter of Oddi and cause acute or relapsing pancreatitis.

D. Primary sclerosing cholangitis (PSC) is a rare disorder characterized by diffuse fibroinflammatory narrowing of the bile ducts, usually affecting both the extrahepatic and intrahepatic ducts.

1. Pathogenesis. PSC origination and development are unknown. Most patients with PSC also have ulcerative colitis; some patients also have other inflammatory and sclerosing disorders, such as diffuse retroperitoneal fibrosis, Riedel's disease, sarcoidosis, and orbital inflammatory pseudotumor, suggesting a general disturbance of fibrous tissue, perhaps immunologically mediated.

2. Clinical features
a. Some 70% of patients with PSC are men, and over two-thirds of these are less than 45 years old. From 75% to 100% of patients have associated idiopathic inflammatory bowel disease, which almost always is ulcerative colitis and rarely is Crohn's disease. (However, only 3% to 4% of patients with ulcerative colitis develop PSC.)

b. Most frequently, patients present with progressive fatigue and pruritus, which are followed by jaundice.

3. **Diagnosis**
   a. Current radiographic techniques, particularly endoscopic retrograde cholangiopancreatography (ERCP), typically demonstrate short annular strictures separated by round or slightly dilated duct segments, giving the extra- and intrahepatic bile ducts a beaded appearance (Figure 14-3).
   b. PSC must be distinguished from secondary bile duct strictures, which result from choledocholithiasis, postoperative (usually postcholecystectomy) strictures, *Cryptosporidium,* Microsporida, and CMV infection in AIDS patients, and other causes.

4. **Pathology**
   a. **Macroscopic findings.** The bile duct is thickened and cordlike, and the involvement is diffuse or segmental. The duct lumen is narrowed and the wall grossly thickened (up to eight times normal). The gallbladder may be involved in the fibrotic process.
   b. **Microscopic findings**
      (1) The duct mucosa most often is intact, although hyperplasia or squamous metaplasia occasionally may be noted. Chronic inflammation and fibrosis involve mainly the subepithelial and subserosal layers. When the periluminal glands are distorted by fibrosis and inflammation, histologic distinction from adenocarcinoma may be extremely difficult.
      (2) The liver shows obstructive changes, with variable loss and duplication of bile ducts. Some intrahepatic ducts are replaced by fibrous cords (fibrous–obliterative cholangitis). Biliary cirrhosis usually results.

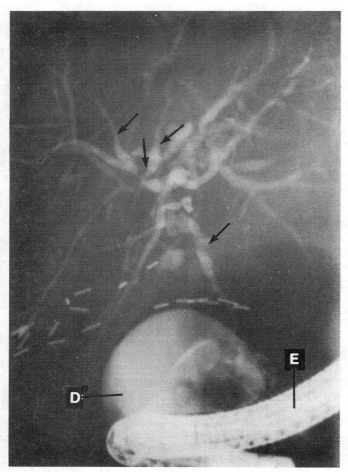

Figure 14-3. The appearance of primary sclerosing cholangitis (PSC) at the time of endoscopic retrograde cholangiopancreatography (ERCP). There is prominent narrowing (stricture) with adjacent dilatation of both the intrahepatic and extrahepatic bile ducts as indicated by the *arrows*. The most distal intrahepatic branches have the appearance of a pruned tree. The endoscope (*E*) is in the duodenum (*D*). (Courtesy of Craig Aronchick, MD; Pennsylvania Hospital, Philadelphia.)

B

5. Treatment and prognosis

a. Mean survival is about 7 years, with the patient's demise usually related to biliary cirrhosis, portal hypertension, and cholangitis. Bile duct carcinoma (either intra- or extrahepatic) may develop in up to 10% of patients with PSC.

b. Hepatic transplantation is the treatment of choice for patients with end-stage disease, the 5-year survival rate is 70%.

E. Tumors of the bile ducts

1. **Benign tumors** are rare and usually are **adenomas;** other nonepithelial lesions (e.g., granular cell tumor, fibroma, leiomyoma) also occur.

2. **Bile duct carcinoma.** Although bile duct carcinoma may occur at any point along the extrahepatic ducts, most tumors (60%) arise near the confluence of the right and left hepatic ducts (Klatskin tumor) and the adjacent common hepatic duct.

   a. **Clinical features**

      (1) The ratio of men to women shows a slight predominance of men. Both women and men are most commonly in the seventh decade of life. Patients with ulcerative colitis (and PSC) have a tenfold increased risk of developing bile duct cancer, which usually presents in the fourth or fifth decade.

      (2) Typical **symptoms** are abdominal pain, jaundice, and weight loss.

   b. **Pathology**

      (1) **Macroscopically,** the tumors may be nodular, papillary, or diffusely infiltrative and vary from one to several centimeters in diameter. Extension into adjacent soft tissue is common.

      (2) **Microscopically,** the tumor often extends a greater distance along the duct than can be discerned grossly. Nearly all of the tumors are found to be **adenocarcinoma,** often at least focally well differentiated. Since the tumor incites a dense fibrotic reaction, distinction from sclerosing cholangitis can be difficult at times.

   c. **Treatment and prognosis.** Metastases to regional lymph nodes and liver are present in 50% of patients at the time of presentation. The 5-year survival rate is about 5% to 10%; however, radical surgery occasionally may prolong life. Local radiation with placement of biliary stents is used for palliation.

F. Lesions of the ampulla of Vater

1. **Gallstones** may become impacted in this region, causing inflammation and fibrosis and, hence, the formation of a stricture. Jaundice, acute pancreatitis, or both may result.

2. **Neoplasms**

   a. **Villous adenomas** may arise in the periampullary region and cause biliary obstruction. In most cases, careful study of resected lesions discloses foci of invasive adenocarcinoma arising in the adenoma. Patients with familial adenomatous polyposis, including Gardner's syndrome, are at increased risk.

   b. **More advanced adenocarcinomas** also may arise in the ampulla, adjacent duodenal mucosa, or the terminal portion of the bile duct (Figure 14-4). Since the precise site of origin may not be discernible, the term, **periampullary carcinoma** often is used. Patients usually present with biliary obstruction. In contrast to carcinoma of the head of the pancreas or in the more proximal bile ducts, periampullary carcinoma shows a significant (30% to 60%) survival rate after surgical resection by Whipple's operation (pancreatoduodenectomy). Recently, wide local excision has been used as an alternative treatment.

III. EXOCRINE PANCREAS. (The endocrine pancreas is discussed in Chapter 20 V.)

A. Normal anatomy and histology

1. The exocrine portion of the pancreas comprises 80% of the organ. Each day, it secretes 1.5 to 3 L of fluid, which is rich in proteases, lipase, and amylase.

   a. The main excretory duct of the pancreas (**duct of Wirsung**) usually joins with the common bile duct to form a common channel just proximal to the ampulla of Vater.

   b. The accessory duct (**duct of Santorini**) in most cases drains only the anterior–superior part of the head of the pancreas. It empties into the accessory papilla, which is proximal to the ampulla.

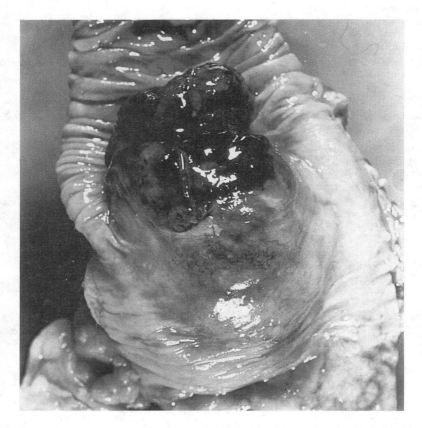

Figure 14-4. Polypoid, hemorrhagic tumor projecting into the duodenal lumen. It proved to be an adenocarcinoma of the ampulla.

    2. Microscopically, the exocrine pancreas is divided into lobules composed of acini; these acini consist of basophilic pyramid-shaped cells that contain numerous zymogen granules. The ductal system is lined with epithelial cells that range from cuboidal to columnar and contain mucin.

B. Congenital disorders

    1. Congenital malformations or abnormal locations of pancreatic tissue may not become clinically apparent until adult life and may even remain totally asymptomatic.

        a. Ectopic pancreatic tissue (acini, ducts, and, less frequently, islets) usually is asymptomatic and is found in approximately 3% of autopsies. The most frequently involved sites are the stomach and duodenum, followed by the jejunum, a Meckel's diverticulum, and the ileum. Symptoms, if they occur, usually result from gastrointestinal obstruction by the ectopic tissue. Gastrointestinal bleeding and intussusception are other complications.

        b. Annular pancreas. In this congenital anomaly, a ring of pancreatic tissue originating from the head of the pancreas encircles the descending part of the duodenum. This ring results from failure of the ventral pancreatic anlage to migrate to its posterior position. The anomaly causes intermittent or permanent duodenal stenosis in infants, with vomiting and failure to thrive as the first symptoms. It may be associated with other congenital anomalies, including duodenal atresia and Down syndrome.

        c. Pancreas divisum occurs when the ducts of the embryologic dorsal and ventral pancreatic anlagen fail to fuse. As a consequence, the majority of the pancreas is drained by the accessory duct. The most common congenital anomaly of the pancreas, it is seen in 1% to 10% of autopsies. The condition may increase the risk of chronic pancreatitis.

    2. Cystic fibrosis. This autosomal recessive disorder is the most common inherited disease of whites (occurring in about 1 in 2000 live births). The systemic disorder affects all exocrine glands, in that a biochemical abnormality of exocrine secretions causes the viscid secretions to be impacted in the exocrine ducts. The genetic defect responsible for cystic fibrosis resides on the long arm of chromosome 7. Thus, the abnormal gene product (cystic fibrosis transmembrane regulator; CFTR) causes abnormal transmembrane ionic transport.

  a. **Clinical features and diagnosis**
    (1) Some 80% of affected children have overt pancreatic exocrine insufficiency, manifested by steatorrhea or malabsorption. Diabetes mellitus due to pancreatic endocrine insufficiency may also be found. Chronic pulmonary disease, cirrhosis, and intestinal obstruction are other important clinical problems.
    (2) A **positive sweat test** (increased sweat chloride) is still the mainstay of diagnosis.
  b. **Pathology.** In the pancreas, the impacted viscid secretions cause inflammation and scarring, which lead to atrophy of ductal and acinar tissue with consequent insufficiency of exocrine function.
  c. **Treatment and prognosis.** Cystic fibrosis is a lifelong disease.
    (1) The nutritional complications of this disorder are treated by pancreatic replacement therapy accompanied by a diet that is normal for the age of the patient. The pulmonary complications are managed with antibiotics and with agents used to remove the thick inspissated secretions in the airways (expectorants, bronchodilators). Gene therapy may be the treatment of the future.
    (2) The prognosis for patients with cystic fibrosis depends primarily on the extent of pulmonary disease. Currently, 80% to 90% of patients survive to beyond 20 years of age.

C. Inflammatory disorders

  1. **Acute (hemorrhagic) pancreatitis**
    a. **Etiology.** Although the cause is unknown, a variety of clinical conditions appear to be important (Table 14-2), most notably biliary tract stones and alcoholism. The frequency of the associated disorders depends on the specific population studied; series from large urban hospitals show a higher percentage of cases associated with alcohol than with gallstones. About 20% of cases are idiopathic.
    b. **Pathogenesis.** Two major pathways may lead to intrapancreatic activation of digestive enzymes, with subsequent pancreatic "autodigestion."
      (1) **The duct obstruction–reflux model.** The reflux of bile and duodenal contents into the pancreas secondary to ampullary obstruction (e.g., by a stone) causes pancreatic damage.
        (a) The pancreatic enzymes trypsinogen and trypsin activate other proteases, initiating a destructive cycle. Lecithin in bile is converted to toxic lysolecithin by phospholipase A. Elastase activation causes blood vessel destruction and consequent hemorrhage.
        (b) In 75% to 80% of patients with cholelithiasis and pancreatitis, a stone is found impacted near the ampulla of Vater. Perhaps in the remainder of these patients, the stone is dislodged and passes into the duodenum after damaging the sphincter and leading to reflux of duodenal contents and bile.

Table 14-2. Conditions Associated with Acute Pancreatitis

Condition	Proposed Mechanism
Common associated conditions	
Gallstones	Duct obstruction; reflux
Alcoholism	Duct obstruction; reflux
Rare associated conditions	
Trauma	Acinar cell injury
Viral infection (mumps)	Acinar cell injury
Toxins (various drugs)	Acinar cell injury
Vasculitis	Acinar cell injury
Pancreatic carcinoma	Duct obstruction
Hyperparathyroidism	Unknown (? Ca^{2+} activation of trypsinogen)
Hypertriglyceridemia	Unknown (? toxicity of free fatty acids)

        (c) Chronic ethanol abuse may increase the protein concentration of pancreatic se-
cretions, leading to obstructive proteinaceous plugs within pancreatic ducts. Alcohol may induce spasm of the sphincter of Oddi. A similar sequence to that just
described for gallstones may then ensue.

    (2) **The acinar cell injury model.** Direct acinar cell damage may result from a variety of
insults, including viruses, toxins, ischemia, and trauma. Pancreatic enzyme leakage
ensues, resulting in pancreatitis.

  c. **Clinical features, diagnosis, and complications.** Patients are most often middle-aged; they
are most commonly men in alcohol-related cases and women in stone-related cases.

    (1) **Signs and symptoms**

        (a) Pain may be mild to marked and often radiates to the back; other symptoms in-
clude nausea, vomiting, and, occasionally, jaundice and fever.

        (b) Shock may result from blood loss, electrolyte disturbance, or release of vasoactive
substances such as bradykinin or prostaglandins.

        (c) Discoloration of the loin (**Turner's sign**) and around the umbilicus (**Cullen's sign**)
occurs rarely but always indicates severe and extensive disease.

    (2) **Laboratory data** may show leukocytosis, increased serum amylase and lipase levels,
increased serum bilirubin, and transient diabetes mellitus; hypocalcemia is a grim
prognostic sign.

    (3) **Complications.** Secondary bacterial infection may cause abscess formation. The ap-
pearance of an abdominal mass heralds the development of an abscess, a pseudocyst
[see III C 2 d (1)], or an area of fat necrosis in the omentum.

  d. **Pathology.** Acute pancreatitis is an autodigestive disease; the gland is "cannibalized" by
its own enzymes. The fundamental lesion is tissue destruction by proteases (proteolysis of
pancreatic substance), lipases (fat necrosis), and elastases (vascular necrosis and hemorrhage), with accompanying inflammatory reaction.

    (1) **Macroscopically,** the appearance of the pancreas depends on the duration and sever-
ity of the illness.

        (a) If the insult is mild, interstitial edema alone occurs (**interstitial pancreatitis**); the
pancreas appears edematous and the changes are fully reversible.

        (b) With more severe injury, small foci of hemorrhage, gray–white foci of parenchy-
mal necrosis, and chalky white areas of fat necrosis are noted. Extensive zones of
necrosis with blood clots may be found, and abscess formation may be seen.

    (2) **Microscopically,** acinar and endocrine cells develop a cloudy appearance and sub-
sequently undergo coagulative necrosis, usually with a neutrophilic infiltrate. Fat necrosis is characterized by outlines of fat cells containing a pink granular precipitate,
usually associated with foci of basophilic calcium salts and foamy macrophages. Vascular necrosis and hemorrhage are commonly found.

  e. **Treatment and prognosis**

    (1) Mild cases of pancreatitis generally are treated with supportive care and measures to
minimize pancreatic secretions.

    (2) More severe cases are more difficult to manage, and early death may occur from car-
diovascular collapse, adult respiratory distress syndrome, intraabdominal hemorrhage, acute renal failure, or sepsis.

    (3) The patient who recovers from a first attack of acute pancreatitis has a 25% to 60%
chance of **recurrence** in the next 1 to 2 years. Clinical, laboratory, and morphologic
signs of pancreatitis should cease if the primary cause or factors are eliminated.

2. **Chronic pancreatitis** is characterized by pancreatic damage, either anatomically or clinically
defined, which persists even if the primary causes or factors are eliminated. Very often the
course of the disease is inexorably progressive.

  a. **Etiology and pathogenesis**

    (1) Chronic ethanol abuse probably is responsible for the overwhelming majority of cases.
Gallstone-associated pancreatitis appears less likely to progress to chronic pancreatitis.

    (2) Other associated conditions include hyperparathyroidism, hypertriglyceridemia,
trauma, cystic fibrosis, and pancreas divisum.

    (3) A hereditary predisposition has been described in a few families (**hereditary pancre-
atitis**), and members of these families appear to be at increased risk for developing
pancreatic adenocarcinoma.

    (4) In some series, up to 40% of cases of chronic pancreatitis are idiopathic.

(5) Some investigators believe that an inherited or acquired defect of the biosynthesis of pancreatic stone protein (lithostatin), which normally inhibits stone formation, is the basic defect in chronic calcifying pancreatitis. This contention is controversial.

b. Clinical features

(1) Pain, either intermittent or chronic, is the predominant symptom of this disorder. The pain may be dull or sharp, and it frequently radiates to the back.

(2) Fat and protein malabsorption (causing steatorrhea and azotorrhea, respectively) do not occur until at least 90% of pancreatic secretory capacity is lost. Both conditions are present in up to 70% of patients beginning at 8 years after onset of symptoms. Malabsorption and anorexia lead to weight loss.

(3) Diabetes mellitus is present in 70% of patients by the time radiographic calcifications are noted.

(4) Fever, usually secondary to infection of a pseudocyst, may occur.

c. Pathology. Two morphologic types have been described.

(1) Chronic calcifying pancreatitis (Figure 14-5) is seen most commonly in alcoholics.

(a) Macroscopically, the gland is firm. Multiple ductal calculi (calcium carbonate) are often present, and calcification may be noted radiographically.

(b) Microscopically, the lesions have a lobular distribution, with lobular atrophy, fibrosis, and chronic inflammation. Intralobular and interlobular ducts often contain amorphous eosinophilic protein plugs that frequently calcify.

(2) Chronic obstructive pancreatitis has been described in association with impacted gallstones; but any cause of ampullary obstruction, such as carcinoma, may produce this histologic pattern. The destruction or fibroinflammatory damage is nonlobular; ductal protein plugs and calcified stones are rare. The head of the pancreas is most severely affected.

(3) Superimposed acute inflammatory changes may be seen in both patterns. Islets may appear relatively spared or may be focally increased or decreased in number.

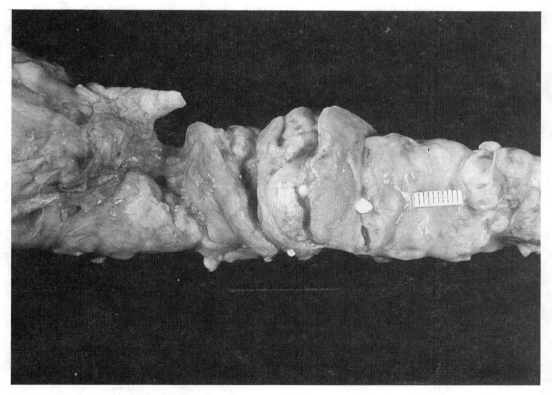

Figure 14-5. Fibrotic, narrowed pancreas with numerous calcified stones involving the main duct system. The patient, a 38-year-old man with a long history of alcoholism, died of complications of cirrhosis.

d. Complications

(1) **Pancreatic pseudocysts** are encapsulated collections of fluid with a high concentration of pancreatic enzymes, including amylase. The pseudocysts may be found within the pancreas itself, in the lesser omental sac, or, less frequently, at other sites. The pseuodocyst wall is composed of fibroinflammatory tissue, and an epithelial lining is lacking. Pseuodocyst formation requires disruption of the ductal system in the presence of an actively secreting pancreas.

    (a) In adults, acute or, more commonly, chronic pancreatitis is the cause of pseudocysts in approximately 75% of cases, trauma accounting for the remainder. Occasionally, pseudocysts may be the first presentation of chronic pancreatitis. In children, trauma is the major cause of pseudocysts.

    (b) The natural history of any individual pseudocyst is difficult to predict. A pseudocyst may resolve spontaneously within 6 weeks. Those present for longer periods usually require surgical intervention, because complications such as hemorrhage, rupture, compression, fistulization or rupture into adjacent viscera, splenic vein thrombosis, or abscess formation may occur.

(2) **Retention cysts** occur when the main duct or one of its larger branches has become occluded. The cysts, which contain serous pancreatic secretions, are lined by a flattened epithelium and hence are **true cysts**.

(3) **Bile duct strictures** may occur, leading to biliary cirrhosis.

D. Tumors of exocrine pancreas

1. Cystadenomas

a. Microcystic (glycogen-rich, serous) cystadenoma is a rare benign neoplasm usually occurring in the body and tail of the pancreas in elderly women.

(1) **Macroscopically,** this multilocular tumor often is 10 cm in diameter. It frequently is an incidental finding, but its presence in the head of the pancreas may be associated with gastrointestinal bleeding.

(2) **Microscopically,** the tumor has a honeycomb pattern and is lined by flattened cuboidal epithelium. The clear cytoplasm is rich in glycogen but lacks mucin.

b. Mucinous cystadenoma occurs chiefly in women in the fifth to seventh decades, and typically in the body or tail of the pancreas. Because small foci of carcinoma in situ or even invasive carcinoma may be found in a largely benign-appearing mucinous cystadenoma (**mucinous cystadenocarcinoma**), some authors have advocated the designation **mucinous cystic neoplasm** to indicate the uncertain malignant potential of these tumors.

(1) **Macroscopically,** these neoplasms are most commonly multilocular, large, and filled with sticky mucus.

(2) **Microscopically,** the cysts are lined by tall mucus-producing columnar epithelium.

2. Solid and cystic neoplasm of the pancreas is a rare pancreatic tumor found most commonly in adolescent and young women. The cell of origin is unknown but appears to be an uncommitted cell with occasional exocrine or endocrine differentiation. Most patients fare well after limited resections. Metastases rarely occur.

a. Macroscopically, the tumor is generally large (greater than 10 cm) and encapsulated, demonstrating a hemorrhagic or necrotic center.

b. Microscopically, sheets, pseudopapillary structures, and cystic spaces are lined by small- to medium-sized cells with oval bland nuclei and a moderate amount of cytoplasm.

3. Carcinoma. Nearly all pancreatic malignancies are **adenocarcinomas** arising from ductal epithelium. From 60% to 70% of the tumors arise in the head of the pancreas, 10% to 15% in the body, 5% to 10% in the tail, and the remaining 5% to 25% diffusely involve the pancreas.

a. Epidemiology. The incidence of carcinoma of the pancreas appears to be increasing in all age-groups. In the United States, about 25,000 new cases are diagnosed yearly, and it is the fourth leading cause of death from cancer among men and the fifth among women. Men are more commonly affected, and the peak incidence is in the seventh decade.

b. Etiology and pathogenesis of pancreatic cancer are obscure. Several **etiologic factors** have been suggested, including cigarette smoking, diet, diabetes mellitus, chronic pancreatitis, and certain carcinogens, but none have been proven. Patients with hereditary pancreatitis are at increased risk for pancreatic cancer. Most pancreatic adenocarcinomas demonstrate *ras* oncogene mutations.

c. **Clinical features.** Symptoms do not develop until the tumor is well advanced. Generally, patients with tumors localized to the head present earlier than those with tumors located in the body and tail.

(1) The majority of patients complain of midepigastric pain, back pain, or both as well as weight loss and vomiting. On rare occasions (fewer than 5%), patients present with acute pancreatitis or migratory thrombophlebitis (**Trousseau's sign**). If the tumor invades the duodenum or stomach, hematemesis or melena may result.

(2) **Jaundice** is present in over 50% of patients. The majority have a large mass in the head of the pancreas; this mass invades the distal common bile duct. Jaundice is uncommon (less than 10%) in patients with carcinoma of the body and tail; when present, it often is associated with a large tumor mass or hepatic metastases.

(a) **Courvoisier's sign** (i.e., painless jaundice associated with a palpable, distended gallbladder) is due to obstruction of the common bile duct or ampulla by a neoplasm rather than choledocholithiasis. In the latter condition, inflammatory scarring of the gallbladder apparently precludes its distention.

(b) Carcinoma of the pancreatic head is associated with Courvoisier's sign in 10% to 20% of cases. Occasionally this sign may be the only manifestation of small localized tumors of the pancreatic head.

(3) In 25% of patients with pancreatic carcinoma, a large, palpable abdominal mass is found on examination.

d. **Pathology.** Extension into mesenteric vessels, nerves, peritoneal and retroperitoneal tissues, and adjacent viscera has frequently occurred by the time of clinical presentation.

(1) **Macroscopically** (Figure 14-6), the tumors often are poorly demarcated and are yellow to gray–white; they usually range from 2 to 7 cm in diameter. Carcinomas in the head often infiltrate the distal bile duct and main pancreatic duct, giving rise to characteristic findings on ERCP. Rarely, purely intraductal (noninvasive) carcinomas are found.

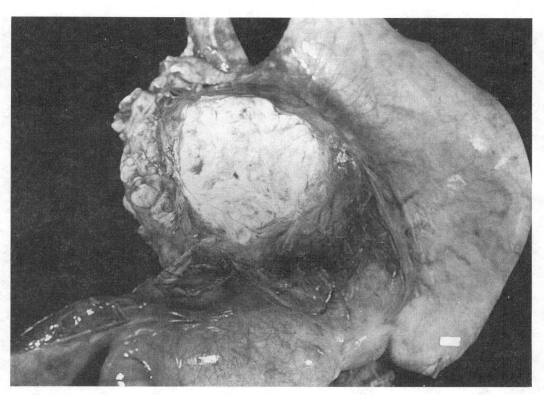

Figure 14-6. Large adenocarcinoma occupying the tail and a portion of the body of the pancreas and protruding into the lesser curvature of the stomach.

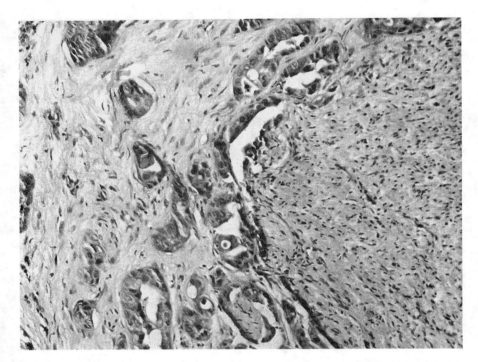

Figure 14-7. Common histologic pattern of pancreatic adenocarcinoma, moderately differentiated. Perineural invasion (*right*) is a common microscopic finding (high-power view).

    (2) Microscopically (Figure 14-7), about 90% of the tumors are **adenocarcinomas,** which often are quite well differentiated. Perineural invasion by the tumor often is quite conspicuous. Occasionally, **adenosquamous** and **pleomorphic giant cell carcinoma** may be found. **Mucinous cystadenocarcinoma** has been described in III D 1 b.

  e. Prognosis

    (1) Early detection of pancreatic carcinoma is extremely difficult because of the lack of characteristic symptoms. By the time of diagnosis, most tumors are quite advanced. Even with surgical intervention (Whipple's operation), the 5-year survival rate usually is less than 5%, although selected patients with very small tumors have prolonged survival. The survival rate for pancreatic cancer is notably poorer than the 30% to 60% 5-year survival rate for tumors arising in the distal common bile duct and periampullary region. Mucinous cystadenocarcinomas are associated with a better prognosis; patients often survive more than 5 years after diagnosis.

    (2) Metastases are found at autopsy in the majority of patients with pancreatic carcinoma, most commonly in the liver, regional lymph nodes, peritoneum, and lung.

STUDY QUESTIONS

Directions: Each of the numbered items or incomplete statements in this section is followed by answers or by completions of the statement. Select the **one** lettered answer or completion that is **best** in each case.

1. A 16-year-old girl with a family history of hereditary spherocytosis enters the hospital for splenectomy as primary therapy for her disease. She had intermittently complained of right upper quadrant pain. Surgery is most likely to disclose which finding?

(A) Chronic pancreatitis
(B) Duodenal ulcer
(C) Cholelithiasis
(D) Gastric ulcer
(E) None of the above

2. A 32-year-old man with known AIDS presents with fever and right upper quadrant pain. Total serum bilirubin level is 2.5 mg/dl (normal < 1.5), and serum alkaline phosphatase level is 850 IU/L (normal < 150). An abdominal ultrasound demonstrates slight dilatation of the common bile duct with a normal gallbladder, while endoscopic retrograde cholangiopancreatography (ERCP) showed multiple bile duct strictures. Which of the following statements is the most likely explanation for this patient's biliary tract disorder?

(A) Primary sclerosing cholangitis (PSC)
(B) Choledocholithiasis
(C) Cytomegalovirus (CMV), cryptosporidial cholangitis, or both
(D) Pancreatic carcinoma
(E) Bile duct carcinoma

3. Which statement concerning gallbladder cancer is true?

(A) Curable cases usually involve a tumor that is an incidental finding at cholecystectomy
(B) The tumors typically are found in patients in the fifth decade of life
(C) Most gallbladder cancers are squamous cell carcinomas
(D) Patients are asymptomatic in most cases
(E) Men are affected more often than women

4. Which statement about gallstones is true?

(A) Cholelithiasis is more common in those living in third world countries
(B) Cholesterol-rich stones result from oversecretion of bile salts by the liver
(C) Pigment stones are more common than cholesterol stones
(D) In 90% to 95% of cases of acute cholecystitis, a gallstone is impacted in the gallbladder neck or cystic duct
(E) More than 80% of gallstones are radiopaque

5. In most cases, acute (hemorrhagic) pancreatitis is associated with

(A) hyperparathyroidism or drug toxicity
(B) normal serum amylase levels
(C) autodigestion of the pancreatic parenchyma by activation of disaccharidases and pepsinogen
(D) ductal obstruction or direct toxicity to pancreatic acinar cells
(E) pancreatic carcinoma

6. Primary sclerosing cholangitis (PSC) has which characteristic?

(A) It frequently is seen in patients with ulcerative colitis
(B) It usually occurs in young females
(C) It has a normal caliber duct that typically demonstrates *Cryptosporidium* microscopically
(D) It can result from operative trauma to the biliary tract
(E) Its most common neoplastic complication is hepatocellular carcinoma

---

1-C   4-D
2-C   5-D
3-A   6-A

7. Which statement about primary sclerosing cholangitis (PSC) is true?

(A) It is caused by prior surgical trauma to the bile ducts
(B) It occurs most commonly in elderly females
(C) It has a strong association with ulcerative colitis
(D) It has no association with other fibroinflammatory disorders
(E) It involves only the intrahepatic ducts

8. All of the following statements about chronic cholecystitis are true EXCEPT

(A) emphysematous cholecystitis refers to dystrophic calcification within the gallbladder wall of affected patients
(B) Rokitansky-Aschoff sinuses are common microscopic findings
(C) women are more commonly affected than men
(D) an association with cholelithiasis is typical
(E) the gallbladder wall may become markedly thickened

9. All of the following pathologic features may be found in pancreatic pseudocysts EXCEPT

(A) hemorrhage
(B) fistulization into the stomach
(C) amylase-rich fluid
(D) mucinous epithelial lining
(E) fibrous tissue in its wall

10. All of the following statements about gallbladder tumors are true EXCEPT

(A) the cholesterol polyp is the most common form of benign gallbladder polyp
(B) adenomyoma typically is found in the fundus
(C) gallstones frequently are found in association with gallbladder carcinoma
(D) gallbladder carcinoma usually is localized to a small region of the gallbladder wall at the time of diagnosis
(E) adenomas are uncommon gallbladder neoplasms

11. All of the following statements about pancreatic adenocarcinoma are true EXCEPT

(A) it locally invades adjacent structures but rarely metastasizes to more distant sites
(B) it may present as acute pancreatitis
(C) jaundice often is present, particularly with tumors of the pancreatic head
(D) back pain is a common symptom
(E) migratory thrombophlebitis (Trousseau's sign) may occur

12. All of the following statements about black pigment gallstones are true EXCEPT

(A) pigment stones are usually multiple and multifaceted
(B) pigment stones have a cholesterol content that does not exceed 20% by weight
(C) black stones are the most common type of pigment stone seen in the United States
(D) they are common in young people
(E) pigment stone formation requires calcium bilirubinate

7-C   10-D
8-A   11-A
9-D   12-D

Directions: The group of items in this section consists of lettered options followed by a set of numbered items. For each item, select the **one** lettered option that is most closely associated with it. Each lettered option may be selected once, more than once, or not at all.

Questions 13–17

Match each disorder of the pancreas or biliary tract to the associated condition.

(A) Ulcerative colitis
(B) Sickle cell anemia
(C) Diabetes mellitus
(D) Alcoholism
(E) Trauma during cholecystectomy

13. Cystic fibrosis of the pancreas

14. Primary sclerosing cholangitis (PSC)

15. Isolated bile duct stricture

16. Acute pancreatitis

17. Pigment gallstones

13-C   16-D
14-A   17-B
15-E

ANSWERS AND EXPLANATIONS

1. The answer is C *[I C 3 b (1)].*
Splenectomy for hereditary spherocytosis is most likely to disclose cholelithiasis. Patients with hemolytic anemias, such as that characterizing hereditary spherocytosis or sickle cell anemia, form black (pigment) calcium bilirubinate stones. The excess bilirubin chronically generated from the hemolytic process predisposes to the formation of this type of gallstone. Neither pancreatitis nor ulcers would be expected findings.

2. The answer is C *[II D 3 b].*
Patients with AIDS may develop a syndrome that clinically mimics primary sclerosing cholangitis (PSC); however, it is caused by infection of the biliary tree with cytomegalovirus (CMV), *Cryptosporidium,* or both. Recently, Microsporida has also been incriminated as an etiologic agent in this clinical setting.

3. The answer is A *[I F 2 f].*
Overall, curable cases of gallbladder cancer usually involve a tumor that is an incidental finding at cholecystectomy. Gallbladder cancer is associated with a dismal prognosis; very few patients can be cured. Gallbladder carcinoma is uncommon, representing only 1% to 3% of all gastrointestinal cancers. These tumors primarily are adenocarcinomas; squamous cell cancers rarely are found. In most cases, patients experience abdominal pain that is similar to the pain associated with cholecystitis and cholelithiasis. Women are affected more frequently than men, and the peak incidence is in the seventh decade of life.

4. The answer is D *[I C].*
An impacted gallstone is found in the gallbladder neck or cystic duct in 90% to 95% of patients with acute cholecystitis. Gallstones are more common in women, affecting about 20% of all women and 8% of all men in the United States. Cholesterol-rich stones are caused by failure of the liver to provide enough bile salts and lecithin or by increased hepatic synthesis of cholesterol, with resulting supersaturation of bile with cholesterol. Of all gallstones, cholesterol stones account for 85% and pigment stones account for 15%. Only 10% to 20% of all gallstones are radiopaque.

5. The answer is D *[III C 1; Table 14-2].*
Acute (hemorrhagic) pancreatitis most often is associated with biliary tract stones or alcoholism; in rare cases, hyperparathyroidism, drug toxicity, or some other factor accounts for this disorder. About 20% of cases are idiopathic. Patients typically are middle-aged men (in alcohol-related cases) or women (in stone-related cases). Ductal obstruction or acinar cell injury can lead to activation of proteases, lipases, and elastases, which destroy the pancreatic parenchyma. Both serum amylase and lipase levels are elevated in most patients. Patients with pancreatic cancer rarely exhibit acute pancreatitis.

6. The answer is A *[II D].*
Up to 70% of patients with primary sclerosing cholangitis (PSC) have associated idiopathic inflammatory bowel disease, which nearly always is ulcerative colitis. PSC is a rare disorder characterized by fibroinflammatory narrowing of the bile ducts, typically affecting both the extrahepatic and intrahepatic ducts. About 70% of patients are men, and over two-thirds of these are under 45 years of age. The characteristic annular bile duct strictures are best demonstrated by endoscopic retrograde cholangiopancreatography (ERCP). Secondary sclerosing cholangitis may be caused by postoperative strictures, choledocholithiasis, infection (*Cryptosporidium*, Microsporida, cytomegalovirus (CMV)] in patients with acquired immune deficiency syndrome (AIDS), and other causes.

7. The answer is C *[Chapter 13 II D].*
Although only 3% to 4% of patients with ulcerative colitis develop primary sclerosing cholangitis (PSC), 70% of patients with PSC have or develop ulcerative colitis. PSC is a disorder characterized by fibroinflammatory narrowing of the biliary tree. Patients most commonly are males under the age of 45. PSC most often diffusely or segmentally involves the biliary tree, causing multiple strictures. Usually, both extrahepatic and intrahepatic ducts are affected. Secondary sclerosing cholangitis may follow surgical trauma to the ducts or other etiologies, but no cause for PSC is known. However, the fact that patients often have other inflammatory and fibrotic disorders suggests a general disturbance of collagenous or fibrous tissue, perhaps on an immunologic basis. Bile duct carcinoma is a potential complication.

8. The answer is A *[I D 2]*.
Emphysematous cholecystitis indicates the presence of gas within the gallbladder wall or lumen. This uncommon manifestation of acute cholecystitis results from gas-forming bacteria, most notably *Clostridium perfringens*. Chronic cholecystitis nearly always develops in the setting of gallstones and is much more common in women than in men. Microscopically, chronic cholecystitis is typified by the presence of Rokitansky-Aschoff sinuses (i.e., outpouchings of the mucosa). Dystrophic mural calcification may develop in affected patients and is termed porcelain gallbladder. Occasionally the gallbladder wall becomes quite thick. The radiopaque calcium deposits render the gallbladder visible on abdominal radiographs.This condition is associated with an increased risk for developing gallbladder carcinoma.

9. The answer is D *[III C 2 d (1)]*.
A pancreatic pseudocyst represents an encapsulated collection of fluid that is rich in amylase; it results from the ravages of pancreatitis. No epithelium is present, but a fibrous tissue lining is found. Hemorrhage and fistulization to adjacent organs are potential complications of a pancreatic pseudocyst.

10. The answer is D *[I F 1, 2]*.
Gallbladder cancer often involves the greater portion of the organ at the time of diagnosis. In most cases, the tumor has extended well beyond the mucosa, generally through the muscular layer into the perimuscular connective tissue and often directly into the liver. Gallstones are found in 75% of gallbladders that contain carcinoma. Of the benign tumors of the gallbladder, cholesterol polyps are the most common. Adenomyoma is a benign tumor typically found in the fundus of the organ. Gallbladder adenomas are uncommon.

11. The answer is A *[III D 3 c–e]*.
Pancreatic adenocarcinoma is an aggressive, metastasizing tumor. Tumor extension into mesenteric vessels, nerves, peritoneal and retroperitoneal tissues, and adjacent structures typically has occurred by the time the tumor is clinically evident. Metastasis to the liver, regional lymph nodes, and lung is most common in patients with adenocarcinoma of the pancreas. Jaundice, back pain, acute pancreatitis, and thrombophlebitis may be present in patients with such cancers.

12. The answer is D *[I C 3 b]*.
Brown gallstones are relatively common in Asia and quite rare in the United States. This type of gallstone has a strong association with infected bile (particularly due to *Escherichia coli* and anaerobes). Black pigment stones are small, multiple, and multifaceted. In comparison to the more common cholesterol stones, which are at least 60% cholesterol by weight, pigment stones have a relatively low cholesterol content (usually less than 20% by weight). Calcium bilirubinate is an important component of black pigment stones. Black stones are by far the most common form of pigment stone in the United States. Patients with chronic hemolytic anemia (from hereditary spherocytosis, sickle cell anemia, or a prosthetic aortic valve) or with cirrhosis are predisposed to the formation of black stones, but most patients with this type of gallstone are elderly men without these disorders.

13–17. The answers are: 13-C *[III B 2 a (1)]*, **14-A** *[II D 1, 2 a]*, **15-E** *[II D 3 b]*, **16-D** *[III C 1 a]*, **17-B** *[I C 3 b (1) (a)]*.
The destruction of the exocrine pancreas in patients with cystic fibrosis may extend to the islet cells, and diabetes mellitus may result. Chronic pulmonary disease, cirrhosis, and intestinal obstruction are additional clinical features of cystic fibrosis.

Although primary sclerosing cholangitis (PSC) is found in only rare cases of inflammatory bowel disease (particularly ulcerative colitis), in many patients with PSC, ulcerative colitis is or has been present. Isolated bile duct strictures most commonly result from operative mishaps during cholecystectomy (i.e., suturing or transection of the bile duct).

Acute pancreatitis may have many causes. However, the major factors are gallstones and alcoholism. The exact mechanism whereby alcohol abuse produces pancreatitis remains unclear, but the strong association of the two conditions is a clinical fact.

Patients with sickle cell anemia or other chronic hemolytic anemias are at an increased risk for developing black pigmented gallstones. Cirrhosis is another predisposing factor. Most black pigment gallstones occur in older patients with no predisposing illness. Brown pigment stones generally arise on a background of biliary tract sepsis.

15
Liver
Scott H. Saul

I. NORMAL STRUCTURE AND FUNCTION

A. Anatomy. The liver lies in the right upper quadrant of the abdomen, where it is almost completely protected by the rib cage. The largest visceral organ in the body, it weighs 1400 to 1600 g and has a span of 10 to 12 cm. The liver is unique for its **dual blood supply**. The portal vein provides 60% to 70% of hepatic blood flow, and the hepatic artery supplies the remainder. Because of this dual blood supply, liver infarction is rare.

B. Histology

1. **Hepatocytes** are polygonal cells with prominent granular eosinophilic cytoplasm and round, centrally located nucleoli. These cells measure approximately 30 μ in diameter. **Bile canaliculi** form by close apposition of hepatocyte cell membranes, which are joined by tight junctions. (Routine light microscopy commonly fails to demonstrate these canaliculi, however.)

2. **Sinusoids** are vascular spaces about 20 to 30 μ wide, which are lined with endothelial cells and **Kupffer (reticuloendothelial) cells**.

3. **Plasma flow.** Fenestrated sinusoids allow plasma to enter the perisinusoidal **space of Disse,** a narrow channel around the hepatocyte. This channel permits free contact of the plasma with the hepatocyte surface. Plasma then flows into the portal lymphatics.

4. **Supportive framework.** The supportive framework of the lobule is found in the space of Disse. It is composed of types I and III collagen (as demonstrated with a reticulin stain) and fibronectin. Stellate perisinusoidal (Ito) cells are found in the space of Disse, where they store fat and vitamin A and potentially act as facultative fibroblasts.

5. **Bile ducts** are lined with cuboidal to columnar epithelium.

6. **Hepatic lobule.** The classic hepatic lobule is conceptualized as a polyhedral or hexagonal cylinder traversed by a **central vein** (also called the **terminal hepatic venule** or **efferent vein**). The central vein is the terminal tributary of the hepatic veins.
   a. At the periphery of the lobule lie **portal tracts** containing supportive collagen, lymphatics, and a **portal triad**. The latter consists of branches of the portal vein, hepatic artery, and bile duct. Blood flows from the portal vessels into the sinusoids, then into the central vein.
   b. The **limiting plate** represents the first hepatocyte layer, which directly adjoins the portal tract. Other one-cell thick hepatocyte plates radiate from this region to the area of the central vein.
   c. Lobule regions include the **centrilobular, midlobular,** and **periportal regions**.
   d. Bile **canaliculi** within the lobules drain bile secreted by hepatocytes. In the portal region, canaliculi empty into cholangioles, which, in turn, drain into the interlobular bile ducts.

7. **Hepatic acinus.** The hepatic acinus has recently gained acceptance as the functional unit of the liver. According to this model, the hepatic afferent microcirculation divides the liver into acini. The portal tract lies at the center of the acinus; two or more terminal hepatic venules lie at the periphery. The regions of the acinus are as follows: zone 1, periportal; zone 2, midlobular; zone 3, centrilobular.

C. Functions. The liver plays an essential role in intermediary metabolism and the synthesis of serum proteins (except immunoglobulins). It also has storage, catabolic, detoxification, and excretory functions.

II. STRUCTURAL ANOMALIES

A. Congenital hepatic fibrosis

1. **Etiology.** Congenital hepatic fibrosis is a rare disorder inherited as an autosomal recessive trait. Bile duct proliferation may result from preexisting Meyenburg's complexes (see XIII A 2 a) or a related lesion known as the ductal plate malformation; fibrosis probably arises as a secondary phenomenon. Congenital hepatic fibrosis commonly is associated with Caroli's disease (see II B 2).

2. **Clinical features.** Patients typically are between age 5 and 20 and present with gastrointestinal bleeding caused by ruptured esophageal varices. Most patients also have ectatic renal collecting tubules similar to those seen in medullary sponge kidney (see Chapter 16 II D 2 e); however, renal function usually is normal. No evidence of hepatic failure generally appears.

3. **Pathology.** In most cases, the liver is enlarged and firm. Portal spaces contain numerous, commonly ectatic, bile ducts filled with inspissated bile. Bands of fibrous tissue connect adjacent portal tracts, carving the hepatic parenchyma into regularly shaped islands resembling pieces of a jigsaw puzzle. Except with superimposed cholangitis, inflammation is absent.

4. **Treatment and prognosis.** Endoscopic sclerosis of the esophageal varices may be performed or a portacaval shunt may be constructed surgically. Recurrent bleeding occurs over the course of the disease and is the most common cause of death. Cholangiocarcincoma is a rare complication.

B. Congenital hepatic cysts occur in two forms.

1. **Noncommunicating cysts** may be single or multiple and, by definition, do not communicate with the biliary tree (Figure 15-1).
   a. **Etiology.** The cysts probably are derived from the persistence and obstruction of Meyenburg's complexes, which lose their connection with the biliary tree.
   b. **Clinical features.** Although the cysts may cause abdominal pain, they frequently are asymptomatic. Multiple cysts are considered part of the spectrum of adult (autosomal dominant) polycystic kidney disease (see Chapter 16 II D 2 a).

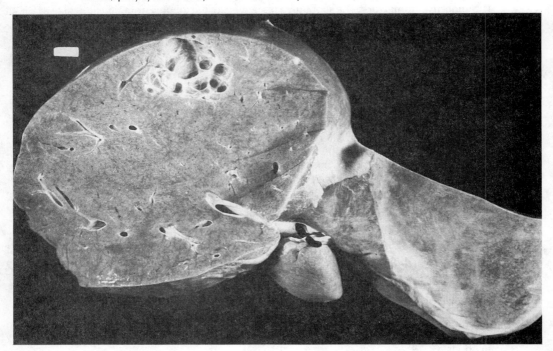

Figure 15-1. Benign, noncommunicating hepatic cyst.

    c. Pathology. Cyst size is quite variable. The cysts are unilocular and are lined by a flattened layer of biliary epithelium with little supportive connective tissue.

  2. Communicating cysts (also known as **Caroli's disease**) are multifocal dilatations of the intrahepatic bile ducts and are caused by weakening of the duct walls and obstruction.

    a. Etiology. The cause of communicating cysts is unknown.

    b. Clinical features. Patients usually present in the first several decades of life with recurrent bouts of cholangitis and, occasionally, bacteremia, which cause fever and abdominal pain.

    c. Pathology

      (1) Macroscopically, the cystic dilatations are 1 cm to 4.5 cm in diameter and may be separated by segments of normal-appearing duct. Calculi may be present.

      (2) Microscopically, the ducts demonstrate prominent chronic inflammation and fibrosis, with variable acute inflammation and mucosal erosion.

    d. Treatment and prognosis. Symptomatic treatment is with antibiotics. Patients with recurrent cholangitis often die within 5 to 10 years after the onset of this complication. With disease localized to one part of the liver, partial hepatectomy can be performed. Transplantation should be considered for patients with diffuse disease.

    e. Complications. Cholangiocarcinoma complicates this disorder in 7% to 14% of patients.

III. HYPERBILIRUBINEMIA AND CHOLESTASIS

  A. General concepts

    1. Hyperbilirubinemia

      a. Definition. Hyperbilirubinemia refers to an increased serum bilirubin concentration (i.e., > 1.2 mg/dl). At serum bilirubin concentrations above 2 to 2.5 mg/dl, the skin and sclerae turn yellow—a condition known as **jaundice** or **icterus**.

      b. Classification

        (1) Unconjugated hyperbilirubinemia. This disorder is characterized by elevated serum levels of unconjugated bilirubin; levels of conjugated bilirubin are within normal limits. This finding typifies conditions associated with increased red blood cell (RBC) destruction (e.g., hemolytic anemia, ineffective erythropoiesis), reduced hepatic bilirubin uptake (e.g., as from such drugs as rifampin), and impaired bilirubin conjugation (e.g., Crigler-Najjar and Gilbert's syndromes, discussed in III B). These disorders usually are not associated with cholestasis.

        (2) Conjugated hyperbilirubinemia. Levels of both conjugated and unconjugated bilirubin rise in this disorder. Intrinsic liver disease and extrahepatic biliary obstruction are the underlying causes of conjugated hyperbilirubinemia. Cholestasis is usually, but not always, present.

    2. Cholestasis may be defined in several ways.

      a. Clinically, cholestasis refers to the presence of jaundice and pruritus in addition to elevated serum levels of conjugated bilirubin, cholesterol, bile acids (which normally accumulate only in the bile), and alkaline phosphatase.

      b. Physiologically, cholestasis refers to decreased hepatocytic secretion of bilirubin, bile acids, and water, accompanied by decreased bile flow through the bile canaliculi.

      c. Pathologic identification

        (1) Macroscopic findings. Cholestasis is identified by green or greenish-black hepatic discoloration.

        (2) Microscopic findings. The presence of brownish-green bile pigment within hepatocytes and bile canaliculi (bile plugs or thrombi) typifies cholestasis. Early-stage cholestasis appears in the centrilobular region (zone 3), regardless of etiology.

          (a) Feathery degeneration is a common hepatocyte injury accompanying cholestatic conditions. Affected cells are swollen with stringy, bile-impregnated cytoplasm, which may appear foamy. Necrosis of a group of such cells is called a **bile infarct**.

          (b) With **chronic cholestasis,** periportal (zone 1) hepatocytes typically show feathery degeneration and may contain Mallory's hyalin [see IV D 5 b (1) (a)] and increased amounts of copper. These histologic changes presumably stem from the detergent action of retained bile acids in periportal hepatocytes.

          (c) Large bile duct obstruction (extrahepatic cholestasis). Histologic analysis often can distinguish cholestasis caused by intrinsic liver disease (intrahepatic cholestasis) from cholestasis caused by large bile duct obstruction (extrahepatic cholestasis).

(i) With extrahepatic cholestasis, features include portal tract edema, proliferation of bile ducts (which occasionally contain inspissated bile), and periductal neutrophils, in addition to the general histologic features of cholestasis previously mentioned.

(ii) Occasionally, large periportal bile infarcts and portal accumulation of extravasated bile (bile extravasates) are evident.

(iii) Neutrophils within large bile ducts indicate obstruction with ascending biliary tract infection, a condition known as **cholangitis.**

(iv) Radiographic imaging techniques, such as computed tomography (CT) and endoscopic retrograde cholangiopancreatography (ERCP), have greatly reduced the need for percutaneous liver biopsy to differentiate intrahepatic and extrahepatic cholestasis.

B. Disorders associated with decreased bilirubin conjugation and unconjugated hyperbilirubinemia

1. **Crigler-Najjar syndrome (congenital hyperbilirubinemia).** This rare inherited disorder results from deficiency of uridine diphosphate (UDP)–glucuronyl transferase, the hepatic enzyme responsible for bilirubin conjugation.

   a. **Classification.** Crigler-Najjar syndrome occurs in two forms.
      (1) **Type I disease,** the more severe form, is characterized by complete absence of UDP-glucuronyl transferase. The serum bilirubin level may rise as high as 50 mg/dl, reflecting severe unconjugated hyperbilirubinemia. The bile is colorless.
      (2) **Type II disease,** the milder form, is characterized by only partial enzyme deficiency. Typically, the serum bilirubin level is 6 to 20 mg/dl.

   b. **Etiology.** Type I disease is inherited as an autosomal recessive trait. Type II disease possibly is inherited as an autosomal dominant trait with incomplete penetrance.

   c. **Clinical features**
      (1) Type I disease often causes severe neurologic disturbances (bilirubin encephalopathy) reflecting **kernicterus** (toxic bilirubin accumulation in the brain).
      (2) Type II disease often causes jaundice during adolescence but only rarely causes bilirubin encephalopathy.

   d. **Pathology.** With both disease forms, the liver is histologically normal except for rare unexplained canalicular bile plugs.

   e. **Treatment and prognosis.** Type I disease is invariably fatal; however, liver transplantation and enzyme replacement may prove to be useful treatment modalities. The majority of cases of type II disease have a benign course and respond to treatment with phenobarbital.

2. **Gilbert's syndrome.** This chronic abnormality is characterized by mild, persistent unconjugated hyperbilirubinemia (the serum bilirubin level rarely exceeds 6 mg/dl). It affects roughly 3% to 7% of the population.

   a. **Etiology and pathogenesis.** Gilbert's syndrome usually is inherited as an autosomal dominant trait. Because patients have reduced levels of UDP–glucuronyl transferase, some researchers believe that the pathogenesis of this disorder resembles that of type II Crigler-Najjar syndrome.

   b. **Clinical features.** Gilbert's syndrome typically is diagnosed after puberty—from laboratory determination of an increased serum unconjugated bilirubin level. Most patients are asymptomatic or have nonspecific complaints; about half have mild hemolysis of uncertain etiology. Jaundice is common and may be exacerbated by fever, infection, prolonged fasting, or excessive exercise.

   c. **Pathology.** Light microscopy shows normal liver cells.

   d. **Treatment and prognosis.** Phenobarbital may reduce the serum bilirubin level. Patients have an excellent prognosis, with no long-term sequelae.

C. Disorders associated with selective defects in intracellular transport of conjugated bilirubin and conjugated hyperbilirubinemia

1. **Dubin-Johnson syndrome.** Chronic or intermittent jaundice occurs in this syndrome, in association with conjugated hyperbilirubinemia.

   a. **Etiology and pathogenesis.** This autosomal recessive disease involves defective hepatocyte excretion of conjugated bilirubin and other organic anions into the bile canaliculus. Coproporphyrin metabolism also is impaired.

    b. Clinical features. Patients commonly are asymptomatic or have vague symptoms. The conjugated hyperbilirubinemia may be exacerbated during pregnancy or with the use of oral contraceptives.

    c. Pathology

      (1) Macroscopic findings. The liver appears black or gray.

      (2) Microscopic findings. Dark-brown melaninlike pigment is detected primarily in the cytoplasm of zone 3 hepatocytes; electron microscopy shows the lysosomal location of the pigment. Pigment origin and significance are unknown. Otherwise, the liver appears normal, with **no histologic evidence of cholestasis**.

    d. Treatment and prognosis. Dubin-Johnson syndrome generally is innocuous and carries an excellent prognosis.

  2. Rotor's syndrome. This form of chronic conjugated hyperbilirubinemia also is characterized by impaired hepatic excretion of conjugated bilirubin and other organic anions. Like Dubin-Johnson syndrome, it is inherited as an autosomal recessive trait. Unlike the former, however, Rotor's syndrome is not characterized by hepatic pigmentation.

IV. ACUTE HEPATITIS

A. General concepts. Acute hepatic dysfunction usually suggests one of six disorders—viral hepatitis, chemical hepatitis, alcoholic liver disease, ischemic and congestive hepatopathy, or extrahepatic biliary obstruction. Viral, chemical, and alcoholic forms of acute hepatitis are by far the most common; these disorders and the general concepts of hepatic failure are discussed in this section. Vascular hepatic disorders and extrahepatic biliary obstruction are discussed in V and III A 2 c (2) (c) [see also Chapter 14 II B 1], respectively.

  1. Clinical features and diagnosis

    a. Signs and symptoms typically include anorexia, malaise, nausea, fever, jaundice, brownish urine (bilirubinemia), and abdominal discomfort.

    b. Laboratory findings

      (1) Viral and chemical hepatitis usually cause marked elevation in serum transaminase levels (10 to 100 times normal) and a normal or slightly elevated serum alkaline phosphatase level.

      (2) With viral hepatitis, the ratio of serum aspartate aminotransferase (AST) to serum alanine aminotransferase (ALT) typically is less than 2:1.

      (3) The serum bilirubin level may increase with all forms of acute hepatitis.

  2. Complications of acute hepatitis

    a. Fulminant hepatic failure is a rare but frequently fatal complication. Defined as hepatic failure accompanied by encephalopathy (see XII C 1 c), this disorder typically is associated histologically with one of the forms of **confluent hepatic necrosis** discussed in IV B 4 b (2) (b). It also commonly complicates cirrhosis.

    b. Hepatorenal syndrome is a form of unexplained progressive renal failure that accompanies liver disease. Death usually occurs shortly after onset.

      (1) The kidneys are morphologically normal and, when transplanted into patients with chronic renal failure, function normally.

      (2) The renal defect seems to be linked with decreased renal blood flow, which, in turn, reduces the glomerular filtration rate (GFR).

      (3) Defective hepatic production of a substance that normally increases the GFR (or failure to metabolize these substances) may be the underlying cause of hepatorenal syndrome.

      (4) Usually irreversible, hepatorenal syndrome causes death shortly after onset.

B. Acute viral hepatitis

  1. General description. In this viral infection of hepatocytes, hepatocellular necrosis and inflammation lead to characteristic biochemical, immunoserologic, morphologic, and clinical features.

  2. Etiology and epidemiology (Tables 15-1 and 15-2)

    a. In industrialized countries, 95% of cases of acute hepatitis are caused by one of the four **hepatotrophic viruses**: hepatitis A virus (HAV), hepatitis B virus (HBV), hepatitis C virus (HCV), and hepatitis D virus (HDV; delta agent). The typical course of a case of acute hepatitis B is depicted in Figure 15-2. HCV accounts for the overwhelming majority of cases

Table 15-1. Acute Viral Hepatitis: Comparative Features of Five Hepatotrophic Viruses

Feature	Hepatitis A	Hepatitis B	Hepatitis C	Hepatitis D	Hepatitis E
Agent	HAV	HBV	HCV	HDV (delta agent)	HEV
Family	Picornavirus	Hepadenovirus	Flavivirus	Satellite virus	Calicivirus
Particle size	27 nm	42 nm	30–60 nm	40 nm	27–32 nm
Genome	RNA	DNA	RNA	RNA; needs HBV "helper"	RNA
Antigens	HAAg	HBsAg, HBcAg, HBeAg	HCAg	HDAg	HEAg
Antibody	Anti-HAV*	Anti-HBs, anti-HBc, anti-HBe	Anti-HCV	Anti-HDV	Anti-HEV
Transmission	Fecal–oral	Parenteral, perinatal, sexual	Parenteral, possibly sexual	Parenteral, possibly sexual	Fecal–oral
Incubation period	15–45 days	40–180 days	15–150 days	30–50 days	21–63 days
Mortality	0.2%	0.2%–1%	0.2%	2%–20%	0.2%
Progression to chronic hepatitis	0%	5%–10%	50%–70%	2%–70%	0%
Increased risk for hepatocellular carcinoma	No	Yes	Yes	Possibly	No

Adapted with permission from Hoofnagle JH and DiBisceglie AM: Serologic diagnosis of acute and chronic viral hepatitis. *Semin Liver Dis* 11:74, 1991.
HAAg = hepatitis A antigen; HAV = hepatitis A virus; HBcAg = hepatitis B core antigen; HBeAg = hepatitis B e antigen; HBsAg = hepatitis B surface antigen; HBV = hepatitis B virus; HCAg = hepatitis C antigen; HCV = hepatitis C virus; HDAg = hepatitis D antigen; HDV = hepatitis D virus; HEAg = hepatitis E antigen; HEV = hepatitis E virus.
*The presence of IgM anti-HAV is considered diagnostic of acute hepatitis A.

previously designated as non-A, non-B hepatitis. Another virus, the hepatitis E virus (HEV), is a common cause of sporadic and epidemic hepatitis in underdeveloped countries. Each of these viruses can affect people of any age and may cause sporadic or epidemic disease. Acute hepatitis E has a high mortality in pregnant patients. Hepatitis B vaccine can prevent infection with this virus.

b. While HAV and HCV may be directly cytopathic, hepatocyte damage related to HBV usually is considered secondary to host immune response.

c. In rare cases, acute hepatitis may stem from other viruses, such as Epstein-Barr virus (EBV) or cytomegalovirus (CMV).

3. Clinical features. The clinical spectrum of the hepatitis viruses ranges from inapparent and asymptomatic infection (the most common presentation) to fulminant and possibly fatal disease (rare). Fulminant hepatitis B is more likely when the virus has undergone mutation in the precore region (precore mutants) and fails to secrete hepatitis B e antigen (HBeAg) or when there is associated HDV infection.

Table 15-2. Hepatitis A, B, and C: Epidemiologic Features

Clinical Forms of Viral Hepatitis	Hepatitis A	Hepatitis B	Hepatitis C
Sporadic hepatitis	20%	60%	20%–40%
Posttransfusion hepatitis	0%	5%	95%
Traveler's hepatitis	80%	15%	5%
Hepatitis in drug addicts	10%	40%–50%	40%–50%
Fulminant hepatitis	5%	60%	35%*

*Reported as non-A, non-B hepatitis. Exact frequency for serologically-proven hepatitis C virus requires further data.

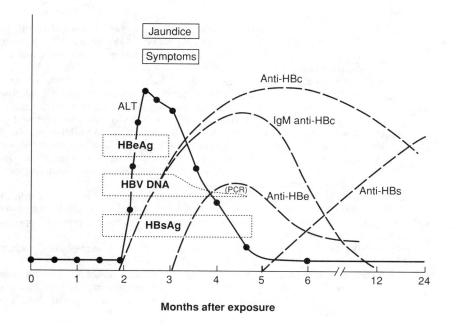

Months after exposure

Figure 15-2. Typical course of a case of acute hepatitis B. Initially, HBV DNA can be detected by blot hybridization, but as the disease resolves, only low levels (detectable by polymerase chain reaction) can be detected. *ALT* = alanine aminotransferase; *anti-HBc* = antibody to hepatitis B core antigen; *anti-HBe* = antibody to HBeAg, *anti-HBs* = antibody to HBsAg; *HBeAg* = hepatitis B e antigen; *HBsAg* = hepatitis B surface antigen; *HBV DNA* = hepatitis B virus deoxyribonucleic acid; *PCR* = polymerase chain reaction. Adapted with permission from Hoofnagle JH and DiBisceglie AM: Serologic diagnosis of acute and chronic viral hepatitis. *Semin Liver Dis* 11:75, 1991.

4. Pathology
  a. Macroscopic findings
      (1) The liver is swollen and red with a bulging capsule; sometimes it is intensely yellow or green because of marked cholestasis. Necrotic foci commonly result in scattered depressed areas.
      (2) With fulminant hepatitis, the liver usually is shrunken and soft with a wrinkled capsule from extensive hepatic parenchymal loss. If the patient survives an episode of fulminant hepatitis, regenerative nodules often are found under the capsule and scattered throughout the liver weeks or months after onset of the illness.
  b. Microscopic findings. Because the histopathologic features of the hepatitis viruses are nearly identical, **serologic evidence** is needed to identify the specific etiologic agent. Also, certain forms of drug-induced hepatic injury are histopathologically indistinguishable from viral hepatitis.
  (1) Basic histologic features
      (a) Hepatocellular injury. This injury may occur in any part of the acinus but generally is most severe in zone 3. It has two basic forms.
          (i) Acidophilic degeneration results in the formation of **acidophilic (Councilman) bodies**. These shrunken, eosinophilic hepatocytes may possess pyknotic nuclear remnants and are found within hepatocyte plates, free within the sinusoids, or within Kupffer cells.
          (ii) Ballooning degeneration (also known as **lytic necrosis**) results from hepatocyte swelling. Cells are enlarged, rounded, and pale. Swelling reflects dilatation of the endoplasmic reticulum (ER).
      (b) Inflammatory infiltrate. Composed mainly of lymphocytes and macrophages, the inflammatory infiltrate contains a variable number of plasma cells, neutrophils, and eosinophils.
          (i) Inflammatory cells generally occur within the lobule, preferentially in regions of **hepatocyte necrosis.** Kupffer cells commonly contain brown pigment, representing phagocytized bile, lipofuscin, or iron.

      (ii) Lymphocyte infiltration between the wall of the central vein and adjacent liver cell plates—known as **central phlebitis**—is characteristic of acute viral hepatitis. Portal inflammation, although consistently present, usually is less marked than lobular inflammation.

      (iii) In some cases, however, the portal infiltrate extends destructively through the limiting plate into the lobule—a condition termed **piecemeal necrosis**. Although characteristic of chronic active hepatitis, piecemeal necrosis also may occur in acute hepatitis; consequently, its presence does not rule out the latter.

    (c) Hepatocyte regeneration. This process develops early in the disease. Nuclei enlarge, and nucleoli become more prominent. Multinucleate hepatocytes, hepatocyte mitotic figures, and hepatocyte thickening indicate regeneration. Ongoing necrosis, regeneration, and inflammation of the lobule give rise to a disordered appearance, termed **lobular disarray**.

  (2) Basic histologic patterns. The degree of hepatocellular necrosis varies with disease severity, the patient's age and immunologic status, and the presence of preexisting liver disease. Several basic patterns of necrosis may occur; more than one may be present in any given case.

    (a) Spotty (focal) necrosis, the basic and most common lesion of classic acute viral hepatitis, is typified by individual hepatocyte necrosis.

    (b) Confluent necrosis is characterized by necrosis of groups of adjacent hepatocytes.

      (i) In **bridging confluent necrosis,** bands of necrotic hepatocytes link vascular structures. Examples include portal–central, portal–portal, and central–central bridging necrosis.

      (ii) In **panacinar confluent necrosis,** complete or near-complete hepatocyte loss occurs in a given acinus, with marked collapse of the reticulin framework (Figure 15-3). Inflammatory infiltrate may be minimal. When most of the liver is affected this way, **massive necrosis** results; **submassive necrosis** refers to lesser degrees of panacinar necrosis.

C. Chemical hepatitis (Table 15-3)

  1. General concepts. Many chemical agents (e.g., drugs, industrial toxins, anesthetics) can produce liver injury when ingested, inhaled, or administered parenterally. Often, only mild hepatotoxicity occurs, resulting in triglyceride accumulation within hepatocytes (**steatosis or fatty change**), transient **cholestasis,** or mild **acute hepatitis**. However, chemical injury may account for extensive hepatic necrosis and causes up to 25% of cases of fulminant hepatic failure in the United States.

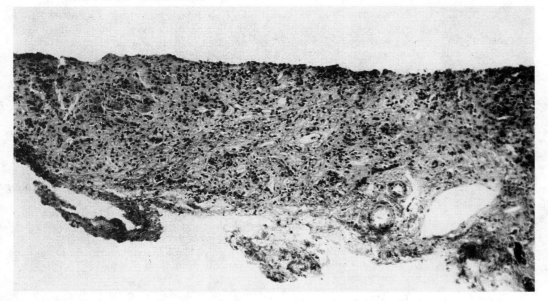

Figure 15-3. Liver biopsy from a patient with fulminant hepatic failure, demonstrating acute hepatitis with panacinar necrosis (× 250).

Table 15-3. Drug or Toxin-Induced Hepatotoxicity: Types of Hepatic Injury and Selected Causative Agents

Primary Type of Injury	Example
Hepatocellular	
Acute hepatitis	
Focal, spotty	Isoniazid, ketoconazole
Zonal*	Zone 1: inorganic phosphorus
	Zone 3: acetaminophen, carbon tetrachloride, halothane
Chronic hepatitis or cirrhosis	Isoniazid, methyldopa, methotrexate
Steatosis	
Macrovesicular	Ethanol, methotrexate
Microvesicular	Tetracycline, valproate
Steatohepatitis	Ethanol, amiodarone
Cholestasis	Erythromycin, OCS, androgens
Neoplasm	
Hepatocellular adenoma	OCS
Hepatocellular carcinoma	Thorotrast, possibly OCS, possibly androgens
Intrahepatic bile ducts	
Chronic cholestasis	Chlorpromazine, amitriptyline
Cholangiocarcinoma	Thorotrast
Vascular	
Sinusoidal dilatation	OCS, cytotoxic drugs
Venoocclusive disease	Pyrrolizidine alkaloids, cytotoxic drugs
Hepatic or portal vein thrombosis	OCS
Peliosis hepatis	Androgens, estrogens, azathioprine
Angiosarcoma	Thorotrast, polyvinyl chloride, arsenic, androgens
Granulomas	Allopurinol, phenytoin, quinidine

OCS = oral contraceptive steroids.
*The same agents that cause zonal acute hepatitis may also cause massive hepatic necrosis.

2. **Etiology and pathogenesis.** The etiology and pathogenesis of chemical hepatitis vary with the causative agent.
   a. **Predictable (intrinsic) hepatotoxicity** results from an agent that is intrinsically hepatotoxic and **injurious to most people** who are exposed to it. The degree of injury is dose-dependent and, with direct hepatotoxins, can be reproduced experimentally. **Zonal necrosis** typically results from predictable hepatotoxins; it appears to correlate with the location of drug-metabolizing enzymes. Predictable hepatotoxins fall into two categories.
      (1) **Direct hepatotoxins** or their metabolic products damage the hepatocyte and its organelles by a direct, nonselective physicochemical effect that distorts or destroys the basic structural framework of the cell and its organelles. Tissue injury, commonly mediated by peroxidation of membrane lipids, leads to metabolic defects. Necrosis and steatosis are histologic features of direct hepatotoxicity.
         (a) **Carbon tetrachloride** is the prototype of direct hepatotoxins, causing centrilobular necrosis and steatosis. Necrosis apparently results mainly from the effects of a free radical generated from carbon tetrachloride biotransformation by the mixed function oxidase (MFO) system (including its principal member, cytochrome P-450).
         (b) **Yellow phosphorus** causes periportal (zone 1) necrosis and steatosis by an unknown mechanism.
      (2) **Indirect hepatotoxins** or their metabolites cause injury by selectively interfering with a specific metabolic pathway or structural process. Necrosis, steatosis, or cholestasis may result.
         (a) High-dose **intravenous tetracycline** can lead to microvesicular steatosis.
         (b) **Acetaminophen toxicity** usually results from a single, large, deliberately ingested dose (typically more than 15 g) of the drug. Generation of large amounts of toxic metabolite by the MFO system outpaces the detoxifying capacities of glutathione, resulting in covalent binding of the substance to tissue macromolecules and

centrilobular necrosis. Smaller acetaminophen doses may have similar effects in chronic alcoholics or in patients receiving other drugs that stimulate the MFO system (e.g., phenobarbital).

(c) Toxins of the poisonous mushroom *Amanita phalloides* may cause steatosis and centrilobular necrosis; erythromycin and anabolic or contraceptive steroids may induce cholestasis.

(d) **Ethanol toxicity** and related disorders—also examples of indirect hepatotoxicity—are discussed in IV D.

b. **Unpredictable (idiosyncratic) hepatotoxicity** stems from exposure to an agent that causes hepatic **injury in only a small number of exposed people**. It is not dose-dependent. Most hepatotoxic reactions to drugs are idiosyncratic. The offending agents cause **nonzonal but occasionally massive hepatic necrosis**. Reactions to unpredictable hepatotoxins fall into two main categories.

(1) **Hypersensitivity-related injury.** This damage occurs shortly (1 to 5 weeks) after exposure, with prompt recurrence upon drug readministration. Frequently, fever, rash, peripheral eosinophilia, and atypical lymphocytosis develop. The liver may show a prominent eosinophilic infiltrate, granulomas, or both. Although the clinical features of this reaction suggest the importance of immunologic mechanisms, efforts to document such mechanisms have been inconclusive. Examples of agents causing hypersensitivity-related hepatotoxicity include **phenytoin, chlorpromazine, sulfonamides, and halothane**.

(2) **Metabolic aberration.** This hepatotoxic reaction results when an aberrant metabolic pathway for drug metabolism results in accumulation of toxic metabolites in a susceptible patient. The latent period before development of overt hepatic injury varies greatly (1 week to 12 months), and the response to a challenge dose may be delayed many days or weeks. No clinical features of hypersensitivity appear. The prototype agent for this type of injury is **isoniazid**. Liver biopsy findings may be indistinguishable from those seen with acute viral hepatitis. Chronic active hepatitis and cirrhosis also have developed from this type of reaction.

3. **Clinical features.** Like other forms of acute hepatitis, chemical hepatitis typically causes jaundice. Other manifestations may include fever, arthralgia, nausea, vomiting, dark urine, and abdominal pain. Carbon tetrachloride poisoning may cause headache, drowsiness, and dizziness.

4. **Pathology.** Chemical hepatitis often is morphologically indistinguishable from acute viral hepatitis. Steatosis also may be a manifestation of chemical hepatitis.

a. **Steatosis** most commonly appears as a single large fat droplet within the hepatocyte (**macrovesicular steatosis**), although numerous small droplets (**microvesicular steatosis**) or mixed types can occur. Microvesicular steatosis, which may be difficult to detect on routinely processed sections, can be confirmed with a stain for neutral fat (oil red O) on frozen tissue sections.

b. **Microvesicular steatosis** may be seen with valproate, intravenous tetracycline, or ethanol toxicity, although it also can result from such conditions as Reye's syndrome (see VII), fatty liver of pregnancy, obesity, and viral hepatitis.

5. **Treatment and prognosis.** The offending agent must be withdrawn or removed. However, the disease may progress even after withdrawal. Potential sequelae of chemical forms of liver injury include chronic hepatitis, cirrhosis, vascular disorders, and hyperplastic and neoplastic hepatic nodules.

D. **Alcoholic liver disease**

1. **General concepts.** The spectrum of liver disease induced by chronic excessive consumption of alcohol (ethanol) includes **steatosis (fatty liver), alcoholic hepatitis,** and **cirrhosis**. These disorders may occur as single conditions or in various combinations.

2. **Epidemiology.** Alcoholism and alcohol-related diseases affect more than 10 million Americans and, after heart disease and cancer, represent the third largest health problem in the United States. The amount of ethanol consumption required to produce clinically significant liver disease varies with such factors as age, sex, race, and body size.

a. In most cases, alcoholic liver disease follows long-term ingestion of more than 80 g/day of ethanol (equivalent to eight 12-ounce beers, 1 L of wine, or a half-pint of 80-proof whiskey).

b. However, some studies show an increased risk of cirrhosis with ingestion of as little as 40 to 60 g/day in males and 20 g/day in females.

3. **Pathogenesis.** Because ethanol is hepatotoxic, it can cause liver disease even in the absence of the malnutrition that often accompanies alcoholism.

   a. The **alcoholic dehydrogenase (ADH) system,** present in the cytosol, accounts for 90% of ethanol metabolism. Nearly all the remaining ethanol is degraded by the inducible microsomal ethanol oxidizing system (MEOS)—a mixed-function oxidase system located in the smooth ER.

   b. **Acetaldehyde** and, possibly, free radicals produced by ethanol oxidation may be cytotoxic. Alcohol may change the physical state and lipid composition of the cell membrane and, therefore, impair cell function. Immunologic mechanisms also have been postulated as the cause of cell injury.

   c. **Stimulation of Ito cells** to produce collagen may be an important mechanism of the fibrosis seen in alcoholic liver disease.

   d. Multiple **defects in fat metabolism** lead to steatosis. Ethanol-induced microtubular injury may result in defective secretion of export proteins; along with retained water and fat, this defect causes the cellular enlargement and the increased liver weight that characterize steatosis.

4. **Clinical features and diagnosis.** Alcoholic liver disease may result in a wide range of clinical manifestations.

   a. With **steatosis,** hepatomegaly may be the only apparent sign.

   b. Patients with **alcoholic hepatitis** may be asymptomatic or may have symptoms mimicking viral hepatitis, such as nausea, vomiting, jaundice, and hepatomegaly. With advanced disease, hepatic encephalopathy (manifested by confusion, lethargy, hallucination, coma, and asterixis) may develop. The ratio of serum AST to ALT frequently exceeds 2:1.

   c. **Cirrhosis** may cause ascites, wasted extremities, jaundice, bleeding esophageal varices, testicular atrophy, and hepatic encephalopathy.

5. **Pathology.** Steatosis, alcoholic hepatitis, and cirrhosis may occur as single conditions or in various combinations.

   a. **Steatosis**—the earliest and most common manifestation of alcoholic liver disease—is found in the liver biopsies of over 90% of chronic alcoholics.

   (1) The liver appears yellowish-tan and may be several times its normal size.

   (2) Initially, zone 3 (centrilobular) hepatocytes are involved.

   (3) Most commonly, steatosis is macrovesicular; however, microvesicular steatosis (**alcoholic foamy degeneration**) sometimes appears.

   (4) Rupture of fatty hepatocytes may lead to lipogranuloma formation.

   (5) Fat disappears from hepatocytic cytoplasm within 2 to 4 weeks after ethanol intake ceases.

   b. **Alcoholic hepatitis** is characterized by steatosis, hepatocyte injury, a neutrophil-rich inflammatory infiltrate, and perivenular fibrosis (Figure 15-4). These changes are most prominent in zone 3.

   (1) **Ballooning (hydropic) degeneration** is the most common form of hepatocyte injury, although scattered acidophilic bodies may appear.

   (a) **Mallory's hyalin** (also called **Mallory's bodies** or **alcoholic hyalin**) are irregularly shaped masses of deeply eosinophilic hyaline material found in clumps , strands, or perinuclear rings in the hepatocyte cytoplasm of 50% to 75% of alcoholic hepatitis patients. The hyaline material consists of cytokeratin filaments.

   (b) Although neutrophils generally predominate within the lobule, lymphocytes and plasma cells occasionally are the most conspicuous inflammatory cells.

   (2) **Perivenular fibrosis** and associated thickening of the terminal hepatic venule (**phlebosclerosis**) frequently occur in alcoholic hepatitis (this finding is a hallmark of all forms of alcoholic liver disease).

   (a) Collagen initially deposited in the space of Disse causes a chicken wire–like microscopic appearance as it extends along the sinusoids and traps individual hepatocytes.

   (b) Dense fibrotic perivenular areas (**central hyaline sclerosis**) results from progressive hepatocyte dropout and more extensive fibrous obliteration of the sinusoids and efferent veins.

   c. **Cirrhosis** (see XI)

   d. **Other morphologic features of alcoholic liver disease** may include mild parenchymal iron overload, cholangiolitis, cholestasis simulating extrahepatic biliary obstruction, portal fibrosis, and piecemeal necrosis resembling that seen in chronic active hepatitis.

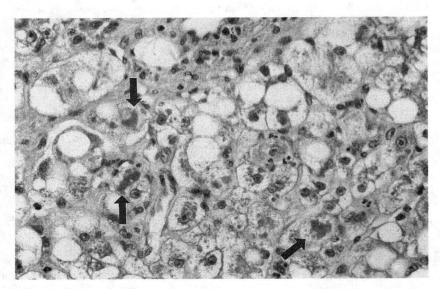

Figure 15-4. Liver demonstrating alcoholic hepatitis. Steatosis and neutrophil-rich inflammatory infiltrate are evident. Hepatocytes show ballooning degeneration; several contain Mallory's hyalin (*arrows*).

    e. Other conditions showing characteristic histopathology of alcoholic hepatitis or cirrhosis include obesity, diabetes mellitus, drug toxicity (e.g., from amiodarone, perihexilene maleate, estrogens), or post-jejunoileal bypass surgery or gastropexy for obesity. Therefore, the more general terms **steatohepatitis** or **steatonecrosis** may be used. **Mallory's bodies** also may occur in Wilson's disease, Indian childhood cirrhosis, certain hepatocellular tumors, and disorders associated with chronic cholestasis (e.g., primary biliary cirrhosis).

6. Treatment and prognosis
    a. Steatosis usually resolves when the patient stops drinking.
    b. Alcoholic hepatitis and cirrhosis warrant long-term supportive care as well as abstinence from alcohol. Specific measures are directed at such complications as bleeding esophageal varices and ascites.
    c. The overall mortality rate from alcoholic hepatitis is 15% to 30%. More than one-third of surviving patients who continue to consume alcohol progress to cirrhosis within 1 to 2 years. Of patients who abstain, roughly 20% eventually progress to cirrhosis.

V. VASCULAR HEPATIC DISORDERS

A. Acute and chronic passive liver congestion. These circulatory abnormalities typically reflect right-sided heart failure.

    1. Etiology. Hepatic congestion may result from any condition in the systemic venous circulation—from the level of the liver to the heart—that increases pressure within hepatic venules and sinusoids.
        a. Severe right-sided heart failure and constrictive pericarditis are by far the most common causes.
        b. Thrombosis of large hepatic veins (Budd-Chiari syndrome) is a rare cause. Frequently idiopathic, this syndrome may accompany such conditions as myeloproliferative disorders (apparent or subclinical); hypercoagulable states; adrenal, renal, or hepatocellular carcinoma; radiation damage or oral contraceptive use.
        c. Occlusion of hepatic venules (venoocclusive disease) initially was described from sequelae of ingestion of herbal teas containing pyrrolizidine alkaloids. More recently, it has been associated with radiotherapy and with administration of azathioprine and cytotoxic agents in recipients of bone marrow and renal transplants. These agents appear to damage the endothelium of the terminal venules and sinusoids.

2. **Clinical features.** In most cases, hepatic congestion is an incidental autopsy finding. However, an occasional patient presents with abrupt onset of an enlarged, tender liver sometimes associated with ascites. With markedly elevated serum transaminase levels (i.e., > 1000 U/L), the disorder may be misdiagnosed as acute hepatitis.

3. **Pathology**
   a. **Macroscopic findings.** Hepatic congestion appears as a diffuse parenchymal mottling, with reddish-purple perivenular areas surrounded by paler regions. (From this appearance, which resembles the cut surface of a nutmeg, comes the term **nutmeg liver**.)
   b. **Microscopic findings.** Congestion and dilatation of efferent veins and centrilobular sinusoids are evident.
      (1) Hepatocyte plates in the affected regions appear atrophic and may disappear altogether, leaving a collapsed reticulin framework. Zone 2 hepatocytes may demonstrate fatty change.
      (2) Chronic and typically severe venous outflow obstruction may lead to linking of adjacent perivenular areas by fibrous septa—a pattern called **reverse lobulation**. Less commonly, portal–central septa result. The terms cardiac fibrosis and cardiac cirrhosis sometimes are used for these advanced states of liver injury.
      (3) Fibrin thrombi in hepatic veins characterize Budd-Chiari syndrome; obliteration of terminal venules in the absence of fibrin thrombi or other causes of venous outflow obstruction typifies venoocclusive disease.

B. **Ischemic hepatocellular necrosis**

1. **Etiology and pathogenesis.** This abnormality may stem from systemic hypotension or any disorder that causes hepatic congestion. Cirrhotic nodules, whose blood supply comes mainly from hepatic artery branches, are predisposed to infarction when peripheral hypotension occurs.

2. **Pathology**
   a. Findings include centrilobular necrosis and hemorrhage without sinusoidal dilatation (in cases of peripheral circulatory failure without outflow obstruction).
   b. True hepatic infarction generally is very rare because of the liver's dual blood supply. The so-called **Zahn infarct,** which appears as a wedge-shaped area with its base along Glisson's capsule, is not really an infarct but an area of sinusoidal dilatation stemming from occlusion of intrahepatic portal vein branches.

VI. NEONATAL HEPATITIS AND CHOLESTASIS (INFANTILE OBSTRUCTIVE CHOLANGIOPATHY)

A. **General concepts**

1. **Terminology**
   a. The terms **noenatal hepatitis** and **neonatal cholestasis** often are used to describe a wide range of disorders characterized **clinically** by conjugated hyperbilirubinemia and variable serum transaminase elevation and **microscopically** by varying degrees of cholestasis, hepatocellular injury, multinucleate hepatocytes (giant cell hepatitis), and inflammation.
   b. Landing first proposed that neonatal hepatitis, choledochal cyst, extrahepatic biliary atresia, and some forms of intrahepatic biliary atresia all might represent manifestations of a single disease process, which he termed **infantile obstructive cholangiopathy**.

2. **Disease spectrum**
   a. **Disorders associated with neonatal hepatitis and cholestasis** include:
      (1) **Certain infections,** including viral diseases (e.g., CMV, hepatitis B, rubella, herpes simplex) and infections caused by *Treponema* and *Toxoplasma* organisms
      (2) **Various metabolic disorders,** including cystic fibrosis, errors of carbohydrate and lipid metabolism, and α_1-antitrypsin deficiency (see VI B for further discussion of α_1-antitrypsin deficiency)
   b. **Disorders of the intrahepatic and extrahepatic bile ducts** include:
      (1) Intrahepatic biliary atresia (see VI C)
      (2) Extrahepatic biliary atresia
      (3) Choledochal cyst
      (4) Caroli's disease (see II B 2)

(5) Congenital hepatic fibrosis (see II A)

(6) Idiopathic neonatal (giant cell) hepatitis, a condition that has no identifiable cause

B. Alpha$_1$-antitrypsin deficiency. The major α_1-globulin found in human plasma, α_1-antitrypsin is synthesized in the liver, where it inhibits several proteolytic enzymes (e.g., trypsin, elastase). More than 70 α_1-antitrypsin variants, designated as **protease inhibitor (Pi)** phenotypes, have been identified. Each allele is inherited codominantly. The normal genotype is PiMM; 3% and 0.07% of the general population have the slower moving (on electrophoresis) PiMZ and PiZZ genotypes, respectively. Those in the homozygous PiZZ state show an 85% to 90% reduction in the serum level of α_1-antitrypsin.

1. **Etiology and pathogenesis**
   a. Liver disease is associated with the PiZZ genotype in both children and adults and, possibly, with the PiMZ genotype in adults. Approximately 10% to 15% of newborns with the PiZZ phenotype develop neonatal cholestasis.
   b. The defect in α_1-antitrypsin deficiency is a selective defect in the transport of α_1-antitrypsin from the ER to the Golgi apparatus of the hepatocyte. This defect appears to result from a single amino acid substitution (lysine for glutamic acid at position 342), an action which leads to misfolding of the protein molecule and an inability to transport it from the ER. The pathogenesis of the liver injury itself is still controversial.

2. **Clinical features.** When associated with α_1-antitrypsin deficiency, neonatal hepatitis usually presents within a few days to weeks after birth. Hepatitis usually resolves by 6 months of age, but in some cases it progresses to cirrhosis. Patients with chronic active hepatitis or cirrhosis may sometimes present for the first time in adulthood. It is estimated that 10% to 20% of all PiZZ patients develop cirrhosis.

3. **Pathology**
   a. When a Z allele is involved, round eosinophilic hyaline globules of α_1-antitrypsin appear within periportal or periseptal hepatocytes. These globules are periodic acid–Schiff (PAS)-positive and resist diastase digestion, reflecting their glycoproteinaceous nature. They reside in dilated saccules of the ER. Immunohistochemistry using specific antibody to α_1-antitrypsin can definitively identify these globulins in tissue sections.
   b. Proliferation of bile ductules may simulate extrahepatic obstruction. With disease progression, histologic features of chronic active hepatitis and cirrhosis appear.

4. **Treatment.** While liver transplantation is the only currently available treatment for patients with end-stage disease, gene replacement therapy is an area of active investigation. Those who develop cirrhosis have an increased risk of hepatocellular carcinoma.

C. Intrahepatic biliary atresia (intrahepatic bile duct paucity)

1. **Classification.** This disorder occurs in two forms—the **syndromic form** (also called **Alagille's syndrome** or **arteriohepatic dysplasia**) and the **nonsyndromic form**.

2. **Etiology and pathogenesis.** Viral infection, chromosomal abnormalities, metabolic errors (including α_1-antitrypsin deficiency) and developmental defects may be important pathogenetic factors. A hereditary predisposition appears to be crucial to the syndromic form. Although some researchers debate whether the initial defect involves hepatocytes or bile ducts, one hypothesis proposes that secondary bile duct involution results from marked impairment of hepatocytic bile excretion into the canaliculi.

3. **Clinical features.** Affected infants are cholestatic and intensely pruritic. In the syndromic disease form, the face shows such classic signs as slight hypertelorism, deep-set eyes, and a broad forehead. Other manifestations include vertebral, ocular, and renal abnormalities and pulmonic stenosis.

4. **Pathology.** Microscopic findings include near absence of the interlobular bile ducts and an associated decrease in the number of portal tracts. In early infancy, bile duct proliferation and portal inflammation may appear.

5. **Treatment and prognosis.** Most patients survive to adulthood. The serum bilirubin typically normalizes; however, pruritus persists (due to serum bile acid elevation) and must be treated symptomatically. Rarely, prominent fibrosis or cirrhosis develops (most frequently with nonsyndromic disease). Liver transplantation should be considered in cirrhotic patients.

VII. REYE'S SYNDROME. This acute disease (also called **fatty liver with encephalopathy**) nearly always occurs in children—most commonly those between the ages of 4 and 12 years.

A. Etiology and pathogenesis

1. Reye's syndrome typically follows **viral infection** (usually influenza A or B or varicella). **Aspirin ingestion** has been implicated in more than 90% of cases. This drug may act as a pathogenetic cofactor. Aspirin is a known mitochondrial toxin—a fact that lends credence to the theory that mitochondrial brain and liver abnormalities are the characteristic, and perhaps major, defects in Reye's syndrome. (Impairment of mitochondrial fatty acid oxidation leads to increased triglyceride synthesis.)

2. A syndrome similar to Reye's may stem from **inborn errors of fatty acid oxidation**. Jamaican vomiting sickness is caused by ingestion of hypoglycin, a substance found in the unripened fruit of the akee tree. This condition results in inhibition of fatty acid oxidation and a Reye-like syndrome.

B. Clinical features and diagnosis. A biphasic disorder, Reye's syndrome is manifested by acute encephalopathy and noniteric hepatic dysfunction. Since the epidemic of 1974, this disorder has become less frequent and now is considered uncommon.

1. After the prodromal febrile illness, the child appears to recover. However, about 1 week after onset of the viral illness comes an abrupt onset of protracted vomiting. The patient may progress rapidly to seizures, coma, and death in the absence of jaundice.

2. Serum transaminase elevation (more than 3 times normal), plasma ammonia elevation, and hypoprothrombinemia are classic laboratory findings.

C. Pathology. The liver is grossly yellow or white, reflecting a high triglyceride content. **Microvesicular steatosis** is striking; necrosis and inflammation are absent. Liver and brain mitochondria are swollen, show fewer cristae, and may have peculiar budding and branching forms.

VIII. CHRONIC HEPATITIS

A. General concepts

1. **Definition.** The term **chronic hepatitis** encompasses a group of disorders characterized by hepatic necroinflammation that persists unabated for at least 6 months. Typically, lymphocytes dominate the inflammatory infiltrate. Chronic hepatitis may precede or accompany cirrhosis.

2. **Disease spectrum.** Generally, chronic hepatitis refers to hepatitis stemming from a virus, drug use, or an autoimmune mechanism. However, other forms of chronic liver disease (Figure 15-5) may meet the clinicopathologic definition of chronic hepatitis at certain stages. These disorders include primary biliary cirrhosis, primary sclerosing cholangitis, Wilson's disease, α_1-antitrypsin deficiency, and even advanced alcoholic liver disease.

B. Classification. Chronic hepatitis should be classified by both morphologic features and etiology.

1. **Morphologic classification.** Regardless of etiology, chronic hepatitis has characteristic histopathologic features.
   a. **Chronic persistent hepatitis.** In this disease form, inflammatory infiltrate (predominantly lymphocytic) is restricted to the portal tract, and **the limiting plate is intact**. Fibrosis, lobular inflammation, and necrosis are minimal.
   b. **Chronic lobular hepatitis.** In this disease form of chronic hepatitis, the lobular features of acute hepatitis persist for more than 6 months. **The limiting plate remains intact.**
   c. **Chronic active hepatitis.** In this form, portal and periportal inflammation appear in association with **piecemeal necrosis** (hepatocyte degeneration and necrosis at the limiting plate). Injured hepatocytes are swollen or shrunken.
      (1) The inflammatory infiltrate typically replaces significant portions of periportal parenchyma. Extension of newly formed collagen strands into the lobule gives the portal tract a stellate or maple-leaf shape.
      (2) In many cases, portal–portal and portal–central fibrous septa form. In patients with bridging or multiacinar necrosis, cirrhosis is common.

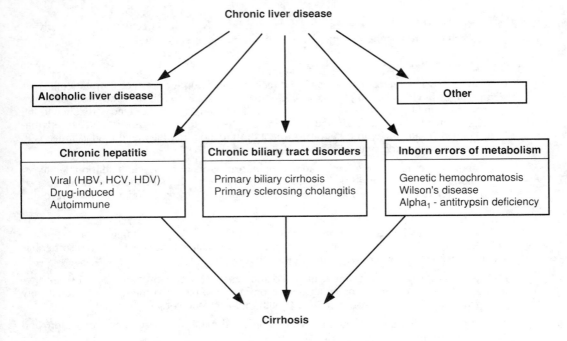

Figure 15-5. Classification of chronic liver disease.

2. **Etiologic classification**

a. **Hepatitis viruses.** Hepatitis B, C, and D viruses can cause chronic hepatitis. In patients with chronic HBV infection, the hepatocyte nucleus may contain HBV DNA in the episomal form, HBV DNA integrated into the host DNA, or both. Mutation of the HBV genome in patients with acute hepatitis B may provide a selective growth advantage—allowing the virus to escape, to some degree, the host response to the virus—resulting in chronic hepatitis B.

   (1) Integrated and episomal HBV DNA correlate with the absence or presence of serum markers of HBV replication, respectively.

   (2) Hepatocytes with "ground glass" cytoplasm or "sanded" nuclei, which demonstrate hepatitis B surface antigen (HBsAg) and hepatitis B core antigen (HBcAg), respectively, are morphologic markers of chronic HBV infection.

   (3) Using immunohistochemical techniques, HDV and HCV antigens may be demonstrated in the nucleus and cytoplasm of the hepatocyte, respectively. In situ hybridization (ISH) and the polymerase chain reaction (PCR) provide other more sensitive methods for looking for viral antigens.

b. **Autoimmune (lupoid) mechanisms.** The etiology of autoimmune chronic hepatitis is undefined. However, autoimmune mechanisms are suggested by the frequent presence of several serum autoantibodies, hypergammaglobulinemia, the relatively high incidence of extrahepatic autoimmune disorders, the preferential incidence of this disease form in women, the prominence of plasma cells in the inflammatory infiltrate in some cases, and the favorable response to corticosteroid therapy.

c. **Drugs.** Methyldopa, nitrofurantoin, oxyphenisatin, isoniazid, and other drugs may cause chronic hepatitis. Serum autoantibodies are detected in some cases of drug-induced chronic hepatitis.

C. **Clinical features and diagnosis**

1. **Chronic HBV infection** may be silent or may manifest as anorexia, abdominal pain, hepatosplenomegaly, ascites, jaundice, and bleeding esophageal varices. Extrahepatic signs (e.g., rash, arthritis, vasculitis) may occur because of circulating HBsAg–anti-HBs immune complexes. The majority of patients are males.

a. Serum transaminase levels remain elevated, and HBsAg generally is still detected in the serum. However, absence of HBsAg does not rule out chronic HBV infection; in some cases, HBV DNA can be detected in the blood and liver by ISH or PCR, or southern blot analysis may reveal that the HBV DNA has been integrated into the host genome.

b. With HDV superinfection, chronic HBV infection commonly shows clinical exacerbation and morphologically shows increased activity of the hepatitis.

2. Chronic hepatitis C often does not cause symptoms. However, up to 25% of patients may progress to cirrhosis.

3. Autoimmune chronic hepatitis (see VIII B 2 b) typically has an insidious onset, although occasionally it may have an acute presentation. This disorder has been classified into three types based on the pattern of autoantibodies found in the serum. It has recently been suggested that HCV may play a role in some cases of autoimmune hepatitis.

    a. Type 1 (classic) autoimmune chronic hepatitis demonstrates anti–smooth muscle (antiactin) antibody (ASMA) and antinuclear antibody (ANA).

    b. Type 2 autoimmune chronic hepatitis demonstrates anti-liver–kidney microsomal (anti-LKM1) antibody.

    c. Type 3 autoimmune chronic hepatitis demonstrates anti-liver soluble antigen (anti-LSA) antibody.

D. Treatment and prognosis

    1. Regardless of the etiology, a significant number of patients with chronic hepatitis (**particularly chronic active hepatitis**) eventually develop cirrhosis.

    2. Interferon-α (IFN-α) is currently used to treat some patients with chronic hepatitis C and B, whereas corticosteroids are often used in patients with chronic autoimmune hepatitis. Patients with drug-induced chronic hepatitis often improve when the offending agent is withdrawn.

IX. OTHER DISORDERS ASSOCIATED WITH CHRONIC LIVER DISEASE

A. Primary biliary cirrhosis (Table 15-4). This chronic cholestatic disorder occurs mainly in middle-aged females.

    1. Etiology. An autoimmune mechanism has been suggested. The characteristic bile duct damage may result from T-cell sensitization to increased expression of class I major histocompatibility (MHC) antigens and aberrant expression of class II MHC antigens on the biliary epithelium.

Table 15-4. Primary Biliary Cirrhosis (PBC) and Primary Sclerosing Cholangitis (PSC): Clinicopathologic Features Helpful in Differential Diagnosis

	PBC	PSC
Histologic feature		
Chronic Cholestasis	Yes	Yes
Granulomatous Cholangitis	Yes	—
Fibrous obliterative cholangitis	−/+	Yes
Large duct obstruction	No	Yes
Lobular granulomas	+ + +	+
Lymphoid aggregates	+ + +	+
Bile duct loss	+ + +	+
Clinical feature		
Age, sex	Middle-aged women	Young to middle-aged men
Associated idiopathic IBD	No	> 70%
↑ Serum alkaline phosphatase	Yes	Yes
↑ Serum immunoglobulin M	Yes	+/−
Positive serum AMA	> 90%	< 5%
Positive serum ANCA*	0	65%
Abnormal ERCP (extrahepatic)	No	Yes

AMA = antimitochondrial antibody; ANCA = antineutrophil cytoplasmic antibody; ERCP = endoscopic retrograde cholangiopancreatogram; IBD = inflammatory bowel disease.

*Perinuclear pattern only. (The specificity of this test requires further evaluation).

2. **Clinical features and diagnosis.** Patients who present with symptoms experience intense, diffuse pruritus and, over the course of the disease, develop jaundice, xanthomas, cutaneous pigmentation, steatorrhea, and bony effects of vitamin D and calcium malabsorption (e.g., osteomalacia, osteoporosis). In some cases, the physician makes the diagnosis in an asymptomatic patient by discovering abnormal laboratory test results.

   a. **Connective tissue disorders** are found with increasing frequency. Particularly common are the **sicca syndrome** (i.e., dry mouth and eyes, with or without the systemic connective tissue disease component that completes Sjögren's syndrome), **scleroderma,** and the milder form of scleroderma referred to as **CREST syndrome** (calcinosis, Raynaud's phenomenon, esophageal dysfunction, syndactyly, and telangiectasia).

   b. **Laboratory findings**
      (1) Markedly elevated levels of serum alkaline phosphatase (in the absence of extrahepatic obstruction), cholesterol, triglycerides, and IgM are characteristic. Serum transaminase levels are only mildly elevated.
      (2) Serum bilirubin elevation is variable but usually is not present early in the disease.
      (3) At least 90% of patients have elevated serum antimitochondrial antibody titers.

3. **Pathology**
   a. Small to medium-sized intrahepatic bile ducts undergo progressive damage and loss when they are surrounded and infiltrated by chronic inflammatory cells. Destruction of bile ducts by epithelioid granulomas (**florid duct lesion**) is nearly pathognomonic of primary biliary cirrhosis. Lobular granulomas may be found.
   b. As with other chronic cholestatic diseases, primary biliary cirrhosis is associated with high tissue copper levels (see III A 2 c for a discussion of the pathologic features of chronic cholestasis).
   c. Four disease stages characterize progressive bile duct damage and hepatic scarring culminating in cirrhosis. The magnitude of these changes varies throughout the liver. Cirrhosis develops only in the late stage of this disorder.

4. **Treatment and prognosis**
   a. Symptomatic patients may receive ursodeoxycholic acid or other drugs; however, the efficacy of these agents has not been proven. Patients with end-stage disease may be candidates for liver transplantation.
   b. Primary biliary cirrhosis carries an extremely variable prognosis. Asymptomatic patients with early-stage disease may survive more than 10 years; late-stage symptomatic disease may cause death within a few years.

B. **Primary sclerosing cholangitis** (see Chapter 14 II D; Table 15-4).

C. **Inborn errors of metabolism** (Table 15-5). These disorders merit consideration in the differential diagnosis of chronic hepatitis with or without cirrhosis.

1. **Genetic (primary, idiopathic) hemochromatosis.** This relatively common inborn error of iron metabolism may lead to massive hepatic deposits (often 50 to 100 times the normal level) of iron as hemosiderin. The resulting cirrhosis is followed by hemosiderin deposits in and impairment of many organs, most notably the pancreas, other endocrine organs, the heart, and salivary glands. Hepatocellular carcinoma is an important complication.

   a. **Classification of iron overload (Table 15-6).** Iron overload may be classified into two major groups: genetic hemochromatosis, which involves a hereditary predisposition to absorb increased amounts of iron from the small bowel, and secondary forms of iron overload, in which oral or parenteral mechanisms may be operative.

   b. **Inheritance**
      (1) Genetic hemochromatosis is inherited as an autosomal recessive trait. About 1 in 200 to 400 people is homozygous for genetic hemochromatosis, but only 20% of homozygotes progress to symptomatic disease. The heterozygote carrier rate is estimated at 1 in 10 persons; heterozygotes do not develop liver disease.
      (2) The gene is located on the short arm of chromosome 6 and is closely linked to the human leukocyte antigen (HLA)-A3 locus, with a weaker relationship to HLA-B7 and B14.

   c. **Pathogenesis**
      (1) In genetic hemochromatosis, increased duodenal iron absorption begins early in life. Although the precise mechanism of iron loading is still unclear, the intestinal epithelial cell is unable to store enough iron to regulate the amount absorbed. This situation

Table 15-5. Chronic Liver Disease: Inborn Errors of Metabolism*

	Genetic Hemochromatosis	Alpha₁-antitrypsin Deficiency	Wilson's Disease
Metabolic defect	↑ Iron absorption	α_1-antitrypsin secretion	Copper excretion
Chromosome	6	14	13
Inheritance	Autosomal recessive	Autosomal co-dominant (ZZ)	Autosomal recessive
Age at presentation	40–60 years	Variable (neonate, adult)	First few decades
Clinical features	Bronze diabetes, liver disease, congestive heart failure, or asymptomatic	Cholestasis, chronic liver disease	Kayser-Fleischer rings, liver disease, neuropsychiatric disturbances
Affected organs	Liver, pancreas, heart, others	Liver, lung	Liver, eye, basal ganglia
Histologic hallmark	Prominent hemosiderin in hepatocytes	Hyaline globules (liver only)	None, other than clinical presentation
Laboratory data	↑ Serum iron ↑ % Saturated transferrin ↑ Ferritin ↑ Iron in hepatic tissue	↓ Serum α_1-antitrypsin	↓ Ceruloplasmin ↓ Serum copper ↑ Urine copper ↑ Copper in hepatic tissue
Therapy	Phlebotomy	Possibly gene therapy	D-penicillamine

*Each of these disorders may result in cirrhosis.

leads to saturation of circulating transferrin with iron. Saturation, in turn, leads to increased delivery of iron—first to hepatocytes via portal blood, then to parenchymal cells of other organs. The mechanism of iron loading is being studied, as are the role and importance of a possible reticuloendothelial blockade to iron storage.

(2) The iron is stored in hepatocytes, first as **ferritin**. As iron stores increase, the ferritin within lysosomes is converted into **hemosiderin**. Iron may be indirectly toxic to hepatocytes and other parenchymal cells since it generates free radicals that cause peroxidation of organelle membranes—leading to their dysfunction and subsequent cell death. A direct role in stimulating collagen biosynthesis is also a possibility.

Table 15-6. Classification of Hepatic Iron Overload

Genetic (primary, idiopathic) iron overload*

Secondary iron overload
    Increased intestinal iron absorption
        Refractory anemias with ineffective erythropoiesis[†]
            Thalassemia major
            Sideroblastic anemia
        Increased oral intake
            In South African blacks (Bantu hemosiderosis)
            Medicinal iron ingestion
        Other inherited diseases
            Porphyria cutanea tarda
            Congenital atransferrinemia
        Alcoholic liver disease

    Parenteral iron overload
        Multiple transfusions
        Parenteral iron administration
        Associated with hemodialysis

    Unknown
        Perinatal (neonatal) hemochromatosis
        Post-portacaval shunt

---

*Mechanism is increased intestinal iron absorption.
[†]Transfusions provide an additional parenteral source of iron.

d. Clinical features and diagnosis
  (1) Signs and symptoms
    (a) Symptomatic patients are usually between age 40 and 60. Typical clinical manifestations include liver disease, diabetes mellitus, cardiac failure, arrhythmias, testicular atrophy, arthropathy, and skin pigmentation.
    (b) Asymptomatic patients are detected by laboratory abnormalities found in screening tests.
  (2) Laboratory findings
    (a) Characteristics of this disorder are elevated serum iron (often exceeding 200 μg/dl), transferrin saturation (usually greater than 70%), ferritin (often exceeding 1000 ng/ml), and serum transaminases (mild elevation). Patients with secondary forms of iron overload, other forms of liver disease, and, sometimes, heterozygotes for genetic hemochromatosis can show such laboratory abnormalities.
    (b) Iron quantitation performed on liver biopsy specimens is the best way to evaluate the degree of iron overload. Hepatic fibrosis or cirrhosis is usually found when levels exceed 20,000 μg/g dry weight liver. A hepatic iron index (μmol Fe per gram dry weight divided by the patient's age) greater than 1.9 appears to separate homozygotes from heterozygotes.
e. Pathology
  (1) In genetic hemochromatosis, marked **hepatocellular hemosiderin deposition**—most prominent in the periportal region—is usually found by the time of diagnosis. Once parenchymal damage (e.g., fibrosis or cirrhosis) occurs, hemosiderin accumulates in the fibrous septa, in proliferated bile ductules, and in Kupffer cells. Hemosiderin deposits are minimal in Kupffer cells early in the disease. Inflammation is nearly absent. Distinction of heterozygotes from homozygotes early in the disease may be impossible if based on biopsy findings alone [see IX C 1 d (2) (b)].
  (2) In cases of parenteral iron overload, hemosiderin first accumulates within Kupffer cells and portal macrophages. In extreme cases of marked hepatocellular overload, distinction from genetic cases may also be impossible.
f. Treatment and prognosis
  (1) **Phlebotomy** is the treatment of choice. It frequently improves symptoms, may cause regression of fibrosis, and prolongs life.
  (2) Hepatocellular carcinoma develops in 10% to 20% of genetic hemochromatosis patients with cirrhosis; cholangiocarcinoma is less common. Phlebotomy can prevent the development of carcinoma if performed prior to the onset of fibrosis or cirrhosis.
  (3) All family members of patients with genetic hemochromatosis should be screened for the disease.

2. Alpha₁-antitrypsin deficiency (see VI B)

3. Wilson's disease (hepatolenticular degeneration). This inborn error of copper metabolism leads to copper accumulation and subsequent injury—first to the liver and then to the brain, kidneys, eyes, and other organs. The disease prevalence is about 1 in 30,000 to 200,000 in the general population, with a heterozygote carrier rate of 1 in 200 to 400 persons.
  a. Etiology and pathogenesis. Wilson's disease is inherited as an autosomal recessive trait; the responsible gene is located on chromosome 13, linked to the esterase D locus (a red cell enzyme). The precise excretory defect and the mechanism of copper-induced cellular injury are unknown.
  b. Clinical features and diagnosis
    (1) Signs and symptoms. Although the clinical presentation varies, slightly more than half the patients have evidence of hepatic disease (acute or chronic hepatitis); the remainder have neurologic signs (tremors, dysarthria, dysphagia, dementia) or behavioral abnormalities.
      (a) In some cases, massive acute hemolytic anemia, sometimes associated with fulminant hepatic failure, is the initial clinical manifestation.
      (b) Most patients are diagnosed in the first few decades of life; however, primary diagnosis may come as late as the seventh decade. Patients presenting by age 10 usually have hepatic manifestations, whereas those diagnosed later typically show neuropsychiatric signs. Renal tubular and glomerular defects and skeletal abnormalities also are present.

(2) Kayser-Fleischer rings—granular deposits of copper pigment in Descemet's membrane in the cornea—are nearly pathognomonic of Wilson's disease. They always are present in patients with neurologic signs but may be absent in asymptomatic patients or in those with hepatic signs only. If they are invisible to the naked eye, slit-lamp ophthalmologic examination should be performed.

(3) Laboratory findings include elevated levels of serum free copper, urine copper, and hepatic copper ($>$ 250 µg/g dry weight); levels of total serum copper and ceruloplasmin (which normally binds nearly all serum copper) generally are decreased. Subnormal ceruloplasmin levels ($<$ 20 mg/dl) alone are insufficient for diagnosis, as heterozygotes occasionally have decreased levels. Serum transaminase levels usually are only mildly elevated.

  c. Pathology. Findings in the precirrhotic liver include spotty hepatocyte necrosis, cholestasis, steatosis, glycogenated hepatocyte nuclei, periportal Mallory's hyalin, or a histologic appearance, indistinguishable from that seen in chronic active hepatitis. Histochemical copper stains are unreliable and, even when positive, yield nonspecific results. Ultrastructural examination shows that copper deposits initially are cytoplasmic; however, with advanced disease, they are confined to lysosomes. Cirrhosis, usually macronodular, is present at the time of diagnosis in half the cases.

  d. Treatment and prognosis. D-Penicillamine, a copper chelator, is the drug of choice, promoting urinary copper excretion and clinical recovery in most patients; treatment must continue for life. Liver transplantation cures patients with end-stage liver disease. The patient's siblings must be screened for asymptomatic disease.

4. Other childhood metabolic diseases. Although these disorders may cause the syndrome of neonatal cholestasis, many progress to chronic liver disease.

  a. Cystic fibrosis (Chapter 10 III B 2). In this disease, hepatic injury worsens with duration of survival. Prominent biliary fibrosis or cirrhosis is characteristic of cystic fibrosis; histologically, this condition is associated with proliferation of bile ductules containing inspissated secretions that are intensely positive with the PAS stain.

  b. Inborn errors of carbohydrate metabolism that may cause progressive liver disease and cirrhosis include glycogenosis (types III and IV), galactosemia, tyrosinemia, and hereditary fructose intolerance.

X. CIRRHOSIS. This disorder represents the end stage of various chronic diseases that cause diffuse parenchymal damage. It is characterized by fibrosis and conversion of the normal hepatic architecture into structurally abnormal nodules; these events lead to abnormal vascular relationships (arteriovenous shunts) and portal hypertension. Regenerative hepatocellular changes may be inconspicuous in early cirrhosis but become more prominent as the disease progresses.

A. Classification. Cirrhosis should be classified according to morphologic features and etiology. Etiologic classification is determined by clinical, epidemiologic, serologic, immunopathologic, and morphologic features.

1. Morphologic classification. Cirrhosis occurs in three macroscopic forms differentiated by the diameter of the overwhelming majority of nodules. The degree of cirrhosis activity depends on whether ongoing piecemeal necrosis and lobular hepatitis exist.

  a. Micronodular cirrhosis (Laënnec's cirrhosis or **portal cirrhosis**) [Figure 15-6]. In this form of cirrhosis, nodule diameter is less than 3 mm.

    (1) Nodules are uniform in size and separated by thin fibrous bands that lack portal tracts and central veins.

    (2) The liver is firm and may be normal, increased, or decreased in size. Steatosis (typical of alcoholic cirrhosis) lends a tan appearance to the liver.

    (3) Micronodular cirrhosis commonly stems from excessive alcohol intake but may result from other conditions, such as genetic hemochromatosis, biliary disease, chronic venous outflow obstruction, hypervitaminosis A, and some forms of chronic active hepatitis.

  b. Macronodular cirrhosis (also called **postnecrotic** or **posthepatic cirrhosis**). Nodule diameter exceeds 3 mm and may measure several centimeters.

    (1) Nodules, which vary in size, may be separated by broad, depressed scars. One or more portal tracts and an excessive number of efferent veins often appear within nodules.

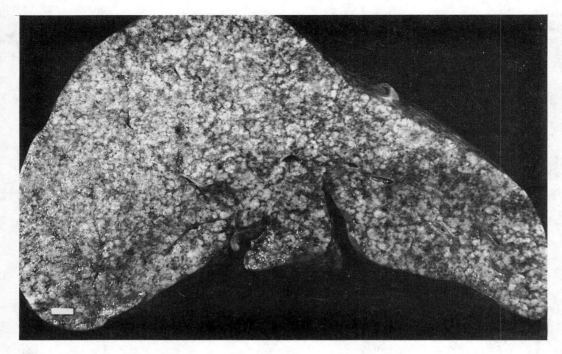

Figure 15-6. Micronodular cirrhosis. Most nodules have a diameter of less than 3 mm.

      (2) The liver appears firm and may be enlarged or shrunken.

      (3) Although macronodular cirrhosis most frequently results from viral or autoimmune forms of chronic active hepatitis, it may have any etiology. It sometimes occurs in alcoholics, particularly after they have stopped drinking.

   c. Mixed cirrhosis. In this disease form, the number of nodules with a diameter of less than 3 mm roughly equals the number of nodules with a diameter exceeding 3 mm.

  2. Etiologic classification. The various disorders that may cause cirrhosis have been discussed in IV D and VIII. However, in 15% to 60% of cases, the etiology has been reported as unknown. A significant proportion of these cases may be related to HCV.

B. Clinical features and diagnosis. Loss of functional parenchyma causes the major clinical consequences of cirrhosis—hypoalbuminemia, clotting abnormalities, jaundice, impaired hepatic drug detoxification, heightened risk of infection, portal hypertension, and increased risk for the development of hepatocellular carcinoma.

  1. The disorder may affect virtually every organ system, causing anemia, parotid gland enlargement, peptic ulcer disease, cutaneous spider angiomas, and palmar erythema.

  2. Many patients have constitutional complaints, such as fatigue, anorexia, and weight loss.

  3. Dupuytren's contracture (palmar fibromatosis), hypogonadism, and gynecomastia are more frequent in alcoholic cirrhosis than in other forms of cirrhosis.

C. Treatment and prognosis

  1. Treatment generally is supportive and includes management of the complications of portal hypertension. Agents that inhibit collagen synthesis (e.g., colchicine) are being used investigationally in an attempt to improve survival and induce fibrosis regression.

  2. Liver transplantation may be considered for patients with decompensated cirrhosis, including those who develop hepatorenal syndrome.

  3. Generally, the prognosis for patients with cirrhosis varies with the cause of the cirrhosis and other factors.

XI. PORTAL HYPERTENSION. This condition is defined as an elevation of the portal vein pressure (i.e., to a pressure exceeding 5 to 10 mm Hg).

A. The mechanisms and classification of portal hypertension are summarized in Figure 15-7.

B. Clinical features. Major manifestations of portal hypertension reflect formation of portosystemic collateral veins (venous shunts), ascites, and congestive splenomegaly.

  1. Portosystemic venous shunts can cause various complications.

    a. Bleeding from esophageal and gastric varices is the most important complication of portal hypertension and cirrhosis; it is associated with a mortality rate of about 50%.

      (1) Dilated venous channels arise as the portal vein communicates with the gastric coronary vein and, thus, the esophageal veins.

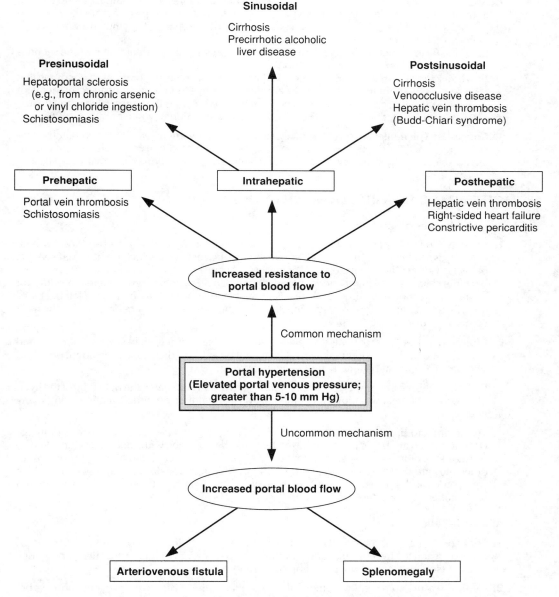

Figure 15-7. The mechanisms and classification of portal hypertension.

      (2) Recent studies show that **endoscopic sclerotherapy** (i.e., injection of a sclerosing solution into or around the varices) frequently stops active variceal bleeding. Surgical portacaval shunt creation is another treatment option.

    b. **Bleeding from rectal varices**—although much less common or life-threatening than esophagogastric variceal bleeding—is an occasional and sometimes persistent complication. Periumbilical collection of venous collaterals (**caput medusae**) occurs on the abdominal wall of many patients with portal hypertension.

    c. **Portosystemic (hepatic) encephalopathy,** a metabolic disorder of the central nervous system (CNS), commonly results from portosystemic venous shunts. Encephalopathic patients experience alterations of consciousness (ranging from drowsiness to coma), impaired intellectual functioning, neuromuscular abnormalities, slowed brain waves, and hyperammonemia. Asterixis (flapping tremor) and fetor hepaticus (sweet breath odor) are other typical signs.

2. **Ascites.** An abnormal accumulation of peritoneal fluid, ascites has a complex pathogenesis. In most cases, it results from portal hypertension of the sinusoidal, postsinusoidal, or posthepatic type. These forms of vascular blockade lead to increased hepatic lymph flow and weeping of lymph from the liver surface into the peritoneal cavity.

    a. Other factors, such as decreased plasma osmotic pressure (hypoalbuminemia) and secondary hypoaldosteronism, may contribute to ascites.

    b. The ascitic fluid may become infected in the absence of bowel perforation—a condition that is known as **spontaneous bacterial peritonitis**. The infection route appears to be hematogenous; usually, a single organism (most commonly *E. coli*) is the cause. Even when treated with antibiotics, this complication is associated with a mortality rate of 60% to 90%.

3. **Congestive splenomegaly** serves as a key sign of portal hypertension. Spleen weight may increase up to 1000 g. Hypersplenism—sequestration of a peripheral blood element in the enlarged spleen—may cause cytopenia, with associated reactive bone marrow hyperplasia.

XII. BACTERIAL AND PARASITIC LIVER INFECTIONS

A. Pyogenic hepatic abscess

1. **Etiology.** The most common cause of pyogenic hepatic abscess is biliary obstruction, which leads to ascending cholangitis (cholangitic abscess). Other causes include bacterial seeding of portal venous blood (**pyelophlebitic abscess,** occurring with intraabdominal sepsis) and bacterial seeding of hepatic arterial blood (accompanying generalized bacteremia or distant localized infections). In about 20% of cases, the bacterial source is unknown. Half the cases involve more than one type of microbe, often including anaerobes; *Escherichia coli* is the most common causative organism.

2. **Clinical features.** Most patients complain of fever, malaise, rigors, night sweats, anorexia, and right upper quadrant abdominal pain (all of recent onset). Jaundice appears in about one-third of cases. The typical patient is middle-aged or older.

3. **Pathology.** Abscesses may be single or multiple and usually appear in the right lobe of the liver. They consist of creamy yellow, foul-smelling, pus-containing, necrotic liver tissue and many neutrophils.

4. **Treatment and prognosis.** Abscesses may be managed with open or percutaneous drainage combined with antibiotics; in some cases, they may be managed with antibiotics alone. Severe sepsis and rupture of the abscess into the chest, peritoneal cavity, intraabdominal organs, or other sites are the more frequent complications. Mortality has dropped to less than 10% in some series and is related to the age of the patient, the severity of the underlying disease, and the number of abscesses.

B. Amebic hepatic abscess

1. **Etiology.** Hepatic abscess is the most common extraintestinal complication of amebiasis. Amebae reach the liver through portal blood. Most patients have recently traveled to or resided in a developing country where amebiasis is endemic.

2. **Clinical features.** Presenting complaints are similar to those seen with pyogenic abscess but have a slower onset. However, patients with amebic abscess generally are younger than those with pyogenic abscess, and men are affected 3 to 10 times more frequently than women. Serologic tests for amebiasis are positive in more than 90% of patients.

3. Pathology. In half of the cases of amebic hepatic abscess, multiple abscesses are found.
   a. The earliest lesions are yellow and firm and demonstrate coagulative necrosis. These foci coalesce into one or more odorless, variable-size cavities containing classic orange-brown, pasty, blood-stained, necrotic hepatic tissue (often described as "anchovy sauce").
   b. Actually, the term abscess is a misnomer, as the cavities contain virtually no neutrophils (except in cases of secondary bacterial infection). Amebic trophozoites usually appear in the periphery of the lesion, near the border of adjacent viable hepatic tissue.

4. Treatment and prognosis. Metronidazole is the treatment of choice. As with pyogenic abscess, rupture is the most serious complication, carrying a poor prognosis. In uncomplicated cases, the fatality rate generally is less than 1%.

C. Echinococcosis (hydatidosis)

1. Epidemiologic features. Echinococcosis is the most common cause of hepatic cysts worldwide, with a particularly high incidence in the Middle East, Greece, Australia, and some parts of South America.

2. Etiology. Echinococcosis is caused by **cestodes** (tapeworms) of the genus *Echinococcus. E. granulosus,* the agent of cystic hydatid disease, is the most common causative species. Infection by *E. multilocularis* (alveolar hydatid disease) is less frequent; this disorder may mimic a solid neoplasm.
   a. The dog is the definitive host for *E. granulosus.* Humans can become infected if they swallow eggs shed in the stool of infected dogs.
   b. In the duodenum, larvae called oncospheres invade the intestinal mucosa, enter portal venous blood, and travel to the liver. Usually, the larvae are retained there and form cysts. However, extrahepatic cysts—particularly those involving the lung—may result if extrahepatic dissemination occurs.

3. Clinical features. Manifestations reflect the mechanical effects of the space-occupying cyst (e.g., abdominal pain), a cyst rupture, or a generalized allergic reaction (which commonly includes shock due to absorption of parasitic products into the blood). Peripheral eosinophilia occurs in 25% of cases. Patients usually are asymptomatic until the cyst diameter reaches 10 cm. Treatment is primarily surgical.

4. Pathology. About 70% of echinococcal cysts are found in the liver, where they most commonly appear as single lesions of the right lobe. The cysts are unilocular, white, and fluid-filled; the germinal layer gives rise to brood capsules attached by a short stalk. Scoleces (future heads of the adult tapeworm) develop within brood capsules; they contain a double row of hooklets. Detached brood capsules are called daughter cysts. Identification of hooklets, which stain red with acid-fast stains, serves as a useful diagnostic feature. Calcification of the cyst's outer wall, occurring in up to 20% of cases, can be detected radiographically.

D. Helminthic hepatic infections

1. Schistosomiasis (bilharziasis)
   a. Etiology. This disorder results from infection by *Schistosoma mansoni* or *S. japonicum.* It leads to obstructive hepatic vascular disease and consequent portal hypertension and esophageal varices.
   b. Clinical features and diagnosis. Liver function remains normal until late in the disease. Common findings include splenomegaly with hypersplenism and pancytopenia.
   c. Pathology. Ova deposition results in obliterative fibrosis of portal vein branches and portal tract fibrosis. These, in turn, cause prominent portal space enlargement, described macroscopically as **"pipestem" (Symmers') fibrosis**.
      (1) True cirrhosis is rare.
      (2) Early in the disease, eosinophilic microabscesses surround the ova. Over time, epithelioid granulomas develop, the ova calcify, and fibrosis becomes more dense.
      (3) Grayish-black schistosomal hemozoin pigment appears in portal macrophages and Kupffer cells.

2. Ascariasis and liver fluke disease (distomiasis)
a. **Etiology.** *Ascaris lumbricoides,* an intestinal roundworm, causes ascariasis; trematode worms (e.g., *Fasciola hepatica, Clonorchis sinensis, Opisthorchis* organisms) cause liver fluke disease.

b. **Disease course and pathology.** These disorders are characterized by bile duct obstruction, commonly complicated by acute cholangitis and cholangitic abscess formation; brown pigment stones are a typical associated finding.

    (1) The bile frequently becomes secondarily infected with *E. coli* organisms, leading to **recurrent pyogenic cholangitis** (Oriental cholangiohepatitis).

    (2) Chronic *C. sinensis* or *Opisthorchis* infection is accompanied by adenomatous hyperplasia of the biliary epithelium—a precursor to cholangiocarcinoma.

XIII. HEPATIC TUMORS

A. Benign hepatic tumors

1. Hepatocellular tumors
a. **Hepatocellular adenoma**

    (1) **Etiology.** About 95% of patients with hepatocellular adenoma are women (mostly between age 30 and 50). In up to 90% of cases, the tumor presumably stems from oral contraceptive use; androgens also may induce these tumors. (The tumor may regress once the drug is discontinued.)

    (2) **Clinical features.** Typically, the patient complains of abdominal pain, most likely resulting from intraperitoneal or intratumoral rupture or an abdominal mass. Only rarely is the tumor detected as an incidental finding.

    (3) **Pathology**

        (a) **Macroscopic findings.** Hepatocellular adenoma usually appears as a solitary subscapular, well-circumscribed, tan-to-white mass in a noncirrhotic liver. Its diameter ranges from 5 to 15 cm. Occasionally, extensive hemorrhagic necrosis causes the tumor to resemble a hematoma.

        (b) **Microscopic findings.** Closely apposed cords of normal-appearing hepatocytes make the tumor appear sheetlike. Cellular pleomorphism and prominent nucleoli are extremely rare. The tumor lacks bile ducts and portal tracts but contains many widespread, thin-walled veins. Peripheral blood vessels commonly show myxoid degeneration and intimal fibrosis.

    (4) **Treatment and prognosis**

        (a) Oral contraceptives should be discontinued and the tumor completely excised if surgically feasible.

        (b) Rare cases of hepatocellular carcinoma have been linked to hepatocellular adenoma, even after oral contraceptives are stopped and the tumor has apparently resolved.

        (c) Deaths related to hepatocellular adenoma are rare and almost always follow tumor rupture.

b. **Focal nodular hyperplasia.** This tumor—which some authorities regard as a hamartomatous malformation and others see as a local hyperplastic response of hepatocytes to a vascular anomaly—typically affects women between age 30 and 50. Only 5% to 15% of patients are men.

    (1) **Etiology.** Oral contraceptives apparently promote focal nodular hyperplasia, although they probably do not cause it on their own.

    (2) **Clinical features.** An abdominal mass is the most common presenting sign; however, the tumor is an incidental finding in 50% to 80% of cases.

    (3) **Pathology**

        (a) **Macroscopic findings.** Focal nodular hyperplasia typically occurs as a solitary, well-circumscribed, subscapular, tannish nodular mass with a diameter of less than 5 cm. Fibrous septa, which divide the lesion into nodules, merge centrally or eccentrically to form a scar.

        (b) **Microscopic findings** include nodules of normal-appearing hepatocytes surrounded completely or partially by fibromyxoid septa; the septa contain a variable number of proliferating bile ductules and inflammatory cells. Numerous thick-walled blood vessels near the fibrous scar may show fibromuscular hyperplasia or myxomatous change.

(4) Treatment and prognosis

(a) Usually, the mass is completely excised, although incomplete excision of a bona fide case of focal nodular hyperplasia has never been associated with an unfavorable outcome.

(b) No studies link incompletely excised tumor with hepatocellular carcinoma.

c. Nodular transformation (also known as **nodular regenerative hyperplasia**). This condition typically affects persons between age 40 and 70. Often confused with cirrhosis, it represents a form of noncirrhotic portal hypertension.

(1) Etiology. Conditions associated with nodular transformation include connective tissue diseases (especially rheumatoid arthritis and the CREST variant of scleroderma) and myeloproliferative and lymphoproliferative disorders. Some patients have a history of cytotoxic or immunosuppressive drug use.

(2) Clinical features. Symptomatic patients typically present with manifestations of portal hypertension, including ascites.

(3) Pathology

(a) Macroscopic findings. Liver weight may be normal, increased, or decreased. Light-tan nodules measuring 0.1 cm to 4 cm in diameter may almost completely replace the hepatic parenchyma. The nodules may be mistaken for cirrhosis or a metastatic tumor.

(b) Microscopic findings. This condition has three basic features: nodules of hyperplastic hepatocytes distributed diffusely throughout the liver, atrophy of internodular hepatocytes with sinusoidal congestion, and absent or minimal fibrosis.

(4) Treatment and prognosis. Portal diversion may successfully treat this disorder. Tumor rupture, hepatic failure, and bleeding esophageal varices are important causes of tumor-related fatality.

2. Bile duct tumors

a. Bile duct hamartoma (Meyenburg's complex) and bile duct adenoma. Hamartomas are much more commonly found than adenomas.

(1) Clinical features. These tumors are always incidental findings.

(2) Pathology

(a) Macroscopic findings. These tumors appear as small, firm, grayish-white, subscapular masses, usually less than 1 cm in diameter. Hamartomas may be multiple; adenomas usually occur as solitary lesions. Multiple hamartomas may grossly simulate metastatic carcinoma, abscesses, or multiple granulomas.

(b) Microscopic findings

(i) Hamartomas are discrete lesions intimately associated with portal tracts. They consist of ectatic, branched bile ducts—often containing inspissated bile—separated by a dense hyalinized, collagenous stroma.

(ii) Bile duct adenomas consist of a compact network of bland ductal structures that usually possess tiny lumina and are ensheathed in a fibrous stroma. No bile appears.

(3) Treatment. These tumors are innocuous and do not warrant treatment.

b. Biliary cystadenoma. These cystic lesions are clinically and pathologically similar to mucinous cystadenomas of the pancreas; the same caveats regarding the development of cystadenocarcinoma apply here (see Chapter 14, III D 1 b).

3. Vascular tumors

a. Cavernous hemangioma. The most common primary hepatic tumor, cavernous hemangioma is found in about 1% of routine autopsies. It most likely represents a hamartomatous malformation rather than a true neoplasm.

(1) Clinical features. Most of these tumors do not cause symptoms and are found incidentally. "Giant" lesions may cause abdominal pain.

(2) Pathology

(a) Cavernous hemangioma typically is a solitary, soft, reddish-purple lesion with a diameter of less than 2 cm to 4 cm. (One with a diameter greater than 4 cm to 10 cm is termed a **giant cavernous hemangioma**.)

(b) Microscopically, hepatic cavernous hemangiomas are identical to those found in other sites (see Chapter 10 IV A).

(3) Treatment and prognosis. Symptomatic patients may require surgical excision or another ablation procedure. Spontaneous rupture and thrombocytopenia are rare complications of giant lesions.

    b. Infantile hemangioendothelioma. This vascular tumor is the most common mesenchymal liver tumor among children.

        (1) Clinical features. Nearly 90% of patients are less than 6 months old at the time of diagnosis; in about half the cases, the tumor is found incidentally. Common presenting signs in patients with symptoms include an abdominal mass and high-output cardiac failure.

        (2) Pathology

            (a) Macroscopic findings. The tumor may be solitary or multicentric, with a nodule diameter ranging from 0.2 cm to 15 cm. The mass may be firm or soft and may appear tan to red.

            (b) Microscopic findings. An orderly proliferation of small, irregularly dilated vascular spaces appears; the spaces are lined with flattened endothelium (or, occasionally, more plump and pleomorphic endothelial cells). Bile ductules may be numerous and frequently are interspersed among blood vessels.

        (3) Treatment and prognosis

            (a) The tumor may regress spontaneously.

            (b) Lesion number or size usually rules out surgical resection.

            (c) Congestive heart failure (CHF) secondary to AV shunting or hepatic failure may cause death; however, better medical management of CHF has increased recent survival rates.

            (d) Rarely, transformation to angiosarcoma occurs.

    c. Peliosis hepatis

        (1) Etiology. Initially linked with such wasting diseases as tuberculosis and cancer, peliosis hepatis more recently has been associated with anabolic and contraceptive steroid use and has been found in AIDS patients (bacillary peliosis hepatis).

        (2) Clinical features. Usually, this disorder is an incidental autopsy finding. However, in some patients, it leads to severe hepatic dysfunction, hepatic rupture, and even death.

        (3) Pathology

            (a) Macroscopic findings. Multiple reddish-purple, blood-filled spaces measuring 0.2 cm to 5 cm in diameter give the liver a honeycomb appearance.

            (b) Microscopic findings. Blood lakes are bordered by hepatocyte cords (which usually lack an endothelial lining). Adjacent sinusoidal dilatation typically occurs. (Direct toxicity to the sinusoidal endothelium and hepatocellular necrosis may be initiating events.) In bacillary peliosis hepatis in AIDS patients, Warthin-Starry stain can detect the etiologic agent (*Rochalimaea henselae*).

        (4) Treatment. Peliosis hepatis is untreatable.

  4. Mesenchymal hamartoma. This congenital malformation is the second most common benign liver tumor of childhood.

    a. Pathology. The tumor, measuring 5 cm to 23 cm, usually shows both solid and cystic areas. It is made up of bland stellate cells embedded in a myxoid stroma, angular bile ducts, hepatocyte plates, and proliferated blood vessels.

    b. Treatment and prognosis. The tumor is surgically resected. No cases of malignant transformation have been reported.

B. Primary malignant hepatic tumors

  1. Hepatocellular carcinoma

    a. Epidemiology

        (1) Hepatocellular carcinoma accounts for about 85% of all primary hepatic malignancies in adults and 30% to 40% of those in children. Although relatively uncommon in North America and Western Europe, it may be the most common malignant tumor worldwide.

        (2) In regions of low incidence, it affects two to three times as many men as women and typically occurs in people between the ages of 50 and 70. In regions of high incidence, such as sub-Saharan Africa and Southeast Asia, a greater male predominance exists, and the tumor often affects people between the ages of 20 and 40.

    b. Etiology and pathogenesis. Chronic liver injury leads to sustained hepatocyte hyperplasia, increased susceptibility to various carcinogens, and greater risk of chromosomal damage—and, hence, the possibility of hepatocellular carcinoma. Evidence of chronic liver injury (usually cirrhosis) of varied etiology is found in 90% of patients. Only 10% of cases of hepatocellular carcinoma occur in otherwise normal livers. Macroregenerative nodules

(> 1 cm in diameter) in the cirrhotic liver may represent an important precursor lesion for hepatocellular carcinoma. Factors implicated in the pathogenesis of hepatocellular carcinoma are summarized in Table 15-7.

c. **Clinical features and diagnosis**

    (1) Approximately 85% of patients present with abdominal pain, fullness, or an abdominal mass or have manifestations resembling those of cirrhosis. (Decompensated cirrhosis suggests hepatocellular carcinoma.)

    (2) Various **paraneoplastic syndromes,** including erythrocytosis, hypercalcemia, and hypoglycemia, may be associated findings.

    (3) **Serum alpha-fetoprotein (AFP)** is elevated in 80% of patients; the level usually exceeds 400 ng/ml and may even exceed 1000 ng/ml. However, elevated serum' AFP is not diagnostic for hepatocellular carcinoma, as it occurs in other neoplastic and some nonneoplastic conditions. Ultrasonography and monitoring of serum AFP levels can detect subclinical tumors (usually smaller than 3 to 5 cm) in regions where incidence of hepatocellular carcinoma is high.

Table 15-7. Factors Implicated in the Pathogenesis of Hepatocellular Carcinoma

---

Chronic hepatic injury (60%–90%)
    Chronic hepatitis
    Cirrhosis, particularly macronodular

Specific etiologies
  High frequency of associated hepatocellular carcinoma (> 15%)
    Chronic hepatitis C infection*
    Chronic hepatitis C hepatitis*
    Hemochromatosis, genetic (primary) type
    Hereditary tyrosinemia
    Thorotrast
    Porphyrias
    Hypercitrullinemia

  Intermediate frequency of associated hepatocellular carcinoma (5%–15%)
    Alcohol*
    Alpha$_1$-antitrypsin deficiency
    Chronic autoimmune hepatitis

  Low to rare frequency of associated hepatocellular carcinoma (< 5%)
    Primary biliary cirrhosis
    Primary sclerosing cholangitis
    Hereditary fructose intolerance
    Glycogenosis (types 1 and 3)
    Allagille's syndrome
    Progressive intrahepatic cholestasis (Byler's disease)
    Ataxia telangiectasia
    Wilson's disease
    Oral contraceptive steroids
    Cardiac cirrhosis
    Possibly anabolic steroids[†]
    Exposure to various chemicals or toxins[‡]

Adapted with permission from Saul SH: Masses of liver. In *Diagnostic Surgical Pathology, 2nd edition.* Edited by Sternberg S. New York, Raven Press. In press, 1994.

*Most important specific etiologies associated with hepatocellular carcinoma worldwide. For alcohol, highest risk of hepatocellular carcinoma is with advanced (macronodular) cirrhosis.

[†]Although hepatic tumors associated with anabolic steroid usage may have the histologic appearance of hepatocellular carcinoma, biologically malignant behavior is either poorly documented or not reported.

[‡]While aflatoxin has been associated with the occurrence of hepatocellular carcinoma in areas of high incidence and in experimental animals, its role as a carcinogen has not been proven in man. Chronic exposure to vinyl chloride, pesticides, herbicides, and other organic chemicals have occasionally been reported in association with hepatocellular carcinoma. Cigarette smoking may be a risk factor.

d. Pathology
  (1) Macroscopic findings. Classic hepatocellular carcinoma may be multinodular or appear as a single large mass (referred to as **massive hepatocellular carcinoma**); in rare cases, it presents as multiple diffuse nodules.
   (a) Debate centers over whether multiple nodules result from intrahepatic metastases or a multicentric origin.
   (b) The masses are soft and appear grayish-tan or green (bile-stained). Commonly, they invade the portal veins; less commonly, the hepatic veins or bile duct.
   (c) The tumor may extend via the hepatic veins into the inferior vena cava and right atrium.
  (2) Microscopic findings
   (a) The tumor almost always grows, at least focally, in a **trabecular (sinusoidal) pattern** resembling the normal liver pattern. Tumor cells resemble hepatocytes histologically, although they have more prominent nucleoli and coarser chromatin. Bile production or detection of bile canaliculi is diagnostic for hepatocellular carcinoma. Hyaline globules (commonly representing α_1-antitrypsin or AFP) and Mallory's hyalin are occasional findings.
   (b) Variants. Architectural and cytologic variants of hepatocellular carcinoma include the fibrolamellar pattern, pseudoglandular (adenoid) pattern, pleomorphic (giant cell) pattern, and clear cell pattern. The **fibrolamellar variant** of hepatocellular carcinoma is the only histologic variant with prognostic significance; it carries a much better prognosis than the other forms.
    (i) A single mass often is found, sometimes containing a fibrous scar. The mass is characterized by nests and sheets of large polygonal cells with abundant granular eosinophilic cytoplasm (oncocytes), vesicular nuclei, and large nucleoli. Cells are separated by parallel hyalinized bands of acellular collagen (hence, the term "fibrolamellar").
    (ii) The fibrolamellar variant occurs mainly in adolescents and young adults with an otherwise normal liver and no known risk factors for hepatocellular carcinoma.
 e. Treatment and prognosis. The typical patient survives only a few months after diagnosis.
  (1) The few patients whose tumors are resectable have a median survival of 1 to 2 years. Among patients with the fibrolamellar variant, however, the 5-year survival rate after resection is nearly 60%.
  (2) Autopsy reveals metastases in about half the patients; most commonly, metastases affect the hilar lymph nodes and lungs.

2. Intrahepatic cholangiocarcinoma (bile duct carcinoma). Bile duct tumors can arise from any portion of the biliary tree—from the bile ductule to the ampulla of Vater. Accounting for 8% to 25% of primary malignant hepatic tumors, intrahepatic cholangiocarcinoma may develop in the hepatic hilum or the liver periphery. (Because tumors arising in the hepatic hilum share clinicopathologic features with extrahepatic bile duct cancers, they also are discussed in Chapter 14 II E 2.)
 a. Etiology. In about 90% of cases, the cause of intrahepatic cholangiocarcinoma remains unknown. In the remaining 10%, the tumor is associated with such disorders as chronic ulcerative colitis (which typically occurs with primary sclerosing cholangitis), Caroli's disease, congenital hepatic fibrosis, clonorchiasis, opisthorchiasis, genetic hemochromatosis, and Thorotrast administration. Less than 10% of patients with intrahepatic cholangiocarcinoma have cirrhosis. The cholangiocarcinoma has no association with HBV infection.
 b. Clinical features. Most patients complain of abdominal pain, malaise, fever, and weight loss. Typically, the tumor is diagnosed in people between the ages of 50 and 70.
 c. Pathology
  (1) Macroscopic findings. The tumor may be multinodular, massive, or diffuse. Usually, the lesion is large, firm, and grayish-white.
  (2) Microscopic findings. More than 95% of these tumors are adenocarcinomas; however, squamous cell differentiation appears in rare cases. Most tumors contain a moderate amount of densely fibrotic stroma. Histologically, intrahepatic cholangiocarcinoma cannot be distinguished from metastatic adenocarcinoma.
 d. Treatment and prognosis. Most patients die within 1 year of diagnosis; those who undergo tumor resection may have a longer survival. Autopsies show metastasis (most commonly to the hilar lymph nodes, peritoneal surfaces, and lung) in about 75% of patients.

3. **Combined hepatocellular–cholangiocarcinoma.** This tumor, characterized by both hepatocellular and bile duct differentiation, accounts for less than 5% of primary hepatic malignancies. The two elements may form separate nodules, may be contiguous, or may intermingle. Patients with these tumors have manifestations resembling those of hepatocellular carcinoma.

4. **Hepatoblastoma.** Rare overall, this tumor is the most common primary malignant hepatic tumor among children. Generally, it develops before age 3 and affects twice as many boys as girls.
   a. **Etiology.** In about one-third of the patients, hepatoblastoma is associated with such congenital anomalies as renal and cardiac malformations and hemihypertrophy. Like Wilms' tumor, it appears to represent both a malformation and a neoplasm developing during gestation.
   b. **Clinical features and diagnosis.** The most common signs are abdominal enlargement (from hepatomegaly), failure to thrive, and vomiting. In a few cases, ectopic production of human chorionic gonadotropin (hCG) causes virilization. The serum AFP level is elevated in about 85% of cases and usually shows very high titers.
   c. **Pathology**
      (1) **Macroscopic findings.** Hepatoblastoma appears as a solitary, well-circumscribed, grayish-tan mass. It may be smooth or lobulated, solid or cystic. Average lesion diameter is 10 cm but in some cases reaches 20 cm. Necrosis and hemorrhage are common; cirrhosis is extremely rare.
      (2) **Microscopic findings.** Hepatoblastoma has an epithelial component, frequently accompanied by a mesenchymal component.
         (a) The **epithelial component** shows fetal, embryonal, and anaplastic patterns.
            (i) With the **fetal pattern,** the tumor cells form cords resembling the fetal liver.
            (ii) With the **embryonal pattern,** cells are poorly cohesive and appear in sheets, ribbons, acini, or papillary formations.
            (iii) With the **anaplastic pattern,** cells occur in sheets and nests. Small and uniform, they resemble the cells of neuroblastoma.
         (b) The **mesenchymal component** consists of spindle-shaped cells that may be associated with osteoid deposits.
   d. **Treatment and prognosis**
      (1) Successful outcome depends mainly on complete tumor excision, which now can be achieved in up to 75% of patients. With complete resection, up to 50% of patients have long-term survival.
         (a) Preoperative chemotherapy may allow excision of tumors that previously would have been inoperable.
         (b) Pure fetal tumors carry the best prognosis; pure anaplastic tumors, the worst.
      (2) In half the cases, autopsy reveals metastasis (usually to the hilar lymph nodes and lung).

5. **Angiosarcoma.** Overall, hepatic sarcoma is rare. Angiosarcoma, the most common form of hepatic sarcoma, typically occurs in men between age 50 and 70.
   a. **Etiology.** About one-third of these tumors are associated with such agents as thorotrast, vinyl chloride, arsenic, and anabolic steroids. The latent period between exposure to the agent and tumor development averages 20 to 25 years.
   b. **Clinical features.** Most patients present with abdominal pain, fatigue, weight loss, or an abdominal mass. Hematologic abnormalities [e.g., anemia, disseminated intravascular coagulation (DIC)] are common.
   c. **Pathology**
      (1) **Macroscopic findings.** Multiple tumor foci involving both liver lobes appear in 75% of cases. Individual foci are spongy and hemorrhagic and vary greatly in size.
      (2) **Microscopic findings.** Pleomorphic spindled and epithelioid cells are found lining anastomosing blood-filled spaces. Frequently, extramedullary hematopoiesis is detected.
   d. **Treatment and prognosis.** No treatment is available. In nearly all cases, patients die within 2 years of diagnosis—typically from hepatic failure and intraabdominal bleeding. Metastases appear in 60% of autopsied patients.

6. **Epithelioid hemangioendothelioma.** This rare hepatic endothelial malignancy has an unknown etiology and affects females more often than males. Compared to angiosarcoma, it affects younger patients and carries a better prognosis (5-year survival is nearly 30%). Until recently, such tumors often were misdiagnosed as cholangiocarcinoma because of their vacuolated cells and dense stromal fibrosis.

7. **Other sarcomas,** such as **leiomyosarcoma** and **rhabdomyosarcoma,** are very rare and are identical microscopically to sarcomas arising at other sites. **Undifferentiated (embryonal) sarcoma,** a primitive tumor, is rare in adults but accounts for nearly 10% of all childhood hepatic tumors.

C. **Metastatic hepatic tumors.** These tumors account for 98% of all hepatic malignancies. In most cases, they develop from carcinoma of the lung, breast, colon, or pancreas; lymphomas and leukemias also may metastasize to the liver.

1. In nearly every case, tumor deposits are multiple; often, they are quite large.

2. Necrosis causing central umbilication is a common feature of metastatic solid tumors, particularly those derived from the colon.

STUDY QUESTIONS

Directions: Each of the numbered items or incomplete statements in this section is followed by answers or by completions of the statement. Select the **one** lettered answer or completion that is **best** in each case.

1. A 45-year-old woman with a long history of depression is taken to the emergency room after ingesting a large quantity (20 g) of acetaminophen. Which one of the following statements is true?

(A) Her serum transaminase levels are likely to be within normal limits

(B) Spotty nonzonal foci of hepatocellular necrosis would be an expected finding on liver biopsy

(C) Acetaminophen is classified as a predictable hepatotoxin; the degree of injury is dose-dependent

(D) Acetaminophen hepatotoxicity results from direct binding of the drug to Kupffer cells, resulting in selective Kupffer cell necrosis

(E) Chemical hepatic injury is a rare cause of fulminant acute hepatitis

2. Which hyaline masses are often seen in the cytoplasm of hepatocytes in patients with alcoholic hepatitis?

(A) Councilman bodies

(B) Negri bodies

(C) Mallory's bodies

(D) Michaelis-Gutmann bodies

(E) Rotor's bodies

3. Constrictive pericarditis is most likely to produce which histologic finding in the liver?

(A) Macronodular cirrhosis

(B) Portal lymphocytic infiltrate

(C) Bile duct proliferation

(D) Sinusoidal dilatation

(E) Mallory's hyalin

4. Which statement regarding chronic hepatitis is correct?

(A) Hepatitis A progresses to chronic hepatitis in 5% to 10% of cases

(B) Chronic persistent hepatitis is characterized histologically by the presence of piecemeal necrosis

(C) Chronic active hepatitis is characterized histologically by an intact limiting plate

(D) Autoantibodies are detected in the serum of some patients with drug-induced chronic hepatitis

(E) Chronic persistent hepatitis often progresses to cirrhosis

5. Which liver tumor is most commonly associated with the use of oral contraceptives?

(A) Bile duct adenoma

(B) Bile duct hamartoma

(C) Focal nodular hyperplasia

(D) Hepatocellular carcinoma

(E) Hepatocellular adenoma

6. Which histologic description is most typically seen in patients with alcoholic liver injury?

(A) Massive centrilobular hepatocyte necrosis with numerous Councilman bodies

(B) Prominent portal chronic inflammation with minimal damage to the hepatic lobule

(C) Steatosis, Mallory's hyalin, centrilobular fibrosis, and a lobular inflammatory infiltrate with a conspicuous component of neutrophils

(D) Mallory's hyalin, an inflammatory infiltrate rich in eosinophils, and many Councilman bodies

(E) Thrombosis of the hepatic veins causing venous outflow obstruction

---

1-C   4-D
2-C   5-E
3-D   6-C

7. Which statement accurately describes the primary route of transmission of the various forms of acute viral hepatitis?

(A) Hepatitis A is transmitted by the parenteral route
(B) Hepatitis B is transmitted by the parenteral route
(C) Hepatitis C is transmitted by the fecal–oral route
(D) Hepatitis D is transmitted by the fecal–oral route
(E) Hepatitis E is transmitted by the parenteral route

8. Which feature is most characteristic of genetic hemochromatosis?

(A) Selective hemosiderin deposition in Kupffer cells, leading to cirrhosis
(B) Selective copper deposition in Kupffer cells, leading to cirrhosis
(C) Kayser-Fleischer rings
(D) A decreased saturation of plasma transferrin
(E) An increased risk for developing hepatocellular carcinoma

9. Which disorder causes hepatic venous outflow obstruction?

(A) Reye's syndrome
(B) Crigler-Najjar syndrome
(C) Schistosomiasis
(D) Budd-Chiari syndrome
(E) Rotor's syndrome

10. Findings on liver biopsy that might suggest large bile duct (extrahepatic) obstruction include all of the following EXCEPT

(A) bile duct proliferation
(B) portal tract edema
(C) bile ducts with inspissated bile
(D) the absence of bile within hepatocytes and bile canaliculi
(E) neutrophils adjacent to proliferated bile ducts

11. Conditions that are viewed as significantly increasing the risk for developing hepatocellular carcinoma include all of the following EXCEPT

(A) alcohol-related cirrhosis
(B) hepatitis B virus (HBV)-related cirrhosis
(C) genetic hemochromatosis-related cirrhosis
(D) primary biliary cirrhosis
(E) hepatitis C virus (HCV)-related cirrhosis

12. Parasitic infections that are likely to involve the liver or bile ducts include all of the following EXCEPT

(A) filariasis
(B) echinococcosis
(C) amebiasis
(D) schistosomiasis
(E) clonorchiasis

13. Hepatocellular carcinomas commonly spread to all of the following EXCEPT the

(A) central nervous system (CNS)
(B) lungs
(C) lymph nodes in the porta hepatis
(D) portal vein
(E) hepatic vein

14. Conditions that can be associated with neonatal hepatitis and cholestasis include all of the following EXCEPT

(A) galactosemia
(B) cystic fibrosis
(C) extrahepatic biliary atresia
(D) alpha$_1$-antitrypsin deficiency
(E) Reye's syndrome

15. Histopathologic features that are often found in chronic active hepatitis include all of the following EXCEPT

(A) portal inflammation
(B) bridging necrosis
(C) fibrous tissue septa
(D) piecemeal necrosis
(E) hepatic vein thrombosis

7-B	10-D	13-A
8-E	11-D	14-E
9-D	12-A	15-E

Directions: Each group of items in this section consists of lettered options followed by a set of numbered items. For each item, select the **one** lettered option that is most closely associated with it. Each lettered option may be selected once, more than once, or not at all.

Questions 16–20

Match each morphologic feature with its related hepatic disorder.

(A) Chronic hepatitis B
(B) Amebiasis
(C) Alpha₁-antitrypsin deficiency
(D) Primary biliary cirrhosis
(E) Dubin-Johnson syndrome

16. Decreased number of bile ducts

17. Hyaline globules in periportal hepatocytes

18. Ground-glass hepatocyte cytoplasm

19. Abscesslike cavities

20. Grossly black liver

Questions 21–25

Match each microscopic finding with its associated hepatic disorder.

(A) Acute viral hepatitis
(B) Echinococcosis
(C) Reye's syndrome
(D) Genetic hemochromatosis
(E) Alcoholic hepatitis

21. Mallory's hyalin

22. Microvesicular steatosis

23. Lobular disarray, often with acidophilic bodies

24. Marked hemosiderin deposition in hepatocytes

25. Unilocular fluid-filled cysts

16-D	19-B	22-C	25-B
17-C	20-E	23-A	
18-A	21-E	24-D	

ANSWERS AND EXPLANATIONS

1. The answer is C *[IV C 2 a (2) (b)]*.
Acetaminophen is a predictable hepatotoxin when it is ingested in large doses (i.e., more than 15 g). Chemical forms of hepatic injury are common, accounting for up to 25% of the cases of fulminant hepatic failure in the United States. Hepatic injury by chemical agents usually results in marked elevation of the serum transaminase levels; levels greater than 1000 U/L would be typical in an acetaminophen overdose patient. Acetaminophen overdose results in extensive zone 3 (centrilobular) necrosis because the hepatocellular mixed function oxidase (MFO) system that is responsible for the generation of toxic metabolites is located in this area. Massive hepatic necrosis may also occur in the most severe cases.

2. The answer is C *[IV D 5 b (1) (a)]*.
Mallory's hyalin (also known as alcoholic hyalin or Mallory's bodies) represents eosinophilic hyaline material that is found in clumps, strands, or perinuclear rings in the cytoplasm of swollen hepatocytes of alcoholic hepatitis patients. This material actually consists of cytokeratin filaments, which normally have a role in the structural support of the cell. Although Mallory's hyalin is characteristic of alcoholic hepatitis, it can be found in other conditions and, therefore, is not pathognomonic of ethanol-induced liver disease. Councilman bodies are shrunken, acidophilic hepatocytes found in the liver in acute viral or toxic hepatitis. Negri bodies are seen in neurons infected with rabies virus, and Michaelis-Gutmann bodies are found in malacoplakia—a rare lesion of the genitourinary tract.

3. The answer is D *[V A 3 b]*.
Hepatic venous outflow obstruction, which most commonly is caused by congestive heart failure (CHF) and constrictive pericarditis, causes dilatation and congestion of the efferent veins and sinusoids. Hepatocyte atrophy often results, with collapse of the supportive reticulin framework. The macroscopic appearance is termed "nutmeg liver." It is characterized by red or purple perivenular areas surrounded by paler, often fatty, regions. When outflow obstruction is severe and prolonged, fibrous septa may form, linking adjacent perivenular areas. Less commonly, portal–central septa result. The term cardiac fibrosis, rather than cardiac cirrhosis, is most appropriate for this form of advanced disease, as a true cirrhosis only rarely occurs.

4. The answer is D *[VIII B 1–2, D 4 Table 15-1]*.
Chronic hepatitis may be classified by etiology or by morphologic features. Causes of chronic hepatitis include hepatitis viruses (i.e., HBV, HCV and HDV; HAV and HEV infections never advance to chronic hepatitis), autoimmune mechanisms, and certain drugs. In some patients with drug-induced hepatitis, serum autoantibodies may be detected. Morphologically, chronic hepatitis is classified as one of three types. The chronic persistent type is characterized histologically by an inflammatory infiltrate that is restricted to the portal tract; the limiting plate is intact, and necrosis is minimal. The chronic active type is characterized histologically by portal and periportal inflammation that appears in association with piecemeal necrosis (i.e., hepatocyte degeneration and necrosis at the limiting plate). The third morphologic type is chronic lobular hepatitis. Chronic persistent hepatitis rarely progresses to cirrhosis.

5. The answer is E *[XIII A 1 a (1)]*.
Hepatocellular adenoma, although an uncommon hepatic neoplasm, is the most common liver tumor associated with the use of oral contraceptives. Roughly 95% of cases of hepatocellular adenoma occur in women between age 30 and 50, most (90%) of whom use oral contraceptives. This neoplasm is prone to hemorrhage and necrosis, which lead to pain in the right upper quadrant of the abdomen. Intraperitoneal rupture may occur, with shock and death being potential complications. Focal nodular hyperplasia is somewhat less frequently associated with the use of oral contraceptives. In this disorder, the steroid use is believed to promote tumor growth rather than to cause its initiation, as is believed to be the case for hepatocellular adenoma. Whether oral contraceptive use may play a role in the pathogenesis of a small subset of hepatocellular carcinomas is controversial. These steroids have no relationship to the development of biliary tumors.

6. The answer is C *[IV D 5 b]*.
Alcoholic hepatitis is characterized by prominent ballooning degeneration of hepatocytes that often contain Mallory's hyalin. An occasional acidophilic (Councilman) body may be seen. The lobular inflammatory infiltrate usually demonstrates an abundance of neutrophils, which sometimes cluster around the cells containing the Mallory's hyalin. Steatosis (i.e., fatty change) and centrilobular fibrosis typically are present. Continued consumption of alcohol frequently leads to the development of cirrhosis.

7. The answer is B *[IV B 2–3; Tables 15-1, 15-2]*.
Hepatitis B, C, and D are transmitted by the parenteral route. Initially, it was believed that transmission of hepatitis B virus (HBV) required infected blood via percutaneous exposure; however, it has become clear that exposure via sexual contact with infected semen and saliva is also an important mode of transmission. HBV evidently gains access to the blood by way of small breaks in the mucous membrane (inapparent parenteral transmission). Hepatitis A and E are transmitted by the fecal–oral route.

8. The answer is E *[IX C 1]*.
Hepatocellular carcinoma develops in 10% to 20% of patients. Genetic (idiopathic or primary) hemochromatosis is a disorder of iron metabolism, which is inherited as an autosomal recessive trait. It is associated with an increased frequency of certain human leukocyte antigens (HLAs); the strongest association is with HLA-A3, although HLA-B7 and HLA-B14 frequencies also are increased. The responsible gene is located on the short arm of chromosome 6. Although the precise molecular defect is unknown, hepatocytes accumulate massive amounts of hemosiderin in the presence of a relatively minimal increase in reticuloendothelial iron. Patients usually present with cirrhosis from age 40 to 60, although asymptomatic patients can be detected with biochemical screening. Laboratory findings in affected patients include elevated serum levels of iron and ferritin and an increased percent saturation of plasma transferrin. Kayser-Fleischer rings are corneal deposits found in patients with Wilson's disease, an inherited disorder of copper metabolism.

9. The answer is D *[V A 1 b]*.
Budd-Chiari syndrome is a rare condition caused by thrombosis of the major hepatic veins. It often is idiopathic but may occur in association with several other conditions, including a myeloproliferative disorder (e.g., polycythemia vera); a hypercoagulable state; an adrenal, renal, or hepatocellular carcinoma; or radiation damage. Hepatic venous thrombosis usually causes marked sinusoidal congestion of the liver, resulting in postsinusoidal portal hypertension and, often, ascites. Marked elevation of serum transaminase levels may lead to a clinical misdiagnosis of acute viral hepatitis. Patients often complain of abdominal pain, and hepatomegaly typically is present.

10. The answer is D *[III A 2 c (2) (c)]*.
Initially, all forms of cholestasis demonstrate changes in the centrilobular region (zone 3). The changes are characterized histologically by the presence of brown or green pigment within hepatocytes and bile canaliculi. Extrahepatic biliary obstruction is suggested when the biopsy also shows portal tract edema and a proliferation of bile ducts, which often contain inspissated bile. The bile duct proliferation typically is most conspicuous in the region of the limiting plate (marginal bile duct proliferation), and there often is a periductal neutrophilic infiltrate. Although highly suggestive of extrahepatic obstruction, these features occasionally are seen in its absence. For example, they may be seen with sepsis or in patients who are receiving hyperalimentation.

11. The answer is D *[XIII B 1 a, b; Table 15-7]*.
Although other etiologic factors have been associated with an increased risk for the development of hepatocellular carcinoma, patients with primary biliary cirrhosis, primary sclerosing cholangitis, and Wilson's disease only rarely develop this malignancy. Hepatocellular carcinoma is by far the most common primary malignancy of the liver. Although it is relatively uncommon in North America and Western Europe, it is perhaps the most common tumor worldwide. Areas of high incidence include sub-Saharan Africa and Southeast Asia. In 90% of cases there is evidence of some form of chronic liver disease— usually cirrhosis. The most important etiologic factor worldwide appears to be hepatitis B virus (HBV). In regions with a low incidence of hepatocellular carcinoma, alcohol-related cirrhosis is a frequent association. Recent studies have also suggested an important role for chronic hepatitis C infection.

12. The answer is A *[XII B–D 1]*.
Filariasis is caused by a parasite that enters through the skin, permeates the lymphatics, and localizes in regional lymph node groups, particularly in the lower extremities. The resulting lymphatic obstruction can cause a hypertrophic disorder called elephantiasis. Numerous parasitic infections affect the liver, although many do not occur commonly in the United States. Schistosomiasis, amebiasis, and echinococcosis all can involve the liver. Portal "pipestem" fibrosis, with obliteration of portal vein branches, occurs in response to the portal deposition of ova in schistosomiasis; this fibrosis results in portal hypertension. Amebic involvement of the liver causes the formation of multiple cavities filled with necrotic tissue. *Echinococcus granulosus* probably is the most common cause of hepatic cysts worldwide. Clonorchiasis causes bile duct obstruction and may be complicated by acute cholangitis and abscess formation.

13. The answer is A *[XIII B 1 d (1) (b), e (2)].*
Overall, about 50% of patients with hepatocellular carcinoma have metastases at the time of autopsy, but the central nervous system (CNS) is a rare site. Metastases at the time of autopsy are found more frequently in noncirrhotic than in cirrhotic patients, probably because the former group lives longer with the tumor. The patterns of tumor spread are similar in both cases, with macroscopic portal vein invasion being found quite frequently (in 30% to 80% of cases), hepatic vein involvement being found somewhat less frequently, and the portal hepatis lymph nodes and lung being the most common sites of more distant tumor metastasis. Patients with hepatocellular carcinoma usually survive for less than 1 year. The prognosis is better for noncirrhotic patients, particularly those with tumors of the fibrolamellar histologic variant of hepatocellular carcinoma, which generally is more amenable to surgical resection. About 60% of patients with fibrolamellar variant survive 5 years after resection.

14. The answer is E *[VI A 2, B; VII; Chapter 14 II B 1].*
With the exception of Reye's syndrome, each disorder listed may be responsible for the syndrome of neonatal hepatitis and cholestasis. Congenital absence of galactose-1-phosphate uridyl transferase is a rare disorder that causes galactosemia; it may progress to cirrhosis in late infancy or early childhood if milk or milk products are not withdrawn from the diet. About 5% of all patients with cystic fibrosis and 20% of those who survive into adolescence develop biliary cirrhosis. Amorphous eosinophilic secretions distend the bile ducts. In extrahepatic biliary atresia, the natural history of the disease is to progress to biliary cirrhosis during infancy. Portoenterostomy (the Kasai procedure) and transplantation are methods of treatment. Children presenting with neonatal cholestasis who are found to have α_1-antitrypsin deficiency (PiZZ genotype) frequently progress to cirrhosis by the end of the second decade of life. Patients with PiZZ genotype may present for the first time in adulthood with chronic active hepatitis or cirrhosis. Adults with the PiMZ genotype also may be at increased risk for the development of chronic liver disease. The presence of a Z allele is identified histologically by the presence of periodic acid–Schiff (PAS)-positive, diastase-resistant hyaline globules in periportal hepatocytes that demonstrate immunoreactivity for α_1-antitrypsin.

15. The answer is E *[VIII B 1 c].*
Hepatic vein thrombosis is the cause of the Budd-Chiari syndrome but is not a feature of chronic active hepatitis. The term chronic hepatitis encompasses a group of disorders demonstrating a necroinflammatory process of the liver that continues without improvement for at least 6 months. The most common causes of chronic hepatitis are hepatitis B, hepatitis C, autoimmune factors, and drugs. However, other disorders also may have indistinguishable histopathologic findings at different points in their evolution. Therefore, it is imperative that all clinical, serologic, biochemical, and histologic data be synthesized in order to arrive at the most specific diagnosis. Chronic hepatitis is divided morphologically into two major categories, persistent and active. In chronic persistent hepatitis, the portal chronic infiltrate does not breach the limiting plate; that is, piecemeal necrosis is absent. This disorder generally is mild and progression to cirrhosis is rare. In chronic active hepatitis, piecemeal necrosis is present; that is, portal and periportal chronic inflammation include degeneration and necrosis of hepatocytes of the limiting plate. Lobular inflammation and necrosis may be conspicuous, and bridging necrosis can occur. Cirrhosis frequently occurs in patients who develop bridging necrosis and fibrous septa.

16–20. The answers are: 16-D *[IX A 3 a],* **17-C** *[VI B 3 a],* **18-A** *[VIII B 2 a (2)],* **19-B** *[XII B 3],* **20-E** *[III C 1 c (1)].*
Primary biliary cirrhosis is characterized by nonsuppurative destructive cholangitis. The bile duct damage eventually results in loss of small and medium-sized intrahepatic bile ducts. The granulomatous destruction of bile ducts that occurs in this disorder (referred to as florid duct lesion) is nearly pathognomonic.

Periportal hyaline globules that are periodic acid–Schiff (PAS)-positive and resist diastase digestion, indicting their glycoprotein nature, are characteristic of the presence of at least one Z allele for α_1-antitrypsin. Immunohistochemical analysis can confirm that this material actually is α_1-antitrypsin. Patients with α_1-antitrypsin deficiency and associated liver disease usually are homozygous for the Z allele. Cirrhosis is a frequent result and often is accompanied by emphysema.

Hepatocytes with a ground-glass cytoplasmic appearance often are seen in liver biopsies from patients with chronic hepatitis B. This ground-glass appearance is due to the proliferation of smooth endoplasmic reticulum required for the synthesis of hepatitis B surface antigen (HBsAg). Rarely, drugs that stimulate the proliferation of smooth endoplasmic reticulum can cause the same appearance, but immunohistochemical assay for HBsAg in these cases is negative.

Hepatic amebic abscesses are the most common form of extraintestinal amebiasis. The term "abscess" actually is a misnomer, because neutrophils are absent in these lesions unless there is secondary bacterial infection. The lesions consist of necrotic hepatic parenchyma and blood, with the amebic trophozoites found at the periphery of the lesions.

The Dubin-Johnson syndrome is characterized by chronic or intermittent jaundice associated with conjugated hyperbilirubinemia. The black color of the liver reflects the presence of dark-brown, melaninlike pigment in the hepatocytes. The origin of the pigment is unknown.

21–25. The answers are: 21-E *[IV D 5 b (1)],* **22-C** *[VII C],* **23-A** *[IV B 4 b (1) (c)],* **24-D** *[IX C 1 e (1)],* **25-B** *[XII C 4].*

Hepatitis due to chronic ethanol abuse (i.e., alcoholic hepatitis) characteristically demonstrates steatosis, Mallory's hyalin, an inflammatory infiltrate rich in neutrophils, and perivenular sclerosis. These findings are not entirely specific for alcoholic hepatitis, and the generic term steatohepatitis sometimes is used. Other conditions that can produce steatohepatitis include obesity, diabetes mellitus, a jejunoileal bypass or gastropexy for obesity, and amiodarone therapy—to name a few.

Reye's syndrome is characterized microscopically by microvesicular steatosis. This condition may be difficult to detect on routinely prepared sections; therefore, when microvesicular steatosis is considered, frozen sections should be stained with oil red O to demonstrate the small fat droplets. Other conditions that can cause a similar histologic picture include high-dose intravenous tetracycline administration, acute fatty liver of pregnancy, and valproate therapy.

The liver in acute hepatitis often demonstrates degenerative and regenerative hepatocyte changes and inflammation that give the lobule a disordered appearance referred to as lobular disarray. Hepatocyte degeneration may result in cellular swelling (ballooning degeneration) or cellular shrinkage with nuclear pyknosis and loss (acidophilic, or Councilman, body). The different forms of acute viral hepatitis cannot be distinguished solely on the basis of morphology.

In genetic hemochromatosis, hepatocytes become overloaded with hemosiderin, and the overload results in cirrhosis. The fibrous septa, bile ductules, and, to a lesser extent, the Kupffer cells also may demonstrate hemosiderin deposits. Hemosiderin subsequently is deposited in the parenchymal cells of a number of organs, particularly the heart, pancreas, and endocrine organs.

Echinococcosis is the most common cause of hepatic cysts worldwide. The cysts typically appear as single lesions of the right lobe and are unilocular, white, and fluid-filled. The cysts give rise to brood capsules that contain scoleces, which become the future heads of adult tapeworms.

16
Kidney and Urinary Tract

John E. Tomaszewski

I. NORMAL ANATOMY AND EMBRYOLOGY

A. Kidney structure (Figure 16-1)

1. **General description**
   a. The kidneys are located retroperitoneally in the upper dorsal region of the abdominal cavity. Each adult kidney weighs 120 to 150 g and is covered by a thin capsule of connective tissue. Fatty tissue surrounds the kidney and is delimited by **Gerota's fascia**.
   b. Through the **hilus** of each kidney pass a renal artery and vein, lymphatics, a nerve plexus, and the **renal pelvis,** which divides into three major and several minor **calices**.
   c. On cut section the kidney reveals two sections: the reddish-brown **cortex** and the lighter **medulla**. The medulla is formed into medullary rays and 10 to 20 **pyramids,** whose most distal ends—the **papillae**—project into the calices of the upper collecting system. The cortex covers the base of the pyramids and extends between them to form the **renal columns of Bertin**.

2. **Nephron.** Each kidney is composed of approximately 1 million nephrons, the basic functional unit of the kidney.
   a. **Nephron components.** The primary elements of the nephron follow.
      (1) The **glomerulus** (Figure 16-2), with its afferent and efferent arterioles, consists of a tuft of capillary loops that protrude into **Bowman's capsule**. The glomerular tuft has several components.
         (a) The mesangium is a supporting structure composed of cells and matrix.
         (b) The glomerular capillary loops are endothelial-lined tubes, which are covered with basement membrane and visceral epithelium and held in place by the mesangium.
         (c) The glomerular basement membrane (GBM) and visceral epithelial cells together comprise the ultrafiltration barrier necessary for urine formation.
      (2) The **renal tubule** begins as Bowman's capsule and consists of the proximal convoluted tubule, loop of Henle, distal convoluted tubule, and collecting duct (the last of which conveys urine to the renal pelvis and ureter).
      (3) The **interstitium** is connective tissue consisting of reticular fibers and interstitial cells, lymphatics, and nerves.
   b. **Nephron types.** There are two distinct types of nephrons (see Figure 16-1).
      (1) **Cortical nephrons,** the predominant type, have glomeruli situated in the outer cortex.
      (2) **Juxtamedullary nephrons** have glomeruli located at the corticomedullary junction. These nephrons have long loops of Henle penetrating deep into the medulla.

B. Urinary tract structure. The urinary tract connects to the kidney at the renal pelvis and consists of the ureters, urinary bladder, and urethra.

1. **Transitional epithelium** lines the entire urinary tract. The epithelium rests on a relatively thin basement membrane.

2. **Urethral variations with gender**
   a. The male urethra exits the neck of the bladder, penetrates the prostate gland and urogenital diaphragm, and reaches the urinary meatus at the tip of the glans penis.
   b. The female urethra, which is much shorter, exits the neck of the bladder, extends above the anterior vaginal wall, and penetrates the urogenital diaphragm to reach the urinary meatus.

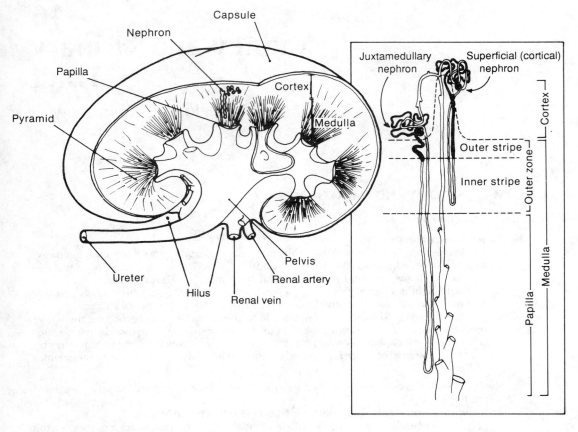

Figure 16-1. Structure of the human kidney, cut open to show the various zones. (Reprinted from Marsh DJ: *Renal Physiology.* New York, Raven, 1983, p 37.) **Inset:** Two principal nephron types and their collecting duct systems. Superficial (cortical) nephrons have their glomeruli near the surface of the kidney and do not possess long loops of Henle. Juxtamedullary nephrons have their glomeruli at the corticomedullary junction. Glomeruli and proximal tubules are shown as *solid black.* The remaining nephron is shown as *white.* (Reprinted from Brenner B, Coe FL, Rector FC: Transfer functions of renal tubules. In *Renal Physiology in Health and Disease.* Philadelphia, WB Saunders, 1987, p 29.)

   C. Kidney and urinary tract origin

   1. The **kidney** has its **origin** in two mesodermal structures: the mesonephros and metanephros.
      a. The renal pelvis, renal calices, collecting tubules, and ureters are derived from the **ureteric bud**—an outgrowth of the **mesonephric duct**.
      b. The glomerulus, Bowman's capsule, proximal and distal convoluted tubules, and loop of Henle are derived from **metanephric blastema**.

   2. The bladder, female urethra, and portions of the male urethra are formed from the **urogenital sinus**.

II. CONGENITAL ANOMALIES OF THE KIDNEY are seen most commonly in pediatric patients. They range widely in severity.

   A. Renal agenesis refers to absence of one or both kidneys. Although bilateral renal agenesis (Potter's syndrome) is incompatible with life, unilateral agenesis is compatible with normal renal function. Renal agenesis may be due to congenital absence of the nephrogenic primordium or failure of the wolffian duct to contact the metanephric blastema.

   B. Renal hypoplasia. A small kidney may be the result either of an acquired disorder that causes kidney atrophy or of congenital hypoplasia. In congenital renal hypoplasia, the renal parenchyma fails to develop to a normal weight, and the number of lobules and calices is reduced. Renal hypoplasia usually is unilateral, and the affected kidney is a frequent site of infection.

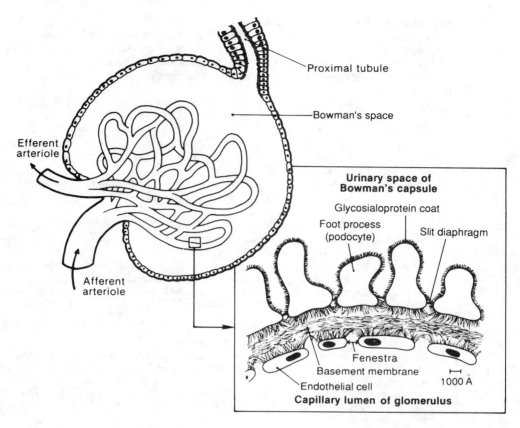

Figure 16-2. Organization of the glomerulus. The afferent arteriole forms a capillary plexus, which then fuses to form the efferent arteriole. The outer lining of the glomerulus, called Bowman's capsule, is continuous with the proximal tubule. (Reprinted from Marsh DJ: *Renal Physiology*. New York, Raven, 1983, p 41.) **Inset:** Glomerular capillary wall in cross-section. The luminal surface is covered by fenestrated endothelial cells. The basement membrane has a middle lamina densa surrounded by lamina rara interna and externa. Overlying this are the foot processes of epithelial cells, separated by small slit diaphragms. (Illustration by Nancy Lou Gahan Markris. Reprinted from Brenner BM, Beeuwkes R III: The renal circulations. *Hosp Pract* 13:35–46, 1978.)

C. **Horseshoe kidney** results from fusion of the blastema and most commonly involves the region of the lower pole, although it can occur in other areas of the kidney. The kidneys are connected by fibrous tissue or by an isthmus of renal parenchyma. Renal function typically is not impaired. Horseshoe kidney is a common finding at autopsy.

D. **Renal cystic disease** refers to a group of related disorders characterized by the presence of cysts in the kidneys. Although some of these disorders represent acquired lesions, most have hereditary associations.

   1. **Simple renal cysts** are considered acquired lesions; they may result from inflammation and scarring that create cystic dilatation of the proximal nephron. The incidence of simple cysts increases with age.
      a. **Clinical features.** Although usually asymptomatic, in rare cases simple cysts may reach a large size and become clinically palpable; thus, they must be distinguished from tumors.
      b. **Pathology.** Simple cysts may be single or multiple and generally they are translucent, 1 to 5 cm in diameter, and lined by a single layer of flattened to cuboidal epithelium.

   2. **Polycystic kidney disease** is the classic renal cystic disease. Most commonly, it is inherited as an autosomal dominant trait with a high degree of penetrance—a form that is seen in adults (also called adult polycystic disease). A rare, autosomal recessive form is seen in infants and children (also called infantile polycystic disease).

a. **Autosomal dominant polycystic kidney disease**
   (1) **Clinical features.** Patients are asymptomatic until the fifth to sixth decade, when they present with renal insufficiency. Enlarging flank or abdominal masses, flank and back pain, and hematuria are characteristic. A significant extrarenal feature is the development of **berry aneurysms,** which frequently lead to intracranial bleeding.
   (2) **Pathology**
       (a) **Macroscopically,** both kidneys are massively enlarged, with the external surfaces completely replaced by innumerable large cysts.
       (b) **Microscopically,** there is visible compression of adjacent nephrons by cysts.
   (3) **Complications and prognosis.** Two-thirds of patients eventually die of renal failure and vascular complications.
b. **Autosomal recessive polycystic kidney disease**
   (1) **Clinical features.** Most often, the disease presents as renal failure in a newborn or infant. Occasionally, the first clinical signs are delayed until later childhood.
   (2) **Pathology**
       (a) The kidneys are bilaterally enlarged and, on cut section, show numerous small dilated channels arranged perpendicularly to the cortical surface. These cysts actually are **massively dilated collecting tubules**.
       (b) Associated liver cysts are common. A peculiar type of hepatic portal fibrosis, termed **congenital hepatic fibrosis,** also may be seen.
   (3) **Complications and prognosis.** Infants with extensive polycystic changes often suffer renal failure. In children, the disease usually progresses to renal failure before adolescence.
c. **Medullary cystic disease** is a condition characterized by progressive tubular atrophy, interstitial fibrosis, and variable numbers of medullary cysts.
   (1) **Clinical features.** The disease is inherited as an autosomal dominant trait and usually presents in the third or fourth decade. Patients have polyuria, polydipsia, sodium wasting, and tubular acidosis.
   (2) **Pathology.** The kidneys are small. Tubular atrophy, interstitial fibrosis, and chronic interstitial inflammation are present. The calices are normal. The number of medullary cysts is variable.
   (3) **Prognosis.** Patients progress to renal failure over several years.
d. **Familial juvenile nephronophthisis** is a disease with a morphology identical to medullary cystic disease (see II D 2 c) but with a different pattern of inheritance.
   (1) **Clinical features.** The disease is inherited as an autosomal recessive trait and presents in childhood. Clinical features are similar to those found in medullary cystic disease but also include severe growth retardation.
   (2) **Pathology** is identical to that of medullary cystic disease.
   (3) **Prognosis** is similar to that of medullary cystic disease.
e. **Medullary sponge kidney** is the term applied to a condition usually discovered incidentally in adults. It is not a true cystic disease.
   (1) **Clinical features.** Unless there is superimposed infection, renal function usually is normal.
   (2) **Pathology.** The papillary ducts of the medulla are dilated to form small cysts lined by cuboidal or transitional epithelium. Radiographs may show numerous minute calcifications within the medullary region.
f. **Cystic renal dysplasia** is characterized by a distorted kidney, with cysts that are lined by a flattened epithelium and surrounded by undifferentiated mesenchyme admixed with heterologous mesodermal tissue (e.g., cartilage). The disease is sporadic and often associated with obstructive abnormalities of the lower urinary tract. Prognosis depends on the extent of parenchymal involvement.

III. MEDICAL NEPHROPATHOLOGY may be considered from various points of view. A purely clinical outlook distributes diseases only by their clinical characteristics. If exact mechanisms for the various disease states were known, then this would be the most logical framework for establishing a nomenclature. Unfortunately, very little is known about the pathogenesis of most diseases. In the absence of such details, pathologists have taken an approach that combines microanatomy, clinical characteristics, and existing knowledge concerning mechanisms. This approach is termed "clinical pathologic correlation." In III A to III D, each microanatomic compartment of the kidney (i.e., glomeruli, tubules, interstitium, vasculature) is examined, and the pathologic changes within that compartment are correlated with clinical and mechanistic information.

A. Glomerular diseases

1. **General concepts**
   a. **Mechanisms of glomerular disease**
      (1) **Immune-mediated glomerular injury**
         (a) **Immune complex–associated injury** is characterized by the presence of antigen–antibody aggregates, which usually are precipitated in the glomerulus. Immune complexes may exist preformed in the circulation and subsequently may be trapped in the glomerulus, or they may arise in situ. In situ formation occurs when antibodies are directed against **endogenous glomerular antigens** or against foreign antigens that have been planted in the glomerulus, inciting an antibody response.
         (b) **Injury associated with antibody to GBM.** This method of injury is caused by antibody directed against components (antigens) that are distributed in a continuous fashion in the basement membrane. Antibody reacts with this antigen in a monolayer fashion and activates the mediators of inflammation, which cause glomerular injury.
         (c) **Complement-associated diseases.** Certain conditions, such as membranoproliferative glomerulonephritis (MPGN) appear to involve a predominant and, perhaps, primary activation of complement via the alternative pathway.
         (d) **Cell-mediated immunologic damage** of the glomerulus is a poorly understood process. This mechanism appears to be important in some experimental models.
      (2) **Loss of glomerular polyanion** effectively destroys part of the charge-selective barrier that is essential to glomerular ultrafiltration. Diseases involving loss of glomerular polyanion are characterized by heavy proteinuria.
      (3) **Hyperfiltration** injury occurs during hemodynamic changes (e.g., increased glomerular blood flow, increased glomerular pressure, and increased single-nephron glomerular filtration). Hyperfiltration may be a final common pathway for the development of progressive glomerulosclerosis.
   b. **Patterns of glomerular response to injury**
      (1) **Cellular proliferation.** Endothelial, mesangial, and epithelial cells all may proliferate. A circumferential proliferation of epithelial cells in Bowman's capsule is referred to as a **crescent**.
      (2) **Leukocytic infiltration** of the glomerulus may include neutrophils, monocytes, and lymphocytes.
      (3) **Thickening of the glomerular capillary loops** can result from:
         (a) The deposition of immune complex
         (b) An increase in GBM material (e.g., expansion of matrix components in diabetes mellitus)
         (c) An infiltrate of abnormal material (e.g., amyloid)
      (4) **Basement membrane reaction** to injury may be represented as epimembranous projections (so-called "spikes") or a splitting of the basement membrane (so-called "double contour").
      (5) **Hyalinosis** is the accumulation of homogeneous, eosinophilic, amorphous material that probably represents precipitated plasma protein. Hyalinosis usually is associated with increased mesangial matrix and collagenosis.
      (6) **Fibrosis** or collagenous scarring can affect a portion or all of the glomerulus and represents irreversible damage.
      (7) **Epithelial cell change.** In conditions associated with heavy proteinuria, the visceral epithelial cells may show swelling of cell bodies and effacement of podocytes. This change often corresponds with a loss of glomerular polyanion.
   c. **Evaluation of glomerular disease**
      (1) **Terminology.** The following terms are used to describe the extent of glomerular injury:
         (a) **Diffuse**—all glomeruli are affected
         (b) **Focal**—some glomeruli are affected
         (c) **Segmental**—part of one glomerulus is affected
         (d) **Global**—the entirety of one glomerulus is affected

- **(2) Techniques**
    - **(a) Light microscopy.** Thin sections and special stains are used to highlight histologic features.
    - **(b) Immunofluorescence.** Antibodies tagged with a fluorochrome are used to localize immunoreactants in the glomerulus.
    - **(c) Electron microscopy.** Ultrastructural studies of the glomerulus are used to show such features as the position of immune complex, basement membane reactions, and epithelial cell changes.
- **d. Clinicopathologic correlations.** Patients with glomerulonephritis may present with **nephrosis, nephritis,** or a mixture of nephritic and nephrotic changes. Clinicopathologic entities within each of these categories are listed in Figure 16-3.
    - **(1) Nephrosis** (or **nephrotic syndrome**) is characterized by marked proteinuria, hypoalbuminemia, hyperlipidemia, and edema. Patients with nephrosis tend to show much less glomerular inflammation and proliferation; the sclerosing glomerulopathies predominate in this group.
    - **(2) Nephritis** (or **acute nephritic syndrome**) is characterized by hematuria with red blood cell (RBC) casts, oliguria, uremia, varying degrees of hypertension, and only mild proteinuria. In general, patients with nephritis have glomerular pathology, predominated by proliferation and inflammation.

2. Nephrotic syndrome is the most common clinical syndrome associated with glomerulonephritis.
- **a. Definition and description**
    - **(1)** Nephrotic syndrome is defined clinically as **heavy proteinuria** (i.e., > 3.5 g/day), hypoalbuminemia, hyperlipidemia, and edema. The syndrome is the result of excessive glomerular permeability to macromolecules.
        - **(a)** Loss of protein in the ultrafiltrate is the primary process.
        - **(b) Hypoalbuminemia and edema** resulting from lower intravascular oncotic pressure are secondary. Hypoalbuminemia may stimulate the liver to synthesize lipoproteins, such as cholesterol-rich low-density lipoprotein (LDL) and triglyceride-rich very low-density lipoprotein (VLDL).
    - **(2) Hyperlipidemia** may increase the risk for development of coronary artery disease. Thrombotic complications (e.g., renal vein thrombosis) result from the concomitant urinary loss of anticoagulant factors, such as antithrombin III. Patients with nephrosis are vulnerable to bacterial infections, perhaps as a result of the urinary loss of immunoglobulin and complement.

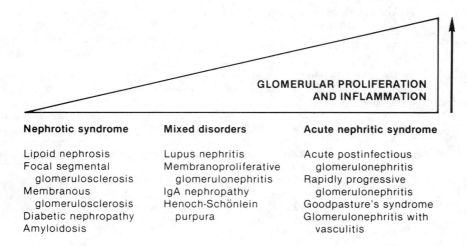

GLOMERULAR PROLIFERATION AND INFLAMMATION

Nephrotic syndrome	Mixed disorders	Acute nephritic syndrome
Lipoid nephrosis	Lupus nephritis	Acute postinfectious
Focal segmental	Membranoproliferative	glomerulonephritis
glomerulosclerosis	glomerulonephritis	Rapidly progressive
Membranous	IgA nephropathy	glomerulonephritis
glomerulosclerosis	Henoch-Schönlein	Goodpasture's syndrome
Diabetic nephropathy	purpura	Glomerulonephritis with
Amyloidosis		vasculitis

Figure 16-3. Clinicopathologic classification of glomerulonephritis. Disorders that are associated with marked proteinuria but minimal glomerular inflammation and proliferation fall under the category of nephrotic syndrome. Those characterized by only mild proteinuria but extensive glomerular inflammation and proliferation are classified as acute nephritic syndrome. As shown, there are several overlap disorders.

b. Lipoid nephrosis (also known as **nil disease** or **minimal change disease**) is the most common cause of nephrotic syndrome in children. The peak incidence is in children between age 2 and 3.

(1) **Etiology.** The cause is unknown. Features that point to a possible immunologic mechanism include a clinical association with immunization and lymphoproliferative disorders, a characteristic response to steroids, an association with atopic disorders, and an increased prevalence in patients with human leukocyte antigen (HLA)-B12 or HLA-Dr7.

(2) **Clinical features.** The disease sometimes follows a respiratory tract infection or immunization. Affected patients have selected proteinuria but otherwise relatively normal renal function.

(3) **Pathology.** The glomeruli are normal by light microscopy. The main ultrastructural change is the uniform and diffuse effacement of the epithelial cell foot processes. Loss of glomerular polyanion seems to correlate with this change. There are no immune complex deposits. The term "lipoid" nephrosis reflects the presence of numerous lipid droplets in tubules and fat bodies in the urine.

(4) **Treatment and prognosis.** The disease is highly responsive to steroid therapy. Nephrosis may recur, and some patients can become steroid-dependent. Renal failure is infrequent in children; however, relapses are more common in adults, and the ultimate prognosis is less favorable.

c. Focal segmental glomerulosclerosis is an idiopathic entity that was first defined in a group of steroid-resistant children with nephrotic syndrome.

(1) **Etiology.** The cause and pathogenesis of focal segmental glomerulosclerosis are unknown. Some authorities believe that it is secondary to primary damage of the glomerular epithelial cells, whereas others suggest that the hemodynamic changes of hyperfiltration injury are responsible.

(2) **Clinical features.** About 80% of patients with focal segmental glomerulosclerosis have nephrosis. Hematuria, reduced glomerular filtration rate (GFR), and hypertension also are common. In many patients, the disease progresses to chronic renal failure.

(3) **Pathology.** Segmental sclerosis may involve only a small minority of glomeruli. Hyalinosis and increases in mesangial cellularity and matrix [see III A 1 b (5)] are common findings. Interstitial fibrosis and tubular atrophy are present in areas of glomerulosclerosis.

(4) **Treatment and prognosis.** Most patients do not respond to steroid treatment. About 20% of patients experience a rapid downhill course, progressing to renal failure within 2 years. Most others suffer a slowly progressive decrease in renal function.

d. Membranous glomerulopathy is said to be the most frequent cause of nephrotic syndrome in adults.

(1) **Etiology.** Most cases are idiopathic, but a small percentage are associated with known factors and conditions, such as infections (e.g., hepatitis B, syphilis, malaria, schistosomiasis), drugs (e.g., gold, penicillamine), autoimmune disease (e.g., lupus), and tumors (e.g., colon and lung carcinoma).

(2) **Clinical features.** The clinical presentation is characterized by severe, nonselective proteinuria, with both albumin and globulins excreted in the urine.

(3) **Pathology**

(a) Diffuse thickening of the capillary walls is seen by light microscopy.

(b) Electron microscopy shows the presence of numerous epimembranous and, in advanced cases, intramembranous electron-dense deposits. Basement membrane reaction to the deposits may take the form of "spikes" and "domes" of material separating and surrounding deposits.

(c) Immunofluorescence studies demonstrate immunoglobulin and, occasionally, complement in a finely granular pattern along all of the capillary loops. Deposits may undergo resolution in the later stages of the disease.

(4) **Treatment and prognosis.** The course of the disease is irregular, but in most patients there is a slow progression to renal failure over several years. A small percentage of patients (perhaps 20%) have a more benign course. Steroid therapy is of questionable benefit. The effectiveness of recently established cytotoxic therapies remains to be proven.

e. Diabetic nephropathy is a term that encompasses a variety of renal lesions, including diabetic glomerulosclerosis, arteriosclerosis, increased susceptibility to pyelonephritis and papillary necrosis.

    (1) Etiology and pathogenesis
        (a) The cause of **diabetic glomerulosclerosis** is not known. Biochemical alterations of the GBM are described, including increased type IV collagen and decreased proteoglycans. Nonenzymatic glycosylation may increase permeability. Hyperfiltration may accelerate the sclerotic process.
        (b) Atherosclerosis and arteriosclerosis are accelerated in diabetes. Atheromas may cause generalized ischemia or focal infarcts. Arteriosclerosis can affect both afferent and efferent arterioles.
        (c) Pyelonephritis and papillary necrosis are more common in patients with diabetes. Papillary necrosis may be related to the impaired microvasculature.
    (2) Clinical features. The renal lesions of diabetic glomerulosclerosis usually occur after 10 to 20 years of clinical disease and are accompanied by other microangiopathic manifestations, such as retinopathy, coronary artery disease, and peripheral vascular insufficiency. The predominant renal symptoms are proteinuria, glucosuria, and a progressive decrease in renal function. Dependent edema and hypertension may be late manifestations.
    (3) Pathology. Diabetic glomerulosclerosis refers to morphologic changes in the glomeruli, which may include isolated capillary basement membrane thickening, diffuse diabetic glomerulosclerosis, and nodular glomerulosclerosis. Pathologic changes likely progress over time from isolated membrane thickening to nodular glomerulosclerosis.
        (a) Capillary basement membrane thickening occurs in virtually all diabetics and is the earliest form of diabetic microangiopathy; it can be recognized only by electron microscopic studies. Capillary basement membrane thickening may begin as early as a few years after the clinical onset of juvenile diabetes. There is simultaneous thickening of tubular basement membranes.
        (b) Diffuse glomerulosclerosis refers to overall widening of the mesangial space by an increase in mesangial matrix. The increase in matrix appears to lag behind the basement membrane thickening but always is associated with it. Immunofluorescent studies may show weak linear staining with immunoglobulins and albumin, as plasma proteins bind to the GBM.
        (c) Nodular glomerulosclerosis (also called **Kimmelstiel-Wilson lesion**) arises on a background of diffuse glomerulosclerosis. The diagnostic feature is a nodular accentuation of the increased matrix material. Also, the number of mesangial cells found within the nodules is increased, and there is microaneurysm dilatation of the adjacent peripheral capillary loops.
  f. Amyloidosis. Renal involvement is one of the most common and serious manifestations of amyloidosis. The kidneys may be affected in both primary and secondary amyloidosis.
    (1) Clinical features. Patients with renal amyloidosis usually present with proteinuria and a variable degree of renal failure. Kidneys that are slightly enlarged or normal in the setting of renal failure suggest the diagnosis of amyloidosis.
    (2) Pathology
        (a) Macroscopically, the kidneys are normal in size or somewhat enlarged and have a waxy appearance.
        (b) Microscopically, the amyloid deposits are brightly eosinophilic and homogeneous on hematoxylin-eosin (H and E) stain. The deposits are seen first in the mesangium and capillary loops and later may appear in the blood vessels, tubular basement membranes, and interstitium. The amyloid material has a characteristic apple-green birefringence under polarized light after staining with Congo red stain.
        (c) Ultrastructurally, electron microscopy shows an accumulation of small fibrils that are less than 100 Å in diameter.
    (3) Treatment and prognosis. There is no effective treatment for amyloidosis, and prognosis is poor.

3. Acute nephritic syndrome is the second major clinical syndrome associated with glomerular disease. It is characterized by the presence of gross hematuria with RBC casts, oliguria, uremia, varying degrees of hypertension, and mild proteinuria. Edema usually is not a component of acute nephritic syndrome.
  a. Acute postinfectious glomerulonephritis
    (1) Etiology and epidemiology. Acute postinfectious glomerulonephritis is a fairly common glomerular disease that usually occurs 2 weeks after a streptococcal infection of

the pharynx or, less commonly, the skin. It occurs most often in children but can be seen in adults. Only certain strains of group A β-hemolytic streptococci are nephritogenic. Other infectious agents (e.g., *Staphylococcus aureus*) also may cause a similar picture.

    (2) Clinical features and diagnosis. Acute postinfectious glomerulonephritis is characterized by an abrupt onset of hematuria, usually with associated edema and hypertension. A clinical diagnosis can be established in patients with nephritis and rising titers to one or more streptococcal exoenzymes.

    (3) Pathology. Postinfectious glomerulonephritis is the prototypical immune complex–associated glomerulonephritis.

        (a) Electron microscopy reveals large immune complexes on the epithelial side of the basement membrane. These complexes contain immmunoglobulin and, most likely, the causative streptococcal antigen.

        (b) Complement also can be demonstrated by immunofluorescent techniques. Leukocytes infiltrate the glomeruli and incite an inflammatory response to these deposits. The glomeruli react with endothelial and mesangial proliferation, giving the histologic picture of a diffuse proliferative glomerulonephritis.

    (4) Treatment and prognosis. Over 95% of children recover spontaneously or respond to a short course of steroids. The recovery rate is lower among adults. In a small minority of patients, the disease may develop into rapidly progressive glomerulonephritis.

b. Rapidly progressive ("crescentic") glomerulonephritis represents a heterogeneous group of glomerulonephritides with different etiologies and pathogenetic mechanisms. This form of glomerulonephritis may be found in streptococcal infection, lupus, Goodpasture's syndrome, vasculitis, or cryoglobulinemia, or it may be idiopathic.

    (1) Clinical features. Patients present with nephritis, severe oliguria, or anuria and, without appropriate therapy, may succumb to irreversible renal failure within weeks.

    (2) Pathology. The characteristic finding is extensive crescent formation in the glomeruli. Crescents are a circumferential proliferation of epithelial cells and monocytes in Bowman's space, which occurs in response to fibrin leaked from damaged capillary loops. The immunofluorescent and electron microscopic studies vary with the etiology.

    (3) Treatment and prognosis. Historically, the prognosis for patients with rapidly progressive glomerulonephritis has been quite poor. However, new treatment protocols, including aggressive immunosuppression, have improved the outlook.

c. Goodpasture's syndrome refers to a disorder defined by the triad of alveolar hemorrhage, glomerulonephritis, and deposition of antibody along the alveolar and glomerular basement membranes.

    (1) Etiology and pathogenesis. Circulating anti-GBM antibodies can be detected in the serum of patients with Goodpasture's syndrome. This antibody reacts with both glomerular and alveolar capillary basement membranes. The triggering cause for antibody formation is unknown.

    (2) Clinical features. Goodpasture's syndrome is characterized by pulmonary hemorrhage and renal failure. Patients present with hemoptysis, anemia, pulmonary infiltrates, and hematuria.

    (3) Pathology

        (a) Early stages may involve focal and segmental proliferation, with necrosis of the glomerular tuft. In later stages, a crescentic glomerulonephritis occurs.

        (b) Immunofluorescent staining shows a linear deposition of immunoglobulin along the GBM, indicating that a monolayer of antibody has been deposited against an antigen that is distributed in a **continuous** fashion along the GBM. This antibody incites an inflammatory reaction, which causes the glomerular injury and subsequent proliferative response.

    (4) Treatment and prognosis. Therapy is directed at eliminating the causative antibody by intensive plasma exchange and immunosuppression. Therapy is most effective when instituted early. If delayed, patients may require dialysis or kidney transplantation.

d. Glomerulonephritis associated with vasculitis. Systemic vasculitic syndromes, including hypersensitivity vasculitis and Wegener's granulomatosis, may be associated with nephritic renal involvement. Focal and segmental glomerulonephritis accompanies the vasculitis. In Wegener's granulomatosis, a granulomatous arteritis may be found on the kidneys, lungs, and respiratory mucosa.

4. Glomerular diseases with combined nephrosis and nephritis
  a. Lupus nephritis refers to glomerulonephritis that occurs as a manifestation of systemic lupus erythematosus (SLE). 50% to 80% of cases of lupus show clinical evidence of renal involvement. If renal biopsy is performed, almost all patients show some evidence of renal damage. The onset of renal disease occurs within 2 years after the appearance of systemic symptoms. The pathogenesis and overall systemic features of this autoimmune disease are detailed in Chapter 6 IV B.
  (1) Clinical features. Patients may have a variable degree of proteinuria, hematuria, and cylindruria.
  (2) Pathology
    (a) Histopathologic classification. Five histologic patterns are described on the basis of light microscopic findings.
      (i) Normal kidneys. In only rare cases does light microscopy reveal normal glomeruli.
      (ii) Mesangial proliferative glomerulonephritis. In this pattern, the mesangium of all glomeruli is hypercellular. Glomerular inflammation, necrosis, and fibrosis are absent.
      (iii) Focal proliferative glomerulonephritis. In this pattern, some of the glomeruli are involved with endocapillary and epithelial proliferation, necrosis, and acute inflammation. Depending on the age of the lesions and their mode of resolution, variable degrees of glomerulosclerosis can be seen.
      (iv) Diffuse proliferative glomerulonephritis. In this pattern, more than 80% of the glomeruli show global proliferative changes, with inflammation and necrosis of the capillary tuft. Capillary loop thrombi and, occasionally, hematoxylin bodies also can be seen.
      (v) Membranous lupus nephritis. This histologic pattern is similar to that seen in idiopathic membranous glomerulopathy (see III A 2 d).
    (b) Immunofluorescent studies show granular deposits of immunoglobulin G (IgG), IgM, IgA, C3, and fibrin. In the mesangial proliferative pattern, deposits are confined to the mesangial space. In focal and diffuse proliferative patterns and the membranous pattern, deposits also are seen along the capillary loops.
    (c) Electron microscopic studies. Ultrastructurally, electron-dense deposits are present in the mesangium and subendothelial spaces. Massive subendothelial deposits correspond with the "wire loops" that can be seen histologically. In membranous forms, epimembranous deposits also are prominent.
  (3) Treatment and prognosis. Patients with normal kidneys or only mesangial proliferative changes have little in the way of clinical symptoms. Patients with diffuse proliferative and focal proliferative histologies involving more than 50% of the glomeruli require aggressive immunosuppression. The prognosis is quite variable and seems to correspond with the chronicity of damage.
  b. Membranoproliferative glomerulonephritis (MPGN) refers to a clinicopathologic entity characterized by a histologic lesion showing irregular thickening of the GBM and cellular proliferation.
  (1) Pathogenesis. There are two types of MPGN. The most prominent clinicopathologic change in both types is serum hypocomplementemia and the prominent glomerular deposition of complement components.
    (a) In type I MPGN, complement activation proceeds via the classic pathway.
    (b) In type II MPGN, activation of complement occurs primarily via the alternative pathway. An antibody against the alternative pathway C3 convertase, known as C3 nephritic factor, stabilizes the convertase and leads to unopposed complement activation. It is unclear how this change might lead to glomerular injury.
  (2) Clinical features. Two-thirds of patients present with nephrotic syndrome. Some patients experience only hematuria. Others present with combined features of nephritis and nephrosis.
  (3) Pathology
    (a) Microscopic findings. Light microscopy reveals glomeruli that are hypercellular due to a prominent increase in mesangial cells. The glomerular capillary loops are thickened by mesangial matrix extending into the subendothelial space of the peripheral capillary loops (i.e., so-called "mesangial interposition"). This change is reflected in the presence of a "double-contour" or "tram-track" appearance on special stains.

(b) **Electron microscopic and immunofluorescent findings** are divided into those characteristic of type I or type II MPGN.

    (i) **Type I MPGN** shows numerous **subendothelial electron-dense deposits** by electron microscopy. Immunofluorescence reveals the presence of complement components (C3, early complement Clq, and C4) and immunoglobulin.

    (ii) **Type II MPGN** ("dense deposit disease") is characterized by the **deposition of electron-dense material in the lamina densa** of the GBM. In type II MPGN, complement is activated by the alternative pathway, so that C3 (but not Clq or C4) is found.

(4) **Clinical course and prognosis.** About 50% of patients develop chronic renal failure within 10 years.

c. **IgA nephropathy (Berger's disease).** This clinicopathologic entity recently was defined with the aid of immunofluorescent microscopy. It affects children and young adults.

    (1) **Pathogenesis.** Circulating IgA immune complex is present in 50% of patients. Defective phagocytic function also is a feature. The familial occurrence as well as HLA associations suggest a genetic influence.

    (2) **Clinical features.** IgA nephropathy is associated with recurrent, gross, or microscopic hematuria and mild proteinuria.

    (3) **Pathology.** The characteristic lesion is diffuse mesangial proliferation with **mesangial IgA deposition**.

    (4) **Clinical course and prognosis.** The initial course usually is benign, although chronic renal failure develops in up to 50% of patients over 20 years.

d. **Henoch-Schönlein purpura** is a disease associated with generalized skin rash, arthropathy, intestinal hemorrhage, hematuria, and proteinuria. The kidney may show lesions varying from mild focal mesangial proliferation, to diffuse mesangial proliferation, to crescentic glomerulonephritis. Although vasculitis occurs in the skin and gastrointestinal tract, it is rare in the kidney. The marked **deposition of IgA** in immune complexes leads to the belief that Berger's disease and Henoch-Schönlein purpura are varying forms of the same disease.

B. Renal tubular disorders

1. **Acute tubular necrosis (ATN)** refers to acute renal failure secondary to destruction of the tubular epithelial cells.

a. **Etiology**

    (1) The **toxic form** of ATN results from ingestion or inhalation of toxic agents, including aminoglycoside antibiotics, cyclosporine, mercury, lead, gold, arsenic, ethylene glycol, pesticides, carbon tetrachloride, and methyl alcohol.

    (2) The **ischemic form** occurs in cases of shock—specifically septic shock.

b. **Clinical features.** Within 24 hours after exposure to the causative agents, oliguria and proteinuria develop, and blood urea nitrogen (BUN) and creatinine levels rise. There is a low specific gravity of the urine, with loss of electrolytes.

c. **Pathology**

    (1) **Macroscopic appearance.** The kidneys are enlarged, swollen, and pale.

    (2) **Microscopic appearance**

        (a) The **toxic form** primarily affects the **proximal convoluted tubules**. The tubular cells may contain acidophilic inclusions in the cytoplasm or appear necrotic and desquamated toward the lumen of the tubule. Lipid deposition within the cells or ballooning of the cytoplasm may occur, depending on the toxic agent. The tubular basement membrane is intact, and the distal tubules are spared.

        (b) The **ischemic form** affects both the **distal tubules** and the loops of Henle, with necrosis of tubular cells and rupture of the tubular basement membrane.

d. **Prognosis** depends on the etiologic agent and the severity of the damage. In most patients, renal failure is reversible, with complete recovery.

2. **Vacuolar nephrosis**

a. **Etiology.** The most common cause is hypokalemia; other diseases involving electrolyte imbalance also may be responsible. Vacuolar nephrosis also is seen in patients who have been administered hypertonic solutions (e.g., mannitol or sucrose solution).

b. **Clinical features.** Vacuolar nephrosis shows the same signs seen in ATN (see III B 1 b).

c. **Pathology.** The proximal convoluted tubule, loops of Henle, and collecting tubules may be affected. Histologically, the hallmark is the presence of **large vacuoles in the cytoplasm,** which fill the entire tubular cell.

    d. Prognosis. Recovery occurs in almost all affected patients whose osmotic disturbance is corrected.

  3. Fanconi's syndrome, an inherited disease affecting children and adults, is characterized by urinary excretion of phosphates, amino acids, and glucose resulting from failure of tubular reabsorption.

    a. Clinical features include skeletal disturbances (e.g., osteomalacia, osteoporosis, propensity to fractures), acidosis, and dehydration.

    b. Pathology. The tubular cells are flattened, and there is an abnormal neck piece in the proximal convoluted tubule.

C. Diseases of the interstitium

  1. Acute pyelonephritis is acute inflammation of the kidney and renal pelvis.

    a. Etiology and epidemiology

      (1) The most common infecting agent is *Escherichia coli;* other causative agents include *Proteus, Pseudomonas,* and *Staphylococcus* species. Most commonly, acute pyelonephritis begins as a urinary bladder infection, which ascends to the kidneys.

      (2) Factors that often contribute to the development of acute pyelonephritis include the use of instruments in the urinary tract, urinary tract obstruction, prostatism in older men patients, vesicoureteral reflux, and diabetes mellitus. Women are more commonly affected than men.

    b. Clinical features. Symptoms include fever, malaise, pain at the costovertebral angle, dysuria, and urinary urgency. Urinalysis shows pyuria and bacteriuria.

    c. Pathology

      (1) Macroscopic appearance. The affected kidney may be enlarged. Small yellowish microabscesses with hyperemic borders are scattered over the renal surface. The pelvic mucosa shows marked granularity and hyperemia.

      (2) Microscopic appearance

        (a) Diffuse suppurative necrosis or abscess formation occurs within the renal parenchyma. The abscesses contain neutrophils and cause tubular destruction.

        (b) Occasionally, the lesion may be severe and produce **renal papillary necrosis,** which is characterized by yellow necrosis of the apical portion of the pyramids. This feature of acute pyelonephritis is seen most often in diabetic patients, in patients with sickle cell disease, and in those with a history of analgesic abuse.

    d. Treatment and prognosis. Antibacterial therapy is the treatment of choice, but surgical therapy may be necessary in severe cases of unilateral renal papillary necrosis. Patients with this complication have a far worse prognosis than patients with uncomplicated acute pyelonephritis.

  2. Chronic pyelonephritis

    a. Etiology and pathogenesis. Chronic pyelonephritis exists in two forms, which develop in different ways.

      (1) Obstructive chronic pyelonephritis occurs in patients with chronic urinary obstruction caused by prostatic enlargement or renal calculi.

      (2) Nonobstructive chronic pyelonephritis probably is produced by a derangement of the vesicoureteral sphincter, which results in reflux of urine and passage of bacteria from the bladder to the ureters.

    b. Clinical features and diagnosis. Patients presenting late in the course of the disease have renal failure and hypertension. Pyelograms are diagnostic, showing the affected kidney asymmetrically contracted, with deformity of the caliceal system.

    c. Pathology

      (1) Macroscopic appearance. The affected kidney appears contracted and has an irregular granular surface. The parenchyma is atrophic and replaced by fat.

      (2) Microscopic appearance. There is chronic inflammation of the kidney and renal pelvis, with papillary atrophy and fibrosis of the caliceal fornices. The tubules have dilated, the lining of the epithelium shows atrophy, and pink material is present in the lumen, giving the kidney a thyroidlike appearance. The vessel walls show marked thickening.

    d. Prognosis. The disease follows a chronic course. With bilateral involvement, tubular damage is followed by glomerular involvement and, in severe cases, may progress to azotemia and death from uremia.

3. **Interstitial nephritis**
   a. **Acute interstitial nephritis** is characterized by the presence of eosinophils in the inflammatory infiltrate. It often is associated with allergic manifestations in other organs and may appear after the administration of a variety of drugs.
      (1) Acute interstitial nephritis causes rapidly progressive renal insufficiency, but this process is reversible following discontinuation of the causative drug.
      (2) If the process is not related to drugs, the rate of progression to renal insufficiency relates to the primary cause.
   b. **Chronic interstitial nephritis** is more common and may follow acute tubulointerstitial disease. Symptoms are related to distal tubular damage and usually are progressive and irreversible.

D. **Hypertensive renal disease.** Vascular disease in the kidney may include aneurysm, vasculitis, metabolic disease, or hypertension. The following discussion refers only to hypertensive renal injury. The other topics are covered in Chapter 10.

1. **General concepts**
   a. Systemic hypertension is a disorder of sustained blood pressure elevation. It may have no identifiable cause (**essential hypertension**), or it may be attributable to an underlying condition (**secondary hypertension**).
   b. Hypertension is the result of an imbalance in the factors that control cardiac output, peripheral resistance, and sodium homeostasis. The renal vasculature may be the primary source of kidney disease as it contributes to a renal cause for hypertension, or **renovascular hypertension**.
   c. The clinical course of hypertension may be chronic and relatively mild (**benign hypertension**), with a slow progression to serious end-organ effects; or it may be acute and severe (**malignant hypertension**), with an accelerated progression to serious (life-threatening) end-organ effects.
   d. The classification, epidemiology, pathogenesis, and cardiac effects of systemic hypertension are described in more detail in Chapter 9 V. The following discussion addresses renovascular hypertension as a cause of systemic hypertension and the renal effects of benign and malignant forms of hypertension.

2. **Renovascular hypertension.** Most often, hypertension is "essential," with no easily definable cause. In 2% to 5% of cases, hypertension is secondary to renal artery stenosis and its hemodynamic effects. Two forms of renovascular hypertension have been defined.
   a. In one form (which is more common in older adults), hypertension develops from atherosclerotic narrowing of the renal artery, which is mediated—to a great degree—by perturbations in the renin–angiotensin system. Recognizing this potentially curable form of hypertension is important, because it often is amenable to surgical therapy.
   b. In the other form (which is more common in younger patients), hypertension develops from fibromuscular dysplasia of the renal artery.

3. **Benign nephrosclerosis** is the term used to identify the renal effects of benign hypertension, which characteristically are associated with hyaline arteriosclerosis [see Chapter 10 I B 3 b (1) for further discussion of hyaline arteriosclerosis].
   a. **Pathology.** Histologically, there is deposition of amorphous hyaline material within the arteriolar wall, disrupting and replacing the elastic membrane and causing gradual narrowing of the lumen. Progression of the process causes atrophy and scarring of the tubules and glomerulus.
   b. **Prognosis.** Progression of the disease may lead to renal insufficiency and cardiovascular complications.

4. **Malignant nephrosclerosis** is the term used to identify the renal effects of malignant hypertension, which frequently are characterized by necrotizing arteriolitis and hyperplastic arteriosclerosis. Malignant hypertension arises de novo or is superimposed on preexisting renal disease, including glomerulonephritis and scleroderma.
   a. **Pathology.** Light microscopy reveals a characteristic necrotizing arteriolitis. The arteriolar medium becomes necrotic and is replaced by fibrin or fibrinoid material. Intimal hyperplasia (hyperplastic arteriosclerosis) reduces the diameter of the vessels. The lumen of the vessel may be obliterated completely, leading to thrombosis and infarction of the parenchyma supplied by the vessel.
   b. **Prognosis.** Progression of the disease leads to renal insufficiency and death.

IV. TUMORS OF THE KIDNEY

A. Benign renal neoplasms

1. **Angiomyolipoma** is a benign tumor composed of a mixture of fat, blood vessels, and smooth muscle tissue. These tumors are of significance because—clinically and radiologically—they often are misdiagnosed as carcinomas.
   a. **Clinical features.** Angiomyolipomas primarily appear in the fourth and fifth decades of life and are twice as common in women as in men. The most common symptom is flank pain, but hematuria and hypertension may be the initial manifestations.
   b. **Pathology**
      (1) **Macroscopic appearance.** Angiomyolipomas range in size from a few centimeters in diameter to quite large. They affect the cortex and medulla equally and have no predilection for the right or left kidney. On cut surface, they exhibit a yellow-to-gray color, depending on fat content.
      (2) **Microscopic appearance.** There is an admixture of mature adipose tissue, thick-walled vessels, and varying amounts of smooth muscle tissue.
   c. **Treatment** consists of complete resection of the lesion, even if a total nephrectomy is required.

2. **Mesoblastic nephroma** (benign nephroblastoma) is a congenital hamartoma that commonly is confused with Wilms' tumor. Most mesoblastic nephromas are diagnosed in the early months of life.
   a. **Pathology**
      (1) **Macroscopic appearance.** Mesoblastic nephromas vary in size and are unilateral. On cut section, they have a characteristic firm, whitish surface that resembles smooth muscle. Necrosis usually is absent, but cystic changes may be present. The tumors lack clear encapsulation.
      (2) **Microscopic appearance.** The predominant features are interlacing bundles of mature connective tissue, which entrap the glomeruli and other renal elements. Rarely, foci of dysplastic cartilage and embryonic mesenchyme may be present.
   b. **Treatment** is complete resection of the tumor and adequate margins of uninvolved tissue.

3. **Adenoma.** Traditionally, this tumor has been defined as a renal epithelial neoplasm that is less than 2.5 cm in size. Most of these lesions are associated with a benign course; however, approximately 10% of the lesions that are between 1 and 3 cm behave in a malignant fashion. These 10% are best considered small renal cell carcinomas of low malignant potential.

B. Malignant renal neoplasms

1. **Wilms' tumor** (nephroblastoma) is a mixed neoplasm composed of metanephric blastema and its stromal and epithelial derivatives at variable stages of differentiation. Wilms' tumor is the most common malignancy of renal origin in children.
   a. **Etiology and pathogenesis.** Very recent work has located a tumor suppressor gene on chromosome 11p13. Thought to repress transcription and designated WT-1, this gene is lost or deleted in sporadic and hereditary Wilms' tumor. WT-1 is expressed in various sites in the developing kidney and gonad. Since Wilms' tumor is often associated with developmental anomalies at these sites, the loss of activity of WT-1 may genetically link certain genitourinary developmental anomalies to Wilms' tumor.
   b. **Epidemiology.** Wilms' tumor occurs with equal frequency in both sexes. The tumors appear at any age, but most cases are diagnosed before age 5, with the peak incidence in the second year of life. Familial cases include those in monozygous twins.
   c. **Clinical features**
      (1) The most common presenting sign is an abdominal mass, which is seen in almost 90% of patients. Other findings include hypertension, nausea, vomiting, hematuria, and, occasionally, leg edema. Arteriography reveals poorly vascularized tumors.
      (2) Nephroblastomas may be combined with several other congenital malformations, such as sporadic aniridia, microcephaly, mental retardation, and spina bifida. Another associated condition is hemihypertrophy of the body.
   d. **Pathology.** Wilms' tumor can be unilateral, bilateral, or multifocal in its involvement of the same kidney.
      (1) **Macroscopic appearance.** The tumors are large, well delineated, and well encapsulated. On cut section, they often appear grayish-white to tan, with areas of hemorrhage

and occasional cystic changes. The junction between the tumor and the kidney is sharp, often with a rim of normal kidney parenchyma. Wilms' tumor coexists with nodular metanephric blastema in 12% to 17% of cases. Diffuse bilateral persistence of metanephric blastema is felt to be a risk factor for the development of Wilms' tumor. The renal pelvis is compressed in Wilms' tumor; and local spread into the perirenal fat, renal vein, and hilar nodes is common.

    (2) **Microscopic appearance.** The lesions are characterized by formation of abortive or embryonic glomerular and tubular structures surrounded by an immature spindle cell stroma. The epithelial elements may be scanty or predominantly tubular. The stroma may show different elements, such as skeletal muscle, cartilage, and fat.

  e. Metastases. The renal hilar and paraaortic lymph nodes are frequent sites of metastatic spread. The lungs, liver, adrenal gland, diaphragm, retroperitoneum, and bones also are commonly involved. The presence of metastases usually is discovered within 2 years after diagnosis of the primary tumor.

  f. Prognosis. Several factors influence the prognosis for patients with Wilms' tumor.

    (1) **Age of patient.** Patients under age 2 have a good 5-year survival rate.

    (2) **Extent of disease.** Capsular permeation, venous extension, and distant metastases are associated with a poor prognosis.

    (3) **Microscopic features.** Marked tubular and glomerular differentiation is associated with a good prognosis. Unfavorable histology includes nuclear pleomorphism and abnormal mitotic figures.

  g. Treatment consists of surgical resection of the lesion and systemic chemotherapy, supplemented by radiation of the affected area.

2. Renal cell carcinoma (hypernephroma) is an adenocarcinoma that arises from the proximal or distal convoluted tubule.

  a. Etiology and pathogenesis. The cause of these tumors remains obscure, but they have been produced in laboratory animals using chemical, physical, and viral agents. The chemicals used include aromatic hydrocarbons, amines, amides, and such aliphatic compounds as aflatoxins or metabolic products of the fungus *Aspergillus flavus*. Partial deletion of the short arm chromosome 3 is a frequent cytogenetic finding in renal cell carcinoma.

  b. Epidemiology. Most cases occur in adults, with the peak incidence around the sixth decade of life. Occasionally, cases involving children are reported. Renal cell carcinoma affects men and women in an approximate ratio of 2:1. Usually, the tumor is not discovered until it is in an advanced stage.

  c. Clinical features include the characteristic triad of hematuria, pain, and a flank mass although this complete triad is found in only a minority of patients. Other symptoms include fever, fatigue, and anorexia.

  d. Diagnosis

    (1) **Laboratory studies.** Approximately 5% of affected patients have polycythemia with erythrocytosis. Other laboratory findings include leukocytosis, thrombocytosis, hypercalcemia, and an elevated erythrocyte sedimentation rate. Anemia is present in up to 25% of patients with these neoplasms.

    (2) **Arteriography.** A selective arteriogram of the kidney demonstrates a mass with increased and irregularly branching vessels.

  e. Pathology. Renal cell carcinoma may affect either kidney and has no predilection for a specific location within the organ.

    (1) **Macroscopic appearance.** The tumor protrudes from the renal cortex as an irregular bosselated mass, which, on cut section, has a characteristic yellow-orange appearance. Hemorrhage and necrosis are commonly seen. At the periphery of the tumor, the normal parenchyma is compressed, forming a pseudocapsule. Foci of myxoid degeneration and calcification may be present (Figure 16-4).

    (2) **Microscopic appearance.** Several patterns can be seen, including papillary, tubular, granular, solid, or sarcomatoid. However, most tumors are composed of clear cells with distinct cytoplasmic membranes, abundant cytoplasm, and eccentric nuclei (Figure 16-5). The lesions are markedly vascularized, with little stroma between the cells; occasionally clusters of histiocytes and inflammatory cells are present. Renal cell tumors frequently show areas of pleomorphism and giant cells and, thus, resemble different types of sarcomas.

  f. Metastases. Renal cell carcinoma metastasizes mainly through the bloodstream although lymphatic spread also is possible. Approximately 95% of affected patients have evidence

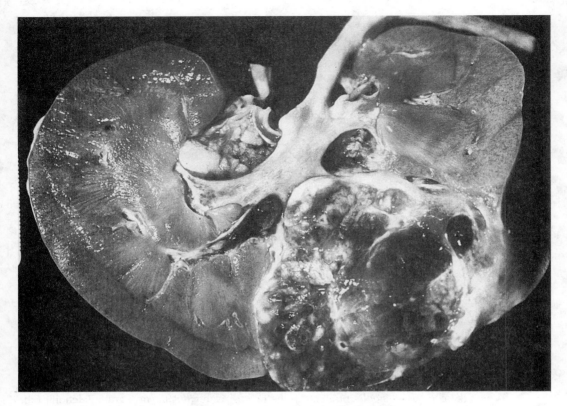

Figure 16-4. Renal cell carcinoma showing compression of the renal pelvis.

of metastatic spread at the time of death. The most commonly affected organs are the lungs, brain, bones, liver, adrenal glands, lymph nodes, and contralateral kidney.

g. Prognosis. Although spontaneous regression of renal cell carcinoma has been reported, these tumors generally are associated with a poor prognosis: 20% 10-year survival rate. The unfavorable prognosis is the result of both the aggressive nature of the tumor and its tendency to be silent until it reaches a large size, frequently having metastasized at the time of presentation.

h. Treatment. The treatment of choice is surgical resection of the lesion, with removal of adjacent lymph nodes. Radiation and chemotherapy have not proven to be successful treatment options.

V. DISORDERS OF THE URINARY TRACT

A. Congenital anomalies

1. **Bladder diverticula** consist of pouchlike eversions of the bladder wall. They may be congenital (due to a failure of development of the normal musculature), or they may be acquired (due to obstruction in the urethra or bladder neck). Bladder diverticula are more common in men than in women—and occur more frequently at sites of urinary stasis, infection, or tumor.

2. **Persistent urachus.** In the fetus, the urachus connects the apex of the bladder with the allantois through the umbilical stalk. Normally, the urachus atrophies and undergoes fibrosis after birth; occasionally, however, it remains patent, creating fistulous tracts between the bladder and the umbilicus. It also may be the site of origin of epithelial malignancies.

3. **Exstrophy of the bladder** is the absence of the anterior musculature of the bladder and is due to a failure of downgrowth of the mesoderm over the anterior surface of the bladder. It commonly is a site of severe infections. Exstrophy usually is associated with other developmental defects in the anterior abdominal wall.

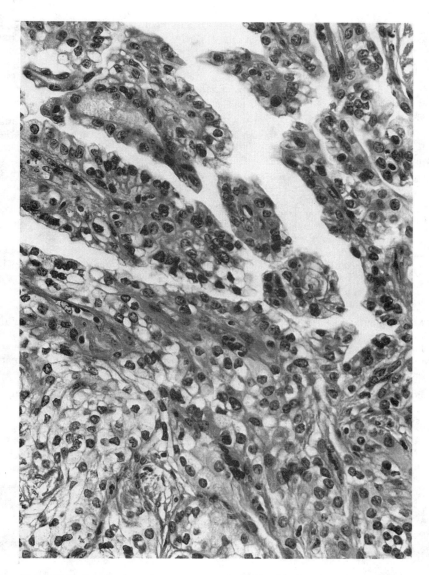

Figure 16-5. Renal cell carcinoma composed of cells with abundant clear cytoplasm.

4. Double ureters is an entity of little clinical significance. The two ureters may unite at some point before the junction to the urinary bladder, or they may pursue separate courses.

B. Benign disorders

1. Urinary tract infection

a. **Clinical features.** Affected patients complain of lower abdominal pain, urinary frequency, and dysuria. Examination reveals mucosal edema, redness, and, occasionally, ulcerations. The urethra is short in women; and since most infections are thought to arise from organisms ascending from the perineum, cystitis (bladder infection) is very common in women.

b. **Pathology**

(1) The transitional epithelium of the urinary tract responds to inflammation by various forms of proliferation or by invagination of the epithelium within the lamina propria of the submucosa, forming nests that eventually lose their continuity with the surface. These changes are referred to as **cystitis** (occurring in the urinary bladder), **ureteritis** (occurring in the ureter), or **pyelitis** (occurring in the renal pelvis).

    (2) Occasionally, there may be metaplasia of the transitional epithelium (e.g., glandular metaplasia, which resembles the epithelium of the large intestine). This change is associated with infections, irritants, or calculi; there is no evidence that implies a premalignant condition if localized.

  c. Treatment is correction of the condition that is causing the inflammation (e.g., obstruction, calculi, prostatic enlargement) by means of specific antibiotics, surgical procedure, or both.

2. Hydronephrosis is the dilation of the renal pelvis due to a partial block of urinary outflow. The obstruction can occur at any level in the urinary tract. The most common causes are nodular hyperplasia of the prostate, calculi, or malignant tumors such as cervical or bladder carcinoma.

  a. Clinical features. The dilation may remain silent for a long time. When present, the symptoms usually are related to the cause of the hydronephrosis.

  b. Pathology

    (1) Macroscopic appearance. The kidneys may show some degree of enlargement. Cut section shows blunting of the renal calices and cortical thinning. The pelvis is dilated massively and is filled with urine (Figure 16-6).

    (2) Microscopic appearance. The tubules may be atrophic, but the glomeruli become hyalinized only in late stages of the disease. Chronic inflammatory cells may be present in the interstitium.

  c. Treatment is directed toward the cause of the hydronephrosis. Nephrectomy is performed for some unilateral cases produced by calculi.

3. Malacoplakia is a rare lesion—produced by *E. coli* and characterized by multiple yellowish thickenings of the mucosa and submucosa. Clinically, this condition may appear as cancer. Histologically, multiple histiocytes with granular cytoplasm accumulate beneath the surface epithelium. Round, concentric, intracytoplasmic inclusions (Michaelis-Gutmann bodies) are present in some of these histiocytes; these inclusions stain positive for calcium and iron.

4. Endometriosis is the presence of ectopic endometrial tissue beneath the intact mucosa. These lesions undergo cyclic changes during the menstrual cycle. Clinically, they may mimic carcinomas.

5. Caruncles are small, red, painful masses in the external urethral meatus of the affected women. Histologically, they are composed of a vascularized stroma covered by squamous or transitional epithelium. The lesions may recur if not completely excised.

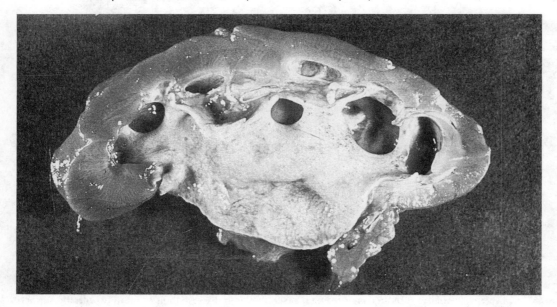

Figure 16-6. Hydronephrosis showing massive dilatation of the renal pelvis.

C. Malignant tumors

1. **Transitional cell carcinoma** of the urothelium has characteristic features that remain the same regardless of the tumor's location along the urinary collecting system. These tumors typically are multifocal and tend to recur.

    a. Incidence. Malignant tumors of the urinary collecting system account for more than 10,000 deaths per year in the United States.

    b. Etiology. Urinary tract carcinomas, especially those involving the bladder, have been linked to environmental factors, such as industrial carcinogens (e.g., aniline dyes), metabolites of tryptophan, cigarette smoking, mechanical irritation (e.g., due to calculi or diverticuli), and parasites. The longer the duration of exposure, the greater the chance that these tumors will develop.

    c. Clinical features. Patients experience painless hematuria.

    d. Pathology (Figure 16-7). On cytoscopic examination, the tumors may appear as papillary lesions or plaquelike ulcers. The region of the trigone in the bladder is the most common location. Histologically, the transitional cell epithelium is thickened, with an increased number of layers of cells, which show varying degrees of nuclear atypia and pleomorphism. The tumors are assigned one of three histologic grades, which are significant for estimating prognosis.

        (1) Grade I is composed of a central core of fibrovascular tissue covered by uniform transitional cells. Pleomorphism and mitoses are rare, and necrosis is absent. The epithelium is 7 to 10 cells thick.

        (2) Grade II tumors are characterized by persistence of the papillary configuration but more crowding of cells, with enlargement and hyperchromatism of nuclei (see Figure 16-7). The epithelium is 15 to 20 cells thick, or more. The number of mitoses varies.

        (3) Grade III tumors have a sessile, cauliflower-like appearance. Necrosis and ulceration are frequent findings. The cell masses form groups; atypia and mitoses are abundant.

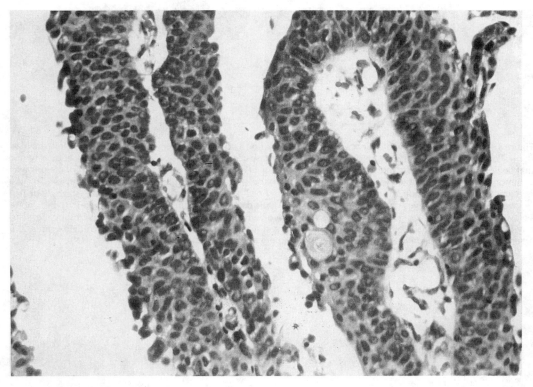

Figure 16-7. Papillary transitional cell carcinoma. Notice the stalk of fibroconnective tissue and the cellular proliferation (× 200).

    e. Prognosis depends on the histologic grade and the stage of the disease. The more undifferentiated the tumor, the worse the prognosis (Figure 16-8).
    f. Treatment is resection of the lesion (local or total cystectomy) followed by radiation.

2. Squamous cell carcinoma of the urinary tract is rare, representing 5% of all bladder tumors.
    a. Epidemiology. These tumors occur in persons living in geographic areas (such as Egypt) where close associations between parasitic infections (e.g., schistosomiasis) and carcinoma are known to occur.
    b. Pathology. Grossly, the tumors appear as ulcerated and necrotic masses. Histologically, they are poorly differentiated, but areas of keratinization may be present.
    c. Prognosis. Squamous cell cancers are associated with a poor prognosis.

3. Adenocarcinoma may arise from urachal remnants, cystitis cystica, cystitis glandularis, or metaplasia of transitional epithelium. Histologically, the glands produce abundant mucin and often are well differentiated.

4. Sarcomas (i.e., malignant mesenchymal tumors) of the bladder are rare. Of these, sarcoma botryoides is the most common. The histologic appearance is identical to that of sarcoma botryoides in the vagina.

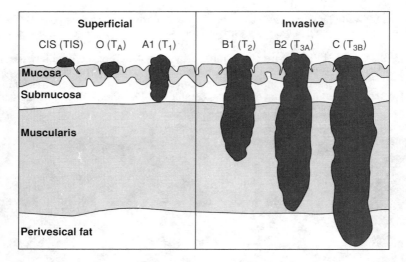

Figure 16-8. Carcinoma of the bladder can be staged according to the depth of penetration of the tumor into the bladder wall and, for advanced disease, by the location of metastases. *Superficial* disease represents the presence of tumors that do not invade the bladder mucosa (carcinoma in situ, or *CIS*; also known as tumor in situ, or *TIS*) or the presence of tumors that extend only into the mucosa (stage *O* or T_A) or only into the submucosa (stage *A1* or T_1). Invasive disease is characterized by extension into the muscle layer (stage *B1* or T_2), deep penetration into the muscle (stage *B2* or T_{3A}), or involvement of the perivesical fat (stage *C* or T_{3B}). Metastatic disease (not pictured) represents spread to lymph nodes below the aortic bifurcation (stage D1 or $T_x N_+ M_O$) or involvement of lymph nodes above the aortic bifurcation or of any bone or soft tissue (stage D2 or $T_x N_+ M_+$). (Reprinted from Garnick MB: Oncology, "Oncologic Cancer." In *Scientific American: Medicine.* New York, Scientific American, 1991, Section 12, subsection IX, p 9.)

STUDY QUESTIONS

Directions: Each of the numbered items or incomplete statements in this section is followed by answers or by completions of the statement. Select the **one** lettered answer or completion that is **best** in each case.

1. A 55-year-old man who is admitted to the hospital with impaired renal function has massive bilateral multicystic masses in the kidneys on ultrasound examination. The patient dies shortly after admission. Autopsy reveals the cause of death as a ruptured aneurysm in the circle of Willis. What is the most likely type of renal cystic disease in this patient?

(A) Medullary cystic disease
(B) Multiple simple cysts
(C) Autosomal dominant polycystic kidney disease
(D) Medullary sponge kidney
(E) Cystic renal dysplasia

2. Lipoid nephrosis of the kidney characteristically produces ultrastructural changes in which renal glomerular element?

(A) Endothelium
(B) Epithelium
(C) Mesangium
(D) Blood vessels
(E) Basement membrane

3. Which statement best characterizes membranous glomerulopathy?

(A) It is the most common cause of nephrotic syndrome in children
(B) Affected patients usually present with acute renal failure
(C) The characteristic pathology is best described as "diffuse proliferative glomerulonephritis"
(D) Electron microscopy demonstrates numerous subepithelial immune-type deposits
(E) It usually is responsive to steroid therapy

4. Which statement about diabetic nephropathy is true?

(A) It is characterized by diffuse thinning of the glomerular basement membrane (GBM)
(B) It usually is accompanied by microangiopathic changes in other organs
(C) Affected patients most often present with nephritis
(D) The disease usually remits after a few years
(E) A granular pattern of glomerular IgG deposits characteristically is seen on immunofluorescent studies

5. A kidney biopsy specimen that shows subendothelial granular electron-dense deposits is characteristic of which disease state?

(A) Rapidly progressive glomerulonephritis
(B) Poststreptococcal glomerulonephritis
(C) Membranous glomerulonephritis
(D) Systemic lupus erythematosus (SLE)
(E) Goodpasture's syndrome

6. Mercury poisoning causes which condition in the kidneys?

(A) Acute tubular necrosis (ATN)
(B) Renal papillary necrosis
(C) Crescentic glomerulonephritis
(D) Acute interstitial nephritis
(E) Renal cell carcinoma

7. In most cases of nonobstructive chronic pyelonephritis, bacteria reach the kidney via

(A) the bloodstream
(B) the lymphatics
(C) Batson's plexus
(D) vesicoureteral reflux
(E) aberrant arteriovenous shunts

1-C	4-B	7-D
2-B	5-D	
3-D	6-A	

8. Malacoplakia of the renal pelvis occurs following infection by which organism?

(A) *Mycoplasma pneumoniae*
(C) *Cryptococcus neoformans*
(C) *Escherichia coli*
(D) α-Hemolytic streptococci
(E) *Staphylococcus aureus*

9. An immunofluorescence-stained kidney specimen from a patient with poststreptococcal glomerulonephritis is likely to show

(A) granular deposits of immunoglobulin G (IgG)
(B) linear deposits of IgG
(C) granular deposits of IgA
(D) linear deposits of streptococcal antigen
(E) granular deposits of streptococcal antigen

10. Which statement is true of a patient with renal cell carcinoma?

(A) Clinical presentation is usually at an early stage
(B) The combination of hematuria, flank pain, and flank mass is found in the majority of patients
(C) The classic histopathology is that of clear cell carcinoma
(D) Metastases are rare and, when present, are usually confined to the perirenal area
(E) The gross morphology of renal cell carcinoma is usually that of a solid gray–white tumor, indicating its low lipid content

11. A patient presents at the physician's office complaining of intermittent hematuria. As a Board-certified urologist, the physician elects to perform a cystoscopic examination as part of this patient's evaluation. He sees several 3-mm exophytic lesions in the left lateral wall of the bladder, decides to biopsy them, then sends them to the surgical pathology laboratory for expert evaluation. Which pathologic description of these lesions would be most ominous for the patient's prognosis?

(A) Papillary tumor lined by seven layers of cytologically bland epithelium
(B) Papillary groups with marked nuclear pleomorphism infiltrating through skeletal muscle
(C) Dense inflammation of lamina propria lifting normal-appearing urothelium and forming polypoid mass
(D) Papillary tumor with moderate nuclear pleomorphism confined to the mucosa
(E) Extensive cystitis glandularis

12. All of the following clinical features are likely to be found in nephrotic syndrome EXCEPT

(A) proteinuria
(B) hypoalbuminemia
(C) red cell casts
(D) hyperlipidemia
(E) edema

13. All of the following statements regarding postinfectious glomerulonephritis are true EXCEPT

(A) the disease follows infection with group A β-hemolytic streptococci
(B) large subepithelial immune-type deposits are seen by electron microscopy
(C) the histologic picture is that of diffuse proliferative glomerulonephritis
(D) the clinical picture is characteristic of acute nephritis
(E) most affected children progress to chronic renal failure

8-C   11-B
9-A   12-C
10-C   13-E

14. All of the following statements about Goodpasture's syndrome are true EXCEPT

(A) patients present with hemoptysis and hematuria

(B) death occurs due to uremia and pulmonary hemorrhage

(C) electron microscopy shows an absence of electron-dense deposits

(D) immunofluorescence reveals granular deposits of immunoglobulin G (IgG) in the glomeruli

(E) immunofluorescence reveals linear deposits of IgG in the glomeruli

15. All of the following are causes of hydronephrosis EXCEPT

(A) chronic renal vein thrombosis

(B) large uterine leiomyoma

(C) renal calculi

(D) benign prostatic hypertrophy

(E) papillary transitional cell carcinoma of the ureter

14-D
15-A

ANSWERS AND EXPLANATIONS

1. The answer is C *[II D 2 a]*.
The presence of cysts in the kidneys, or renal cystic disease, may be an inherited or acquired disorder. Of the several forms of renal cystic disease, the classic form, polycystic kidney disease, is inherited most often as an autosomal trait, which presents in the fifth to sixth decade. Roughly 15% of patients with this disorder have associated berry aneurysms (i.e., saccular aneurysms originating in or near the circle of Willis), which often lead to intracranial bleeding.

2. The answer is B *[III A 2 b (3)]*.
Lipoid nephrosis sometimes is referred to as minimal change glomerulonephritis because of the paucity of histologic findings. Electron microscopic examination, however, reveals accumulation of lipids in the renal tubular epithelial cells and loss of foot processes of the glomerular epithelial cells. Lipoid nephrosis is the most common cause of nephrotic syndrome in children, particularly those under age 15.

3. The answer is D *[III A 2 d (3) (b)]*.
Membranous glomerulopathy is the most common cause of nephrotic syndrome in adults. The salient pathologic feature is the presence of numerous epimembranous immune-type deposits noted on electron microscopic examination. Patients present with severe, nonselective proteinemia, and—although the course is irregular—most experience a slow progression to renal failure. Steroid therapy has not proven to be of much benefit in these patients.

4. The answer is B *[III A 2 e (2)]*.
Diabetic nephropathy usually develops in diabetic patients after many years of clinical diabetes. The renal lesions in diabetic nephropathy usually are accompanied by microangiopathic vascular changes in other organs, especially the eyes. Diabetic nephropathy may show diffuse or diffuse and nodular glomerulosclerosis. A constant feature at the ultrastructural level is diffuse thickening of the glomerular basement membrane (GBM). The course of clinical diabetic nephropathy is progression toward renal failure.

5. The answer is D *[III A 4 a (2) (c)]*.
Granular subendothelial immune deposits and proliferation of mesangial and endothelial cells are characteristic of systemic lupus erythematosus (SLE). In lupus, the immune complexes are often located between the endothelial cells and the glomerular basement membrane (GBM).

6. The answer is A *[III B 1 a (1)]*.
Acute tubular necrosis (ATN) is the destruction of the tubular epithelial cells, which causes acute renal failure. Toxic agents that can produce ATN include mercury, lead, gold, arsenic, ethylene glycol, numerous pesticides, carbon tetrachloride, and methyl alcohol. Because mercury is excreted through the urine, the proximal convoluted tubular cells are damaged, causing disruption of intracellular organelles, breaks in the plasma membrane, and the appearance of curious acidophilic droplets within the cytoplasm.

7. The answer is D *[III C 1 a, 2 a (2)]*.
In the overwhelming majority of cases, pyelonephritis begins as a bladder infection that ascends to the kidneys. Nonobstructive chronic pyelonephritis likely results from vesicoureteral dysfunction, with chronic reflux of urine and passage of bacteria from the bladder to the ureters causing the recurrent kidney infection.

8. The answer is C *[V B 3]*.
Malacoplakia may be related to a defect in histiocytes that prevents degradation of infecting coliforms such as *Escherichia coli*. The term malacoplakia originally referred to a distinctive type of chronic inflammation of the urinary bladder. However, the condition has been shown to occur in several locations along the urinary tract. In the bladder, malacoplakia grossly appears as focal thickenings of the mucosa (and sometimes submucosa), which may be mistaken for cancer. Microscopically, these lesions appear as accumulations of granular histiocytes beneath the surface epithelial cell layer.

9. The answer is A *[III A 3 a (3)]*.
Poststreptococcal glomerulonephritis is a form of immune complex–mediated nephritis that can develop as a result of an immunologic reaction to an infection. Kidney biopsies from patients with this condition show endothelial and mesangial cell proliferation, granular deposits of fibrin, and granular deposits of immunoglobulin G (IgG) and complement component C3; sometimes, other complement components also may be detected. It is difficult to demonstrate the causative streptococcal antigen immunologically, although these antigens are presumed to be present and can be imaged in a small minority of cases.

10. The answer is C *[IV B 2 b–f].*
The histopathology of renal cell carcinoma is most typically that of a clear cell tumor. Renal cell carcinoma is most common in adults, with a peak incidence at about age 50 to 60. It is one of the most frequently metastasizing tumors; about 95% of affected patients have evidence of metastasis at the time of death. In fact, a large number of patients have advanced disease at diagnosis. Renal cell carcinoma patients present with hematuria, pain, and a flank mass, and they may have associated polycythemia and erythrocytosis. The gross morphology is usually that of an irregular yellow–orange mass.

11. The answer is B *[V C 1].*
Transitional cell carcinoma of the bladder is a common malignancy in men. It is linked epidemiologically to smoking and exposure to industrial carcinogens, such as aniline dyes. Transitional carcinoma often has a papillous morphology. Low-grade tumors confined to the mucosa have a good prognosis. High-grade tumors with invasion into the muscle of the bladder wall have a poor prognosis.

12. The answer is C *[III A 1 d (1), 2].*
Nephrosis, or the nephrotic syndrome, is defined as heavy proteinuria (i.e., > 3.5 g/day), hypoalbuminemia, hyperlipidemia, and edema; red cell casts are not a feature of nephrosis, although they are characteristic findings in patients with nephritis. Both nephrosis and nephritis are major clinicopathologic forms of glomerulonephritis. At the nephrosis end of the disease spectrum, glomerular inflammation and proliferation are minimal; at the nephritis end of the spectrum, they are significant.

13. The answer is E *[III A 3 a (4)].*
Acute postinfectious glomerulonephritis develops about 2 weeks after infection with nephritogenic strains of group A β-hemolytic streptococci. The clinical presentation usually is characteristic of acute nephritis. During the most active stage, the histopathology is that of a diffuse proliferative glomerulonephritis. Large subepithelial immune-type deposits are classic findings on electron microscopy. In children, full recovery after resolution of the nephritis is usual.

14. The answer is D *[III A 3 c].*
Goodpasture's syndrome is characterized by proliferative glomerulonephritis and proliferative pulmonary hemorrhage. Patients present with hemoptysis, pulmonary infiltrates, and hematuria. Although the course is variable, some patients develop fulminant disease and die due to renal failure and suffocation by massive pulmonary bleeding. The characteristic pathologic feature of Goodpasture's syndrome is the linear deposition of immunoglobulin G (IgG) and complement along the glomerular basement membrane (GBM), which can be seen with immunofluorescent staining. Electron microscopy fails to show any immune complex electron-dense deposits.

15. The answer is A *[V B 2].*
Hydronephrosis is the term given to dilatation of the renal pelvis due to complete or incomplete obstruction of urine flow from the pelvis. The obstruction may occur at any level in the urinary tract and can result from many causes, including prostatic hypertrophy, pelvic tumors, and the presence of renal calculi. Renal vein thrombosis is not a known cause of hydronephrosis.

17
Male Reproductive System

Maria J. Merino

I. TESTIS, SCROTUM, AND EPIDIDYMIS

A. Normal anatomy and embryology

1. Anatomy

 a. The normal adult **testis** is an ovoid gland, which is approximately 4 to 5 cm long and 2.5 to 3 cm wide and weighs from 10 to 45 g. Both testes normally are situated in the **scrotum,** where they are maintained at a temperature for normal spermatogenesis.

 b. Each testis is surrounded by a thick, dense, fibrous capsule called the **tunica albuginea,** which, in turn, is surrounded by a serous membrane called the **tunica vaginalis.**

 c. At the hilus of the testis is a condensation of fibrous tissue that extends into the testicular stroma and divides it into several compartments. Each compartment contains **seminiferous tubules** and clumps of **interstitial (Leydig) cells.**

 d. The seminiferous tubules, which contain both germinal cells **(spermatogonia)** and nongerminal cells **(Sertoli cells),** are organized into coiled loops, with each loop beginning and ending in a single duct—the **tubulus rectus.** The tubuli recti join to form the **rete testis** and eventually drain into the **epididymis,** which is the primary storage and final maturation site for spermatozoa.

2. Embryology

 a. The **testes and Leydig cells** are mesenchymal derivatives.

  (1) The testicular germ cells originate from the endoderm of the yolk sac and migrate toward the gonadal or genital ridge by active movement of individual cells. At 7 to 9 months' gestation, the testes normally descend through the inguinal rings into the scrotum.

  (2) The Leydig cells are extensive at birth but disappear after about 6 months. Leydig cell production begins again at puberty.

 b. The **male internal genitalia** (including the seminiferous tubules, rete testis, epididymis, vas deferens, ejaculatory duct, and seminal vesicles) arise from the **wolffian ducts.**

 c. The **scrotum** arises from the **genital swelling.**

B. Congenital anomalies

1. Anorchism refers to congenital absence of the testis; this anomaly may be unilateral **(monorchia)** or bilateral **(anorchia).**

2. Cryptorchidism refers to the absence of one testis (most common) or both testes from the scrotal sac. The testes may be retained in the abdominal cavity, inguinal region, or the inguinal canal. Often, the cause of cryptorchidism is not evident.

 a. If not discovered and corrected until after puberty, cryptorchidism results in testicular atrophy (i.e., smaller than normal-sized testes) and, in most cases, lack of normal spermatogenesis.

 b. Undescended testes have a higher tendency to develop malignancies than do normal testes.

3. Bifid scrotum is the presence of two separate scrotal sacs.

C. Disorders associated with infertility

1. Hypospermatogenesis is a condition involving a decreased number of cells of the spermatogenic series; the normal number is about 2 million. The cells that are present appear histologically normal. Clinically, the condition is **oligospermia** (i.e., a decreased number of spermatozoa in the semen).

2. **Maturation arrest** consists of a failure of normal spermatogenesis at some stage and results in either oligospermia or **azoospermia** (i.e., absence of spermatozoa in the semen).

3. **Klinefelter's syndrome** is one of the most common causes of hypogonadism in men.
   a. The condition is characterized by testicular hypoplasia, azoospermia, gynecomastia, eunuchoid build, and elevated urinary gonadotropin levels. Affected men also may manifest mild mental retardation.
   b. Chromosome studies usually reveal 47 chromosomes with an XXY karyotype.

4. **Testicular atrophy** is characterized by testes that weigh less than 10 g and have no histologic evidence of spermatogenesis. **Acquired atrophy** occurs in old age, in conditions such as hypothyroidism and cachexia, and in patients receiving estrogen therapy for prostatic carcinoma.

5. **Germ cell aplasia (Sertoli-cell–only syndrome)** is characterized by the absence of germ cells. The seminiferous tubules are lined only by Sertoli cells, with no evidence of normal spermatogenesis. Leydig cells are present but reduced in number. This disorder is associated with chemotherapy or radiation therapy but also can be idiopathic.

6. **Testicular torsion and infarction.** Free mobility of the testes predisposes to twisting of the spermatic cord, with resultant compression and occlusion of the blood vessels.
   a. **Clinicopathologic features.** The decrease in blood flow leads to hemorrhagic infarction of the testis and epididymis. If only partial or temporary torsion of the cord occurs, the result is hyperemia and edema but not necrosis.
   b. Predisposing factors include anomalies in the insertion of the vas deferens, a wide tunica vaginalis, absence of the scrotal ligaments, or an atrophic testis.

D. Inflammatory disorders

1. **Acute orchitis** refers to an acute inflammation of the testicular parenchyma because of an infectious process that usually reaches the testis and epididymis by ascending through the vas deferens or via lymphatics.
   a. **Etiology and pathogenesis**
      (1) The most **common agents** of acute orchitis are *Escherichia coli,* staphylococci, and streptococci.
      (2) The most **common sources** of acute orchitis are acute urethritis, acute cystitis, and prostatitis. Rarely, the condition occurs as a complication of mumps, affecting patients (postpubescent more commonly than prepubescent) approximately 1 week after the onset of parotitis.
   b. **Clinical features** commonly include fever, pain, tenderness, and swelling of the testis.
   c. **Pathology. Histologically,** a diffuse infiltrate of neutrophils, lymphocytes, and plasma cells involves both the interstitium and the tubules. Edema, vascular dilatation, and hemorrhage are present.
   d. **Complications.** Sterility may result as a consequence of extensive fibrosis, scarring, and damage to the tubules.

2. **Granulomatous orchitis** has an obscure etiology. Trauma and autoimmune disorders have been postulated as causes of the lesion.
   a. **Clinical features.** Granulomatous orchitis is characterized by unilateral testicular enlargement occurring predominantly in middle-aged men.
   b. **Pathology**
      (1) **Histologically,** the hallmark is the presence of epithelioid granulomas with abundant plasma cells, lymphocytes, and neutrophils surrounding ruptured tubules and nests of spermatozoa.
      (2) The condition should be differentiated from tuberculous orchitis, in which necrotizing granulomas containing acid-fast bacilli can be demonstrated.

3. **Tuberculous epididymitis**
   a. **Pathogenesis.** This condition can result from hematogenous spread from diseased kidneys or lungs. The inflammation usually begins in the interstitial tissue and then spreads to the testis.
   b. **Pathology. Histologically,** the hallmark is the presence of caseating granulomas, in which acid-fast bacilli can be demonstrated either by culture of the tissue or by special stains.

4. **Spermatocytic granuloma** is a granulomatous reaction to a lipid fraction released by the sperm. It can occur in the vas deferens or epididymis.

    a. Pathogenesis. The lesion probably is the result of inflammation or trauma that damages the tubular epithelium and basement membrane. Spermatocytic granulomas are common in men who have had vasectomies.

    b. Pathology. Histologically, a prominent histiocytic reaction intermixes with numerous spermatozoa.

5. Dermatologic disorders of the scrotum include scabies, pediculosis, eczema, and prurigo.

E. Testicular tumors

    1. Germ cell tumors. Approximately 95% of malignant testicular neoplasms are of germ cell origin.

        a. General features of germ cell tumors

            (1) Incidence. Germ cell tumors are one of the most common forms of cancer in men between age 15 and 34; however, they account for only about 1% of cancer-related deaths in males.

            (2) Etiology and pathogenesis. The cause is unknown, although several predisposing factors have been identified.

                (a) Patients with **undescended testes** have a greatly increased (up to 14-fold) risk of developing malignant tumors, when compared to those whose testes descended.

                (b) Infection and **trauma** are other known predisposing factors.

                (c) A **genetic influence** is suggested by the increased occurrence of testicular tumors in siblings and other family members of affected patients.

            (3) Classification. Germ cell tumors can be classified into six histologic types: intratubular germ cell neoplasia, seminoma, teratoma, embryonal cell carcinoma, infantile embryonal cell carcinoma, and choriocarcinoma. In more than 40% of cases, germ cell tumors exhibit more than one histologic type.

        b. Intratubular germ cell neoplasia is a proliferation of abnormal germ cells within the seminiferous tubules. The tumor also is called **in situ germ cell neoplasia,** since the tumor cells have not infiltrated through the tubular basement membrane.

            (1) Incidence. Intratubular germ cell neoplasia occurs in association with cryptorchidism, testicular dysgenesis, infertility, and germ cell tumor in the contralateral testis.

            (2) Pathology

                (a) Histologically, the seminiferous tubules are filled with round cells that have abundant clear cytoplasm and irregular nuclei with prominent nucleoli. Tubule involvement varies in degree and may have a patchy distribution.

                (b) The tumor cells stain positive for **placental alkaline phosphatase,** an enzyme found in germ tumors and fetal cells.

            (3) Prognosis. The tumor may progress to invasive germ cell cancer if untreated.

        c. Seminoma is the most common testicular tumor and the one most likely to occur in an undescended testis. It accounts for approximately 70% of primary germ cell tumors of the testis.

            (1) Clinical features. Seminoma occurs predominantly in the third to fifth decades of life and only rarely is encountered in children. Enlargement of the testis, with or without pain, is the most common symptom. In about 2% of cases, the tumor is bilateral.

            (2) Pathology

                (a) Gross appearance (Figure 17-1)

                    (i) The involved testis maintains its normal contour and configuration, although it is enlarged. The tunica albuginea is intact, and frequently the epididymis and spermatic cord are spared.

                    (ii) On cut section, the tumor shows a bulging, white-gray, homogeneous mass with a firm consistency. Hemorrhage and necrosis are not present.

                (b) Histologic appearance (Figure 17-2)

                    (i) Seminomas consist of sheets of uniform, polyhedral cells with large hyperchromatic nuclei and abundant clear cytoplasm that is rich in glycogen.

                    (ii) Strands of fibroconnective tissue and lymphocytes are common, interspersed with tumor cells. Chronic inflammatory cells may surround the tumor cells.

                    (ii) Occasionally, multinucleate giant cells are present. These cells represent syncytiotrophoblastic cells capable of producing **human chorionic gonadotropin (hCG).**

                    (iv) Approximately 10% of seminomas show marked anaplasia and increased mitotic activity **(anaplastic seminoma).** According to some authorities, these tumors are more aggressive than ordinary seminomas.

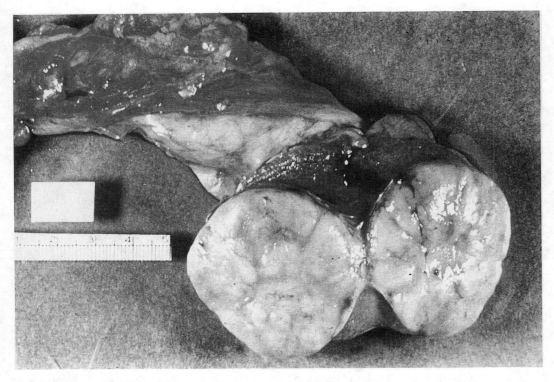

Figure 17-1. Cross section of a testis involved by a seminoma, showing an encapsulated homogeneous tumor and compressed normal testicular parenchyma.

    (3) Metastasis to regional lymph nodes and viscera can occur.
    (4) Treatment. The treatment of choice is orchiectomy followed by radiation therapy, chemotherapy, or both.
    (5) Prognosis. The tumors are associated with a good prognosis, with a 5-year survival rate of 90% to 98%.
    (6) Spermatocytic seminoma accounts for up to 10% of seminomas and occurs in older patients.
        (a) Pathology. Histologically, it is characterized by three types of cells. Medium-sized cells with round nuclei and abundant eosinophilic cytoplasm constitute the main population. The other cells are large mononuclear or multinucleate cells and small cells that resemble spermatocytes.
        (b) Prognosis. Patients with seminoma have an excellent prognosis.
  d. Teratoma is characterized by the presence of elements from the three germinal layers: ectoderm, endoderm, and mesoderm. It accounts for about 30% of testicular tumors.
    (1) Clinical features. Teratomas can occur at any age but are most common in the first to third decades of life. The symptomatology is identical to that of other testicular tumors.
    (2) Pathology
        (a) Gross appearance
            (i) The testis is enlarged, the tunica is distorted, and, occasionally, the lesion extends beyond the capsule.
            (ii) Cut section of the tumor reveals a lobulated, soft to firm, partly cystic mass surrounded by a rim of compressed normal testicular tissue.
            (iii) Areas of calcification, hemorrhage, and necrosis are present.
        (b) Histologic appearance
            (i) A variety of heterogeneous tissues are present, including bone, cartilage, and neural elements and gastric, respiratory, and squamous epithelium.
            (ii) Immature elements may be present, and sarcomatous transformation may occur.

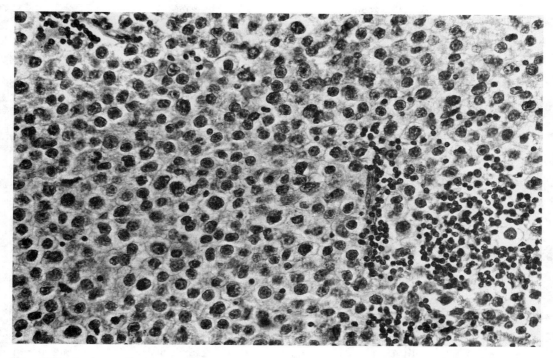

Figure 17-2. Seminoma, showing sheets of uniform germ cells with clear cytoplasm and prominent nuclei as well as occasional lymphocytes (high power).

        (iii) Elements from other germ cell tumors (e.g, seminoma, embryonal cell carcinoma) also may be present.

    (3) Metastasis via lymphatics or blood vessels can occur even when no histologic evidence of malignant transformation can be demonstrated. Metastases can be composed of one or several histologic patterns, which may be poorly or well differentiated.

    (4) Treatment. The treatment of choice is orchiectomy followed by chemotherapy and radiation therapy.

    (5) Prognosis. The 2-year mortality rate for patients with teratoma is about 30%.

  e. Embryonal cell carcinoma accounts for 15% to 20% of testicular germ cell tumors. It occurs predominantly in the second and third decades of life.

    (1) Clinical features. Gradual swelling of the testis, with or without pain, is the most common clinical complaint.

    (2) Pathology

      (a) Gross appearance

        (i) The tumors usually are small, with no evidence of encapsulation; they produce asymmetrical distortion of the testis.

        (ii) On cut section, the tumor reveals nodules, with extensive areas of hemorrhage and necrosis.

        (iii) Infiltration of the tunica albuginea, spermatic cord, and epididymis is common.

      (b) Histologic appearance

        (i) The tumors consist of pleomorphic epithelial cells that vary in size and shape. The cells have large nuclei, prominent nucleoli, and abundant eosinophilic cytoplasm.

        (ii) The tumor cells can appear in a variety of patterns (e.g., glandular, papillary, tubular) or be solid sheets of cells.

        (iii) Mitosis, hemorrhage, and necrosis are common.

    (3) Metastasis. Embryonal cell carcinomas are far more aggressive than seminomas, and metastasis to lymph nodes and viscera (e.g., lungs, liver) is common. About one-third of affected patients have evidence of metastasis at the time of diagnosis.

(4) Treatment. Orchiectomy always should be performed, usually followed by cisplatin-based chemotherapy.

(5) Prognosis. The 5-year mortality rate for patients with embryonal cell carcinoma is about 65%.

f. **Infantile embryonal cell carcinoma** (also called **yolk sac tumor**) is so named because it resembles the endodermal sinus and amniotic cavity of a yolk sac. The tumor occurs predominantly in children; it is rare in adults.

    (1) Clinical features. Serum alpha-fetoprotein (AFP) levels are elevated in affected patients.

    (2) Pathology

        (a) Histologically, the hallmark of this tumor is the presence of organoid structures that simulate embryoid (Schiller-Duval) bodies. A variety of patterns are recognized, including solid, papillary, cystic, hepatoid, and alveolar.

        (b) In adults, endodermal sinus tumor usually is combined with other germ cell elements.

    (3) Treatment. Chemotherapy is the treatment of choice.

    (4) Prognosis. This highly aggressive neoplasm is associated with a 5-year mortality rate of 50%.

g. **Choriocarcinoma** is the most malignant of the testicular tumors, accounting for about 1% of germ cell neoplasms. It occurs predominantly in men age 15 to 25.

    (1) Clinical features

        (a) Enlargement of the testis is common; however, the presenting symptoms at times are those produced by metastasis of the tumor. Some patients may have gynecomastia.

        (b) Serum and urine levels of hCG are elevated.

    (2) Pathology

        (a) Gross appearance

            (i) The tumor either can be very small and difficult to identify or involve the entire testis, producing distortion and nodularity.

            (ii) On cut section, extensive hemorrhage and necrosis are present, with small foci of white-gray, well-preserved tissue interspersed among hemorrhagic areas.

        (b) Histologic appearance

            (i) For the diagnosis of choriocarcinoma, two types of cells must be present—the **syncytiotrophoblast** and the **cytotrophoblast.** Syncytiotrophoblasts are large multinucleate cells with abundant eosinophilic cytoplasm and, occasionally, vacuolated cytoplasm. Cytotrophoblasts are cuboidal cells with dark nuclei and clear cytoplasm, arranged in sheets or cords.

            (ii) In some instances, these cells are arranged around stalks of fibroconnective tissue, resembling the normal architecture of the mature placenta.

            (iii) Extensive hemorrhage always is present, and foci of other germ cell tumors may be found.

    (3) Treatment. These tumors are sensitive to chemotherapy, which usually is given after orchiectomy.

    (4) Prognosis. The poor prognosis associated with these neoplasms (i.e., 2-year survival rate of less than 5%) often is ascribed to their tendency to invade blood vessels and disseminate to viscera (e.g., lungs, liver, brain).

2. **Tumors of specialized gonadal stroma.** The testicular stroma has the capacity to differentiate into a variety of patterns and to elaborate androgens, estrogens, or both. The **Leydig cell tumor** originates from the interstitial cells of the testis and accounts for about 1% of all testicular neoplasms.

a. **Clinical features**

    (1) Most Leydig cell tumors occur in the second to sixth decades of life, but they have been reported in males of all ages.

    (2) The symptoms are due to the tumor's ability to produce hormones.

        (a) If the tumor occurs before puberty, the clinical manifestations are those of precocious puberty because of androgen production.

        (b) In adults, bilateral gynecomastia and feminization resulting from excess estrogen are the main symptoms, present in up to 35% of patients.

b. **Pathology**

    (1) Gross appearance. Most Leydig cell tumors consist of several nodules that are 1 to 2 cm in diameter and yellow-brown. Hemorrhage and necrosis are rare.

    (2) Histologic appearance

        (a) The tumor consists of a fairly uniform population of cells with round nuclei and abundant eosinophilic cytoplasm.

        (b) A cigar-shaped structure—**Reinke's crystal**—is present in the cytoplasm, as are lipid vacuoles and brown pigment.

    c. Treatment consists of orchiectomy.

    d. Prognosis. The tumor usually behaves in a benign fashion, but malignancies can develop in up to 10% of cases. Malignancy is determined by the presence of invasive or metastatic spread to the lymph nodes, liver, lungs, or bones.

  3. Metastatic tumors to the testis are rare; malignant lymphoma and leukemia are the most common tumors to involve the testis.

F. Tumors of the epididymis are rare and usually are of mesenchymal origin. They can occur at any age, but predominantly affect men in the third to fifth decades of life. They manifest clinically as asymptomatic nodules that usually are discovered as incidental findings on routine physical examination.

  1. Adenomatoid tumor is a benign neoplastic growth of mesothelial origin.

    a. Grossly, the tumor is a small, white, solitary, well-demarcated nodule.

    b. Histologically, it consists of acidophilic cells arranged in solid cords. The cells are low, columnar, and cuboidal with a vacuolated cytoplasm. Variable amounts of stroma and smooth muscle fibers are present.

  2. Papillary cystadenoma originates in the efferent ducts and may be unilateral or bilateral. It is a common finding in patients with von Hippel-Lindau disease. **Histologically,** prominent papillae are lined by columnar cells with abundant, clear cytoplasm.

II. PROSTATE GLAND

A. Normal anatomy and embryology

  1. Anatomy

    a. Lobes. The prostate gland is divided into five lobes: an anterior, a middle, and a posterior lobe and two lateral lobes. These lobes are purely anatomical, without functional significance.

    b. Glands. There are three major types of glands in the prostate gland: the **periurethral glands,** which are the smallest; the **submucosal glands;** and the **external glands,** which comprise the largest portion of the prostate.

    c. Cells. The glands consist of two layers of cells: **flat cuboidal cells,** which are found in the basal layer, and **tall columnar cells,** which are oriented toward the lumen of the gland. The glands are surrounded by an eosinophilic basement membrane.

  2. Embryology. The prostate gland is formed by evagination from the posterior urethra and, therefore, is considered to be of endodermal origin. Normal development depends on endocrine stimulation.

B. Congenital anomalies of the prostate gland usually are associated with malformations of the urogenital system. The prostate may be **small or absent,** or **abnormal communications** may develop between the prostate and the ureter, the urethra, or both. Such communications may form cavities called **diverticula,** which resemble cysts in the prostate.

C. Inflammatory disorders

  1. Acute prostatitis usually results from local extension of an inflammatory process in the urethra or bladder. It may follow a local operative maneuver, such as urethral catheterization. The inflammatory process may involve the entire organ or entail only localized abscesses.

    a. Etiology. For a long time, *Neisseria gonorrhoeae* was considered the most common cause. However, other organisms, such as *E. coli,* staphylococci, and streptococci, recently have become the leading causes of acute prostatitis.

    b. Clinical features. Fever and lower abdominal pain are common.

    c. Pathology. Histologic examination reveals neutrophilic infiltration of both the stroma and glands.

2. Chronic prostatitis is clinically more significant than acute prostatitis because of its high rate of recurrence. It probably is the most common cause of relapsing urinary tract infection (UTI) in men.

   a. Etiology and pathogenesis. Both a bacterial and a nonbacterial form of the condition exist.

   (1) In most cases, bacterial prostatitis occurs insidiously and is not a sequela of acute prostatitis, although the causative organisms are the same as for the acute infection. Bacterial prostatitis predisposes to UTIs.

   (2) Nonbacterial prostatitis, in some cases, is thought to have a viral origin. It does not predispose to UTI.

   b. Clinical features. Chronic prostatitis predominantly affects older men and can cause low back pain, dysuria, urinary frequency and urgency, and prostatic enlargement and tenderness, although it often can be entirely asymptomatic. The clinical manifestations are similar for both bacterial and nonbacterial forms of the condition.

   c. Pathology

   (1) Histologically, chronic prostatitis causes an inflammatory reaction characterized by the aggregation of numerous lymphocytes, plasma cells, macrophages, and neutrophils within the glandular acini and fibrotic stroma. **Corpora amylacea** (i.e., large laminated calcifications) commonly are contained within the glands.

   (2) The nonspecific aggregations of lymphocytes that occur as part of the normal aging process should not be diagnosed as chronic prostatitis unless other inflammatory cells exist.

3. Granulomatous prostatitis occurs in two forms.

   a. In the first form, nonspecific granulomas occur secondary to either acute or chronic prostatitis, and authorities believe that their cause is retained prostatic secretions. **Histologically,** inflammatory cells accompany well-circumscribed granulomas of epithelial giant cells with few eosinophils.

   b. The second form represents tuberculosis of the prostate gland, usually following tuberculosis of the genitourinary tract.

4. Malacoplakia is a rare inflammatory reaction caused by *E. coli.* It can affect the prostate gland and urinary tract. The lesion predominantly consists of histiocytes and small calcified **Michaelis-Gutmann bodies.**

D. Benign nodular hyperplasia (also known as **benign prostatic hypertrophy, or BPH)** is an enlargement of the prostate that usually affects men over age 40. It occurs in more than 95% of men over age 70. The cause is not known, but it is believed to be due to certain hormonal changes, such as decreased androgen and increased estrogen production.

1. Clinical features. Benign nodular hyperplasia produces symptoms in only a small percentage of affected patients.

   a. When symptoms do occur, they are **secondary effects related to compression of the urethra or to retention of urine in the bladder.** These two problems, in turn, may be further complicated by distention and hypertrophy of the bladder, hydroureter, hydronephrosis, prostatitis, cystitis, renal infections, calculi, and infarctions.

   b. Hyperplasia does not predispose to prostatic cancer, according to most authorities.

2. Pathology

   a. Gross appearance

   (1) The enlarged prostate gland is firm and rubbery and weighs more than 50 g. (A normal prostate weighs 20 to 30 g.)

   (2) The middle lobe appears to be most commonly affected. This condition is in contrast to carcinoma of the prostate, which often involves the posterior lobe.

   (3) On cut section, the prostate may disclose numerous closely packed nodules exuding small amounts of milky fluids. Cystic changes may be present.

   (4) In nodules that are primarily glandular, the tissue is yellow–pink, soft, and fairly discretely demarcated. In those nodules that are primarily fibromuscular, the tissue is pale gray, tough, fibrous, and less clearly demarcated.

   b. Histologic appearance of the nodules varies greatly, depending on whether the nodules consist of only glandular structures, equal amounts of glandular and stromal elements, or predominantly smooth muscle and connective tissue.

E. Malignant prostatic tumors

1. **Prostatic carcinoma** is a malignant tumor of the glandular epithelium. Although it is the third most common cause of cancer-related death in men over age 50, it also is commonly an incidental finding at autopsy.

   a. **Etiology.** The cause of prostatic cancer is unknown, although certain predisposing factors have been suggested.

      (1) A clear association with advancing age (over age 50) has been established, as has a relationship with certain racial backgrounds (a high prevalence in blacks and a low prevalence in Asians).

      (2) Some studies suggest the possibility of an endocrine influence; other factors, such as viral infection and environmental influences (e.g., cadmium exposure), also have been contemplated as causes.

   b. **Clinical features**

      (1) Carcinoma of the prostate may arise in any lobe, but it most commonly originates in the posterior lobe, near the outer margins.

      (2) The clinical diagnosis of prostatic carcinoma usually is based on the rectal examination finding of an indurated area in the gland.

      (3) Small (occult) cancers are asymptomatic, and urinary symptoms appear only after the tumors have spread. Pain is a late symptom, reflecting involvement of capsular perineural spaces.

      (4) Patients with prostatic cancer can have elevated serum levels of prostatic-specific antigens, which can be used as tumor markers to detect recurrences and metastases.

   c. **Diagnosis**

      (1) **Laboratory findings.** Sensitive immunoassay techniques to test for an elevated level of serum acid phosphatase (specifically of prostatic origin) can detect prostatic carcinoma in many cases before it has extended beyond the capsule.

      (2) **Bone scan and x-ray** may reveal multiple osteoblast metastatic lesions in the pelvis, ribs, skull, and spine when the disease has spread beyond the prostate gland.

   d. **Pathology**

      (1) **Gross appearance.** Prostatic carcinomas characteristically appear as nodular, ill-defined areas of a stone-hard consistency, from gray-white to yellow.

      (2) **Histologic appearance.** Most prostatic cancers are adenocarcinomas, consisting of glandular structures.

         (a) Two types of cells may be seen: **clear cells** with abundant foamy cytoplasm or **dark spindle cells** with condensed cytoplasm. The cells have prominent nucleoli, and different degrees of anaplasia can be present (Figure 17-3).

         (b) The normal lobular architecture is destroyed because the **malignant acini** grow irregularly.

         (c) **Perineural invasion** is a common finding.

   e. **Grading** prostatic carcinoma is based on the degree of glandular differentiation and the pattern of growth in relation to the stroma (**Gleason classification).**

   f. **Treatment** includes antiandrogenic therapy (i.e., orchiectomy and estrogen therapy), radiotherapy, and chemotherapy.

   g. **Prognosis.** Tumors that are well differentiated and have not metastasized are associated with a good 5- to 15-year survival rate. Eventually, however, relapse occurs and the disease spreads, with the most frequent sites of metastases being regional lymph nodes, bones, lungs, liver, and brain.

2. **Sarcomas** are uncommon tumors of the prostate gland, which usually have a rapid growth and a high malignant potential. They are predominantly of two types.

   a. **Rhabdomyosarcomas** most commonly affect children.

   b. **Leiomyosarcomas** most commonly affect adults.

III. PENIS

A. Normal anatomy and embryology

1. **Anatomy**

   a. The **body** of the penis is composed of two lateral **corpora cavernosa** and one medial **corpus spongiosum,** which contains the urethra. These three bodies are bound together by a

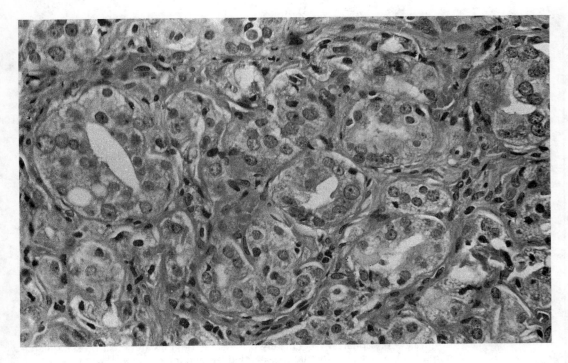

Figure 17-3. Prostatic adenocarcinoma, showing glandular formation (high power).

tough, fibrous connective tissue capsule known as the **tunica albuginea,** and they are covered by pigmented skin that folds at the distal extremity to form the **prepuce.**

b. The **glans** of the penis is formed by the distal molding of the three corpora.

c. The **cavernous bodies** of the penis consist of erectile tissue that expands and becomes rigid when filled with blood.

2. **Embryology.** The **genital tubercle** forms the penis, and the **urethral folds** unite to form the majority of the penile urethra.

B. Congenital anomalies

1. **Hypospadias and epispadias**

a. In **hypospadias,** the most common developmental anomaly of the penis, the urethral meatus is on the underside (ventral surface) of the penis. Ventral curvature, known as **chordee,** usually is present.

b. In **epispadias,** the urethral opening is on the upper (dorsal) surface of the penis.

2. **Phimosis** is constriction of the orifice of the prepuce so that the prepuce cannot be retracted over the glans. This condition often is associated with **balanitis,** a chronic inflammation of the glans penis.

C. Inflammatory disorders. A variety of infections may specifically involve the glans and prepuce (e.g., herpes, syphilis, granuloma inguinale, and lymphogranuloma venereum).

D. Tumors of the penis

1. **Benign condyloma acuminatum** is a papillary excrescence in the coronal sulcus and inner surface of the prepuce. It is caused by human papillomavirus (HPV).

a. **Clinical features.** The lesions usually occur on the glans penis and prepuce, although the urethra and, less commonly, the bladder and ureters may be affected.

b. **Pathology**

(1) **Gross appearance.** The tumors look like a cauliflower.

(2) **Histologic appearance.** A complicated papillary structure characterized by pronounced acanthosis and hyperplasia of the prickle cell layer is present. The basement membrane of the lesion always is intact.

2. Malignant tumors
   a. Erythroplasia of Queyrat is a form of epithelial dysplasia, which may range from mild cellular changes to carcinoma in situ (i.e, **Bowen's disease);** it usually is found on the glans penis and prepuce. In Bowen's disease, the malignant cells are well confined to the basement membrane, with no evidence of invasion. Pathologically, the lesions appear as well-defined, reddish, and shiny plaques.
   b. Squamous cell carcinoma (SCC) of the penis accounts for about 1% to 2% of all cancers of the male genital tract. It occurs most commonly in men between age 40 and 70.
      (1) Etiology. As with most cancers, the etiology is unknown; however, chronic inflammation and accumulations of smegma have been postulated as predisposing factors.
      (2) Clinical features. SCC of the penis is most common in uncircumcised men and presents as an ulcerated, painful lesion that bleeds easily.
      (3) Pathology
         (a) Gross appearance. The lesion appears as exophytic, ulcerated masses of variable dimensions.
         (b) Histologic appearance. The tumor is identical to the SCC that occurs in the skin, tending to be well differentiated and keratinized (see Chapter 24 VIII B 2 b).
      (4) Metastasis. Although it grows slowly, the lesion metastasizes to regional lymph nodes.
      (5) Treatment consists of amputation.
      (6) Prognosis. Patients have a 5-year survival rate of 50%.

STUDY QUESTIONS

Directions: Each of the numbered items or incomplete statements in this section is followed by answers or by completions of the statement. Select the **one** lettered answer or completion that is **best** in each case.

1. Acute orchitis refers to an acute inflammation of the testicular parenchyma. Which statement concerning this condition is true?

(A) It is a common complication of mumps
(B) It is associated with a relatively high incidence of testicular cancer
(C) It is more common in patients with cryptorchidism
(D) It may result from epididymal infection
(E) The presence of acid-fast bacilli on culture specimens is diagnostic

2. Which tumor is associated with the best 5-year survival rate?

(A) Choriocarcinoma
(B) Seminoma
(C) Embryonal cell carcinoma
(D) Teratoma
(E) Yolk sac tumor

3. Leydig cell tumors of the testis have a unique histologic feature, which is referred to as a

(A) Michaelis-Gutmann body
(B) Schiller-Duval body
(C) psammoma body
(D) Reinke's crystal
(E) oxalate crystal

4. A grossly apparent, well-circumscribed white nodule in the epididymis of a patient undergoing testicular surgery is most likely to be which lesion?

(A) Tuberculous granuloma
(B) Adenomatoid tumor
(C) Spermatocytic granuloma
(D) Congenital malformation
(E) Focal infarct

5. Which statement is true of prostatic cancer?

(A) It most commonly arises in a periurethral location
(B) It is associated with an elevated human chorionic gonadotropin (hCG) serum level
(C) Bone is a common metastatic site
(D) Most prostate cancers are sarcomas
(E) Androgen supplementation is indicated

6. Which prostatic lobe is most often affected by benign nodular hyperplasia?

(A) Anterior lobe
(B) Posterior lobe
(C) Lateral lobe
(D) Middle lobe

7. What is the most common type of testicular germ cell tumor?

(A) Seminoma
(B) Embryonal cell tumor
(C) Yolk sac tumor
(D) Choriocarcinoma
(E) Teratoma

8. Which condition probably is the most common cause of recurrent urinary tract infections (UTIs) in men?

(A) Immunodeficiency disorders
(B) Malacoplakia
(C) Chronic prostatitis
(D) Kidney stones
(E) Syphilis

9. Which tumor marker has been associated with the yolk sac tumor of the testis?

(A) Carcinoembryonic antigen (CEA)
(B) Acid phosphatase
(C) human chorionic gonadotropin (hCG)
(D) Alpha-fetoprotein (AFP)
(E) Alpha$_1$-antitrypsin

1-D	4-B	7-A
2-B	5-C	8-C
3-D	6-D	9-D

10. A 25-year-old man presents with lower abdominal pain, high fever, and shaking chills. Digital rectal examination elicits an extremely painful response from the patient, and a diffusely enlarged boggy prostate is palpated. In addition, a purulent urethral discharge is noted. The etiologic agent of the patient's condition is most likely

(A) human papillomavirus (HPV)
(B) herpes simplex virus type III
(C) gram-negative diplococci
(D) Reinke's crystals
(E) corpora amylacea

11. A 60-year-old man complains of difficulty with urination. Physical examination reveals a smooth, diffusely enlarged prostate gland. A biopsy reveals benign prostatic hypertrophy (BPH). Which is the most likely etiology of the patient's urinary symptoms?

(A) Perineural invasion of local nerves
(B) Compression of sacral nerve roots
(C) Infiltration of prostatic tissue into the bladder wall
(D) Urethral compression
(E) Papillomatosis of urethral epithelium

12. All of the following are congenital abnormalities of the male genitourinary tract EXCEPT

(A) bifid scrotum
(B) anorchia
(C) malacoplakia
(D) hypospadias
(E) epispadias

13. Klinefelter's syndrome includes all of the following conditions EXCEPT

(A) hypogonadism
(B) infertility
(C) gynecomastia
(D) absence of germ cells

14. All of the following statements concerning prostatic carcinoma are generally accepted as true EXCEPT

(A) serum acid phosphatase levels can be elevated
(B) it is linked to environmental exposure to certain compounds
(C) metastatic bone disease is a common outcome
(D) it most often originates in the anterior lobe of the gland

10-C   13-D
11-D   14-D
12-C

ANSWERS AND EXPLANATIONS

1. The answer is D *[I D 1].*
Acute orchitis is an acute inflammation of the testis, which often involves the epididymis as a result of infectious organisms (most commonly *Escherichia coli*) ascending through the vas deferens or via lymphatic vessels. The most common sources of infection are acute urethritis, acute cystitis, and prostatitis; only rarely is acute orchitis a complication of mumps. Acute orchitis does not increase the likelihood of later testicular malignancy. The presence of caseating granulomas that demonstrate acid-fast bacilli is the hallmark of granulomatous orchitis.

2. The answer is B *[I E 1 c (5)].*
Of patients with testicular malignancies, those with seminomas have the best prognosis for survival. Survival of patients with seminomas is 90% to 98% at 5 years; with teratomas, 70% at 2 years; with embryonal cell carcinomas, 35% at 5 years; with infantile embryonal cell or yolk sac tumors, 50% at 5 years; and with choriocarcinoma, less than 5% at 2 years.

3. The answer is D *[I E 2 b (2)].*
The interstitial, or Leydig, cell tumor originates from the Leydig cells of the testis. Symptoms resulting from this tumor usually are related to the ability of the tumor to produce hormones. Histologically, Leydig cell tumors consist of uniform sheets of cells with eosinophilic cytoplasm. A cigar-shaped inclusion—Reinke's crystal—is present in the cytoplasm, along with lipid vacuoles and brown pigment.

4. The answer is B *[I F 1].*
Adenomatoid tumor is a benign neoplasm of the epididymis, which is thought to originate from mesothelial cells. Its typical gross appearance is that of a small, white, solitary tumor that is well circumscribed. Multiple confluent tubercles with caseous necrosis are present in tuberculous epididymitis. Spermatocytic granuloma is presumed to be the result of an inflammatory reaction toward a component of semen or spermatocytes. Infarction of the epididymis is not likely to result in a well-circumscribed nodule but, more typically, a fibrous scar.

5. The answer is C *[II E 1 c].*
Bone is a common site of distant metastases of prostate cancer, and these metastases are normally osteoblastic, showing up on areas of increased density on skeletal x-rays. Prostate cancer can involve any portion of the gland, but most commonly arises in the periphery. Most prostate cancers are adenocarcinomas (epithelial origin), not sarcomas (of mesenchymal origin), and such cancers are associated with elevated serum levels of prostate-specific antigen and prostatic acid phosphatase, not human chorionic gonadotropin (hCG). This cancer is treated with anti-estrogenic therapy; hence, androgen supplements are contraindicated.

6. The answer is D *[II D 2 a].*
Benign nodular hyperplasia occurs most commonly in the middle lobe of the prostate gland. By contrast, adenocarcinoma of the prostate most often involves the posterior lobe. Most authorities agree that benign nodular hyperplasia does not predispose to prostatic cancer.

7. The answer is A *[I E 1 c].*
Seminomas are the most common testicular tumor and account for approximately 70% of primary germ cell neoplasms of the testes. Teratomas are the second most common testicular tumor, accounting for only 20% to 25%. Yolk sac tumors, choriocarcinomas, and embryonal cell tumors occur much less frequently.

8. The answer is C *[II C 2].*
Chronic prostatitis, usually resulting from extension of an inflammatory process in the urethra or bladder, is a troublesome condition because of its tendency to recur. It probably is the most common cause of relapsing urinary tract infections (UTIs) in men. It is true that immunodeficient individuals are predisposed to recurrent UTIs; however, immunodeficiency diseases are relatively rare in the population. Malacoplakia is an unusual inflammatory reaction produced by *Escherichia coli* infections of the urinary bladder and prostate gland; it is characterized by large numbers of histiocytes and Michaelis-Gutmann bodies.

9. The answer is D *[I E 1 f (1)].*
The infantile embryonal cell carcinoma often is referred to as a yolk sac tumor because of its resemblance to the endodermal sinus and amniotic cavity of a yolk sac. It is predominantly a testicular tumor of children and is identified by the presence of elevated serum levels of alpha-fetoprotein (AFP) in affected patients. Human chorionic gonadotropin (hCG) is a marker for choriocarcinoma—the most malignant of testicular tumors.

10. The answer is C *[II C 1].*
The patient's symptoms and findings on physical examination are most consistent with acute bacterial prostatitis. *Neisseria gonorrhoeae* (gram-negative diplococci) is one of the common pathogens of this disorder. Neither of the viruses listed causes acute prostatitis and purulent urethritis. Reinke's crystals are microscopic cytoplasmic inclusions found in the Leydig cells of the testis—a normal finding. Corpora amylacea are laminated calcifications found in prostate glands in patients with chronic prostatitis, but they are a secondary effect of this process and in themselves are thought to be harmless.

11. The answer is D *[II D].*
The most common symptoms of benign prostatic hypertrophy (BPH) are decreased urine flow and urinary retention resulting from external compression of the urethra by an enlarged prostate gland. Sacral nerve roots are too far away to be involved. Perineural and bladder wall invasion are properties of carcinoma and are not seen in benign nodular hyperplasia. Urethral epithelium is transitional epithelium and does not become hyperplastic in BPH.

12. The answer is C *[I B 1, 3; II C 4; III B].*
Malacoplakia is an inflammatory process thought to be secondary to chronic bacterial infection. The other choices are congenital abnormalities of the male genitourinary tract: scrotum, testes, and penis.

13. The answer is D *[I C 3].*
Klinefelter's syndrome is characterized by testicular hypoplasia, azoospermia, gynecomastia, eunuchoid habitus, and, sometimes, mental retardation. Individuals with this syndrome have 47 chromosomes with an XXY karyotype. In germ cell aplasia (also called Sertoli-cell–only syndrome), germ cells are absent from the seminiferous tubules, so normal spermatogenesis also is absent.

14. The answer is D *[II E 1].*
Prostatic carcinoma is the most common malignancy in the male population beyond the fifth decade of life. An endocrine cause as well as various viral and environmental causes (e.g., cadmium exposure) have been postulated as etiologic explanations. Sensitive assays for the elevation of serum acid phosphatase levels of prostatic origin have helped in the early diagnosis of prostatic cancer; unfortunately, however, bone metastases as well as metastases to the lymph nodes, lungs, liver, and brain still account for significant morbidity. Nearly 75% of prostatic carcinomas are thought to originate in the posterior lobe of the gland.

18
Female Reproductive System
Maria J. Merino

I. CONDITIONS ASSOCIATED WITH DECREASED FERTILITY

A. Gonadal agenesis and dysgenesis

1. **General considerations.** Abnormalities in the formation of the ovaries include complete or partial failure of development and the presence of both ovarian and testicular structures in the same person. Phenotypic females may be genotypically abnormal (i.e., instead of an XX karyotype, they may have an XO, an XY, or a mosaic karyotype).

2. **Turner's syndrome** (usually an XO genotype). Persons with this condition have infantile external genitalia, short stature, webbed neck, and various skeletal abnormalities. Typically, the uterus is small. The gonads are represented by fibrous tissue or ovarian stroma without germ cells (**streak gonads**).

3. **XY dysgenetic syndromes**
   a. **Pure gonadal dysgenesis.** Patients with this rare syndrome have a normal female habitus with primary amenorrhea. The gonads may be streak gonads or ovotestes. A uterus is present.
   b. **Testicular feminization.** Certain persons with a feminine appearance have bilateral undescended, very immature testes lying in an intraabdominal or inguinal location. No uterus or vagina is present. The patient's chief complaint is amenorrhea or sterility. Some 30% of patients develop gonadal neoplasms, one-third of which are malignant.

B. Endometriosis is defined as benign but displaced endometrial tissue (glands and stroma) occurring outside the uterine fundic mucosa (Figure 18-1).

1. **Location.** The condition can occur anywhere in the pelvis or, less often, in extrapelvic sites. Endometriosis most often affects the uterine tubes, ovaries, cervix, and vagina. Adenomyosis is endometriosis in the wall of the uterus. Extragenital sites include the urinary bladder, intestines, appendix, laparotomy scars, and hernia sacs.

2. **Pathogenesis**
   a. **Sampson's theory** postulates that endometriosis is caused by **reflux menstruation** through the fallopian tubes and beyond into the ovaries and pelvis, with implantation of endometrial tissue.
   b. **Novak's theory** suggests that any part of the müllerian system may undergo a change to endometrial tissue via a **metaplasia** of the specialized surface epithelium (mesothelium). Most modern investigators favor this theory.
   c. Others have postulated that lymphatic or bloodborne **emboli** are responsible. This theory offers the best explanation for endometriosis in rare sites, such as the retroperitoneal lymph nodes and the lungs.

3. **Clinical features**
   a. Pelvic endometriosis is most common in women who delay childbearing. The major symptom is pain. Abnormal uterine bleeding also is common; it occurs because the ectopic endometrial tissue responds to the hormonal variations of the menstrual cycle.
   b. The response of the ectopic endometrium to cyclic hormonal changes can lead to smooth muscle hypertrophy and fibrosis in some affected organs (e.g., the intestine), which, in turn, may become obstructed. In scars and hernia sacs, monthly swelling and pain can result; and in the bladder, endometriosis can cause hematuria.

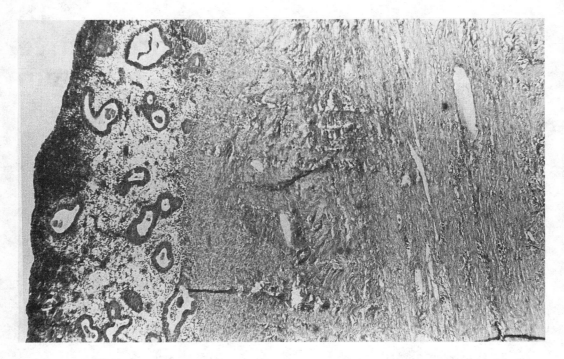

Figure 18-1. Endometriosis. Note the glands and stroma of endometrial type (*left*) in the ovary (low power).

    c. Infertility may develop because the uterine tubes are involved in almost all cases, and the response of the endometrial tissue to cyclic changes can lead to fibrosis and distortion or narrowing of the tubes.

  4. Pathology
    a. Grossly, endometriosis appears as tiny to large blue cysts, often on peritoneal surfaces. In the ovary, large "chocolate" cysts can occur as a result of repeated hemorrhage.
    b. Microscopically, endometrial glands and stroma are found, frequently surrounded by hemorrhage, hemosiderin, and fibrosis.

C. Pelvic inflammatory disease (PID) is an inflammatory (predominantly infectious) condition of the fallopian tubes (**salpingitis**) and paratubal tissues. It can lead to fibrosis, scarring, and obstruction of the tubes, with consequent risk of infertility or ectopic pregnancy.

  1. Etiology and pathogenesis
    a. Multiple factors or pathogens are frequently the cause of the disease; however, the causative infection most often is gonorrhea, usually venereally transmitted.
    b. Coliform organisms, especially *Escherichia coli,* also may be responsible. Recently, coliform organisms producing salpingitis have been found with increasing frequency in women wearing intrauterine devices (IUDs).
    c. Tubal tuberculosis is a rare cause of chronic salpingitis in the western hemisphere.

  2. Clinical features. Fever, pain, and other signs of infection are common. Although therapy may allow the infection to subside, damage to the tubal epithelium is irreversible, and **chronic salpingitis** ensues.

  3. Pathology
    a. The **acutely** inflamed fallopian tube is red and swollen; microscopically, the capillaries are congested, and pus is present in the lumen, wall, and serosa.
    b. As the infection continues, the tubal plicae adhere to each other. The infection extends outside the tube, producing paratubal and tuboovarian abscesses. Both tube and ovary become incorporated into an inflammatory mass, adhered by a fibrinopurulent exudate.
    c. In **chronic salpingitis,** the adherent plicae fuse, and fibrosis occurs. Adhesions may obliterate the lumen of the tube, leading to pyosalpinx or hydrosalpinx. The adhesions and stenosis produced are major causes of sterility and tubal pregnancy.

D. Ovarian causes of sterility

1. **Stein-Leventhal (polycystic ovary) syndrome** is characterized by infertility, hirsutism, obesity, and secondary amenorrhea in young women with enlarged, cystic ovaries. Some patients with this syndrome develop endometrial hyperplasia and, rarely, carcinoma.
   a. **Etiology.** The cause is unknown. The common finding is a persistent failure to ovulate. Biochemically, 17-ketosteroid production usually is normal, follicle-stimulating hormone (FSH) is normal, and androgens are found in excessive quantity in cyst fluid and urine.
   b. **Pathology**
      (1) **Grossly,** the ovaries are large (4 to 6 cm), their pale gray color produced by a thick fibrous capsule. Beneath the capsule are many small cystic spaces containing clear, watery fluid.
      (2) **Histologically,** normal structures are visible, but the pattern is abnormal. The capsule consists of dense fibrous tissue, which is markedly thicker than usual. The cysts are graafian follicles, developing or atretic. The theca layer is overly luteinized, although the granulosa layer is not. Ova are present, generally in normal numbers. The stroma, especially in the medulla, is prominent.

2. **Hyperthecosis and stromal hyperplasia** tend to be more masculinizing than the Stein-Leventhal syndrome and may cause true virilism. Onset of these conditions may not occur until middle-age or later, in contrast to the Stein-Leventhal syndrome, which affects young women.
   a. **Etiology.** The etiology and biochemical changes involved are unknown.
   b. **Pathologically,** the ovaries are large and solid, lacking cysts. Large, luteinized theca cells are distributed in groups throughout hyperplastic ovarian stroma.

II. CONDITIONS ASSOCIATED WITH FERTILITY, PREGNANCY, AND CONTRACEPTION

A. The menstrual cycle. The various hormonal changes that occur during the ovarian cycle lead to characteristic histologic alterations in the endometrium, affecting glands and stroma. Through endometrial biopsy, the stage of the menstrual cycle can be evaluated and, thus, ovulation estimated.

B. Disorders associated with pregnancy

1. **Spontaneous abortion** may result from trauma, blighted ova, viral infections, fetal death, or, most commonly, unknown reasons.

2. **Problems of labor and delivery** for an intrauterine pregnancy at or near term often are mechanical and chiefly involve fetal position, cephalopelvic disproportion, or abnormal placental implantation sites.

3. **Conditions affecting the placenta**
   a. **Multiple-gestation placentas.** With monozygotic twins, there may be a single placenta or two individual ones. When there is only one placenta, gross and histologic examination of the placental membranes at the separation zone will disclose, with a high degree of accuracy, whether the pregnancy is mono- or diamniotic as well as whether it is mono- or dichorionic.
   b. **Preexisting maternal vascular disease** often is reflected in an extremely vascular placenta. Maternal hypertension, diabetes, systemic lupus erythematosus (SLE), and renal disease all may cause vascular abnormalities. Such lesions may be accompanied by degenerative changes and hyalinization of chorionic villi and placental infarcts.
   c. **Placental abruption (abruptio placentae)** is separation of the placenta from the uterine wall before delivery of the infant.
      (1) **The separation,** which may extend for only a few millimeters or be complete, impedes normal postpartum vascular constriction, and bleeding results (**retroplacental hemorrhage**).
      (2) **Clinically,** although mild abruption may be asymptomatic, severe abruption produces uterine rigidity, severe abdominal pain, shock, and occasional disseminated intravascular coagulation (DIC) in the mother as well as severe fetal distress or fetal death.
      (3) **Abruption** is associated with preexisting **maternal hypertension** in 25% to 50% of cases; it is the **most common recognizable cause of fetal death**.
   d. **Placenta previa** is the condition in which the placenta develops in the lower uterine segment and partially or completely covers the internal os, requiring delivery of the placenta before the fetus. Painless vaginal bleeding is the most common symptom. Because the abnormality compromises the infant at birth and predisposes to maternal hemorrhage, its presence generally compels delivery by cesarean section.

e. Placenta accreta, a rare condition, is implantation of the placenta in the myometrial surface; chorionic villi may penetrate the uterine muscle (**placenta increta**), or they may penetrate the entire myometrial wall and extend into the uterine serosa (**placenta percreta**).

    (1) Placenta accreta and its variants occur in a uterus that previously has been scarred by infection or trauma, and they implant in areas of denuded endometrium that lack normal decidua.

    (2) These lesions can cause hemorrhage both during and after delivery because the placenta cannot separate normally from the uterus.

f. Chorioangioma is a true hemangioma of the placenta. Found in only 1% of pregnancies, it is still the most common benign tumor of the placenta. It rarely is large (usually under 5 cm) and has no clinical manifestations unless it expands to a size that compromises the placenta by replacement.

4. Ectopic pregnancy. Pregnancy outside the uterus can occur in the ovary or pelvic peritoneum, but it affects the **fallopian tubes** in over 95% of cases (Figure 18-2).

    a. The incidence of ectopic pregnancy is increased in women who have a history of PID. Tubal pregnancies comprise about 2% of all pregnancies; but if a patient has one such pregnancy, her chance of having another is 1 in 10.

    b. As a tubal pregnancy progresses, the wall of the tube is distended and weakened by infiltration of chorionic villi. With progressive enlargement, tubal rupture and hemorrhage become inevitable. Most tubal pregnancies progress for 6 to 12 weeks and then rupture.

    c. Ectopic pregnancy is life-threatening to the mother and requires surgical treatment.

5. Preeclampsia and eclampsia (toxemia of pregnancy)

    a. Etiology. The cause is unknown.

    b. Clinical features. In the last trimester of pregnancy, about 6% to 7% of women develop hypertension, edema, albuminuria, and salt retention, a syndrome known as preeclampsia. Eclampsia is the more severe form of the syndrome, in which the preceding symptoms are accompanied by convulsions. Eclampsia is a frequent cause of maternal and fetal mortality. The condition tends to occur in young primigravid women.

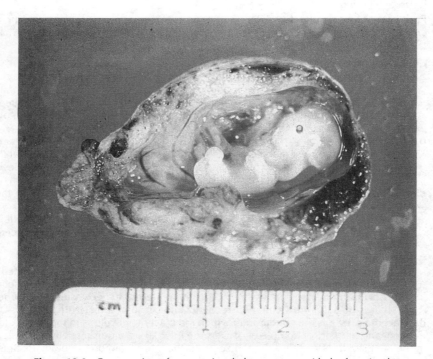

Figure 18-2. Cross section of an ectopic tubal pregnancy, with the fetus in place.

c. **Pathology.** The pathologic findings are similar to those in the generalized Shwartzman reaction (which occurs after endotoxin doses administered 24 hours apart), suggesting that degenerative products of necrotic decidua or the trophoblast may be an inciting factor. Maternal autopsies have shown hemorrhage, necrosis, and fibrin deposition in the liver, kidneys, and brain. The placenta shows aging changes, necrosis, trophoblastic degeneration, and large infarcts.

6. **Disorders of the trophoblast**

   a. **Hydatidiform mole** results from the missed abortion of a pathologic ovum. The condition occurs when the death of an embryo at 3 to 5 weeks' gestation is followed by hydropic changes in the vascular villi; because the trophoblast survives the embryo, the villi accumulate fluid and swell.

      (1) **Incidence.** In the United States, hydatidiform mole occurs in 1 in 2000 pregnancies; in the Orient, it occurs in 1 in 125 to 250 pregnancies. Poor nutrition, consanguinity, and either very young or very old maternal age seem to increase the incidence.

      (2) **Clinically,** the uterus often enlarges more rapidly than normal, and serum levels of human chorionic gonadotropin (hCG) are elevated.

      (3) **Pathology**

         (a) **Grossly,** when the mole aborts, a large mass of edematous tissue with grapelike bulbs of hydropic villi is found.

         (b) **Microscopically,** the hydropic villi are sparsely cellular and avascular; a syncytiotrophoblast covers them. Occasionally, highly proliferative trophoblastic lesions appear.

      (4) **Prognosis.** In 80% of affected patients, the condition has a benign course after uterine evacuation. The remainder of patients eventually manifest evidence of an aggressive malignant lesion, with invasion of the myometrium or extrauterine tissues.

   b. **Choriocarcinoma of gestational origin** is a rare neoplasm composed of malignant trophoblasts. Of these lesions, 50% are preceded by molar pregnancy, 25% by abortion, 22% by normal pregnancy, and 3% by ectopic pregnancy.

      (1) **Pathology.** Choriocarcinoma consists of soft (possibly necrotic) hemorrhagic nodules, microscopically showing admixtures of syncytiotrophoblastic and cytotrophoblastic cells and vascular invasion.

      (2) **Prognosis and treatment**

         (a) Actinomycin D or methotrexate can cure patients with intrauterine tumors, and combination chemotherapy with the two drugs plus cyclophosphamide often is effective for patients with widespread metastases. Overall, chemotherapy is associated with a 75% to 80% cure rate. Hysterectomy is not needed; moreover, normal pregnancies with viable offspring are not unusual in women cured of choriocarcinoma.

         (b) The tumor produces hCG, and its measurement is used clinically to follow response to therapy and determine prognosis.

C. **Disorders associated with oral contraceptives and intrauterine devices**

1. **Oral contraceptives**

   a. Most **endocervical changes** produced by oral contraceptives are recapitulations of the microglandular hyperplasia seen in pregnancy.

   b. In the endometrium, oral contraceptives can produce **atypia** in glandular epithelium and hyperplasia. Recently, **adenocarcinoma of the endometrium** (usually a disease of postmenopausal women) has occurred with abnormally high frequency in young women who take sequential oral contraceptives.

   c. For a discussion of how oral contraceptives affect other body systems, see Chapter 4 V C 4 c.

2. **IUDs.** In the endometrium, **squamous metaplasia** and **chronic endometritis** are found in about 1 in 5 women using IUDs. The incidence of tuboovarian infections (and possibly of ectopic pregnancies) appears to increase in women using IUDs.

III. INFECTIOUS DISEASES

A. **Viral diseases**

1. **Herpes genitalis** is caused by herpes simplex virus type 2 (HSV-2), which is venereally transmitted.

   a. Clinical features. In over 90% of cases, the infection is subclinical. If symptomatic, painful focal vesicles or blisters are found on the cervix, vagina, and vulva. Associated dysuria, fever, and malaise may occur. The herpetic lesion usually resolves spontaneously in 1 to 3 weeks, but recurrences are common.

   b. Pathology

   (1) Grossly, the lesions are 1-mm vesicles surrounded by an erythematous base; focal ulceration may be present.

   (2) Microscopically and on **Papanicolaou (Pap) smears,** the hallmark is the finding of multinucleate giant epithelial cells with homogeneous intranuclear inclusions.

   c. Complications

   (1) The possibility of a relationship between herpesvirus infection and **cervical cancer** is discussed in IV B 6 c (2).

   (2) Active herpetic infection in a pregnant woman usually demands cesarean section to avoid systemic, possibly fatal, **disease in the newborn infant**.

2. Condyloma acuminatum (Figure 18-3) is a human papillomavirus (HPV) infection. Extremely common in women with multiple sex partners, it is an incidental finding in 2% to 10% of Pap smears and usually is asymptomatic.

   a. Pathology

   (1) Grossly, 2% to 4% of affected women have verrucous (warty) papillary tumors on the cervix, vagina, or vulva. However, according to recent evidence , most HPV infections cause flat lesions that especially involve the cervix.

   (2) Microscopically, the affected epithelium is thickened, with superficial cells showing large crinkled nuclei surrounded by clear cytoplasm (**balloon cells, koilocytosis**).

   b. Complications. Studies have shown that 20% to 30% of affected women have a coexistent cervical dysplasia. A possible etiologic association with cervical cancer is discussed in IV B 6 d (3).

B. Syphilis. Caused by the spirochete *Treponema pallidum,* syphilis is transmitted either by venereal contact or, transplacentally, by an infected mother to her unborn child (**congenital syphilis**).

1. Clinical features. Three stages of the venereally transmitted disease are recognized.

   a. Primary syphilis is characterized by the development of a painless, hard-based ulcer, the **chancre,** at the point of inoculation, usually in the genital area. However, this stage is often asymptomatic.

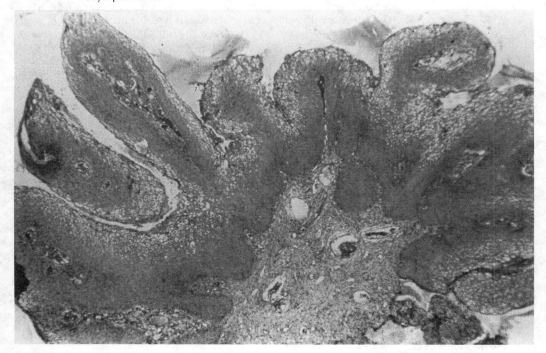

Figure 18-3. A papillary condyloma of the cervix (low power).

    b. Secondary syphilis, usually occurring 1 to 4 months later, is characterized by a diffuse **skin rash** and generalized (especially inguinal) **lymphadenopathy,** often accompanied by fever and malaise. The rash may develop into condylomata lata in moist areas.

    c. Tertiary syphilis, often appearing after latent periods of 1 to 30 years, affects the cardio-vascular system and central nervous system (CNS). Other areas, especially the liver, bones, and joints, may be affected by **gummas**.

  2. Pathologically, the lesions in the three stages are different.

    a. A **chancre** is a grossly shallow ulcer. Microscopically, the epithelium is ulcerated, and the ulcer base shows an intense, predominantly plasmacytic infiltrate, accompanied by an obliterative endarteritis. Spirochetes are numerous.

    b. Skin biopsies from the **rash** of secondary syphilis show a subepidermal, mononuclear-cell (plasmacytic) infiltrate, chiefly perivascular; spirochetes may be found. The lymph nodes demonstrate an extensive capsular fibrosis and plasmacytic perivasculitis.

    c. The cardiac and CNS lesions of tertiary syphilis are described in Chapter 9 V C and Chapter 21 III A 3, respectively.

  3. The **diagnosis** of syphilis is made either by dark-field examination of material from the primary chancre (when present) or by serologic tests.

C. Gonorrhea. The most common venereal disease in the United States, gonorrhea is caused by the diplococcus *Neisseria gonorrhoeae*. This organism has surface pili that preferentially attach to endocervical and fallopian tube epithelium, allowing the organism access into host cells.

  1. Clinical features. Vaginal discharge and dysuria are the most common symptoms, but up to 50% of infected women are asymptomatic. Constitutional symptoms—fever, abdominal pain, and vomiting—are indicative of acute salpingitis with pelvic peritonitis (**PID**). Gonorrheal infection is responsible for about 50% to 65% of cases of PID.

  2. Pathology

    a. The initial involvement may affect Bartholin's glands or the endocervix and often is followed by ascending infection that reaches the fallopian tubes. The tubal epithelium is exquisitely sensitive to the gonococcus, and acute salpingitis with purulent exudate (**pyosalpinx**) results.

    b. Extension into the ovaries and pelvic peritoneum may ensue, with formation of adhesions and decreased fertility.

  3. Diagnosis of gonorrhea requires identification of the organism either by gram-stained direct smears of infected material or by appropriate bacteriologic cultures.

D. Chlamydial infections. Chlamydial organisms are considered to be bacteria although they undergo obligate intracellular development in the cytoplasm of infected cells. Some subtypes of *Chlamydia trachomatis* cause lymphogranuloma venereum; other subtypes produce nonspecific urethritis and cervicitis.

  1. Lymphogranuloma venereum is much less common in the United States than the venereal diseases just described.

    a. Clinical features. Lymphogranuloma venereum is characterized by transient genital or anal ulcers (often overlooked by the affected patient), followed 2 to 6 weeks later by regional lymphadenitis. The lymph node involvement is associated with abscesses and fistula formation, often including the rectal, vaginal, and inguinal areas; at later stages, these lesions heal by scarring and can produce strictures.

    b. Diagnosis usually is made by serologic testing (microimmunofluorescent antibody testing or complement fixation).

  2. Other chlamydial genital infections (e.g., cervicitis, salpingitis) usually are asymptomatic in women and are brought to clinical attention by a concomitant asymptomatic venereal disease.

    a. Clinical features. The greatest importance in recognizing these chlamydial infections lies in their possible **transmission to neonates** at parturition, resulting in neonatal conjunctivitis and pneumonia.

    b. Diagnosis can be made by finding characteristic intracytoplasmic inclusion bodies in cervicovaginal cytologic smears.

E. Chancroid. Caused by *Haemophilus ducreyi,* this venereal disease is endemic in tropical countries; it is of minor significance in the United States.

1. **Clinical features**
   a. One or, more frequently, multiple painful, soft ulcers are noted at the site of inoculation after an incubation period of 3 to 5 days. Early, rapid enlargement of regional lymph nodes may occur; inguinal nodes may develop a fluctuant abscess (**bubo**). Acute, tender, suppurative **lymphadenitis** is found, often unilaterally, in draining nodes.
   b. The disease usually is self-limited, eventually resulting in **scarring** of affected lymph nodes and ulcer sites.

2. **Pathology.** The chancroid ulcer shows superficial necrosis, with underlying granulation tissue and fibrosis.

3. **Diagnosis.** Specific diagnosis requires isolation of *H. ducreyi* from an ulcer or bubo.

F. **Granuloma inguinale.** Caused by the organism *Calymmatobacterium (Donovania) granulomatis,* this presumedly venereally transmitted disease is most common in tropical areas and is rare in the United States.

   1. **Clinically,** at the site of inoculation, an initial papule gives rise to a large serpiginous ulcer. Many satellite lesions may occur and become infected. Regional lymphadenopathy may ensue.

   2. **Pathologically,** signs of acute and chronic inflammation are present. The characteristic vacuolated macrophages containing the causative organisms (**Donovan bodies**) are demonstrable by Giemsa stain.

   3. **Diagnosis** requires identification of Donovan bodies in smears, scrapings, or biopsies of active lesions.

G. **Candidiasis (moniliasis).** This infection is the most common type of vulvovaginitis. The causative fungus, *Candida albicans,* normally is a commensal organism but can become pathogenic under certain conditions (e.g., pregnancy, diabetes, cancer, immunosuppression, ingestion of oral contraceptives or systemic antibiotics).

   1. **Clinically,** affected patients present with intense vulva pruritus. The vulva and vagina may be reddened, and characteristic white patches may be present. Vaginal secretions usually have a white, curdled appearance.

   2. **Diagnosis** is made on clinical grounds, although cytologic smears can confirm it by demonstrating the causative fungus.

H. **Trichomoniasis** is a vaginal infection occurring in women of reproductive age.

   1. **Clinically,** the major symptom is a copious, malodorous, greenish-yellow or gray vaginal discharge, sometimes accompanied by pruritus. The prevalence of asymptomatic infection is high, especially in men.

   2. **Diagnosis** often can be made by clinical examination and can be confirmed by cytologic smears or wet-mount preparations. Atypia in cervicovaginal epithelium may be noted in cytologic preparations.

IV. INFLAMMATORY AND NEOPLASTIC UTERINE DISORDERS

A. **Tumors of the myometrium**

   1. **Leiomyomas (fibroids)** are extremely common benign tumors found in 30% to 60% of women at autopsy (Figure 18-4). Usually multiple, these tumors arise from uterine muscle and may be found in subserosal, intramural, or submucosal locations.
      a. Usually asymptomatic, leiomyomas may undergo degenerative changes leading to pain; if submucosal, they may cause bleeding.
      b. Leiomyomas are hormone-dependent and may increase in size during pregnancy or in women using oral contraceptives. Rarely, they may produce mechanical problems at the time of delivery.
      c. Leiomyomas can interfere with conception.

   2. **Leiomyosarcomas** comprise only 0.5% to 1% of mesenchymal uterine tumors but are the most common sarcoma of the uterus.
      a. **Pathologically,** it is doubtful that leiomyomas undergo malignant change. Most leiomyosarcomas arise de novo.

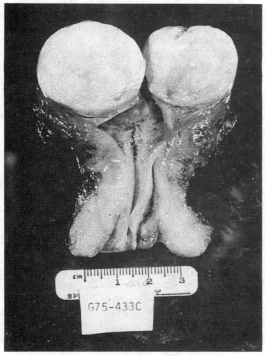

Figure 18-4. Leiomyoma of the uterus, showing a circumscribed homogeneous mass in the wall of the uterus.

  b. Prognosis depends on the extent of the lesion, the size, and mitotic activity. With well-differentiated leiomyosarcomas, a 40% to 50% 5-year survival rate follows surgery and chemotherapy. Premenopausal women fare better than older patients.

B. Disorders of the cervix

 1. Acute cervicitis may be associated with ulceration, especially following trauma at parturition or after specific bacterial infections. The endocervical glands may proliferate in response to inflammation; the lumina of the glands may become occluded, resulting in cystic dilation of the glands and, thus, **nabothian cysts**.

 2. Chronic cervicitis with **squamous metaplasia** is found almost universally in postmenopausal women. The inflammation varies considerably in severity.

 3. Cervical erosion is characterized by extension of the endocervical mucosa beyond the external os onto the exocervix, where it overgrows destroyed squamous epithelium. This process probably is not inflammatory, but is either a congenital condition or a response to a factor, such as vaginal pH.

  a. In a reparative attempt, the squamous epithelium of the exocervix grows back over the eroding endocervical mucosa, in a process called **epidermization**. Also, squamous cells may originate from reserve cells of the endocervix, giving rise to squamous metaplasia.

  b. These competing processes may alter the position of the squamocolumnar junction in the so-called **transformation zone**.

 4. Pregnancy or the use of oral contraceptives may stimulate glandular hyperplasia, leading to what has been called the **"pill tumor."** This florid pattern of hyperplasia must be differentiated from adenocarcinoma.

 5. Endocervical polyp is an overgrown fold of endocervical mucosa. The lesion may have a papillary pattern and contain cystic glands. It is extremely vascular and bleeds easily; it is never malignant, and it is common in postmenopausal women.

6. Cancer of the cervix
   a. Classification
      (1) Cervical intraepithelial neoplasia comprises premalignant changes, such as dysplasia and carcinoma in situ.
      (2) Squamous cell carcinoma (SCC) represents 95% of cervical cancers.
      (3) Adenocarcinoma of endocervical glands represents about 5% of cervical cancers.
      (4) Clear cell carcinoma is a rare form of cervical cancer.
   b. Pathogenesis. The **single cell theory** is the most widely accepted pathogenetic theory concerning cervical SCC and the premalignant states of dysplasia and carcinoma in situ.
      (1) Studies of glucose-6-phosphate dehydrogenase isoenzymes suggest that, in 95% of cases, dysplasia and carcinoma in situ originate in one cell.
      (2) Thus, cancer of the cervix is believed to begin as mild dysplasia in a single cell at the squamocolumnar junction, to pass through a carcinoma in situ stage, and then to involve the transformation zone and the endocervix.
   c. Epidemiology
      (1) A positive epidemiologic relationship exists between cancer of the cervix and the following factors:
         (a) Early age at first coitus
         (b) Multiple sexual partners
         (c) Low socioeconomic status
         (d) Multiparity, which suggests that birth trauma may play a role
         (e) Poor hygiene (smegma may be a factor, as the incidence of cervical intraepithelial neoplasia is low in Jews and Moslems, who practice circumcision)
      (2) Women who have had an **HSV-2** infection have a higher incidence of cervical cancer than those in control populations; women who have cervical cancer have a higher incidence of antibodies to the HSV than women in control populations.
         (a) In vitro experiments have shown the oncologic potential of HSV-2. Recently, hybridization studies have demonstrated part of the HSV genome incorporated within the genetic makeup of cervical cancer cells.
         (b) Proof of causation requires further evidence, however; and it should be noted that a high incidence of two coexisting diseases may occur without a causal relationship between them.
      (3) Recent studies suggest an association between cervical intraepithelial neoplasia and condyloma (HPV) infection of the cervix and vagina. Further studies are needed for adequate interpretation of this relationship.
   d. Cervical intraepithelial neoplasia
      (1) Clinical features. The entire stage of cervical intraepithelial neoplasia has a mean duration of 12 to 15 years from mild dysplasia to carcinoma in situ.
      (2) Diagnosis. Because these two premalignant changes produce no gross visible effects, diagnosis depends on biopsy or exfoliative cytology (the Pap test).
         (a) Biopsy may be directed by use of Lugol's solution (which fails to stain dysplastic areas) or by colposcopy (which identifies abnormal areas by changes in vascular pattern).
         (b) Cytology has the advantage of being atraumatic and easy to repeat.
      (3) Pathology
         (a) Dysplasia usually refers to a combination of nuclear atypia, focal hypercellularity of the epithelium, and loss of cellular polarity involving only part of the epithelial thickness (thus preserving some evidence of normal cellular maturation toward the surface).
         (b) Carcinoma in situ (preinvasive cancer) implies a high mitotic rate, marked cellularity, and loss of polarity and maturation throughout the full thickness of the cervical epithelium (Figure 18-5).
      (4) Prognosis for patients with cervical intraepithelial neoplasia is 100% cure with treatment.
   e. Squamous cell carcinoma
      (1) The stage after carcinoma in situ is **microinvasive cancer,** an invasion of less than 3 mm in depth. This stage is followed by **invasive cancer,** which appears as a granular, papillary, or ulcerated lesion that bleeds easily and is near the external os.
      (2) When **invasion** begins, the cells penetrate into the stroma, keratinize, and may reach the lymphatics. From there, they disseminate first to parametrial, iliac, and hypogastric nodes; later to sacral and obturator nodes; and finally to lumbar and inguinal nodes.

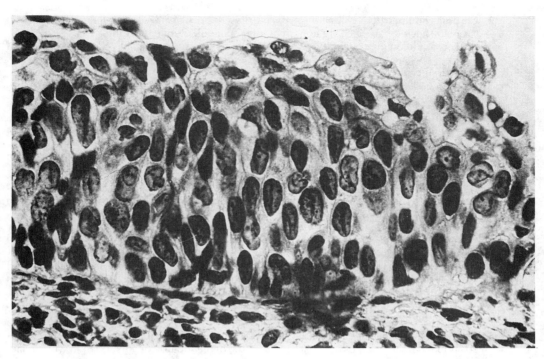

Figure 18-5. Carcinoma in situ of the cervix, showing full-thickness mucosal involvement by neoplastic cells (low power).

    (3) The **average age at diagnosis** of invasive cancer is 40 to 50 years, which is 8 to 10 years later than the average age at diagnosis of carcinoma in situ.

    (4) The **incidence** of invasive cervical cancer has been halved in the past 25 years as a result of routine cytologic screening (i.e., Pap testing), which allows identification of dysplasia, the presumed precursor of the lesion. Invasive cervical cancer now occurs in about 2% of all women in the United States. Previously, carcinoma of the cervix was 20 times more common than endometrial cancer; now the incidence is roughly equal.

    (5) **Prognosis** is related to the clinical stage, with lymphatic spread being the most important consideration. For stage I lesions with negative nodes, the 5-year survival rate is almost 90%; for stage IV lesions, it is closer to 10%.

    (6) **Treatment** consists of hysterectomy for the microinvasive stage and radiotherapy for the frankly invasive stage.

  f. **Adenocarcinoma of endocervical glands** is roughly comparable to SCC in its behavior and degree of malignancy because its lymphatic spread is similar.

    (1) **Clinically,** patients with endocervical adenocarcinoma resemble those with endometrial carcinoma more than they resemble those with SCC. They tend to be postmenopausal, nulliparous (or have few children), obese, hypertensive, and diabetic.

    (2) **Prognosis** depends on the degree of differentiation and the extent of the lesion.

  g. **Clear cell carcinoma,** a rare form of cervical cancer, may occur in all age-groups, although it predominates in young females.

    (1) **Pathology. Microscopically,** clear cell carcinoma is characterized by the formation of glands and papillae lined by clear cells with abundant cytoplasm (the so-called **hobnail cells**).

    (2) **Prognosis** for patients with clear cell carcinoma is favorable; the 5-year survival rate is 40%.

C. Disorders of the endometrium

  1. **Acute endometritis** usually is caused by a bacterial infection of the endometrium in association with septic abortion. Occasionally, a virus [e.g., cytomegalovirus (CMV)] or fungus (e.g., *Aspergillus*) may be responsible.

2. Chronic endometritis is characterized by the presence of plasma cells in inflamed endometrial stroma. Affected patients have abnormal, often painful, uterine bleeding.
   a. The condition may occur following abortion, post partum (especially if retained placental fragments are present), in the presence of an IUD, and after instrumentation of the endometrial cavity.
   b. Over 50% to 60% of cases have no known cause, which may reflect an immunologic response, possibly to sperm.

3. Polyps of the endometrium occur at or near the time of menopause and may cause bleeding.
   a. The polyps are composed of endometrial glands and stroma and represent a portion of basalis endometrium that is unresponsive to the hormonal cycle.
   b. The polyps may become necrotic at their tips, ulcerate, and bleed. Rarely, they contain carcinoma.

4. Hyperplasia of the endometrium is found in patients with relative or absolute **hyperestrogenism,** as accompanies obesity, functioning ovarian tumors, exogenous estrogen intake, and Stein-Leventhal syndrome.
   a. Cystic hyperplasia is characterized by the presence of ectatic glands that are lined by plump, benign endometrial cells. It carries a 1% to 2% risk for progression to endometrial adenocarcinoma.
   b. Adenomatous hyperplasia is characterized by an increase in the number of glands (and hence in the gland-to-stroma ratio), with budding and a new gland formation. The risk of cancer is 10%.
   c. Atypical adenomatous hyperplasia is characterized by the presence of cytologic atypia in the individual glandular cells. The risk of cancer is 20% to 25%.

5. Metaplastic changes in endometrial glandular tissue may be squamous, tubal, papillary, or eosinophilic. The changes occur around the time of menopause or after, often in women taking exogenous hormones, and may be in association with various degrees of hyperplasia. Metaplastic changes have been misinterpreted as adenocarcinoma of the endometrium, from which the changes differ in their lack of cytologic atypia.

6. Adenocarcinoma of the endometrium
   a. Incidence. The incidence of endometrial adenocarcinoma has increased over the past 25 years and now is roughly equal to that of cervical cancer (12 to 15 cases per 100,000). The highest incidence occurs at the age of endometrial atrophy (i.e., postmenopausally) in middle-class, often obese, women.
   b. Etiology. Unopposed **estrogen action** during prolonged anovulatory cycles premenopausally appears to lead to endometrial hyperplasia, which is a possible precursor of endometrial cancer. The etiologic role of estrogen is supported by an increased incidence of endometrial cancer, both in women who have functioning ovarian tumors, Stein-Leventhal syndrome, or delayed menopause and in those who have received prolonged exogenous estrogen therapy.
   c. Pathology
      (1) Microscopically, endometrial adenocarcinoma can be well differentiated (Figure 18-6) or poorly differentiated. About 25% of these tumors show benign squamous metaplasia (**adenoacanthoma**); 25% have malignant squamous elements (**adenosquamous cancer**).
      (2) In 70% of cases, the cancer is confined to the uterine corpus at the time of diagnosis; in 3%, it has spread outside the pelvis.
   d. Prognosis. Prognostic features include the extent of the tumor, histologic differentiation, depth of myometrial invasion, size of the uterine cavity (decreased survival with increasing size), age of the patient, and presence of metastases. The average 5-year survival rate is 63%.
   e. Treatment consists of surgery, usually combined with radiotherapy.

7. Carcinosarcoma and **mixed müllerian tumors** are lesions that show a variety of histologic patterns, often combining sarcomatous and carcinomatous patterns. They usually occur in postmenopausal women. The 5-year survival rate is 15%.

8. Stromal tumors
   a. A **stromal nodule** is a benign circumscribed nodule resembling a leiomyoma; it usually is an incidental finding.
   b. Endolymphatic stromal myosis is a low-grade malignant tumor of endometrial stromal

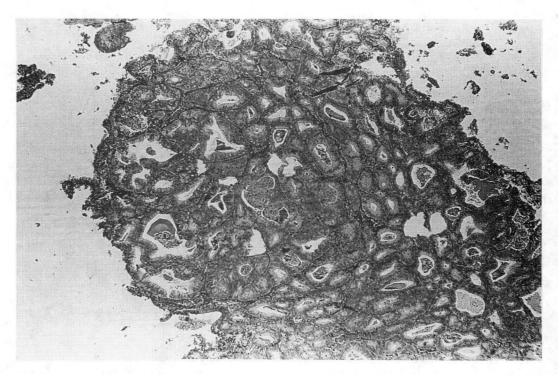

Figure 18-6. Well-differentiated adenocarcinoma of the endometrium (low power).

cells, which have a peculiar propensity to invade the myometrial wall and vascular spaces. Although the 5-year survival rate is fairly high, recurrences and death usually occur within 10 to 15 years of onset.

   c. Stromal sarcomas resemble leiomyosarcomas in terms of clinical features and prognosis. These fully malignant tumors are associated with a 5-year survival rate of less than 50%.

V. TUMORS OF THE OVARIES.
Neoplastic lesions of the ovaries (Table 18-1) are the most diverse group of tumors affecting any organ in the human body. Although malignant tumors of the ovaries occur less frequently than malignant tumors of the cervix or endometrium, they are the fifth most common cause of cancer death in American women (ranking after cancer of the breast, lung, colon, and pancreas).

A. Epithelial tumors

  1. General considerations

    a. Incidence and epidemiology. Epithelial tumors are by far the most common tumors of the ovaries, comprising about 60% of ovarian neoplasms. Epidemiologic studies suggest the following **predisposing factors**:

      (1) White race

      (2) Age over 40 years

      (3) Family history of ovarian cancer

      (4) Low parity

      (5) Environmental factors (e.g., use of talc)

    b. Classification. Epithelial tumors are classified according to **epithelial type** (see Table 18-1). Most tumors are further categorized as **benign, borderline,** or **malignant**.

    c. Clinical features. Epithelial tumors usually come to attention as large abdominal masses, often incidental findings during routine pelvic examination. Presentation is nonspecific; affected patients may complain of abdominal discomfort, distention, constipation, urinary frequency, or abnormal bleeding.

Table 18-1. Classification of Ovarian Tumors

Epithelial (60%)
    Serous tumors
    Mucinous tumors
    Brenner tumors
    Endometrioid carcinomas
    Clear cell carcinomas
    Mixed mesodermal tumors

Germ cell (15% to 20%)
    Teratomas
        Benign dermoid cysts (mature cystic teratomas)
        Immature teratomas
    Dysgerminomas
    Endodermal sinus (yolk sac) tumors
    Mixed germ cell tumors

Gonadal stromal (5% to 10%)
    Thecomas (theca cell tumors) and fibrothecomas
    Granulosa cell tumors
    Sertoli cell tumors
    Lipid cell tumors

Metastatic (5% to 10%)

2. Serous tumors account for about 20% to 50% of ovarian tumors.
  a. General features. Serous tumors arise from the surface epithelium of the ovary and are characterized by ciliated epithelial cells that resemble the epithelium of the fallopian tube. Serous tumors may occur at any age but predominate in women between age 30 and 60. They occur bilaterally in as many as 50% to 60% of affected patients.
  b. Benign serous cystadenomas comprise 20% of serous tumors and usually are unilateral. They can become very large but rarely attain huge dimensions.
    (1) Pathology
      (a) Grossly, these tumors are uni- or multilocular thin-walled cysts filled with yellow, clear fluid. The surface of the ovary is smooth and lacks papillae.
      (b) Microscopically, the cysts are lined by a single layer of ciliated cuboidal epithelium. There is no mitosis, pleomorphism, or necrosis. Occasionally, the cyst lining is not identified.
    (2) Prognosis and treatment. Oophorectomy usually is curative.
  c. Borderline serous tumors (carcinomas of low malignant potential) constitute 9% to 15% of all serous tumors. They are bilateral in 25% of cases.
    (1) Pathology
      (a) Grossly, these lesions are recognizable by the firm papillary excrescences, which may involve the serosal surface of one or both ovaries and are present within the cavity of a cyst. Yellow, clear fluid fills the cystic spaces.
      (b) Microscopically (Figure 18-7), the epithelium reveals complicated papillae lined by stratified epithelium, generally not exceeding two or three layers of cells, with variable degrees of cellular atypia. A cribriform pattern may be present, but true stromal invasion is absent. Calcified psammoma bodies are found in 25% of cases.
    (2) Prognosis
      (a) These tumors often spread beyond the ovary, especially in the form of peritoneal implants (present in up to 40% of cases). The implants may regress, remain stationary, or progress and become invasive. True metastases to viscera or lymph nodes, however, do not occur.
      (b) The stage (degree of spread) appears to be the most important prognostic factor. The 10-year survival rate is about 90%, but recurrences may develop after this period.
    (3) Treatment. Typically, bilateral salpingo-oophorectomy, hysterectomy, and omentectomy remove as much of the tumor as possible. Treatment may be more conservative if the patient is young and wants to preserve fertility and if there is no biopsy-proven involvement of the opposite ovary.

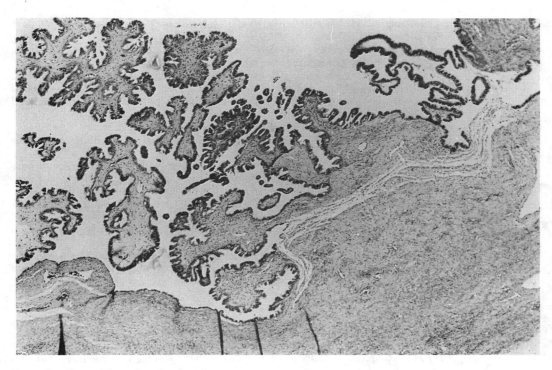

Figure 18-7. Papillary serous tumor of borderline malignant potential. No invasion of the stroma is noted (low power).

   d. Serous cystadenocarcinomas represent at least 65% of serous tumors and are the most common of all malignant ovarian tumors, about 40% of this group. In as many as two-thirds of cases, the tumors are bilateral.
   (1) Pathology
      (a) Grossly, these carcinomas range from predominantly cystic and papillary lesions to entirely solid masses with areas of hemorrhage and necrosis. The ovarian surfaces usually are covered with diffuse papillary excrescences.
      (b) Microscopically, serous carcinomas are characterized by obvious invasive growth, the formation of papillary structures lined by pluristratified epithelium, and abundant calcified psammoma bodies. These poorly differentiated carcinomas may grow in solid sheets of cells that show marked cellular pleomorphism, atypia, and abnormal mitoses.
   (2) Prognosis and staging
      (a) The overall 5-year survival rate is 20% to 30%, with most deaths occurring within the first few years after diagnosis. However, the prognosis depends on the stage of the tumor at the time of initial treatment.
       (i) Stage I tumors involve one or both ovaries.
       (ii) Stage II tumors involve one or both ovaries, with pelvic extension.
      (iii) Stage III tumors involve one or both ovaries, with intraperitoneal metastases outside the pelvis, positive retroperitoneal nodes, or both.
      (iv) Stage IV tumors involve one or both ovaries, with distant metastases (e.g., to lung or liver parenchyma).
      (b) Peritoneal and omental implants occur rapidly, and only 20% of patients have stage I lesions at the time of diagnosis.
   (3) Treatment consists of bilateral salpingo-oophorectomy and hysterectomy, followed by radiation or chemotherapy, according to the stage of the disease.
3. Mucinous tumors account for 15% to 20% of all ovarian tumors.
   a. General features. Mucinous tumors are believed to originate from metaplasia of the coelomic epithelium of the ovary. They are characterized by the presence of tall columnar epithelial cells with abundant intracytoplasmic mucin. The cells resemble the epithelium that lines the endocervix and the intestine. Mucinous tumors occur most frequently in the third to sixth decades of life.

b. Benign mucinous cystadenomas are bilateral in fewer than 5% of cases.
 (1) Pathology
   (a) Grossly, these neoplasms tend to form very large masses (15 to 30 cm), which may have a single loculus or may be polycystic on cut section. The cysts are filled with mucoid, gelatinous material. Papillae are rare, and the surface is always smooth.
   (b) Microscopically, the cysts usually are lined by a single layer of well-differentiated epithelium. The cells have one nucleus toward the base, and the cytoplasm is filled with mucin. Atypia and mitoses are absent.
 (2) Prognosis and treatment. Oophorectomy is curative.
c. Borderline mucinous cystadenocarcinomas are bilateral in up to 20% of cases.
 (1) Pathology
   (a) Grossly, these tumors appear as multiloculated cysts with common intracystic papillary projections. Solid zones are seen in some cases and may contain foci of hemorrhage and necrosis. The ovarian surface is involved in fewer than 10% of cases.
   (b) Microscopically, the tumors are characterized by an overgrowth or papillary projection lined by mucinous epithelium (not more than three layers thick), with moderate atypia and stratification of the nucleus. No invasion of adjacent stroma is noted.
 (2) Prognosis is similar to that associated with the serous counterparts of these tumors.
 (3) Treatment usually consists of bilateral salpingo-oophorectomy and hysterectomy, but a more conservative approach may be taken in young women to preserve fertility.
d. Mucinous cystadenocarcinomas represent about 10% of mucinous tumors and constitute approximately 15% of malignant epithelial tumors.
 (1) Pathology
   (a) Grossly, the tumors exhibit large solid areas with differing amounts of hemorrhage and necrosis. Intracystic papillae frequently are present.
   (b) Microscopically, the tumors are characterized by numerous irregular, glandular structures lined by multilayered, atypical epithelium with numerous mitoses. The stroma is infiltrated by cords and malignant glandular epithelium. Some authors believe that the diagnosis of mucinous carcinoma can be applied in the absence of frank invasion if the atypical lining of the epithelium is more than four cell layers thick.
 (2) Prognosis depends on the stage of the lesion; the overall 5-year survival rate is less than 60%.
e. Pseudomyxoma peritonei is a condition that accompanies 3% to 5% of ovarian mucinous neoplasms. It consists of gelatinous masses scattered throughout the peritoneal cavity as a result of the implantation of cells that secrete abundant mucus.
 (1) Etiology. These cells are thought to originate either from the epithelium of benign or low-grade, malignant, mucinous, ovarian tumors or from mucoceles of the appendix, conditions that commonly coexist. They are believed to reach the peritoneum by spillage or rupture of these tumors at the time of surgery or by spontaneous rupture of the tumors.
 (2) Microscopic appearance. Although histologically benign, pseudomyxoma can compromise vital structures by local spread and cause death.
 (3) Prognosis and treatment. The 5-year survival rate is about 45%. Treatment consists of surgical excision (often repetitive because of recurrences).

4. Brenner tumors are rare, about 1.7% of all ovarian neoplasms.
 a. General features
  (1) Brenner tumors are epithelial tumors that are characterized by the presence of a transitional type of epithelium embedded in dense fibrous connective tissue. Rarely, these tumors secrete hormones. The tumors are associated with mucinous cystadenomas and cystic teratomas in 5% to 10% of cases.
  (2) The age of affected patients ranges from 6 to 81 years, with a mean age at diagnosis of 50 years. Most tumors are incidental findings, but some patients may present with an abdominal mass or complain of irregular menstrual bleeding. Approximately 7% of Brenner tumors are bilateral.
 b. Benign Brenner tumors
  (1) Pathology
   (a) Grossly, these tumors are solid and firm, with a gray–white, whorled, cut surface. They vary in size from microscopic (in about 50% of cases) to 10 cm. They are encapsulated, and there are no papillary excrescences.

        (b) Microscopically, the tumors consist of solid to partly cystic, epithelial nests of polygonal cells, with oval nuclei and distinct nucleoli that have a longitudinal groove ("coffee-bean" appearance) embedded in a dense proliferative stroma. These nests resemble the transitional type of epithelium in the urinary bladder and may undergo mucinous metaplasia.

    (2) Prognosis and treatment. Benign Brenner tumors can be treated by resection or oophorectomy; the prognosis is excellent.

  c. Proliferative Brenner tumors

    (1) Pathology

        (a) Grossly, these lesions form large tumor masses characterized by large cystic spaces into which polypoid tissue projects.

        (b) Microscopically, an exuberant proliferation of papillae is lined by 8 to 20 layers of transitional epithelium, with only mild focal atypia. Occasionally, normal mitoses are present, but there is no evidence of stromal invasion. Adjacent areas may be typical of benign Brenner tumors. Proliferative Brenner tumors resemble grade I transitional-cell tumors of the urinary bladder.

    (2) Prognosis. The malignant potential of these tumors has yet to be determined.

    (3) Treatment varies from unilateral salpingo-oophorectomy to total hysterectomy with bilateral salpingo-oophorectomy in postmenopausal patients.

  d. Malignant Brenner tumors

    (1) Pathology. Microscopically, the transitional-cell type of epithelium is markedly atypical, and areas of hemorrhage and necrosis are identifiable. Foci of squamous metaplasia and frank squamous carcinoma may be present.

    (2) Diagnosis is based on frank evidence of malignancy (i.e., abnormal mitosis, pleomorphism, necrosis), the presence of a benign Brenner tumor, and demonstrable stromal invasion.

    (3) Prognosis and treatment. In most instances, the tumors are treated by total hysterectomy and bilateral salpingo-oophorectomy. The 5-year survival rate is about 50%.

5. Endometrioid carcinomas account for 10% to 25% of primary ovarian adenocarcinomas.

  a. General features. Endometrioid carcinomas of the ovaries are histologically identical to endometrial adenocarcinomas or adenoacanthomas. They may arise in association with preexisting ovarian endometriosis. The mean age of affected patients is 53 years; and at the time of surgery, 30% to 50% of patients have bilateral tumors.

  b. Pathology

    (1) Grossly, the tumors appear as multilocular cystic structures, partly filled with soft papillary tumor tissue.

    (2) Microscopically, the tumors are glands that are arranged in a cribriform pattern similar to that of endometrial cancer, although this pattern may not be easy to identify in poorly differentiated tumors. In some cases, benign endometriosis may be present in areas adjacent to the tumor.

        (a) In about 50% of cases, the glandular component contains benign squamous elements, warranting the diagnosis of adenoacanthoma.

        (b) When the squamous component shows malignant changes, the diagnosis is **adenosquamous carcinoma**.

  c. Prognosis. Endometrioid carcinoma is associated with a 5-year survival rate of about 50%. The prognosis depends on the stage and histology of the tumors; adenosquamous carcinoma, for example, is associated with a lower 5-year survival rate than that for pure adenocarcinoma.

  d. Treatment. Total hysterectomy with bilateral salpingo-oophorectomy, followed by supplementary radiation or chemotherapy, constitutes the major modality of treatment.

6. Clear cell carcinomas constitute 5% to 11% of primary ovarian tumors.

  a. General features. Clear cell carcinoma develops from the surface epithelium of the ovary and is found in association with endometriosis in 25% of cases. The average age of affected patients is 50 to 55 years. The tumors are bilateral in about 5% of cases.

  b. Pathology

    (1) Grossly, the appearance of these tumors is nonspecific; they may be entirely cystic or have a combination of solid or cystic areas.

    (2) Microscopically, the cells are columnar or cuboidal, with abundant clear cytoplasm and large hyperchromatic nuclei. The cells may be arranged in three different patterns:

solid, tubular, or papillary. The nuclei may fill the cytoplasm and bulge into the tubular lamina, imparting a hobnail appearance to the cells.

c. Prognosis. The overall 5-year survival rate is 50% to 55%.

d. Treatment consists of total hysterectomy with bilateral salpingo-oophorectomy, followed by radiation and chemotherapy.

7. Mixed mesodermal tumors are rare.

a. General features. Mixed mesodermal tumors consist of both malignant epithelial and mesenchymal components. They occur predominantly in postmenopausal women; the median age is from 53 to 65 years.

b. Pathology

(1) Grossly, mixed mesodermal tumors tend to be large, with a median diameter of 15 cm. Some are solid, but most are multiloculated cystic neoplasms with solid areas and extensive foci of hemorrhage and necrosis. Approximatelys 50% to 70% of these tumors extend beyond the ovary.

(2) Microscopically, the tumors are of two types.

(a) Mixed mesodermal tumors with homologous elements (carcinosarcomas) consist of an epithelial malignancy (carcinoma) and a sarcoma composed of spindle-shaped cells with nuclear pleomorphism and mitotic activity. The sarcomatous element resembles the stroma of the endometrium.

(b) Mixed mesodermal tumors with heterologous elements contain malignant elements (e.g., striated muscle, cartilage, bone, fat) in addition to the malignant epithelial component.

c. Prognosis for patients with either type is very poor; the median survival time is 6 to 12 months from diagnosis.

d. Treatment consists of total hysterectomy with bilateral salpingo-oophorectomy, followed by radiation or chemotherapy.

B. Germ cell tumors

1. General considerations. Germ cell tumors arise from germ cells, which embryonically originate in the yolk sac and are present in the ovaries at birth.

a. Incidence. These tumors account for 15% to 20% of all ovarian neoplasms and occur primarily in children and young women.

b. Classification. Ovarian germ cell tumors can be divided into five major types (see Table 18-1).

c. Clinical features. The presentation is nonspecific and similar to that of ovarian epithelial tumors.

2. Teratomas

a. Benign dermoid cysts (mature cystic teratomas) are the most common type of benign ovarian neoplasm. They usually occur during the reproductive years and are discovered incidentally.

(1) Pathology

(a) Grossly, benign dermoid cysts are usually unilateral and are of varying sizes. The cut surface reveals a cavity filled with fatty material and hair, surrounded by a capsule of variable thickness (Figure 18-8). The fatty material is similar to normal sebum. Other elements (e.g., bone, teeth, cartilage, fetuslike structures) may be present.

(b) Microscopically, the tumor is characterized by elements from the three germ layers: ectoderm, endoderm, and mesoderm. These elements are histologically benign and mature.

(i) The most frequent elements found are keratinized skin, bronchial and gastrointestinal epithelium, mature glial elements, apocrine glands, and thyroid and salivary glands. (When **thyroid elements** comprise more than 80% of a tumor, the lesion is called **struma ovarii.**)

(ii) The outer portions of dermoid cysts frequently consist of compressed ovarian stroma, which may appear hyalinized or may show inflammation and a foreign-body giant-cell reaction, induced by spillage of the tumor contents into the adjacent stroma.

(2) Prognosis and treatment. Dermoid cysts are benign tumors that can be cured by oophorectomy.

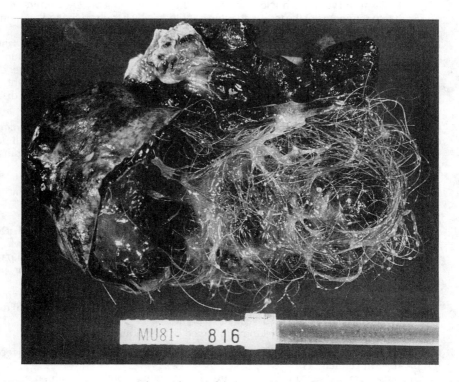

Figure 18-8. Benign cystic teratoma (dermoid cyst) of the ovary. Note the cystic nature of the lesion and the hair.

   b. Immature teratomas constitute about 1% of teratomas and usually occur in young females; the median age at onset is 18 years. These malignant tumors consist entirely or in part of partially differentiated structures that resemble tissues of a developing embryo. They usually are unilateral.
   (1) Pathology
        (a) Grossly, immature teratomas have a median size of 18 cm and generally are more solid than benign teratomas. The external surface is smooth. The cut surface is soft and gray to pink, with areas of hemorrhage and necrosis. Hair, calcifications, and cartilage are present in 40% of the tumors.
        (b) Microscopically, immature teratomas are characterized by elements derived from the three germ layers.
            (i) Immature neural tissue is especially common and is the critical element for diagnosing immature teratomas. The tissue may form tubular structures, rosettes, or solid nests of immature cells. Other elements, such as immature cartilage, may be present.
            (ii) Additionally, histologically mature epithelium may be present, including that of the skin, sweat glands, hair, respiratory and gastrointestinal tracts, muscle, and bone.
   (2) Prognosis is related to the grade and stage of the tumor but in general is poor.
   (3) Treatment consists of surgical removal followed by chemotherapy.
3. Malignant dysgerminomas constitute 50% of germ cell tumors and 2% of all ovarian neoplasms. They occur predominantly in children and in women under 30 years of age. In approximately 15% of cases, the tumors are bilateral.
   a. Pathology
        (1) Grossly, dysgerminomas are solid, fleshy tumors that are well encapsulated and have a homogeneous white-to-tan cut surface. Hemorrhage and necrosis usually are absent.

(2) Microscopically, the tumor consists of large polygonal cells with abundant clear cytoplasm and vesicular nuclei that contain one or more nucleoli. Dysgerminoma is similar to seminoma of the testis and often is infiltrated by lymphocytes and multinucleate giant cells.

b. Prognosis depends on the stage of the disease. The 5-year survival rate is 90% when the tumor is confined to one ovary, and the rate is approximately 40% when the tumor has progressed to an advanced stage. Metatases occur to lymph nodes, bone, and other organs.

c. Treatment. Unilateral oophorectomy is performed in most young female patients, but a total hysterectomy with bilateral salpingo-oophorectomy is necessary when the disease is disseminated, regardless of a patient's age. The tumor is highly radiosensitive.

4. Endodermal sinus tumor (yolk sac tumor) is rare, accounting for about 20% of malignant germ cell tumors. It is characterized by the rapid growth of an abdominal mass; half of all patients have symptoms for 1 week or less before seeking medical attention. The tumor seldom affects patients over age 40.

a. Pathology
(1) Grossly, the tumor is large (median size is 15 cm), with a smooth surface. The cut surface shows a solid mass with extensive hemorrhage and necrosis.
(2) Microscopic appearance
(a) The germ cells may be arranged in several **patterns:** reticular, composed of a loose network of spaces and channels lined by cuboidal cells with scanty cytoplasm; festoon, characterized by glomeruloid structures composed of a central papillary core surrounded by germ cells (Schiller-Duval bodies); alveologlandular; polyvesicular vitelline; and solid.
(b) Hyaline eosinophilic droplets are a common finding; these droplets contain alpha-fetoprotein (AFP) and stain strongly with periodic acid–Schiff (PAS) reagent.

b. Prognosis is poor, with a low 5-year survival rate.

c. Treatment consists of oophorectomy followed by chemotherapy.

5. Malignant mixed germ cell tumors contain two or more malignant components and represent 8% of all germ cell tumors.
a. The most common germ cell tumors are dysgerminoma combined with an endodermal sinus tumor and immature teratoma. Tumors of other cell types, such as **embryonal carcinoma** and **choriocarcinoma,** may occur in the ovary but are rare.
b. Prognosis depends mainly on two factors.
(1) The **size** of the tumor. Those larger than 10 cm have a worse prognosis than smaller ones.
(2) The **cell types** involved. If more than one-third of a mixed germ cell tumor is endodermal sinus tumor, choriocarcinoma, or immature teratoma, the prognosis is poorer than when less malignant elements predominate.

C. Gonadal stromal tumors (stromal tumors of the sex cord) consist of a variety of cells that give rise to neoplasms (e.g., theca granulosa, Sertoli, hilus, or Leydig cell) and fibroblasts of stromal origin, single ones or combinations of two or more types. They arise from the stromal cells of the ovary.

1. General considerations
a. Incidence. As a group, these lesions account for about 5% to 10% of ovarian tumors. They can occur at any age.
b. Classification. Gonadal stromal tumors can be divided into four major types (see Table 18-1).
c. Clinical features. These tumors have the potential to produce steroid hormones, and affected patients may present with clinical manifestations due to the specific hormone produced.

2. Thecomas and fibrothecomas. These tumors consist exclusively of theca cells and fibroblasts of ovarian stromal origin. They almost always are unilateral.
a. Clinical features. These tumors can elaborate estrogen, producing precocious puberty in premenarchal girls and irregular bleeding in women.
b. Pathology
(1) Grossly, the neoplasms range in size from small unpalpable tumors to large, firm, solid masses. Cut sections are a characteristic yellow, most prominent in pure thecomas.
(2) Microscopically, there are two types of cells: a spindlelike cell with a round or oval nucleus and scant cytoplasm, and a round luteinized cell with abundant cytoplasm and a central nucleus. Mitosis almost always is absent. Fat stains usually are positive.

c. **Prognosis and treatment.** Thecomas almost never are malignant. Resection of the tumors by oophorectomy usually is curative.

3. **Granulosa cell tumors.** These tumors commonly are unilateral.
   a. **Clinical features.** Although these tumors affect a wide range, from newborn infant girls to postmenopausal women, most occur after menopause. Granulosa cell tumors can produce a variety of steroid hormones, resulting in either feminizing or virilizing effects. The majority, however, cause signs and symptoms that are related to excessive estrogenic hormones.
   b. **Pathology**
      (1) **Grossly,** the tumors are well encapsulated and vary in size. Cross section shows a solid neoplasm with areas of hemorrhage and necrosis.
      (2) **Microscopically,** the hallmark of these tumors is the presence of a small round or spindle-shaped cell with small amounts of cytoplasm. The nucleus has a longitudinal groove and, occasionally, a small nucleolus.
         (a) The cells may grow in several **patterns**: microfollicular (resembling Call-Exner bodies), macrofollicular, trabecular, and diffuse. A combination of patterns is common.
         (b) Endometrial hyperplasia accompanies the granulosa cell tumors in about 50% of cases, and endometrial adenocarcinoma accompanies the tumors in about 15% of cases.
   c. **Prognosis.** All granulosa cell tumors are thought to be potentially aggressive, but in general the tumors are associated with a good prognosis despite a tendency to recur after long intervals. Poor prognostic factors include advanced tumor stage, age over 40 years, solidity and large size of tumors, bilateral occurrence, and the presence of mitoses or atypia.
   d. **Treatment** consists of hysterectomy with bilateral salpingo-oophorectomy (except when preservation of the reproductive function is a major concern).

4. **Sertoli cell tumors** usually are unilateral.
   a. **Clinical features.** Patients with this type of tumor may have symptoms of virilization or of excess estrogen production.
   b. **Pathology**
      (1) **Grossly,** Sertoli cell tumors are well circumscribed, solitary, and usually large. The cut surface is a characteristic yellow–tan.
      (2) **Microscopically,** they resemble Sertoli tumors of the testis. The cell growth follows three different patterns: simple tubular, complex tubular, and folliculoma lipidique. The patterns are frequently admixed.
   c. **Prognosis.** Most of these tumors are benign.
   d. **Treatment** consists of oophorectomy.

5. **Lipid cell tumors** include **hilus cell** and **Leydig cell tumors**. They account for fewer than 0.1% of all ovarian neoplasms, and they usually are unilateral.
   a. **Clinical features.** Lipid cell tumors predominantly affect adults.
      (1) In 75% to 90% of cases, the tumors have androgenic activity and are virilizing. Patients present with hirsutism, amenorrhea, deepening of the voice, and clitoral enlargement.
      (2) Estrogenic activity occurs in up to 20% of cases.
      (3) About 5% to 10% of patients have associated **Cushing's syndrome**.
   b. **Pathology**
      (1) **Grossly,** lipid cell tumors are lobulated, soft, yellow or brown masses of varying sizes, with areas of hemorrhage and necrosis.
      (2) **Microscopically,** the tumors consist of cuboidal or polyhedral cells that have round nuclei and eosinophilic granular cytoplasm and may contain crystals of Reinke. Areas of fibrosis and hyalinization may be present.
   c. **Prognosis.** The tumors generally are benign, but about 10% to 15% are aggressive and may cause death.
   d. **Treatment** consists of unilateral oophorectomy in most cases; for the rare malignant tumor, more radical surgery is required.

D. **Metastatic tumors.** Tumors metastatic to the ovary from primary tumors elsewhere account for 5% to 10% of ovarian neoplasms and usually are bilateral. They can present a significant diagnostic problem. The most common sites of origin are the stomach (**Krukenberg's tumor**), colon, breast, and genital tract.

VI. TUMORS OF THE FALLOPIAN TUBES

A. Benign tumors of the fallopian tubes are uncommon and frequently confused with inflammatory processes, such as chronic salpingitis or pyosalpinx.

1. **Inclusion cysts** are benign mesothelial inclusions formed by invaginations of the tubal serosa. The cystic cavities are lined by columnar or cuboidal cells and are filled with yellow, clear fluid. They usually are incidental findings of no clinical significance.

2. **Adenomatoid tumors** are benign mesothelial growths identical to those occurring in the testes (see Chapter 17 I F 1). Their only significance resides in their possible confusion with carcinoma.

3. **Leiomyomas** are rare tumors of smooth muscle that arise from the tubal muscularis. They are histologically identical to leiomyomas of the uterus.

B. Malignant tumors

1. **Carcinomas of the fallopian tubes** are rare neoplasms, approximately 0.5% of all gynecologic malignancies.
    a. **Clinical features.** The highest incidence occurs in the fifth and sixth decades of life. The classic symptomatology consists of a clear or serosanguineous vaginal discharge, pelvic pain, and an adnexal mass. The diagnosis of tubal carcinoma is rare prior to surgery.
    b. **Pathology**
        (1) **Grossly,** the tube is swollen because of the neoplastic intraluminal growth, and the serosal surface is congested. On cut section, the lumen is dilated and filled with a papillary or solid tumor, which may infiltrate through the muscularis in advanced cases. The fimbriated end is frequently obliterated.
        (2) **Microscopically,** a complex papillary and solid pattern includes occasional small glandular formations (Figure 18-9).
            (a) The cells pile up and show different degrees of nuclear pleomorphism. Mitosis and

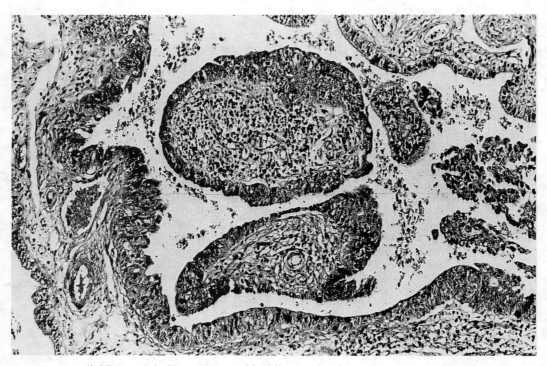

Figure 18-9. Well-differentiated adenocarcinoma of the fallopian tube, showing in situ changes and papillary formation (low power).

necrosis are present. Areas of abrupt transition from normal to neoplastic epithelium may be present, as well as areas of atypical proliferation. The tumor may invade the muscularis and the serosa.
  (b) Primary tubal carcinoma must be differentiated carefully from metastases from
other primary sites (e.g., the ovary) because the histology is very similar.
  c. **Prognosis** depends on the stage of the disease; the overall 5-year survival rate is thought
to be about 19%.
  d. **Treatment** consists of total hysterectomy with bilateral salpingo-oophorectomy, followed
by radiation therapy.

2. **Sarcomas of the fallopian tubes** are very rare. They may be pure or mixed with carcinomatous
elements. The clinical manifestations are identical to those produced by carcinomas, but patients with sarcoma have a poorer prognosis than patients with carcinoma.

VII. VULVAR DISORDERS

A. Benign disorders

1. **Bartholin's cysts** are cystic dilations of Bartholin's glands, and they result from obstruction of
the duct followed by progressive accumulation of secretions. The cyst is filled with mucoid,
clear fluid, and the wall is lined by transitional-type epithelium. Such cysts may be recurrent
and occasionally become infected.

2. A **Bartholin's gland abscess** is an acute process, commonly caused by *N. gonorrhoeae* or *Staphylococcus*. It causes a severe acute inflammation and a purulent exudate. The acute process may
subside and give rise to a chronic form.

3. **Mucinous cysts** usually are located deep in the lamina propria, with no evidence of communication to the surface. The cysts usually are lined by tall columnar cells, similar to those of
the endocervical glands, but occasionally they undergo squamous metaplasia. Mucinous cysts
probably arise from elements of the urogenital sinus, therefore representing examples of dys-
ontogenetic formation.

4. **Papillary hidradenoma,** which is rare before puberty, occurs predominantly in white women.
  a. **Clinical features.** Hidradenomas typically appear as small, firm, well-encapsulated nodules in the labia majora, but they may evert to the surface and look like a cauliflower. They
usually are asymptomatic; but if they ulcerate, they may cause bleeding and soreness.
  b. **Pathology. Microscopically,** these lesions resemble intraductal papillomas of the breast.
They consist of long stalks of connective tissue lined by one or two layers of cuboidal to
columnar cells. Although they may exhibit apocrine metaplasia and some atypia, they are
not malignant.
  c. **Treatment** consists of surgical excision, which is curative.

5. **Vulvar dystrophies** are epithelial disorders that often appear clinically as white, pruritic lesions in the vulva. Any of these lesions may show variable degrees of atypia, but fewer than
10% are thought to progress to invasive or in situ cancers. There are two main **types;** both
forms may affect different areas of the vulva in the same patient.
  a. **Hyperplastic dystrophy** may occur at any age but predominantly affects patients between
age 30 and 60.
    (1) **Clinical features.** The lesions may appear as both white and red patches, and the af-
fected skin surface appears raised and scaly.
    (2) **Pathology. Microscopically,** the lesions show elongation, widening, and confluence
of the rete ridges of the epidermis, with marked hyperkeratosis and parakeratosis. The
dermis is edematous and contains moderate numbers of chronic inflammatory cells.
Normal mitosis may be present in the basal layer.
    (3) **Prognosis and treatment.** Hyperplastic dystrophy is considered to be a benign disor-
der that responds to conservative topical management. Local excision is the preferred
treatment for small lesions.
  b. **Lichen sclerosus** is most common in postmenopausal women but can occur at any age.
    (1) **Clinical features.** This dystrophy can produce gross changes in the vulvar architecture,
with flattening of the labia minora and edema of the preputial folds. The affected area
is white because of avascularity of the superficial layers and may be pruriginous,
which leads to scratching and irritation of the area.

    (2) **Pathology. Microscopically,** the hallmark of lichen sclerosus is sclerosis or homogenization of the upper dermis, which appears markedly edematous and exhibits destruction of the collagen bundles.
        (a) The **epidermis** is thin, with marked keratosis and parakeratosis and loss of rete ridges. Subepidermal bullae may be found.
        (b) The **capillaries** are thin, and there may be extravasation of blood in the dermis.
    (3) **Prognosis and treatment.** The lesion is not considered premalignant, and it responds to topical treatment. Surgery is not recommended because of a high incidence of recurrences.

B. Malignant tumors

  1. Squamous cell carcinoma in situ (Bowen's disease of the vulva)
    a. Clinical features
      (1) The mean age at onset is 41 years, although the lesion may occur at any age. It is more common in black than white women and has a significant association with infectious processes, such as condyloma acuminatum.
      (2) SCC in situ causes asymptomatic, multicentric, raised patchy white plaques that retain toluidine blue dye. Some 30% to 40% of patients have dysplasias or carcinomas in other areas of the genital tract.
    b. Pathology. Microscopically, the lesion is identical to the one in Bowen's disease of the skin.
    c. Treatment for small lesions is local resection. Widespread disease is treated by superficial vulvectomy. Topical chemotherapy has been used with variable success. The lesion usually recurs if it is not completely excised.

  2. Squamous cell carcinoma. This lesion accounts for about 4% of all genital cancers and for more than 90% of all vulvar malignancies.
    a. Clinical features. SCC of the vulva predominantly affects women between age 60 and 90. It appears as either an endophytic or exophytic lesion, usually ulcerated. Pruritus and bleeding may occur. The mass extends progressively to involve the entire vulva, and sometimes the vagina and cervix. It is associated with other primary malignancies in 10% or more of cases.
    b. Pathology. Microscopically, the lesion is identical to the one in SCC of the skin and mucous membranes.
    c. Prognosis and treatment. In general, the 5-year survival rate is about 70%, but the rate drops if inguinal lymph node involvement is present. Total vulvectomy combined with bilateral groin node dissection (even when the tumor is unilateral) is the treatment of choice.

  3. Paget's disease of the vulva
    a. This rare tumor essentially is identical to Paget's disease of other areas, such as the skin or nipple. If the tumor invades the dermis, there is a high likelihood of lymph node metastases. About 14% of patients also have adenocarcinoma of Bartholin's glands and other sites.
    b. Prognosis and treatment depend on the presence or absence of associated carcinomas. Positive lymph nodes worsen the prognosis and reduce the survival rate. Vulvectomy is the preferred treatment; and if an associated invasive cancer is found, regional lymphadenectomy is performed.

  4. Other malignancies (e.g., **melanoma, basal cell carcinoma**) can occur in the vulva. Microscopically, these lesions are identical to the respective tumors occurring in the skin or salivary glands. **Sarcomas** such as leiomyosarcoma, malignant neural tumors, rhabdomyosarcoma, and angiosarcoma also have been reported.

  5. Metastatic tumors. The vulva is infrequently involved during metastatic spread of carcinoma from the cervix or endometrium and even more frequently during metastases from other sites, such as the kidneys or urethra.

VIII. VAGINAL DISORDERS

A. Benign disorders

  1. Adenosis is the presence of ectopic mucinous endocervical glands in the vagina. The disorder has been linked to prenatal exposure to diethylstilbestrol (DES) and predominantly affects girls and young women. Its true incidence is unknown because the condition is probably asymptomatic and not recognized in many patients.

  a. **Pathology. Microscopically,** areas of adenosis do not stain with iodine because the cells do not produce glycogen, but rather mucin. The epithelium usually is tall and columnar but may undergo squamous metaplasia.
  b. Adenosis has been associated with vaginal deformities, such as ridges, hoods, and collars, and with malignant processes, such as clear cell adenocarcinoma.

2. **Gartner's duct cysts** are commonly located in the anterolateral wall of the vagina and originate from vestigial remnants of the wolffian duct. The cysts are lined by low cuboidal epithelium and usually are small.

3. **Fibroepithelial polyps** are polypoid, rubbery lesions covered by vaginal mucosa. They protrude from the introitus as multiple fingerlike projections, which, in children, may be confused with sarcoma botryoides.
  a. **Pathology. Microscopically,** the stroma consists of fibrous connective tissue with dilated capillaries and occasional large atypical cells.
  b. **Treatment.** Surgical resection is curative.

4. **Other benign tumors** of the vagina include leiomyomas, neurofibromas, rhabdomyomas, and granular cell myoblastomas.

B. **Malignant tumors.** Primary malignant tumors of the vagina are very rare and probably account for fewer than 1% of all gynecologic neoplasms.

1. **Epithelial tumors**
  a. The vagina can undergo the same dysplastic and neoplastic changes as the cervix and vulva: dysplasia, carcinoma in situ, and invasive SCC. The last-named affects older patients and has been associated with chronic irritative processes, such as the use of pessaries.
  b. The most common location of a vaginal epithelial tumor is the upper portion of the posterior wall. The 5-year survival rate is about 80% to 90%.

2. **Clear cell adenocarcinoma** is associated with vaginal adenosis and occurs in approximately 0.14 to 1.4 females in 1000 who have been exposed to DES in utero. The tumor chiefly affects young women.
  a. **Pathology. Microscopically,** several patterns can be recognized: solid, tubular (with hobnails), and papillary.
  b. **Prognosis.** The 5-year survival rate is 40% to 50%, similar to that for clear cell adenocarcinoma of the cervix.

3. **Sarcoma botryoides** is a very rare tumor that occurs predominantly in infants and children, with a peak incidence at age 1 or 2. It occurs in other soft tissues as well as the vagina.
  a. **Clinical features.** Vaginal sarcoma botryoides presents as a polypoid, confluent mass resembling a bunch of grapes when it protrudes through the vaginal introitus.
  b. **Pathology. Microscopically,** the lesion originates in the mesenchyma of the lamina propria. A distinct subepithelial zone known as the cambium layer always is present. The cells are round or spindlelike with dark nuclei and scanty cytoplasm. Occasional mitotic figures can be identified. Striated muscle cells may be present.
  c. **Prognosis and treatment.** The 5-year survival rate has been reported at 10% to 35%, although recently it has been improving as patients are treated with pelvic exenteration, regional lymphadenectomy, and vaginectomy, followed by radiation and chemotherapy.

4. The vagina also can be the primary site for other tumors, such as **melanoma** and **leiomyosarcoma**.

STUDY QUESTIONS

Directions: Each of the numbered items or incomplete statements in this section is followed by answers or by completions of the statement. Select the **one** lettered answer or completion that is **best** in each case.

1. Psammoma bodies are most often found in which type of ovarian cancer?

(A) Brenner tumor
(B) Germ cell tumor
(C) Serous cystadenocarcinoma
(D) Mucinous cystadenoma
(E) Mucinous cystadenocarcinoma

2. The most common benign germ cell tumor of the ovaries in premenopausal women is

(A) Brenner tumor
(B) hilus cell tumor
(C) benign dermoid cyst
(D) mucinous cystadenoma
(E) dysgerminoma

3. Which of the following is true of invasive squamous cell carcinoma (SCC) of the vulva?

(A) In this location, it is less common than clear cell adenocarcinoma
(B) It may present as an exophytic lesion
(C) It can be treated topically with success
(D) Inguinal lymph nodes are seldom involved
(E) It is identical to Bowen's disease of the skin

4. The condition in which the placenta partially or completely covers the internal os is known as

(A) abruptio placentae
(B) placenta previa
(C) placenta accreta
(D) placenta increta
(E) ectopic pregnancy

5. Condylomatous cervicitis is most likely to be found in which of the following patients?

(A) An 18-year-old woman with multiple sex partners
(B) A 38-year-old woman with ovarian carcinoma
(C) A 20-year-old woman who is a virgin
(D) A 28-year-old mother of two with chlamydial infection
(E) A 35-year-old multigravida with herpetic vulvitis

6. The endometrial biopsy specimen obtained from a 30-year-old woman shows a proliferative-phase endometrium with evidence of chronic endometritis. This finding most likely represents

(A) a premalignant endometrial lesion
(B) an inadequate luteal phase
(C) a hyperestrogenic state
(D) the effects of an intrauterine device (IUD)
(E) Stein-Leventhal syndrome

7. A 40-year-old woman presents with an ovarian mass. At surgery, a 5-cm cystic mass is found attached to the right ovary. The surface of the cyst is grossly papillary. Which feature distinguishes a borderline serous tumor from a serous cystadenocarcinoma?

(A) Involvement of the other ovary
(B) Involvement of the peritoneum
(C) Cellular atypia
(D) Invasion of ovarian stroma
(E) Psammoma bodies

1-C   4-B   7-D
2-C   5-A
3-B   6-D

8. During a gynecologic examination, a 35-year-old woman is found to have clinically atypical epithelium covering the majority of the cervix and the proximal vagina. The epithelium does not stain with Lugol's iodine. A biopsy of the vagina reveals benign endocervical glands. These findings are consistent with a diagnosis of

(A) chronic cervicitis
(B) condyloma acuminatum
(C) adenosis
(D) cervical intraepithelial neoplasia
(E) endometriosis

9. A 35-year-old woman presents with vague complaints of feeling tired. A low-grade fever, inguinal lymphadenopathy, and a diffuse skin rash are noted. A skin biopsy reveals an intense perivascular lymphocytic infiltrate composed predominantly of plasma cells. Which microorganism is the most likely etiologic agent of the patient's symptoms?

(A) Herpes simplex
(B) *Candida albicans*
(C) *Treponema pallidum*
(D) *Haemophilus ducreyi*
(E) *Neisseria gonorrhoeae*

10. A 17-year-old woman presents with complaints of dysuria. Physical examination reveals multiple small blisters of the labial and periurethral membranes. What is the most likely histologic finding?

(A) Spirochetes
(B) Koilocytes
(C) Multinucleate giant cells
(D) Gram-negative diplococci
(E) Donovan bodies

11. All of the following are associated with endometriosis EXCEPT

(A) infertility
(B) abdominal pain
(C) hematuria
(D) eclampsia
(E) intestinal obstruction

12. Endometrial hyperplasia is typically associated with all of the following clinical settings EXCEPT

(A) acute endometritis
(B) obesity
(C) Stein-Leventhal syndrome
(D) granulosa cell tumor
(E) thecoma

13. All of the following statements about choriocarcinoma are true EXCEPT

(A) it may occur after a normal pregnancy
(B) it can arise in a hydatidiform mole
(C) it consists of malignant trophoblasts
(D) it is treated with hysterectomy and radiation therapy
(E) response to therapy is monitored by human chorionic gonadotropin (hCG) levels

8-C   11-D
9-C   12-A
10-C   13-D

ANSWERS AND EXPLANATIONS

1. The answer is C *[V A 2 d (1)].*
Serous cystadenocarcinoma is the most common of all malignant ovarian tumors, accounting for nearly 40% of ovarian malignancies. Grossly, the tumor is composed of cysts and papillary structures, sometimes with zones of hemorrhage and necrosis. The surface of the tumor is covered with diffuse papillary excrescences, which are formed by pluristratified epithelium with abundant psammoma bodies. Psammoma bodies are small, calcified concentrically laminated structures, which are believed to form degenerated epithelial cells in the papillae.

2. The answer is C *[V B 2 a].*
Benign dermoid cyst, also known as benign cystic teratoma, is the most common ovarian tumor found in premenopausal women. A dermoid cyst originates from the germ cell component of the ovary. The tumor can contain tissues that are characteristic of all three germ cell layers: endoderm, mesoderm, and ectoderm. The dermoid tumor is benign; the malignant counterpart is known as an immature teratoma.

3. The answer is B *[VII B 2].*
Squamous cell carcinoma (SCC) is the most common cancer of the vulva, and it may present as either an exophytic or endophytic lesion. The treatment is radical surgical therapy with regional lymph node dissection since these nodes are the common site of metastasis. Bowen's disease refers to carcinoma in situ (cytologically malignant squamous cells with no evidence of invasion into the underlying dermis).

4. The answer is B *[II B 3 d, e, 4].*
Placenta previa is a serious condition that jeopardizes both infant and mother during a vaginal delivery and, hence, must be diagnosed in the prepartum period. Abruptio placentae refers to premature separation of placenta and uterus, with accompanying hemorrhage. Placenta accreta and increta refer to abnormally deep penetration of the placenta up to and into the uterine myometrium, respectively. Ectopic pregnancy refers to a pregnancy outside the uterine cavity.

5. The answer is A *[III A 2].*
Condylomatous cervicitis is caused by a human papillomavirus (HPV) infection. These infections occur more frequently in women who have multiple sex partners. Also, epidemiologic studies have shown an association between cervical intraepithelial neoplasia and HPV infections of the cervix and vagina.

6. The answer is D *[IV C 2].*
Chronic endometritis is diagnosed by the presence of plasma cells in an inflamed endometrial stroma. The hormonal phase of the endometrium has little to do with the presence of the inflammation; however, the presence of a foreign body, such as an intrauterine device (IUD), is often the cause of chronic endometrial infection. Stein-Leventhal syndrome is associated with hyperestrogenism, which can cause endometrial hyperplasia, but is not a cause of endometritis. A premalignant or malignant endometrial lesion would produce a different endometrial histology, such as hyperplasia.

7. The answer is D *[V A 2 c, d].*
Borderline serous tumors share some but not all characteristics of true carcinomas and are also known by the confusing name of "carcinomas of low malignant potential." Borderline tumors display cytologic atypia, may recur after excision, and may spread throughout the peritoneum by direct seeding. However, this neoplastic process does not have the capacity to invade tissue directly as do serous cystadenocarcinomas and, hence, does not metastasize via lymphatic or hematogenous routes. Ovarian tumors of both borderline and fully malignant types may be bilateral, and both may contain psammoma bodies.

8. The answer is C *[VIII A 1].*
The presence of ectopic endocervical glands in the vagina is consistent with adenosis, an entity associated with prenatal diethylstilbestrol (DES) exposure. Chronic cervicitis is associated with squamous metaplasia of endocervical epithelium in the transition zone. Condyloma acuminatum and cervical intraepithelial neoplasia are disorders of squamous epithelium. Endometriosis involves ectopic endometrial glands and stroma, not endocervical glands.

9. The answer is C *[III B].*
The manifestations of secondary syphilis are protean and may be subtle. The diagnosis is suggested by the plasmacytic perivascular infiltrate in the skin, where rare spirochetes (*Treponema pallidum*) may be seen with special stains. The lesions of herpes are vesicular and painful. *Haemophilus ducreyi* is the

pathologic agent of chancroid, which presents as painful ulcers and lymphadenopathy. *Candida* and *Neisseria* infections are not associated with plasmacellular infiltrates.

10. The answer is C *[III A].*
The clinical findings of multiple small painful vesicles on the genitalia is highly suggestive of herpes simplex infection. The histology will reveal multinucleate giant cells with nuclear inclusions. Spirochetes are seen in syphilis; the genital lesion is a painless chancre. Koilocytes are seen in papillomavirus (HPV) infection; the lesions are condylomatous or flat patches of atypical epithelium. Gram-negative diplococci are seen in *Neisseria* infection (gonorrhea); the genital lesion is a vaginal discharge. Donovan bodies are seen in granuloma inguinale; the genital lesion is a papule or a larger ulcer.

11. The answer is D *[I B; II B 5].*
Eclampsia is a severe complication of pregnancy, usually occurring in young primigravid women and is unrelated to endometriosis. Endometriosis is usually found in older premenopausal multiparous women, with presenting complaints of abdominal pain, infertility, or both. Involvement of other organ systems, with resulting fibrosis and distortion, may cause such disparate symptoms as hematuria and intestinal obstruction.

12. The answer is A *[IV C 1, 4].*
Hyperplasia of the endometrium occurs in states of relative or absolute hyperestrogenism such as seen with the two estrogen-secreting tumors, obesity, and the Stein-Leventhal syndrome. Acute endometritis is not associated with abnormal estrogen levels.

13. The answer is D *[II B 6 b].*
Choriocarcinoma is a tumor composed of malignant trophoblasts that may follow a normal pregnancy, a molar pregnancy, or an abortion. It responds well to chemotherapy, and surgery is not necessarily indicated. The tumor secretes human chorionic gonadotropin (hCG), the serum levels of which may be used to monitor for the presence of residual disease.

19
Breast

Maria J. Merino

I. NORMAL ANATOMY AND PHYSIOLOGY

A. Anatomy and histology

1. The breast consists of an **epithelial parenchyma,** supporting muscular and fascial elements, plus varying amounts of fat, blood vessels, lymphatics, and nerves. The **epithelial component** consists of ducts and acini, which together form **lobules,** the basic structural units of the mammary gland. The number of lobules varies in each female mammary gland; the male breast has no lobules.

2. The **epithelial and mesenchymal elements** are intermingled and are capable of responding to hormonal stimulation.

3. The mammary gland is a **modified sweat gland** that develops from a primitive epidermal thickening of the ectoderm and remains rudimentary in males.

B. Neuroendocrine control. The development and function of the breast are controlled by the neuroendocrine system. The ovaries, the pituitary and adrenal glands, and the hypothalamus are essential members of this system. At puberty, a complex mechanism involving the central nervous system (CNS), pituitary gland, and hypothalamus initiates ovarian function and estrogen production. The estrogens act on the breast, stimulating acini and duct proliferation until the breast reaches maturity.

1. **Changes with age.** The **infantile breast** consists of small ducts scattered in fibrous tissue. **At puberty,** the main lactiferous ducts proliferate, and lobules and acini form. **After menopause,** hormonal stimulation stops, and there is involution of the glandular portion of the breast, with an increase of fat tissue and hyalinization of the intervening connective tissue. Atrophy of acini and ducts accompany these changes.

2. **Pregnancy and lactation.** During pregnancy and postpartum, the breast enlarges, and new ducts and acini are formed. The epithelial cells show marked vacuolization, with luminal secretion of colostrum and milk. The changes are stimulated by the secretion of the hormone **prolactin,** but the mechanism is not completely understood.

II. CONGENITAL ABNORMALITIES

A. Supernumerary breasts constitute the most common congenital anomaly; accessory glands can occur at any site along the embryonal milk line.

B. Amastia (i.e., congenital absence of the breast), although rare, may be unilateral or bilateral and occurs in males as well as females.

III. INFLAMMATORY DISORDERS

A. Acute mastitis almost always is a complication that occurs during lactation (**puerperal mastitis**). The causative agent, usually *Staphylococcus* or *Streptococcus,* enters through fissures in the nipple. The breast is swollen, erythematous, and painful. Histologically, the diffuse infiltration by acute inflammatory cells can destroy ducts, lobules, and surrounding stroma.

B. Chronic mastitis usually is a granulomatous inflammation secondary to a systemic disease such as tuberculosis or sarcoidosis.

C. Duct ectasia occurs predominantly in postmenopausal women. The condition is characterized by dilatation of the collecting ducts in the subareolar region, with periductal fibrosis and the presence of chronic inflammatory cells. In the lumina of the ducts, inspissated amorphous material is present. Clinically, the condition can be misdiagnosed as carcinoma.

D. Fat necrosis is an unusual lesion produced by injury or trauma to the breast. It produces tumoral masses that clinically can simulate carcinomas. Histologically, the adipose tissue is inflamed and necrotic, with areas of saponification and calcification. Chronic inflammatory cells and lipid-filled macrophages are present.

IV. PROLIFERATIVE LESIONS

A. Fibrocystic changes. This most common condition affecting the breast is the reason for more than half of all operations on the female breast.

   1. Etiology. This common condition is believed to be the result of estrogenic hormonal imbalance, because it does not become clinically evident until ovarian function is fully evolved, and it regresses after menopause.

   2. Clinical features. The lesions are commonly bilateral and multiple. Typically, the upper outer quadrant is most commonly involved. The disorder is characterized clinically by dull, heavy pain and by tenderness on palpation. These symptoms increase premenstrually.

   3. Pathology
      a. The **gross appearance** is that of fine fibrofatty tissue with cystic spaces; bluish ones are called **"blue-domed" cysts.**
      b. The **microscopic findings** include:
         (1) Microcysts—cysts that are not visible to the naked eye
         (2) Ductal epithelial proliferation—which, if severe, may form a lacelike pattern filling the ducts
         (3) Apocrine metaplasia—the normal cuboidal epithelium being transformed into columnar epithelium with abundant eosinophilic cytoplasm
         (4) Adenosis—proliferation of acini and ducts in a lobular pattern
         (5) Fibrosis

   4. Relation to breast cancer
      a. **Hyperplasia.** Patients with mild hyperplasia (not more than four layers of cells) do not appear to have an increased risk for carcinoma. Patients with moderate or florid hyperplasia (more than four layers of cells but without atypical changes) may have an increased risk (up to two times) for the development of carcinoma.
      b. **Atypical hyperplasia** refers to lesions with increased numbers of cells and atypical changes suggestive of carcinoma in situ. Patients with these changes have up to five times the risk of developing invasive cancer when compared with normal controls. The risk is significantly increased in those patients who also have a family history of breast cancer.

   5. Treatment. Although no adequate treatment exists for this condition, careful follow-up by the clinician is recommended.

B. Gynecomastia is hypertrophy of the male breast, chiefly ductal and periductal, with stromal proliferation. Gynecomastia is more common unilaterally than bilaterally. Hormonal imbalance, with an increase of estrogenic substances, appears to be the cause. The condition is found most frequently either at puberty or in old age. Patients with testicular tumors or cirrhosis of the liver commonly have gynecomastia. Gynecomastia in cirrhosis is due to decreased capacity of the liver to metabolize estrogens.

V. BENIGN NEOPLASMS

A. Fibroadenoma is the most common benign tumor of the female breast. It develops as the result of increased sensitivity of a focal area of the breast to estrogens.

1. **Clinical features**
   a. **Fibroadenoma** is a disease of youth. The tumor may develop at any time after puberty, most frequently before age 30.
   b. The lesions usually are solitary but occasionally may be multiple. The tumor is easily movable, and neither the overlying skin nor the adjacent axillary lymph nodes show significant changes.

2. **Pathology**
   a. **Grossly,** the tumor is sharply demarcated from the surrounding breast tissue and is seemingly encapsulated, although it does not have a true capsule. The tumor often is 2 cm to 4 cm in size or larger and has a gray-white, firm surface on cut section (Figure 19-1).
   b. **Microscopically,** the tumor consists of two components: a proliferation of the connective tissue stroma and an atypical multiplication of ducts and acini. Both components are histologically benign.

3. **Treatment.** Complete surgical excision of the tumor is curative.

B. Intraductal papilloma

1. **Clinical features.** Intraductal papilloma occurs in women at or shortly before menopause. The neoplasms appear as small masses located in the region of the nipple. Often the lesion is not palpable and is called to a patient's attention by the passage of **bloody fluid** from the nipple. **Nipple discharge** is more common in benign than in malignant lesions, and intraductal papilloma is the most common cause.

2. **Pathology**
   a. **Grossly,** the papillomas appear as small raspberrylike growths attached to the wall of a dilated duct.
   b **Microscopically,** the duct has a thick wall. Within the dilated duct, the intraductal papilloma is recognized by its broad stalk of connective tissue covered by two layers of benign

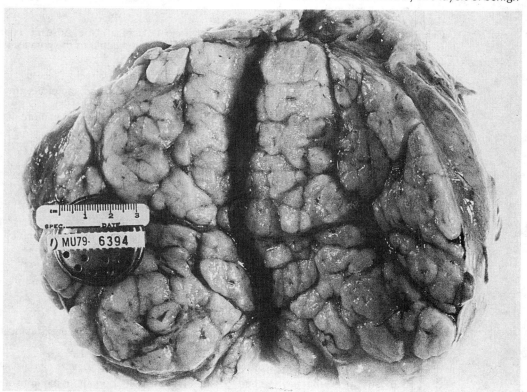

Figure 19-1. Section of a fibroadenoma, showing prominent lobulation and a surrounding pseudocapsule.

epithelial cells. The connective tissue stalk of one papilla may fuse with the fibrous stalk of an adjacent papilla, trapping the epithelium in the process and forming ductlike spaces within the lesion.

3. Treatment is surgical resection of the lesion.

VI. MALIGNANT NEOPLASMS

A. General considerations

1. Incidence
   a. Breast cancer is the leading cause of death in women over age 40. Approximately 1 woman in 13 (nearly 8%) will develop breast cancer during her lifetime.
   b. The incidence of a contralateral breast cancer in those patients with a known breast cancer is greater than the incidence of a primary breast cancer in the general population.

2. Etiology. Although the etiology of breast cancer is unknown, epidemiologic studies indicate certain **risk factors**:
   a. Age over 40 years
   b. Family history of breast cancer
   c. Nulliparity or late age of first pregnancy
   d. Previous cancer in one breast
   e. History of fibrocystic changes (see IV A 4)
   f. Adverse hormonal milieu

3. Clinical features
   a. Clinically, the chief complaints of patients with breast cancer are:
      (1) Palpable lump or mass
      (2) Pain
      (3) Skin symptoms such as edema, redness, and dimpling
      (4) Nipple retraction
      (5) Axillary masses
   b. Carcinomas involve the left breast more frequently than the right, and they arise most commonly in the upper outer quadrant, probably because this area contains the greatest volume of mammary tissue.

4. Pathology
   a. Types. Over 80% of breast cancers arise from the ductal epithelium and, therefore, are adenocarcinomas. The remainder are sarcomas.
   b. Histologic classification of breast cancer is summarized here and discussed in more detail in VI B.
      (1) Ductal carcinoma
         (a) Intraductal (in situ)
         (b) Infiltrating
         (c) Medullary
         (d) Mucinous
         (e) Papillary
      (2) Lobular carcinoma
         (a) In situ
         (b) Infiltrating
      (3) Paget's disease
      (4) Sarcoma
         (a) Cystosarcoma phylloides (or phyllodes)
         (b) Angiosarcoma
      (5) Metastasis from other tumors

5. Prognostic factors. In general, the 5-year survival rate for patients who have breast cancer is about 53%. However, the following factors influence the prognosis.
   a. Stage at diagnosis
      (1) Early diagnosis correlates with a better-than-average prognosis.
      (2) Advanced cancers that have spread to lymph nodes or other organs at the time of diagnosis are associated with a poor prognosis.

     (a) Carcinoma of the breast has a high tendency to metastasize to regional lymph nodes. The presence of four or more positive lymph nodes at the time of diagnosis is associated with a poor prognosis.

     (b) Visceral metastases commonly are found in the lungs, liver, bones, and brain, but any organ can be involved.

b. Histologic features

    (1) Some tumors, such as medullary, papillary, and mucinous ones, seem to be associated with a better prognosis, a lower incidence of lymph node metastasis, and a longer survival rate than other histologic types.

    (2) Certain histologic features, such as an increased number of histiocytes in lymph nodes or the presence of plasma cells and lymphocytes bordering a tumor, are interpreted as favorable signs, related to a better prognosis.

c. Age at onset. The younger the patient, the worse the prognosis is believed to be.

d. Host resistance. The growth and spread of breast cancer depend on the results of the interaction between cancer cells and the host. The tumor–host relationship is not readily assayed, but the fact that breast cancer usually has obtained significant size before it becomes clinically apparent may be a sign of inadequate host resistance.

e. Estrogen-receptor status

    (1) About 50% of breast carcinomas contain **estrogen-receptor proteins** that specifically bind estradiol.

      (a) Few patients whose breast cancers lack estrogen receptors respond to endocrine therapy, whereas more than 50% of patients whose tumors contain estrogen receptors obtain objective remissions from such treatment. Therefore, the results of estrogen-receptor assays provide valuable information for making clinical decisions as to the type of therapy and the prognosis.

      (b) Tumors in premenopausal women have been reported to have a lower incidence of estrogen receptors than tumors occurring in postmenopausal women. This finding has been attributed to the high levels of endogenous estrogens that occupy the receptor sites in younger women.

      (c) At the present time, no histopathologic feature can predict the estrogen-receptor status of a cancer, although it is believed that well-differentiated tumors may have a higher proportion of estrogen receptors than poorly differentiated ones. These proteins are readily detected by radioimmunoassays.

    (2) **Progesterone receptor** is now being used as a marker of a functionally intact estrogen-receptor system. The determination of progesterone-receptor values, alone or in combination with estrogen-receptor assay, provides valuable information on the hormone dependence of a given tumor.

6. Treatment

    a. The treatment of choice has been surgical excision of the breast (**mastectomy**) followed by radiation, chemotherapy, endocrine therapy, or a combination of these three modalities, according to the stage of disease and the estrogen-receptor status.

    b. In the last decade, conservative breast surgery (**lumpectomy**) followed by radiation therapy has been used for the treatment of patients with early breast cancer.

    c. Retrospective studies have shown that in early cancers (i.e., tumors smaller than 2 cm), tumor control can be achieved with surgery and radiation therapy. The disease-free and overall survival rates of patients treated with lumpectomy and radiation are comparable to those of patients who undergo mastectomy.

B. Specific histologic types

1. Ductal carcinoma

    a. Intraductal (in situ) carcinoma represents 5% to 10% of all mammary cancers. The tumor is confined to the duct system, and the ductal basement membrane is intact.

    (1) Pathology

      (a) Grossly, the ducts are thick-walled, dilated, and, in some instances, filled with necrotic material (Figure 19-2).

      (b) Histologically, the epithelial lining has proliferated and shows marked cellular pleomorphism, with hyperchromatic nuclei and mitotic figures. Necrotic debris and histiocytes are present in the lumina (Figure 19-3).

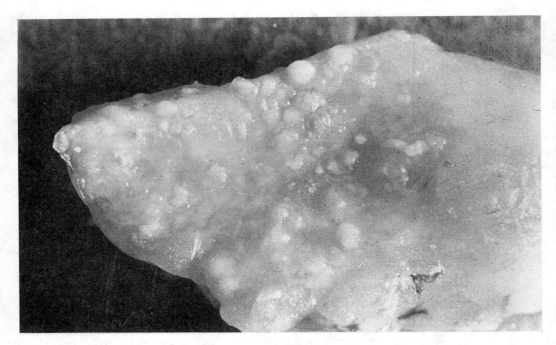

Figure 19-2. Intraductal carcinoma of the breast, showing areas of focal necrosis.

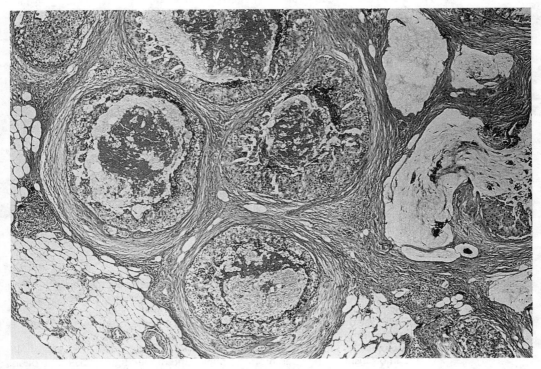

Figure 19-3. Microscopic section of an intraductal carcinoma. The enlarged ducts show epithelial proliferation, with central areas of necrosis.

(2) Prognosis. About 20% to 25% of these in situ tumors eventually break through the duct wall and become invasive.

b. Infiltrating carcinoma accounts for the majority of breast carcinomas. The tumor originates from the ductal epithelium (adenocarcinoma).

    (1) Pathology

        (a) This tumor produces a severe desmoplastic reaction, with abundant connective tissue in which tumor cells can be identified (Figure 19-4.)

        (b) The tumor cells vary in size, are pleomorphic, and have prominent nucleoli. Frequently, they form glandular structures. Necrosis may or may not be present.

    (2) Prognosis. The prognosis for patients with this tumor depends on the prognostic factors discussed in VI A 5.

c. Medullary carcinoma accounts for about 5% of all breast carcinomas.

    (1) Pathology

        (a) Grossly, the lesion is soft and well circumscribed, with a homogeneous gray, moist cut surface. Focal hemorrhagic areas are present.

        (b) Histologically, the tumor is recognized by the large pleomorphic cells and marked lymphocytic infiltration.

    (2) Prognosis. This lesion is believed to behave in a less aggressive fashion than infiltrating ductal carcinoma.

d. Mucinous carcinoma is an uncommon form.

    (1) Pathology

        (a) Grossly, this lesion is a well-circumscribed, soft, glistening tumor characterized by its gelatinous appearance.

        (b) Histologically, large pools of mucin are separated by bands of connective tissue. Suspended in the mucin are clumps of tumor cells.

    (2) Prognosis. This tumor is associated with a better prognosis than that for the ordinary ductal cancer, probably because of a lesser tendency to metastasize.

e. Papillary carcinoma is a very rare form of breast cancer, and can be difficult to differentiate from benign papilloma.

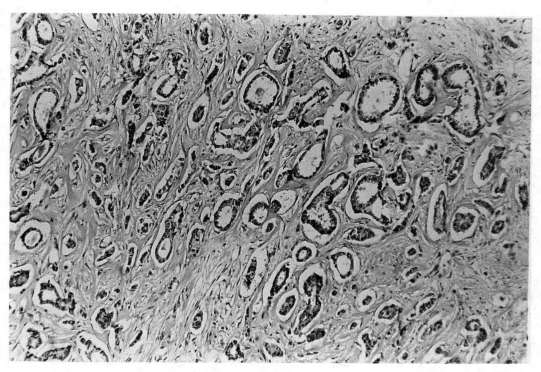

Figure 19-4. Microscopic section of an infiltrating duct carcinoma, with glandular differentiation. Abundant desmoplastic stroma surrounds the epithelial glands.

(1) **Clinical features.** The tumor may first appear as a lump, or an affected patient may complain of hemorrhagic nipple discharge. The lesion frequently is located close to the nipple.

(2) **Pathology**

　　(a) **Grossly,** the tumor is confined within the wall of a duct and appears as a reddish, friable, polypoid mass.

　　(b) **Histologically,** the lesion shows varying degrees of pleomorphism, mitosis, and necrosis.

(3) **Prognosis.** Clinically, the tumor behaves in a benign fashion unless it occurs in association with intraductal carcinoma.

2. **Lobular carcinoma**

　a. **Lobular carcinoma in situ** is a rare variant of breast cancer that occurs in younger (premenopausal) women.

　　(1) **Clinical features.** The tumors are bilateral in up to 20% of cases and are frequently multifocal, involving several areas within the same breast. They do not form a palpable tumor mass and often are discovered as an incidental finding when a breast biopsy is performed for other reasons.

　　(2) **Pathology.** The lesion is confined to the lobules, which appear distended and filled with uniform cells with abundant cytoplasm. The basement membrane of each acinus is intact.

　　(3) **Prognosis.** These tumors do not metastasize but do predispose to the development of invasive carcinomas.

　b. **Infiltrating lobular carcinoma**

　　(1) **Clinical features.** Affected patients are older than those with lobular carcinoma in situ, and the tumor's presentation is similar to that in other forms of carcinoma.

　　(2) **Pathology.** The tumor consists predominantly of small cells, which individually infiltrate the stroma and have a linear ("Indian file") arrangement (Figure 19-5). In about 30% of cases, there is evidence of an in situ lobular component.

　　(3) **Prognosis.** The tumor is associated with the same prognosis as that for infiltrating duct carcinoma.

3. **Paget's disease** accounts for 1% to 2% of all breast cancers.

　a. **Clinical features.** Paget's disease is an eczematous, excoriated lesion that involves the nipple and adjacent skin. The lesion is accompanied, in almost all cases, by intraductal infiltrating carcinoma.

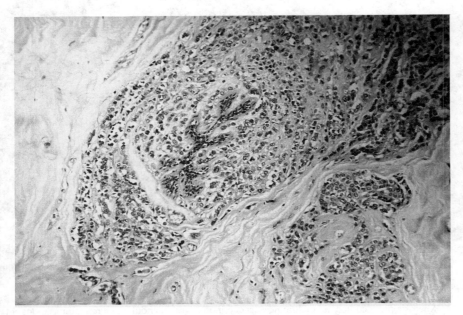

Figure 19-5. Infiltrative lobular carcinoma, with single cells infiltrating the breast parenchyma.

b. Histologically, Paget's cells can be recognized singly or in groups within the epidermis and in the adjacent portions of the mammary duct. The cells have prominent nuclei and abundant periodic acid–Schiff (PAS)-positive, eosinophilic cytoplasm (Figure 19-6).

4. Sarcoma. These tumors arise from the specialized mesenchyma of the breast and account for less than 1% of all breast neoplasms.

  a. Malignant cystosarcoma phylloides (or phyllodes) occurs in older women, who report a rapidly growing tumor mass.

    (1) Pathology

      (a) The **gross features** of the tumor are not characteristic, but, in some instances, the tumor has a fleshy, leaflike appearance. The gross appearance can be confused with that of fibroadenoma.

      (b) Histologically, the hallmark is the presence of a very cellular stroma composed of atypical spindle cells and abundant mitotic figures. Epithelium lines the leaflike processes but is essentially benign.

    (2) Prognosis. The behavior of cystosarcoma cannot be predicted on the basis of a single histologic feature, but, in general, it is accepted that these tumors are locally aggressive and that some have the capacity to metastasize through blood vessels. Large tumors with a high mitotic index and nuclear pleomorphism are associated with the worst prognosis.

    (3) Treatment is surgical resection of the mass. Since cystosarcomas metastasize through the bloodstream, axillary lymph node resection is not necessary.

  b. Angiosarcoma is a highly aggressive neoplasm that accounts for less than 0.5% of breast tumors.

    (1) Clinical features. Most affected patients are in their second or third decade of life. The usual clinical history is that of a lesion that grows rapidly to form a bulky breast tumor.

    (2) Pathology

      (a) Grossly, the lesion consists of an ill-defined infiltrative hemorrhagic mass.

      (b) Histologically, a rich network of communicating vascular channels contains prominent endothelial cells that vary in size and shape. Mitoses are frequently encountered.

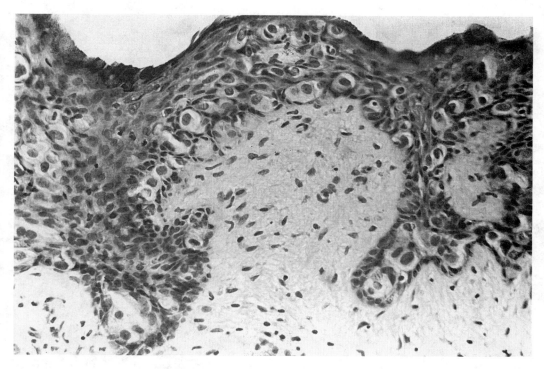

Figure 19-6. Paget's disease of the breast. Large cells with abundant cytoplasm are seen within the epidermis.

        (3) Prognosis. These tumors are associated with a poor prognosis and a high mortality rate. Metastases can occur to any organ; spread is hematogenous and not via lymphatics, as in other forms of epithelial cancer.

        (4) Treatment. Mastectomy is recommended in order to resect the primary tumor mass.

C. Metastases to the breast. The most common tumors to involve the breast secondarily are leukemia, lymphoma, melanoma, lung carcinoma, and endometrial cancer. In general, however, metastases to the breast are rare.

STUDY QUESTIONS

Directions: Each of the numbered items or incomplete statements in this section is followed by answers or by completions of the statement. Select the **one** lettered answer or completion that is **best** in each case.

1. Which histologic feature is the hallmark of invasive lobular carcinoma of the breast?

(A) Its arrangement in pseudoglands
(B) Individual cell infiltration of the stroma
(C) Papillary outgrowths
(D) Pools of mucinous material
(E) Highly cellular stroma with atypical spindle cells

2. Which benign breast disorder has been linked to the development of breast carcinoma in special cases?

(A) Duct ectasia
(B) Fat necrosis
(C) Fibrocystic changes
(D) Fibroadenoma
(E) Intraductal papilloma

3. The primary structural unit of the mammary gland is known as the

(A) ductule
(B) acinus
(C) sinus
(D) lobule
(E) quadrant

4. What is the most common benign breast tumor of premenopausal women?

(A) Cystic fibroma
(B) Fibroadenoma
(C) Lipoma
(D) Intraductal papilloma
(E) Hemangioma

5. A woman who presents with a bloody discharge from one nipple is most likely to have

(A) Paget's disease of the nipple
(B) intraductal papilloma
(C) medullary carcinoma
(D) mucinous carcinoma
(E) intraductal carcinoma

6. Which breast disorder is most likely to occur during lactation and breast-feeding?

(A) Chronic mastitis
(B) Duct ectasia
(C) Fat necrosis
(D) Acute mastitis
(E) Fibrocystic changes

7. Which of the following is the most common type of breast carcinoma?

(A) Intraductal
(B) Medullary
(C) Papillary
(D) Mucinous
(E) Infiltrating ductal

8. Which statement would be true for the diagnosis of lobular carcinoma in situ?

(A) Axillary lymph node dissection is indicated
(B) Excision and radiation therapy are indicated
(C) Careful physical examination will reveal masses in the contralateral breast in 20% of patients with lobular carcinoma in situ in one breast
(D) The patient is at increased risk of invasive breast cancer
(E) This finding is unusual in premenopausal women

9. Presently, in the United States, the most common cause of death in women beyond the fifth decade is

(A) leukemia
(B) myocardial infarction
(C) breast carcinoma
(D) lung carcinoma
(E) cervical carcinoma

1-B	4-B	7-E
2-C	5-B	8-D
3-D	6-D	9-C

10. Which statement is most likely to be true of a patient with cystosarcoma phylloides tumor?

(A) The tumor occurred before menopause
(B) The tumor was a slow-growing mass
(C) The tumor first metastasized to the regional lymph nodes
(D) Distant metastases consisted of malignant stromal cells

11. Important prognostic factors for patients with breast carcinoma include all of the following EXCEPT

(A) age of the patient
(B) histologic tumor type
(C) presence of estrogen receptors in the tumor
(D) presence of metastases
(E) location within the breast

12. All of the following are characteristic of fibrocystic changes EXCEPT

(A) ductal epithelial hyperplasia
(B) microscopic cystic change
(C) apocrine changes of duct epithelium
(D) adenosis
(E) axillary lymphadenopathy

13. All of the following are possible etiologies of a teenager's gynecomastia EXCEPT

(A) lobular hypertrophy
(B) exogenous estrogen
(C) some testicular tumors
(D) puberty
(E) cirrhosis of the liver

10-D   13-A
11-E
12-E

ANSWERS AND EXPLANATIONS

1. The answer is B *[VI B 2 b]*.
Invasive lobular carcinoma of the breast consists predominantly of small cells, which individually infiltrate the stroma in a linear pattern known as "Indian filing." These invasive cells have moderate amounts of eosinophilic cytoplasm and large hyperchromatic nuclei. Pseudoglands are seen in infiltrating ductal carcinoma, papillary outgrowths are observed in benign papilloma and papillary carcinoma, pools of mucin are seen in mucinous carcinoma, and a highly cellular stroma composed of atypical spindle cells and mitotic figures is the characteristic appearance of sarcoma.

2. The answer is C *[IV A 4]*.
The question of whether benign breast disorders represent risk factors for breast cancer has been debated considerably. At present, most authorities agree that benign breast disorders carry little, if any, risk for the development of breast carcinoma, except when accompanying cellular hyperplasia with atypia. Fibrocystic changes of the breast, a disorder that is quite common and variably characterized, may take the form of severe epithelial hyperplasia with atypia and, in these cases, can carry a twofold to threefold increased risk for breast carcinoma. The other benign breast disorders listed (i.e., duct ectasia, fat necrosis, fibroadenoma, and intraductal papilloma) have not been linked with malignant disease of the breast.

3. The answer is D *[I A 1]*.
Clusters of epithelial cells formed into acini are arranged about a ductule to create the lobule, which is the basic structural unit of the mammary gland. Each lobule empties into epithelium-lined ductules and larger ducts, which drain toward the lactiferous sinuses at the nipple. The number of lobules varies in each female mammary gland; the male breast has no lobules.

4. The answer is B *[V A]*.
Fibroadenoma is the most common benign breast tumor. It frequently appears in young women sometime between puberty and age 30. A fibroadenoma consists of proliferated connective tissue and ductal and acinar elements. Cystic fibroma, lipoma, intraductal papilloma, and hemangioma all occur much less commonly.

5. The answer is B *[V B 1]*.
Nipple discharge is encountered more frequently in benign conditions of the breast than in malignant tumors. Intraductal papilloma is the most common cause. This papilloma is a discrete tumor of the connective tissue; it is recognized histologically by its broad stalk of connective tissue, which is covered by two layers of benign epithelial cells. Minor trauma to the delicate, well-vascularized papilloma may be the reason for the intermittent serous or serosanguineous discharge through the nipple.

6. The answer is D *[III A]*.
Acute mastitis usually is produced by a strain of *Staphylococcus* or *Streptococcus,* which enters the breast through fissures in the nipple produced by the minor trauma of breast-feeding. This inflammation, thus, is termed puerperal mastitis. The infection usually can be controlled with antibiotics before severe destruction of breast tissue occurs.

7. The answer is E *[VI B 1 b]*.
Infiltrating ductal carcinoma is the most common form of breast carcinoma, accounting for nearly 70% of breast cancers. Intraductal (in situ) carcinoma and medullary carcinoma each account for about 5% to 10% of cancers of the breast. Papillary and mucinous carcinomas each account for less than 3% of malignant breast tumors.

8. The answer is D *[VI B 2 a]*.
Both lobular carcinoma in situ and ductal carcinoma in situ predispose to the development of invasive cancers. Since lobular carcinoma in situ is not an invasive cancer, further resection, axillary lymph node dissection, and radiation therapy are not indicated. Although lobular carcinoma in situ will be bilateral in 20% of patients with this diagnosis, the microscopic disease usually is an incidental finding and usually occurs in premenopausal women.

9. The answer is C *[VI A 1]*.
At present, carcinoma of the breast is the leading cause of death in women over age 40 in the United States. Although the incidence of lung carcinoma is rapidly increasing in the female population, breast

cancer is even more common; about 1 in 13 women will develop breast carcinoma during her lifetime. Thus far, no screening test to detect breast carcinoma is comparable to the Papanicolaou (Pap) test for early identification of cervical neoplasms.

10. The answer is D *[VI B 4 a].*
Malignant cystosarcoma phylloides are tumors composed of malignant stromal cells and benign epithelial cells; distant metastases consist of the malignant stromal component. Unlike carcinomas of the breast, this tumor does not usually metastasize via lymphatics; hence, regional lymph nodes are spared. This tumor generally occurs in older postmenopausal women and presents as a rapidly growing mass.

11. The answer is E *[VI A 5].*
Although long-term survival for patients with breast carcinoma is difficult to predict precisely, a large number of studies have shown several important prognosticators. These factors include the stage of the cancer at the time of diagnosis, the histologic features of the tumor (medullary, papillary, and mucinous types carry a better prognosis), the age of the patient at the time of diagnosis (the older the patient, the more favorable the prognosis), the estrogen-receptor status (estrogen-positive tumors carry a better prognosis), and the presence or absence of metastases. The location of the primary tumor within the breast has no prognostic significance.

12. The answer is E *[IV A].*
Fibrocystic changes are confined to the breast parenchyma. Axillary lymphadenopathy in a patient with fibrocystic disease should raise the clinical concern of malignancy. Ductal epithelial hyperplasia, microscopic cystic changes, apocrine changes of duct epithelium, and adenosis are typical histologic findings in fibrocystic disease.

13. The answer is A *[IV B].*
Gynecomastia is the proliferation of ductal—not lobular—components (since male breast tissue does not contain lobules) due to hormonal imbalances. It commonly occurs during puberty. Abnormal estrogen levels, from either exogenous or endogenous sources (such as steroid-secreting tumors of the testis) can cause this condition. Gynecomastia is seen in cirrhotic patients because the liver has decreased capacity to metabolize normal estrogenic compounds.

20
Endocrine System
Virginia A. LiVolsi

I. INTRODUCTION: GENERAL CONCEPTS

A. Basic components and functions of the endocrine system. The endocrine system is dispersed throughout the body; its major function is regulation. Endocrine regulation occurs at three sites:

1. The hypothalamus

2. The pituitary gland

3. The endocrine (target) organs (see also Chapter 17 and Chapter 18)

B. Feedback regulation of endocrine function. Negative and positive feedback systems influence the action of the individual target organs and the interaction among the endocrine organs, the hypothalamus, and the pituitary gland. Disturbances of these intricate and delicately balanced feedback systems lead to over- or undersecretion of various hormones and, thus, to clinical syndromes, or endocrinopathies.

C. Not only will lesions in the endocrine system lead to endocrine disease, but disturbed functional states without morphologic abnormalities also can upset this system to such a degree that they create a pathologic lesion. Examples include disorders induced by chemically abnormal neurotransmitters or by overabundant or insufficient amounts of hypothalamic releasing factors.

II. HYPOTHALAMUS AND PITUITARY GLAND

A. Hypothalamus. A part of the brain, the hypothalamus is located just above the pituitary gland.

1. **Function.** The hypothalamus serves as the regulatory center for the endocrine and nervous systems. It integrates incoming neural signals initiated from the body and the environment, and it secretes various releasing or inhibiting factors that invoke specific hormonal responses from the pituitary gland. The most important hypothalamic hormones include:
   a. **Thyrotropin-releasing hormone (TRH),** which stimulates pituitary release of thyrotropin
   b. **Corticotropin-releasing hormone (CRH),** which stimulates pituitary release of adrenocorticotropin
   c. **Prolactin-inhibiting factor (PIF),** which signals the pituitary to halt the release of prolactin

2. **Lesions.** The hypothalamus can be damaged by hamartomas, neoplasms, trauma, or inflammatory conditions (specifically, sarcoidosis). The result of any of these damaging factors is interference with the delicate feedback balance that controls the pituitary gland.

B. Pituitary gland. The pituitary gland is situated in the sella turcica, behind the nose. It is divided into an anterior lobe (the **adenohypophysis**) and a posterior lobe (the **neurohypophysis**).

1. **Anterior lobe.** The adenohypophysis represents approximately 90% of the pituitary gland.
   a. **Function.** Stimulated by hypothalamic hormones, the anterior pituitary produces various tropic hormones that affect the endocrine target glands (thyroid, adrenals, gonads), growth, and lactation.
   b. **Anterior pituitary hyperfunction.** Intrinsic hypersecretion of an anterior pituitary tropic hormone almost always is the result of a neoplasm (usually an adenoma). Uncommonly, it is due to localized areas of hyperplasia or microadenomas. Although functioning adenomas occasionally cause multihormone production, the three most common clinical syndromes are associated with overproduction of a single hormone.

(1) Growth hormone (GH) overproduction
  (a) Clinical features. The effects vary with the patient's age. The causative lesion usually is slow growing, leading to a gradual change in appearance.
    (i) Excessive GH in a child leads to **gigantism**.
    (ii) In an adult, because skeletal epiphyses are closed, **acromegaly** results. The change in appearance consists of a gradual coarsening of the facies, enlargement and swelling of the hands and feet, and thickening of the lips. Because of the influence of GH on glucose tolerance, diabetes mellitus often is found in affected patients.
  (b) Pathology. Gigantism or acromegaly results from an acidophil cell (eosinophilic) pituitary adenoma.
(2) Hyperprolactinemia
  (a) Clinical features. An elevated serum prolactin level associated with spontaneous or inducible galactorrhea has been recognized as a cause of female infertility and secondary amenorrhea (**amenorrhea–galactorrhea syndrome**). This symptom complex has been noted in young women following cessation of oral contraceptives after prolonged use.
  (b) Pathology. The pathologic lesion may be one of a variety of abnormalities ranging from grossly and radiologically visible adenomas to microscopic foci of hyperplasia (microadenomas).
(3) Hypercorticism
  (a) Clinical features. Pituitary hypersecretion of adrenocorticotropic hormone (ACTH) induces adrenocortical hyperfunction; the result is Cushing's syndrome (see VI B). By convention, when this symptom complex is due to ACTH hypersecretion by a pituitary lesion, it is called **Cushing's disease**.
  (b) Etiology and pathology
    (i) Pituitary hypersecretion of ACTH may be caused by hypothalamic overproduction of corticotropin-releasing factor (CRF) or by a tumor of the pituitary gland. Excessive ACTH levels may also be due to ectopic ACTH production by a nonendocrine tumor.
    (ii) The pituitary lesion most frequently found is a **basophil adenoma** or microadenoma. Such tumors usually are quite small and, thus, difficult to detect.
    (iii) After bilateral adrenalectomy for what is clinically considered primary adrenal hyperplasia, some patients develop **Nelson's syndrome,** with extremely high serum ACTH levels and hyperpigmentation; a basophilic pituitary adenoma is then found. This lesion often is locally invasive and difficult to treat.
c. Anterior pituitary hypofunction. Although isolated pituitary hormone deficiencies can occur, **panhypopituitarism** from a destructive pituitary lesion is more common.
  (1) Clinical features. Because of decreases or depletion of pituitary tropic hormones and the resultant nonstimulation of target endocrine organs, affected patients show symptoms of hypothyroidism, hypogonadism, and hypoadrenalism (lethargy, infertility, susceptibility to infection). In children, **dwarfism** also results because of a lack of GH.
  (2) Pathology. Destruction of the pituitary gland may result from:
    (a) A pituitary tumor, either a primary adenoma that compresses the rest of a normal gland or metastasis to the pituitary
    (b) A tumor of a neighboring structure
    (c) Infarction, especially in the peripartum period (**Sheehan's syndrome**)
    (d) Irradiation to the area
    (e) Granulomatous disease, especially sarcoidosis
    (f) The mysterious **empty sella syndrome,** of unknown cause, in which radiologic examination shows the pituitary to be absent or destroyed, although the sella turcica is enlarged
d. Anterior pituitary tumors are nearly always adenomas; carcinomas are very rare. The adenomas can range in size from grossly and radiologically visible to microscopic foci (**microadenomas**).
  (1) Hormonal effects
    (a) Functional adenomas usually are monoclonal and, thus, cause hypersecretion of one anterior pituitary hormone; less commonly, several hormones are produced in excess.
    (b) Nonfunctional adenomas are less common than functional adenomas. When they are large enough to replace the gland, they cause panhypopituitarism.

    (2) Pathology
- **(a)** The **histology** of pituitary tumors is shared by endocrine tumors in general. They usually are composed of groups or nests of uniform, cytologically bland cells encompassed by a delicate vascular network.
- **(b)** Immunohistologic techniques are useful in determining the predominant hormone produced.

2. Posterior lobe. The neurohypophysis is located immediately adjacent to and slightly behind the adenohypophysis.
- **a. Function.** In contrast to the hormone-producing anterior lobe, the posterior pituitary stores and releases two hypothalamic hormones, **oxytocin,** which stimulates uterine contractions and initiates lactation, and **vasopressin** [antidiuretic hormone (ADH)], which regulates the maintenance of serum osmolality.
- **b. Deficiency of vasopressin secretion** leads to **diabetes insipidus,** clinically manifested by the excretion of large volumes of dilute urine (polyuria). Pituitary causes of vasopressin deficiency include compression or destruction of the neurohypophysis by local tumors, radiation, cranial vascular lesions, trauma, or surgery.
- **c. Inappropriate ADH secretion** due to pituitary dysfunction can result from intracranial trauma or infection or from drugs (cyclophosphamide, vincristine). Most other cases are due to ectopic ADH secretion by nonendocrine tumors especially of pulmonary origin.

III. THYROID GLAND

A. Normal anatomy and function. The normal thyroid gland weighs between 20 and 30 g. The **follicle** is the functional unit of the thyroid. It is composed of an epithelium-lined sac filled with colloid, which stores the thyroid hormones in the form of **thyroglobulin.**

B. Thyroid disorders. Goiter is a nonspecific term denoting thyroid gland enlargement. Such increases in gland size and weight may have a variety of causes (Table 20-1). Depending on the underlying cause, patients with an enlarged thyroid gland may be euthyroid, hypothyroid, or hyperthyroid.

1. Inborn defects of thyroid hormone synthesis are rare but can result in congenital goiter. When insufficient thyroid hormone is produced, the pituitary gland responds with increased thyrotropin secretion. This increase stimulates the thyroid follicular epithelium, which then undergoes hyperplasia.

2. Iodine deficiency also can reduce thyroid hormone concentrations, causing the pituitary gland to increase thyrotropin secretion and spur the thyroid gland to hyperplasia. Iodized salt has all but eliminated the problem in the United States, but in certain areas of the world—usually those distant from the sea (and hence from iodine)—endemic goiter occurs in up to 50% of the population.

3. Goitrogens are drugs and foods that interfere with thyroid hormone production and, thus, cause goiter.

4. Nontoxic nodular goiter is an enlargement of the thyroid gland because of repeated or continual hyperplasia in response to a deficiency of thyroid hormone.
- **a. Clinical features.** The thyroid can reach a huge size (250 g or more), extend substernally, and produce respiratory embarrassment. Although nodular goiter involves the entire gland, the nodules may be asymmetrical, or one nodule may dominate the clinical picture and appear to be a thyroid neoplasm.
- **b. Pathology and pathogenesis.** The combination of nodularity, focal hyperplasia, and degenerative changes comprises the entity of nodular goiter.

Table 20-1. Causes of Thyroid Enlargement

Inborn errors of thyroid hormone biosynthesis
Nutritional iodine deficiency
Goitrogenic substances
Nontoxic nodular goiter
Diffuse toxic goiter (Graves' disease)
Thyroiditis
Neoplasms

    (1) In regions where goiter is not endemic, the initial stimulus to nodule formation is unknown. Once an area of hyperplasia is formed, however, intrathyroidal iodine trapping may occur, causing iodine deficiency and promoting the hyperplastic process.

    (2) As hyperplasia continues over years, nodules form. These nodules, which consist of follicles distended with colloid, lie next to zones of microfollicles lined by hyperplastic columnar cells that contain little colloid. Eventually, some of the huge follicles rupture and extrude colloid, inciting an inflammatory reaction.

    (3) Sometimes the foci of hyperplasia are relatively large and circumscribed, resembling a neoplasm (adenoma), and in this case the terms **adenomatous goiter** or **adenomatous hyperplasia in nodular goiter** are used. Occasionally, such a lesion may be associated with clinical hyperfunction, that is, **hyperthyroidism (toxic nodular goiter)**.

  5. Graves' disease (diffuse toxic goiter). This disorder is the most common condition associated with **hyperthyroidism**. Other causes of hyperthyroidism include functioning thyroid adenomas or carcinomas, pituitary tumors that secrete thyrotropin, and choriocarcinomas that secrete thyrotropin-like substances.

    a. Clinical features. Affected patients usually are young females, who exhibit nervousness, tachycardia, sweating, and weight loss. Often exophthalmos also is present. Thyrotropin levels are low to unmeasurable.

    b. Pathology

      (1) Grossly, diffuse toxic goiter is a symmetrical enlargement of the thyroid gland to two or four times the normal size.

      (2) Microscopically, the thyroid shows a diffuse, severe hyperplasia of the follicular epithelium. The follicles are small and contain little colloid. The follicular cells are tall and columnar, with enlarged nuclei. Because the increased numbers of cells do not fit within the follicle in the usual way, papillary infoldings occur (Figure 20-1). The stroma shows marked vascularity, and lymphocytic infiltrates are common.

    c. Pathogenesis. Graves' disease is presumably caused by immunologic mechanisms, but its pathogenesis is unknown.

      (1) The overactivity of the thyroid is caused by excessive stimulation of the gland by thyroid-stimulating immunoglobulins.

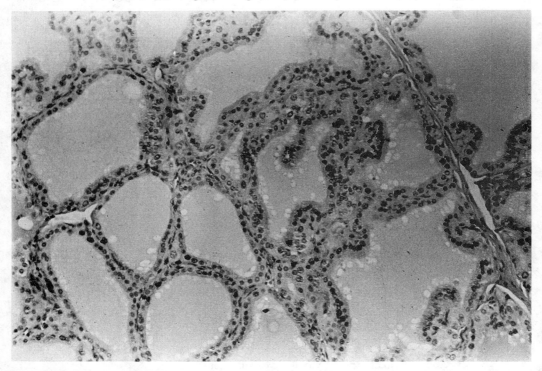

Figure 20-1. Diffuse hyperplasia (Graves' disease) of the thyroid gland. Focal papillary ingrowths into follicles can be seen. Individual cells are enlarged, and their number is increased [hematoxylin and eosin (H and E) stain; low power].

(2) Autoimmune diseases are common in patients with Graves' disease as well as in their close relatives.

6. **Thyroiditis**
   a. **Acute suppurative thyroiditis** is a bacterial infection of the thyroid gland and usually occurs in young children or debilitated patients. It is rare.
   b. **Subacute (granulomatous) thyroiditis** is a self-limited disorder characterized by painful swelling of the thyroid gland, transient hypothyroidism, and recovery in 1 to 3 months. The disorder comprises about 2% of all thyroid disease. The etiology is unknown, but a viral cause is suspected.
      (1) Clinical features. The neck pain begins suddenly and radiates to the jaw or ear. Fever and malaise may be present.
      (2) Pathology
         (a) Grossly, the gland is slightly enlarged. The involved areas are firm and poorly defined, resembling carcinoma.
         (b) Histologically, early in the disease the follicular epithelium degenerates. Colloid leakage from the disrupted follicles accounts for the initial hyperthyroidism and initiates an inflammatory response, which becomes granulomatous. Gland destruction leads to hypothyroidism. Eventually, the follicles regenerate, usually from the edges of the most severely affected areas.
   c. **Chronic thyroiditis (Hashimoto's thyroiditis; struma lymphomatosa; autoimmune thyroiditis)** is a common cause of **hypothyroidism** and is a classic example of autoimmune disease.
      (1) Clinical features. Patients may be euthyroid or, more often, hypothyroid. Hypothyroid (myxedematous) patients often are lethargic, intolerant of cold, and sluggish and have thick skin, bradycardia, and a low body temperature.
      (2) Pathology
         (a) Grossly, the gland is firm and moderately enlarged, from two to four times the normal size. On cut surface, the lobulation of the normal thyroid gland is accentuated and the individual lobules bulge. In the end stage of Hashimoto's thyroiditis, the gland is very small and fibrotic. This pathologic appearance corresponds to the clinical complex of idiopathic myxedema.
         (b) Microscopically, the thyroid follicles are small and atrophic, with sparse or absent colloid (Figure 20-2). Oxyphilic (Hürthle-cell) metaplasia of much or all of the follicular epithelium is common. The most prominent characteristic is infiltration by lymphocytes and plasma cells, with formation of germinal centers. Fibrosis is present and varies in extent.
      (3) Pathogenesis. Although the pathogenesis is unknown, both humoral and cell-mediated immunity are postulated to be involved.
         (a) Affected patients and their close relatives have circulating antibodies to thyroglobulin and to thyroid cell components and surface receptors.
         (b) Patients and their relatives often have other disorders of suspected autoimmune origin as well, including other endocrine disorders.
   d. **Riedel's struma (Riedel's disease)** is not a disorder of the thyroid gland per se, but a connective tissue proliferation that involves the gland. Associated fibrosing processes in the retroperitoneum, orbit, and mediastinum suggest that this disorder is a systemic collagenosis.
      (1) Clinical features. The thyroid compresses the surrounding structures and may obstruct breathing.
      (2) Pathology
         (a) Grossly, the thyroid gland is woody or iron-hard, and the abnormal tissue is adherent to surrounding structures; tissue planes are obliterated.
         (b) Microscopically, fibrous tissue replaces the thyroid. Vasculitis, usually affecting the veins, also is found.

7. **Benign thyroid neoplasms.** All benign tumors of the thyroid gland arise from the follicular epithelium and, thus, are follicular adenomas. The tumors usually are solitary nodules.
   a. **Grossly,** follicular adenomas have the usual well-circumscribed appearance of a benign tumor. Thus, they usually are demarcated from the adjacent normal thyroid tissue and encapsulated (Figure 20-3).

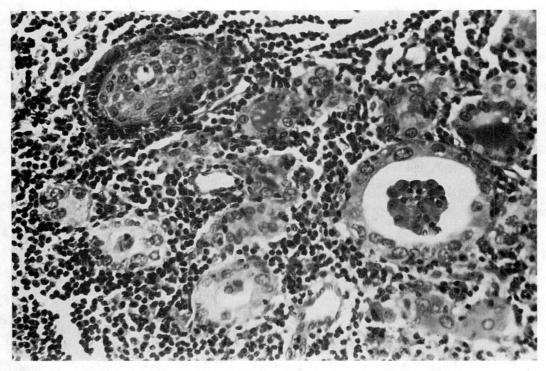

Figure 20-2. Chronic (Hashimoto's) thyroiditis showing follicular atrophy and lymphocytic infiltration [hematoxylin and eosin (H and E) stain; low power].

    b. Microscopically, the encapsulation and the sharp demarcation from the adjacent thyroid tissue are evident. The adjacent thyroid tissue is compressed from the expansile growth of the adenoma.

  8. Thyroid carcinoma
    a. Papillary adenocarcinoma is the most common type of thyroid cancer and accounts for approximately 70% to 80% of all malignant tumors arising in the thyroid.
      (1) Epidemiology. This tumor shows a bimodal distribution: about 50% of patients are under 40, with another peak incidence occurring in the sixth to seventh decade. As with all thyroid cancers, this tumor is more common in women than in men. It has been related to prior head and neck irradiation.
      (2) Clinical features. Thyroid carcinoma presents as an anterior neck mass that usually is painless. On occasion, however, the tumor may present as a cervical lymph node metastasis, with the thyroid gland containing a primary tumor that is too small to be clinically evident.
      (3) Pathology
        (a) Grossly, the appearance varies considerably with the size of the tumor. Small tu-

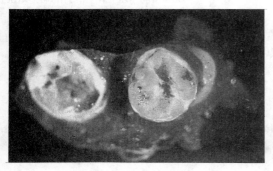

Figure 20-3. A circumscribed nodule of the thyroid gland with a well-developed capsule. The lesion is a benign follicular adenoma.

mors (often called **sclerosing,** or **occult, carcinomas**) resemble minute scars. Large tumors have ill-defined borders, although some show at least partial encapsulation. Cyst formation is common, but the tumor may be solid. Fibrosis and calcification sometimes are extensive.

    (b) Microscopically, the single-layered and well-differentiated tumor epithelium is arranged on fibrovascular stalks. The "ground-glass nuclei" show characteristic clearing. About 40% of papillary carcinomas contain laminated calcific spherules known as **psammoma bodies**.

        (i) Lymphatic invasion by papillary carcinoma is extremely common and probably accounts for the frequency of multiple intrathyroidal foci of the tumor. Metastasis to cervical lymph nodes is so common that 50% of patients already have lymph node involvement at the time of diagnosis.

        (ii) Many papillary carcinomas show follicular differentiation; and for these, some pathologists prefer the term **mixed papillary and follicular carcinoma**. The biologic behavior is similar to that of papillary carcinoma.

  (4) Prognosis. Papillary carcinomas are characterized by their extremely slow growth. The 10-year survival rate is about 95%.

b. Follicular carcinoma accounts for about 5% to 10% of all thyroid carcinomas.

  (1) Clinical features. Adults are affected, with a slight predominance in females. The tumor presents as a nodule. Invasion of blood vessels is common and causes metastases to brain, bones, or lungs. Not uncommonly, the metastatic tumor calls initial attention to the thyroid tumor.

  (2) Pathology

    (a) Grossly, some follicular carcinomas are indistinguishable from follicular adenomas because invasion is not extensive enough to be seen grossly. With other follicular carcinomas, the invasion is grossly evident.

    (b) Microscopically, some tumors are nearly solid, with only abortive attempts at follicle formation; others show neoplastic follicles so well developed that they are indistinguishable individually from normal thyroid tissue.

  (3) Prognosis depends largely on the extent of invasion. If invasion is so minimal that the cancer grossly looks like an adenoma and microscopically shows limited capsular or vascular invasion, the prognosis is very good, with a 5-year survival rate of 85%. Such tumors may take up radioiodine, especially if stimulated with thyrotropin; this characteristic is useful both in diagnosis and in therapy.

c. Medullary carcinoma accounts for 5% to 10% of all thyroid cancers and appears to arise from the **parafollicular (C) cells**. The tumor develops in the upper lateral two-thirds of the thyroid, where these cells are found in highest concentration.

  (1) Clinical features. These tumors usually affect patients over age 40 but occasionally are present in younger adults and in children.

    (a) Parafollicular cells normally secrete **calcitonin,** and the tumors derived from these cells retain this characteristic. Thus, measurement of serum calcitonin is useful as a diagnostic and prognostic tool.

    (b) Medullary carcinoma occurs in familial forms as well as sporadically. In the familial forms, it is a component of multiple endocrine neoplasia (MEN) type II (Sipple's syndrome) and type II b (type III) [see VII and Table 20-4]. In familial cases, medullary carcinoma tends to be multifocal and bilateral.

  (2) Pathology

    (a) Grossly, the tumor typically is a hard, grayish white to yellowish tan mass and usually is well demarcated.

    (b) Microscopically, it contains tumor cells clustered in solid or irregular groups that are separated by a hyaline, **amyloid**-containing stroma.

  (3) Prognosis. Medullary carcinoma can metastasize both by lymphatics and by blood vessels. The prognosis for patients with medullary cancer is not as good as the prognosis for patients with papillary or follicular carcinomas, but it is better than the outlook for patients with undifferentiated carcinoma. The overall 5-year survival rate is 50%.

d. Anaplastic (undifferentiated) carcinoma comprises about 3% to 5% of thyroid carcinomas. It usually is rapidly growing and is one of the most malignant of all cancers.

  (1) Epidemiology. Anaplastic carcinoma occurs almost exclusively in persons over age 60 and, in over 50% of patients, follows a long history of goiter (either benign adenoma or low-grade carcinoma of papillary or follicular type).

(2) **Clinical features.** The tumor presents as a rapidly growing mass that may compromise breathing by compressing the trachea or, on occasion, may ulcerate through the skin.

(3) **Pathology**

(a) **Grossly,** the appearance is that of a typical cancer, with invasion into adjacent areas of the thyroid gland and other structures of the neck. Remnants suggesting a preexisting adenoma or low-grade cancer can be present.

(b) **Microscopically,** the tumor cells are large—often gigantic—and pleomorphism is common.

(4) **Prognosis** is poor. The tumor is nearly always fatal within 1 or 2 years.

IV. PARATHYROID GLANDS

A. Normal anatomy, histology, and function

1. **Anatomy and histology**

   a. About 90% of all persons have four parathyroid glands. These glands usually are located at the superior and inferior poles of the thyroid gland and together weigh 120 to 150 mg.

      (1) In about 5% of people, normal parathyroid tissue is found at ectopic sites, the most common being intrathyroidal, retroesophageal, and intrathymic.

      (2) The superior parathyroids arise from the fourth branchial arch, close to the origin of the thyroid; the inferior parathyroids arise from the third branchial arch, as does the thymus. This embryologic fact explains the occasional presence of ectopic parathyroid tissue and the occasional discovery of intrathymic parathyroid adenomas.

   b. In about 10% of persons, the number of glands varies from the usual number—three to ten (most often five) are found.

   c. The cellularity of the parathyroid glands normally decreases with age; in a normal middle-aged adult, the ratio of cells to fat becomes 1:1.

2. **Function. Parathyroid hormone (PTH),** working in conjunction with vitamin D, calcitonin, and renal mechanisms, plays a major role in calcium homeostasis.

B. Disturbances in calcium homeostasis

1. **Hypercalcemia** is the hallmark of primary hyperparathyroidism.

   a. Hypercalcemia may be due to **other causes** besides an excess of PTH; the mnemonic **MISHAP** provides a useful classification; **m**alignancy (myeloma); **i**ntoxication (vitamin D); **s**arcoidosis; **h**yperparathyroidism (primary and secondary); **a**lkali (milk–alkali syndrome); **P**aget's disease of bone.

   b. **Symptoms** may be absent when hypercalcemia is mild. As serum levels rise above 10 μg/dl, patients develop gastrointestinal, musculoskeletal, cardiovascular, neuropsychiatric, and urinary symptoms. Levels above 18 μg/dl can be lethal.

2. **Hypocalcemia** is much less common than hypercalcemia.

   a. It can result not only from a deficiency of PTH but also from a failure of target organs (bones and kidneys) to respond to PTH, a condition called **pseudohypoparathyroidism.** Other causes of hypocalcemia include vitamin D deficiency, renal disorders, and pancreatitis.

   b. **Symptoms** depend on the degree and duration of the hypocalcemia and are chiefly neurologic: anxiety, depression, functional psychoses, neuromuscular irritability. Severe hypocalcemia causes tetany.

3. **Screening for calcium disturbances.** Serum calcium levels are routinely measured in multichannel screening tests, so many cases of asymptomatic hypo- or hypercalcemia are now being identified. PTH levels can be determined by radioimmunoassay.

C. Primary hyperparathyroidism is a relatively common disorder. It occurs sporadically and, less often, in familial forms, chiefly as a component of MEN types I and II (see VII).

1. **Clinical features.** One or more symptoms of hypercalcemia may be present, but many asymptomatic patients now are identified by mass screening techniques.

2. **Pathology.** From 60% to 80% of patients have solitary parathyroid adenomas (Figures 20-4 and 20-5), and 10% to 25% have primary hyperplasia. The hyperplasia and adenomas usually are of the chief-cell type. Frequently, the histologic distinction between adenoma and hyperplasia is difficult if not impossible to determine; hence, the range of percentages given is wide.

3. **Therapy.** A single adenoma is removed surgically. Multiple gland hyperplasia is treated by subtotal parathyroidectomy or by removal of all parathyroid tissue, a portion of which is then implanted in an arm muscle.

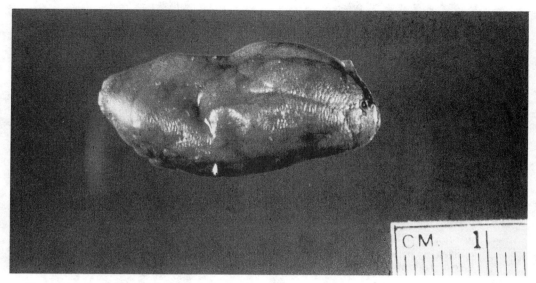

Figure 20-4. A 2.5-cm parathyroid adenoma. The patient's other three parathyroid glands were atrophic.

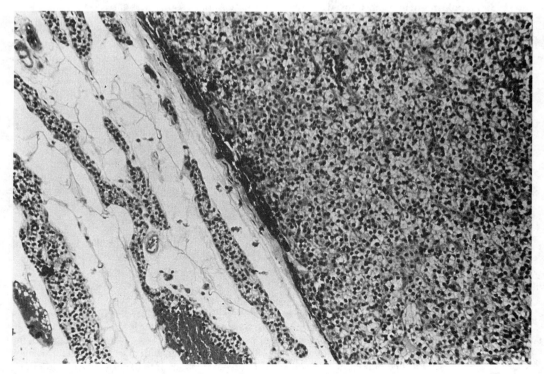

Figure 20-5. Microscopic view of a parathyroid adenoma. Note the cellular area (*right*) abutting the rim of residual normal parathyroid tissue containing few cells and fat (*left*) [hematoxylin and eosin (H and E) stain; low power].

D. Secondary hyperparathyroidism may be caused by renal disease or, more rarely, by malabsorption.

 1. **Clinical features.** Symptoms of the underlying disease will be evident. If the calcium abnormality is not corrected, soft tissue calcification and osteosclerosis develop.

 2. **Pathology.** The parathyroid glands usually show diffuse chief-cell or clear-cell hyperplasia.

 3. **Pathogenesis.** Patients with renal insufficiency cannot synthesize active vitamin D; therefore, they develop hypocalcemia. Some malabsorptive states also cause hypocalcemia. In consequence, a reactive increase in PTH secretion occurs, and parathyroid hyperplasia develops.

E. Hypoparathyroidism usually is an iatrogenic consequence of thyroid surgery, radioiodine therapy, or radical neck dissection. Uncommonly, it is a familial or idiopathic (possibly autoimmune) condition; other infrequent causes are metastases to the parathyroid or iron deposits from long-standing iron-storage disease.

 1. **Clinical features.** Patients have hypocalcemia and hyperphosphatemia, with symptoms related to the degree and duration of the hypocalcemia.

 2. **Pathology.** The pathologic features depend on the cause. Hence, in iatrogenic hypoparathyroidism, no parathyroid tissue is present. In idiopathic hypoparathyroidism, lymphocytes infiltrate and destroy the glands. Metastatic tumors also replace and destroy the parathyroid glands.

F. Parathyroid neoplasms

 1. A solitary **adenoma** is the most common primary disorder of the parathyroid glands (see IV C 2).

 2. **Carcinoma** of the parathyroid glands is very rare, accounting for approximately 1% to 3% of cases of primary hyperparathyroidism. **Clinically,** these tumors are frequently large enough to be palpable and result in severe hypercalcemia. **Pathologically,** mitoses, local invasion, and metastases (usually functional) characterize the lesion.

 3. **Neoplasms of nonparathyroid origin** (usually carcinomas) sometimes can produce substances that mimic the actions of PTH and hence cause hypercalcemia. This condition is known as **ectopic hyperparathyroidism,** or **humoral hypercalcemia of malignancy (HHM).** Recently, **parathyroid hormone-related protein (PTH-rP)** has been characterized. It can cause hypercalcemia by mimicking native parathyroid hormone on end organs involved in calcium homeostasis. The tumors which commonly produce it include squamous cell carcinomas (SCCs) especially of lung origin, renal carcinoma, and certain ovarian cancers.

V. ENDOCRINE PANCREAS

A. Normal anatomy and function. The **islets of Langerhans** are scattered throughout the pancreas but are most numerous in the distal portion (tail). These rounded cellular masses contain several types of endocrine cells. Beta cells produce insulin, α cells produce glucagon, and a variety of other cells secrete somatostatin, vasoactive intestinal polypeptide (VIP), and other hormones. The type of cell that secretes a particular hormone is determined by immunohistochemical staining, which localizes a hormone in a cell.

B. Diabetes mellitus is characterized by glucose intolerance and other metabolic derangements, which result from inadequate secretion of insulin or target-tissue resistance to its action and lead to vascular changes and neuropathy affecting a number of organs.

 1. **Clinical features**
  a. **Types.** Diabetes mellitus has two principal forms.
   (1) **Insulin-dependent (juvenile-onset, or type I) diabetes (IDDM)** comprises only 20% of cases. Often beginning before the patient is age 15, IDDM is characterized by abrupt onset; weight loss; requirement for insulin injections to prevent ketoacidosis; difficulty in maintaining blood sugar levels within normal limits, with marked fluctuations in the blood sugar concentration (this condition has been referred to clinically as brittleness); a less conspicuous genetic pattern than type II diabetes; and a more conspicuous association with histocompatibility antigens. The onset may follow a viral illness.

(2) **Non–insulin-dependent (maturity-onset, or type II) diabetes (NIDDM)** constitutes 80% of cases. Patients may need insulin therapy for control of symptoms but do not require it for survival. In this form, the principal problem may be in the delivery of endogenous insulin or a resistance to it, rather than in its synthesis, especially in obese patients.

b. **Symptoms.** The classic symptoms of diabetes mellitus are polyuria (an obligatory, glucosuric, osmotic diuresis), polydipsia (due to the polyuria), and, particularly in IDDM, polyphagia with a paradoxic weight loss. In uncontrolled IDDM, life-threatening ketoacidosis can develop.

c. **Complications** of diabetes include:

(1) Susceptibility to infections, including tuberculosis, pneumonia, pyelonephritis, and mucocutaneous candidiasis

(2) Peripheral and autonomic neuropathy, manifesting as sensory loss, impotence, postural hypotension, constipation, and diarrhea

(3) Vascular disorders (chiefly from microangiopathy in IDDM and from arteriosclerosis in NIDDM), including:

(a) Retinopathy (the most common cause of blindness in the United States)

(b) Renal disease, notably glomerulosclerosis

(c) Atherosclerosis, causing coronary artery disease, stroke, and gangrene of the lower extremities as well as nephropathy

2. **Etiology and pathogenesis.** Hyperglycemia and diabetes can follow surgical resection of the pancreas, severe pancreatitis, carcinoma of the body or tail of the pancreas, and hemochromatosis (bronze diabetes), but in most cases the pathogenesis of diabetes is not known.

3. **Pathology**

a. **Islets.** Histologic changes in the islets range from complete hyalinization and fibrosis with occasional lymphocytic infiltration to no discernible changes.

b. **Small blood vessels.** Diabetic microangiopathy affects the small arteries and capillaries. The major early morphologic features are the disappearance of pericytes and a thickening of the basement membrane, visible in muscle, skin, retina, kidney, and other tissues.

c. **Medium-sized and large blood vessels.** Precocious development of arteriosclerosis in medium-sized arteries is almost invariably encountered. Lesions are especially common in the coronary, cerebral, mesenteric, renal, and femoral arteries.

d. **Kidneys.** The most common characteristic lesion is nodular glomerulitis, with focal thickening of the capillary basement membrane and an exudative accumulation of hyaline material.

e. **Eyes.** In diabetic retinopathy, the microcirculation exhibits leaky microaneurysms, new formation of capillaries, and hemorrhage into the vitreous.

C. Neoplasms of the endocrine pancreas

1. **General concepts**

a. **Islet cell tumors** are relatively uncommon compared to adenocarcinoma of the pancreas and may be benign or malignant, functioning or nonfunctioning. Most islet cell tumors make themselves known clinically by some type of functional abnormality.

b. **Malignancy of islet cell tumors**

(1) Islet cell tumors are considered benign if they are circumscribed or encapsulated and if no metastases are demonstrated. Neoplasms without metastases but with infiltrative borders, mitoses, or vascular invasion are considered borderline lesions. To diagnose an islet cell carcinoma, metastases to nodes or liver are needed.

(2) Malignant behavior may be noted many years after the initial diagnosis because these lesions usually follow a prolonged course.

c. **Therapy**

(1) Therapy for benign or locally confined islet cell tumors consists of surgical resection.

(2) Therapy for functioning unresectable malignant tumors is directed at the hormonal effects produced, rather than at the tumor, because many patients succumb to the hormonal problems before the tumor replaces vital organs.

2. **Specific tumors**

a. **Benign, nonfunctional islet cell adenomas** do not produce clinical problems and usually are found incidentally at autopsy.

b. Insulinoma. Insulin-producing islet cell tumors are of β-cell origin. They most commonly are found in the distal two-thirds of the pancreas but may be seen in the head of the pancreas or in ectopic locations, such as the duodenal wall. Insulinomas produce large quantities of insulin, most often intermittently.

    (1) Clinical features. Symptoms are related to hypoglycemia and include dizziness, weakness, bizarre behavior, seizures, and coma. Some patients learn to avoid attacks by eating, which leads to obesity.

    (2) Pathology and pathogenesis

        (a) About 90% of insulinomas are benign (including 10% morphologically suspicious for malignancy); thus, 10% are malignant. Most insulinomas are solitary, but approximately 5% of patients have MEN type I (see VII).

        (b) Insulinomas have an endocrine or organoid pattern, with nests and cords of cells supported by fibrovascular stroma (Figure 20-6). Evidence of malignancy includes blood vessel and capsular invasion, numerous mitoses, and metastases to regional lymph nodes and the liver.

        (c) In general, the tumors grow much more slowly than adenocarcinomas of the pancreas. Patients may have hepatic metastases for many years before replacement of liver tissue is extensive enough to cause liver failure. Typically, patients die because of the effects of the hypoglycemia produced by an unresectable tumor.

    (3) Therapy consists of surgical resection of the tumor and, if feasible, resection of hepatic metastases.

c. Gastrinoma. Gastrin-producing islet cell tumors are found in the pancreas or the duodenal wall. These tumors cause the **Zollinger-Ellison syndrome**. The gastrin from the tumor leads to stimulation and hyperplasia of the gastric parietal cells, which then produce 10 to 20 times the normal amount of gastric acid.

    (1) Clinical features. Patients present with intractable peptic ulcer disease (see Chapter 12 II D and E). The ulcers frequently are multiple and may be in atypical locations.

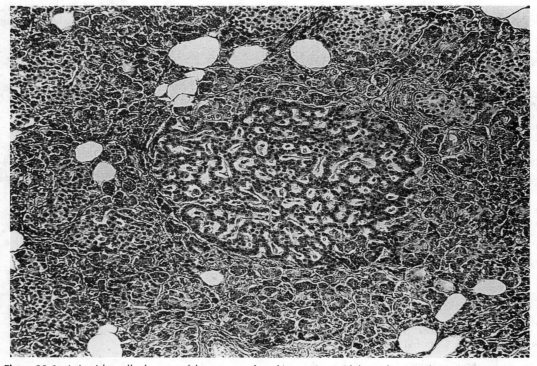

Figure 20-6. A tiny islet cell adenoma of the pancreas found in a patient with hypoglycemia [hematoxylin and eosin (H and E) stain; low power].

(2) **Pathology.** About 60% to 70% of gastrinomas are malignant; thus, about 30% are benign. From 5% to 10% of patients have MEN type I (see VII). **Grossly** (Figure 20-7) and **histologically,** gastrinomas are similar to insulinomas in appearance and present the same difficulties in differentiating benign from malignant tumors.

(3) **Therapy.** Gastrinomas usually are slow-growing, even when in the liver. The major threat to a patient's life is not the tumor itself but complications of peptic ulcer disease. Therefore, when gastrinomas are unresectable, patients are treated by total gastrectomy to remove the target organ of gastrin—that is, the acid-producing parietal cells.

d. **VIPoma.** Islet cell tumors that produce VIP cause a syndrome known as **pancreatic cholera** (also known as **Verner-Morrison syndrome,** or **watery diarrhea, hypokalemia, and achlorhydria (WDHA) syndrome**). The severe electrolyte imbalance caused by these tumors can be fatal. Pathologically, about 80% of these tumors have been classified as malignant.

e. **Glucagonoma.** Glucagon-producing tumors are of alpha cell origin. These tumors are responsible for an unusual clinical syndrome characterized by diabetes mellitus, necrotizing skin lesions, stomatitis, and anemia. Most of these tumors are malignant.

f. **Nonfunctional islet cell carcinomas** produce no hormones and, thus, make themselves known clinically by their malignant behavior, simulating adenocarcinomas. Affected patients may present with obstructive jaundice, hepatic metastases, or a large mass in the abdomen. **Histologically,** an endocrine or organoid pattern may be seen in these tumors, as opposed to the glandular or ductal pattern of adenocarcinoma. About 60% of nonfunctioning islet cell tumors are malignant.

g. **Nesidioblastosis** is a condition usually found in newborns who present with uncontrollable hypoglycemia. Cells similar in morphology to islet cells are found as nodules close to the pancreatic exocrine ducts. Subtotal pancreatectomy often is needed for cure.

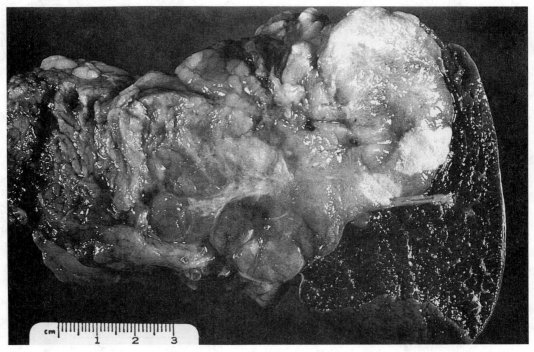

Figure 20-7. A 3-cm malignant islet cell tumor (carcinoma) [a malignant gastrinoma], which produced Zollinger-Ellison syndrome. Invasion of the spleen (*right*) should be noted.

VI. ADRENAL GLANDS. The adrenal cortex and the adrenal medulla have different origins and produce different substances. Therefore, the effects of adrenal disorders depend on where the lesion is and on whether the lesion causes an over- or underproduction of secretions.

A. Normal anatomy and function

1. **The adrenal cortex** has **three zones,** all of which produce **steroid hormones:** the outermost zona glomerulosa produces **mineralocorticoids** (e.g., aldosterone); the intermediate zona fasciculata produces **glucocorticoids** (e.g., cortisol); the innermost zona reticularis produces **androgens** and **progestins**. Some lesions that affect the adrenal cortex produce an excess of steroid hormone; others cause a hormone deficiency.

2. **The adrenal medulla,** which lies within the cortex, originates from the neural crest. The **chromaffin cells** of the medulla produce epinephrine and other **catecholamines**. (Similar chromaffin cells occur in extraadrenal sites, such as the paraganglia.) The adrenal medulla may undergo hyperplastic or neoplastic changes, producing catecholamine excess.

B. Hypercortisolism. Cushing's syndrome results from prolonged exposure to an excess of glucocorticoids.

1. **Etiology and classification.** Cushing's syndrome may be divided into two main groups depending on whether or not the condition results from exposure to excessive ACTH.
   a. ACTH-dependent causes
      (1) Iatrogenic conditions result from administration of excessive doses of ACTH or a synthetic analog.
      (2) Pituitary conditions result from hypersecretion of ACTH, causing bilateral adrenocortical hyperplasia [often called Cushing's disease; see II B 1 b (3)].
      (3) Ectopic ACTH syndrome results from secretion of ACTH by a malignant or benign tumor of nonendocrine origin (see VI B 4).
   b. Non–ACTH-dependent causes
      (1) Iatrogenic conditions result from administration of excessive doses of corticosteroids.
      (2) Adrenal conditions result from adenoma or carcinoma of the adrenal cortex.

2. **Clinical features.** Whatever the cause, an excess of cortisol (or its congeners) produces truncal obesity and redistribution of truncal fat, with a characteristic "buffalo hump"; rounded facies; striae; mild glucose intolerance; mild hypertension; immunologic changes, causing increased susceptibility to infection; thinning of the skin; osteoporosis; and mild electrolyte changes, notably mild hypokalemia. The normal diurnal variation in plasma cortisol (high in the morning and low in the evening) is lost, and plasma levels remain high.

3. **Pathology**
   a. Depending on the cause of the adrenocortical hyperfunction, three **types of lesions** may be seen in the adrenal cortex; their incidence is listed in Table 20-2.
      (1) ACTH-dependent causes are responsible for most cases. Bilateral adrenal hyperplasia, with widening of the zona reticularis, is seen.
      (2) Adrenal adenomas are responsible for the development of Cushing's syndrome in about 10% of cases. These tumors affect women more commonly (80% of cases) than men.
      (3) Adrenal carcinoma also is responsible for about 10% of cases in adults, but is the most common cause of Cushing's syndrome in children.
   b. The malignancy of adrenal neoplasms cannot be diagnosed morphologically because the usual criteria—mitotic activity and vascular or capsular invasion—frequently are absent and also can occur in benign growths. The only accepted criterion is the demonstration of distant metastases.

Table 20-2. Incidence of Adrenal Lesions in Cushing's Syndrome

	Incidence (%)	
Adrenal Lesion	**Adults**	**Children**
Hyperplasia	81	35
Adenoma	9	14
Carcinoma	10	51

    c. In the presence of a functioning adenoma or carcinoma, the contralateral adrenal gland becomes grossly and functionally atrophic.

4. Ectopic ACTH syndrome

    a. A substance similar to ACTH functionally and immunologically may be secreted by non-endocrine tumors, usually small-cell (oat-cell) carcinoma of the lung (accounting for 60% of cases).

    b. Most tumors producing the ectopic ACTH syndrome are rapidly growing malignancies. Often an affected patient does not manifest the typical clinical features of Cushing's syndrome because these features require time to develop. The major abnormalities found are electrolyte disturbances, which may be severe and difficult to control.

C. Hyperaldosteronism

1. Etiology and classification

    a. Primary aldosteronism (Conn's syndrome) is due to a lesion of the adrenal gland and accounts for approximately one-third of all cases of adrenocortical hyperfunction. The aldosterone excess produces sodium retention, increased total plasma volume, increased renal artery pressure, and inhibition of renin secretion.

    b. In **secondary aldosteronism,** the increased secretion of aldosterone is due to extraadrenal causes, chiefly renal hypertension or edematous states, and relates to renin hypersecretion.

2. Clinical features. Most patients with primary aldosteronism are women aged 30 to 50 who present with hypertension. A hypokalemic alkalosis almost always is present.

3. Pathology

    a. The most common lesion in Conn's syndrome is a single, benign **adrenal adenoma** (Figure 20-8). **Grossly,** the tumor is typically a circumscribed, encapsulated lesion with a distinctive golden-yellow cut surface. **Histologically,** the most common cellular pattern consists of large lipid-laden clear cells.

    b. Rarely, an adrenal carcinoma or bilateral adrenal hyperplasia is responsible for the hyperaldosteronism.

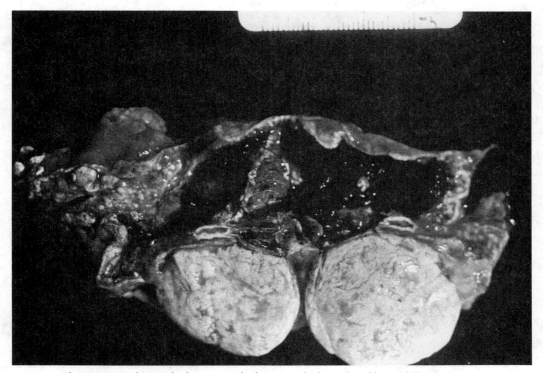

Figure 20-8. A bisected adrenocortical adenoma, which produced hyperaldosteronism.

D. Adrenogenital syndromes

1. **Congenital adrenal hyperplasia** is a term used to describe several **inborn enzyme defects** that inhibit cortisol synthesis. The result is a feedback overproduction of ACTH, causing adrenal hyperplasia and overproduction of the adrenal hormones that are not affected by the enzyme deficiency. Each of these inborn errors of metabolism appears to be caused by an autosomal recessive gene, which is manifested only in the homozygous state, with varying degrees of expression.

   a. **Clinical features.** In the most common forms (Table 20-3), the most striking effect is an increase in adrenal androgens, with **virilizing** consequences. These features are usually apparent at birth, but in some forms do not develop until later.

   b. **Pathology.** Adrenocortical hyperplasia (with weights up to 15 g) is seen. Histologically, the cortical cells are eosinophilic with finely granular cytoplasm, reflecting the effect of elevated levels of circulating ACTH.

2. In adults, **adrenal virilism** can be caused by adrenal hyperplasia, adrenal carcinoma, or, rarely, an adenoma.

E. Adrenocortical insufficiency

1. **Etiology and classification**
   a. **Primary adrenal insufficiency (Addison's disease)** results from destruction of the adrenal cortex.
      (1) In recent years, 60% of cases have been idiopathic, probably autoimmune in nature. The autoimmune basis is supported by the presence of antiadrenal autoantibodies in most patients with idiopathic Addison's disease. In addition, other disorders associated with antibodies coexist with Addison's disease, such as:
         (a) Chronic lymphocytic thyroiditis and Addison's disease (**Schmidt's syndrome**)
         (b) Pernicious anemia and Addison's disease
         (c) Idiopathic hypoparathyroidism, gonadal failure (with antiovarian antibodies), and Addison's disease
      (2) Before effective control of tuberculosis, tuberculous granulomas caused over 50% of cases of adrenal failure. Other causes (e.g., metastatic tumors, amyloidosis, hemorrhage, arterial emboli, fungal diseases) account for only a small proportion of cases.
   b. **Secondary adrenal insufficiency** results from decreased secretion of ACTH, which can be due to destructive lesions of the pituitary gland or the hypothalamus or can be the result of corticosteroid therapy.

2. **Clinical features**
   a. **Acute adrenal insufficiency (adrenal crisis)** is a rapidly progressive illness (over hours or days) presenting clinically as shock. Such an illness may occur in septicemia, especially meningococcemia (**Waterhouse-Friderichsen syndrome**). The septic state, with its associated disseminated intravascular coagulation (DIC), produces multiple vascular thrombi and hemorrhagic infarcts in many organs.
   b. **Chronic adrenal insufficiency** can vary from a complete failure of hormone production to a minor impairment of adrenal reserve capacity. Symptoms develop insidiously and include malaise, weight loss, skin pigmentation, hypotension, loss of body hair, and menstrual irregularities.

Table 20-3. Virilizing Adrenogenital Syndromes

Syndrome	Defect	Symptom Complex
Lipoid hyperplasia	Conversion of cholesterol to pregnenolone	Pseudohermaphroditism in males
Salt-losing syndrome	21-Hydroxylase defect	Precocious virilism in males; pseudohermaphroditism in females; salt loss
Eberlein-Bongiovanni syndrome	11-β-Hydroxylase defect	Virilism, hypertension

3. **Pathology**
   a. In idiopathic Addison's disease, the adrenal cortex loses its normal three-layered architecture. The adrenocortical cells are reduced to islets surrounded by increased fibrous tissue, and lymphocytic infiltration is present.
   b. Adrenal destruction by infarcts, tuberculosis, fungi, or metastatic tumors shows the same pathologic patterns as destruction by such lesions elsewhere in the body.

F. **Adrenal medullary disorders**

1. **Pheochromocytoma.** This uncommon chromaffin cell tumor is a treatable cause of hypertension. Approximately 90% of pheochromocytomas occur in the adrenal medulla; of these, about 10% are malignant and 10% are bilateral. Pheochromocytomas may occur alone or as a component of MEN type II or II b (type III) [see VII].
   a. **Variants**
      (1) About 10% of pheochromocytomas are **extraadrenal,** occurring in other tissues of neural crest origin.
      (2) **Adrenal medullary hyperplasia** (bilateral or unilateral) causes symptoms similar to those of a pheochromocytoma. Although this condition may occur sporadically, most affected patients are from families with MEN type II.
   b. **Clinical features**
      (1) The catecholamines released into the circulation by a pheochromocytoma cause paroxysmal or sustained hypertension, angina, cardiac arrhythmias, headache, and carbohydrate intolerance. If the tumor is untreated, a potentially fatal cerebrovascular accident, congestive heart failure with pulmonary edema, or ventricular fibrillation may result.
      (2) Laboratory findings typically include elevated urinary vanillylmandelic acid (VMA) and norepinephrine levels.
   c. **Pathology**
      (1) **Grossly,** pheochromocytomas usually are circumscribed, gray to brown tumors, ranging in size from 1 to 4 cm or more.
      (2) **Microscopically,** the tumors are composed of nests and cords of large cells with voluminous cytoplasm. Often, nuclear atypia is seen; multiple nuclei may be seen.

2. **Neuroblastoma.** This extracranial malignant solid tumor is the most common in infancy and childhood, comprising about 15% to 50% of neonatal malignancies and 7% to 14% of childhood malignancies.
   a. **Clinical features.** Neuroblastoma is slightly more common in men than in women. The most frequent sites are the adrenal medulla and the cervical, thoracic, and abdominal sympathetic ganglia. Abnormal quantities of catecholamines are present in the urine of about 80% of affected patients, forming the basis of the diagnosis.
   b. **Pathology**
      (1) **Grossly,** neuroblastomas usually are within a pseudocapsule, are nodular in appearance, and have a grayish surface when cut. Frequently, areas of necrosis, hemorrhage, and calcification are present within the tumor.
      (2) **Microscopically,** a typical neuroblastoma is highly cellular, with cells arranged in broad sheets that in some areas form rosette patterns. Mitotic figures often are found in large numbers. The presence of rosettes plus neurofibril formation is pathognomonic.
   c. **Prognosis.** The most important determinants of survival are age at the time of diagnosis (younger patients having better survival rates) and stage of disease (5-year survival rates ranging from 85% for localized disease to 30% for wide metastatic neuroblastoma).

VII. MULTIPLE ENDOCRINE NEOPLASIA (MEN) SYNDROMES

A. Usually familial and genetically induced (autosomal dominant), MEN syndromes include several complexes characterized by neoplasia (benign or malignant), hyperplasia of one or more of the endocrine glands, or both.

Table 20-4. Components of Multiple Endocrine Neoplasia (MEN) Syndromes

Gland	MEN Type I	MEN Type II or IIa	MEN Type III or IIb
Parathyroid	Tumors (usually multiple discrete adenomas or adenomatous hyperplasia)	Adenomas or adenomatous hyperplasia	Occasionally hyperplasia
Pancreas	Islet cell tumors (Zollinger-Ellison, insulinomas, multiple tumors, or diffuse hyperplasia)	. . .	. . .
Pituitary	Adenoma	. . .	. . .
Thyroid	Occasional adenomas	Medullary carcinoma	Medullary carcinoma
Adrenal	Cortical adenomas	Pheochromocytoma (usually multiple and bilateral)	Pheochromocytoma
Other	Occasionally carcinoid tumors (especially bronchial)	Occasional carcinoid tumors	Multiple mucosal and gastrointestinal tract neuromas Melanosis, myopathy, marfanoid habitus

B. Three MEN syndromes have now been defined; their components are listed in Table 20-4. Glands may be affected synchronously or asynchronously in a single patient, or some tumors may occur in some family members whereas others occur in other members. Frequently, multiple endocrine lesions are found at autopsy, although during life the effects of one particular tumor may have dominated.

C. The genes for MEN have been mapped to chromosome 10.

STUDY QUESTIONS

Directions: Each of the numbered items or incomplete statements in this section is followed by answers or by completions of the statement. Select the **one** lettered answer or completion that is **best** in each case.

1. A 32-year-old woman is found to have a non-tender nodule on the side of her neck. Routine examination reveals no symptoms, no other masses, and a normal thyroid gland on palpation. Results of thyroid function tests and scan are unremarkable. Biopsy of the mass reveals pathologically normal-appearing thyroid tissue in an enlarged lymph node. This mass most likely represents

(A) a lateral aberrant thyroid
(B) a thyroid papillary carcinoma
(C) a metastatic thyroid follicular carcinoma
(D) a thyroglossal duct remnant
(E) branchial cleft cyst

2. Diffuse lymphocytic infiltration of the adrenal gland is the pathologic lesion most commonly associated with

(A) Conn's syndrome
(B) Cushing's syndrome
(C) Waterhouse-Friderichsen syndrome
(D) Addison's disease
(E) ectopic adrenocorticotropic hormone (ACTH) syndrome

3. The primary thyroid carcinomas that show multiple intrathyroidal foci are

(A) papillary carcinoma and medullary carcinoma
(B) follicular carcinoma and papillary carcinoma
(C) medullary carcinoma and follicular carcinoma
(D) anaplastic carcinoma and papillary carcinoma

4. Which sequence lists pancreatic islet cell tumors in order, from the most benign to the most malignant?

(A) Gastrinoma, vasoactive intestinal polypeptide (VIP)-producing tumor (VIPoma), insulinoma
(B) Insulinoma, gastrinoma, glucagonoma
(C) Insulinoma, glucagonoma, gastrinoma
(D) Gastrinoma, insulinoma, VIPoma
(E) Insulinoma, VIPoma, glucagonoma

5. All of the following features characterize anaplastic thyroid carcinoma EXCEPT that

(A) it accounts for about 5% of thyroid cancer
(B) the malignancy typically arises in a preexisting tumor
(C) young adults primarily are affected
(D) the tumor typically extends beyond the thyroid capsule at diagnosis
(E) affected patients have a very poor prognosis

6. Carcinoma of the parathyroid gland is characterized by all of the following EXCEPT

(A) the presence of mitoses in the tumor
(B) severe hypercalcemia
(C) extension of the tumor beyond the capsule of the gland
(D) large tumor size
(E) a rim of atrophic parathyroid tissue

7. Multiple endocrine neoplasia (MEN) syndrome type IIb (type III) has all of the following components EXCEPT

(A) pheochromocytoma of the adrenal gland
(B) medullary carcinoma of the thyroid gland
(C) neuromas of the lips
(D) marfanoid appearance
(E) pituitary adenoma

8. All of the following endocrine disorders are pathogenetically grouped as autoimmune diseases EXCEPT

(A) Addison's disease
(B) Hashimoto's disease
(C) Nelson's syndrome
(D) Schmidt's syndrome
(E) Graves' disease

1-B	4-B	7-E
2-D	5-C	8-C
3-A	6-E	

Directions: The group of items in this section consists of lettered options followed by a set of numbered items. For each item, select the **one** lettered option that is most closely associated with it. Each lettered option may be selected once, more than once, or not at all.

Questions 9–12

Match each syndrome with its related pituitary hormone.

(A) Nelson's syndrome
(B) Cushing's disease
(C) Gigantism
(D) Diabetes insipidus

9.   Antidiuretic hormone (ADH)

10. Adrenocorticotropic hormone (ACTH)

11. Growth hormone (GH)

12. Melanocyte-stimulating hormone (MSH)

9-D   12-A
10-B
11-C

ANSWERS AND EXPLANATIONS

1. The answer is B *[III B 8 a].*
Despite the follicular appearance, the mass identified in this woman most likely represents a papillary adenocarcinoma in the primary site. Most papillary cancers have follicles; this fact does not make a papillary lesion a follicular cancer. The biology of these lesions is distinctive.

2. The answer is D *[VI B, C, E 2 a, 3 a].*
In idiopathic Addison's disease, the adrenal cortex is reduced to a few residual adrenocortical cells surrounded by increased fibrous tissue and lymphocytic infiltration. In Conn's syndrome and Cushing's syndrome, the adrenal cortex is hyperplastic rather than destroyed. In Waterhouse-Friderichsen syndrome, the adrenal cortex is destroyed by hemorrhage evoking an acute adrenal crisis; lymphocytes are not part of the pathologic picture. In ectopic adrenocorticotropic hormone (ACTH) syndrome, the adrenal cortex is thickened and hyperplastic; lymphocytes are not a part of the microscopic picture.

3. The answer is A *[III B 8 a (3) (b), c (1) (b)].*
Papillary carcinoma of the thyroid, because of its tendency to invade lymphatics in the gland, can show multiple intrathyroidal foci as a consequence of lymphatic permeation. Medullary carcinoma in the setting of multiple endocrine neoplasia (MEN) type II can present as multiple, bilateral, and apparently separate clonal proliferations of tumor in the gland; this presentation does not occur in sporadic cases. Neither follicular nor anaplastic carcinoma is known to give rise to multiple foci within the gland.

4. The answer is B *[V C 2 b–e].*
Of all pancreatic islet cell tumors, the most frequently benign are those that produce insulin, with 90% of insulinomas being benign. Tumors producing Zollinger-Ellison syndrome, or gastrinomas, have a malignancy rate of 60% to 70%, whereas almost all tumors producing glucagon are malignant. Vasoactive intestinal polypeptide (VIP)-producing tumors (VIPomas), or those associated with pancreatic cholera [also known as the watery diarrhea, hypokalemia, and achlorhydria (WDHA) syndrome], have a malignancy rate of approximately 80%.

5. The answer is C *[III B 8 d].*
Anaplastic thyroid cancer accounts for about 3% to 5% of thyroid carcinomas. The tumor occurs almost exclusively in patients over the age of 60 and typically arises in a preexisting goiter, usually a preexisting benign or low-grade malignant tumor. It often extends beyond the capsule at the time of diagnosis and rarely is confined to the gland. Anaplastic thyroid carcinoma is a rapidly growing tumor that is associated with a very poor prognosis; most affected patients die within the first year following diagnosis.

6. The answer is E *[IV F 2].*
Carcinoma of the parathyroid glands is caused by a solitary, large, often palpable tumor that clinically presents as severe hypercalcemia. Other pathologic features include the presence of mitoses and local invasion into peritumoral soft tissues beyond the capsule of the gland. Since the tumor tends to be large and replaces the gland, a remnant of uninvolved parathyroid tissue is not found.

7. The answer is E *[III B 8 c (1) (b); VII; Table 20-4].*
Patients with type IIb (type III) multiple endocrine neoplasia (MEN) syndrome characteristically present with medullary thyroid carcinoma (which may be multiple and bilateral), pheochromocytoma of the adrenal gland (which may be multiple and bilateral, mucosal neuromas (especially around the head and neck), and musculoskeletal abnormalities (e.g., a marfanoid appearance, myopathy). The associated pituitary lesions are not components of this syndrome but are characteristic of MEN type I.

8. The answer is C *[II B 1 b (3) (b) (iii); III B 5, 6; VI E 1 a (1) (a)].*
Nelson's syndrome reflects the response of a pituitary tumor to removal of its target organ and has not been related to autoimmunity. Addison's, Hashimoto's, Schmidt's, and Graves' diseases have been proven to be of autoimmune etiology or strongly linked with it.

9–12. The answers are: 9-D *[II B 2],* **10-B** *[II B 1 b (3) (a)],* **11-C** *[II B 1 b (1) (a) (i)],* **12-A** *[II B 1 b (3) (b) (iii)].*
Diabetes insipidus results from a lack of vasopressin, or antidiuretic hormone (ADH), which can result from injury to the neurohypophysis.

Cushing's disease is related to a pituitary tumor (basophil adenoma) secreting adrenocorticotropic hormone (ACTH) in large amounts.

Gigantism occurs in children with pituitary adenomas (acidophil type) producing growth hormone (GH).

Nelson's syndrome occurs after bilateral adrenalectomy; the lesion in the pituitary can produce both ACTH and melanocyte-stimulating hormone (MSH) leading to hyperpigmentation.

21
Nervous System
Virginia A. LiVolsi

I. CONGENITAL ABNORMALITIES OF THE CENTRAL NERVOUS SYSTEM are common lesions that vary from minor asymptomatic defects to gross malformations incompatible with life. They are assumed to be due to a transient pathologic state during pregnancy (metabolic, nutritive, toxic, or infective), faulty implantation of the placenta, or genetic abnormalities. Only representative conditions are described.

A. Neural tube defects (posterior midline lesions, dysraphia). These congenital anomalies result from defective closure of dorsal midline structures during early gestational life. They may involve the cranium, brain, and spinal cord as well as the skin, soft tissues of the back, vertebrae, and meninges. Symptoms vary with the severity of the defect.

1. Spina bifida is the most common neural tube defect. The arches and dorsal spines of one or more vertebrae are absent. Spina bifida may hinder or completely preclude walking.

2. Meningocele is a herniation of spinal arachnoid and dura through a vertebral defect. If a spinal root or part of the spinal cord is included in the herniation, it is a **meningomyelocele**. A soft saclike swelling is palpable beneath the skin in the midline of the back. The overlying skin may ulcerate, with leakage of cerebrospinal fluid (CSF) followed by entry of bacteria and suppurative leptomeningitis.

3. Arnold-Chiari malformation is the caudal displacement of the medulla and cerebellum into the cervical region of the vertebral canal; it often accompanies lumbar spina bifida and hydrocephalus.

4. Anencephaly, the most severe dysraphia, is incompatible with life. The vault of the skull usually is missing, and the cerebral hemispheres, diencephalon, and midbrain are absent. A mass of undifferentiated vascular tissue is exposed.

B. Hydrocephalus. In this condition, the CSF is under increased pressure in the ventricles of the brain, with dilation of these cavities (**internal hydrocephalus**).

1. Clinical features. In late prenatal life and early infancy, before the bony sutures of the skull close, hydrocephalus leads to abnormal enlargement of the head. The sutures are widely separated, and the fontanelles are large and tense.

2. Pathology. The brain is large, with dilated ventricles, flattened gyri, and narrowed sulci. The walls of the cerebral hemispheres are thinned, the central white matter is atrophied, and the basal ganglia and thalamus are compressed.

3. Pathophysiology
a. In **noncommunicating hydrocephalus,** there is a partial or complete obstruction of the flow of fluid. The obstruction may be within the ventricles or in the subarachnoid space above the exit from the fourth ventricle. No communication remains between the ventricles and the spinal subarachnoid space, and the entire ventricular system proximal to the block is dilated.
b. In **communicating hydrocephalus,** no point of obstruction is found, and, thus, free communication exists between the ventricles and the spinal subarachnoid space. The cause of interference with CSF flow is not always known, but it may be due to malformation of subarachnoid spaces, overproduction of fluid by the choroid plexus, or deficient filtration through the arachnoid granulations.

C. Agenesis of the corpus callosum is a congenital malformation of unknown cause. It may be complete or partial. The hemispheres are connected only at the brain stem level. Affected patients may have no symptoms or only minor psychiatric dysfunction.

D. Tuberous sclerosis (Bourneville's disease), an autosomal dominant disorder, affects both the central nervous system (CNS) and the skin.

1. **Clinical features.** Patients have epileptic seizures, mental retardation, and facial eruptions (adenoma sebaceum).

2. **Pathology.** Smooth nodules composed of glial fibers, malformed astrocytes, and nerve cells are found in the walls of the ventricles and cerebral gyri. These nodules grow slowly, producing mass effects. Neoplasms of the heart, liver, kidney, or pancreas also may occur.

E. von Recklinghausen's disease, or neurofibromatosis, is a hereditary disorder characterized by cutaneous café au lait spots and superficial neurofibromas. Multiple tumors of nerve sheath origin (neurofibromas, schwannomas) can arise in any nerve. Benign and malignant lesions can occur.

1. **Peripheral neurofibromatosis** (or neurofibromatosis, type 1) consists primarily of skin lesions as well as dermal and peripheral nerve tumors. The gene for this disorder has been recently cloned and is located on chromosome 17.

2. **Central neurofibromatosis** (or neurofibromatosis type 2) is characterized by bilateral schwannomas of the acoustic nerve, meningiomas, gliomas, and neurofibromas. The gene for this form of the disease is located on chromosome 22.

F. Degenerative heredofamilial disorders comprise a large, uncommon group of diseases in which the **clinical course** is chronic, with progressive deterioration of motor and mental functions and finally death in months or years. **Pathologically,** these disorders all show degeneration and disappearance of nerve cells and fibers in various parts of the nervous system.

1. **Huntington's disease** is an autosomal dominant familial dementia in which psychopathic disorders, involuntary movements, and grimacing are common; the defect involves the basal ganglia. The average age at onset is about 50 years; the course lasts 10 to 15 years and is ultimately fatal.

2. **Wilson's disease,** an autosomal recessive disease, is due to a biochemical abnormality of copper metabolism.
   a. Copper accumulates in the brain, the eyes (**Kayser-Fleischer rings**), and the liver; the normal copper-carrying protein, ceruloplasmin, is decreased, absent, or defective.
   b. The disease begins in adolescence, with movement disorders and hepatic dysfunction. Treatment with copper-chelating agents has dramatically improved the outlook.

3. **Lipid storage diseases. Tay-Sachs disease** and **Niemann-Pick disease** are discussed in Chapter 8 VIII B 3 and 4. In the nervous system, accumulation of the abnormal lipid in nerve cells results in diffuse dysfunction, with mental retardation and early death.

4. **Friedreich's ataxia** is an autosomal recessive trait in some families and, less commonly, autosomal dominant in others. Both forms cause degeneration of the spinal cord, kyphosis, and optic atrophy.

II. VASCULAR DISORDERS OF THE CENTRAL NERVOUS SYSTEM

A. Intracranial hemorrhage. The classification and pathogenesis of hemorrhagic disorders are based on the natural partition of the intracranial space into **four anatomic compartments:** the brain parenchyma, the subarachnoid space, the subdural space, and the epidural space. Each has distinctive lesions.

1. **Intraparenchymal hemorrhage** is diverse in pathogenesis, size, and clinical expression. It produces lesions predominantly in three locations, with the following approximate incidences: in the basal ganglia and thalamus, 65%; in the pons, 15%; and in the cerebellum, 10%.
   a. **Clinical significance of size.** Minute lesions (**petechiae**) are less harmful per se than the obstruction of the associated small vessel. Large hematomas, as masses, have the potential to produce focal neurologic deficits and to initiate lethal transtentorial herniation.

  b. Etiology

    (1) Hypertension (see II D 2) is a prominent cause of intraparenchymal hemorrhage.

    (2) Hematomas accompany **leukemia,** particularly when the neoplastic cells engorge and obstruct the small vessels. The thrombocytopenia associated with leukemia and its therapy also is significant.

    (3) Berry aneurysms and **arteriovenous (AV) malformations** (see II B 1 and II C 1) may rupture and produce intracerebral hematomas.

    (4) Primary and metastatic **neoplasms** within the brain may bleed.

    (5) Intracerebral hemorrhages that result from **trauma** usually are multiple and are associated with adjacent superficial cortical contusions.

    (6) Coagulation disorders and **vasculitis** are other causes of intraparenchymal hemorrhage.

  c. Clinical features

    (1) The patient suffering a cerebral hemorrhage (**cerebrovascular accident, hemorrhagic stroke**) suddenly loses consciousness and falls. The head is thrown back, the face is congested, breathing is hard, and the limbs on one side are paralyzed (**hemiplegia**). Urinary and fecal incontinence may develop.

    (2) If hemorrhage appears toward the surface of the brain, irritation of the cerebral cortex may give rise to **convulsions**.

    (3) Coma may occur and deepen, and death may occur in a few hours or days.

    (4) If the hemorrhage is small and is resorbed and the edema subsides, the patient may recover completely or have a neurologic deficit, with manifestations depending on the site of the hemorrhage.

  d. Pathology. Acute massive hemorrhage in the brain usually occurs in hypertension, embolism, or vasculitis and is due to the rupture of an abnormal vessel wall.

    (1) Gross appearance (Figure 21-1) When the hemorrhage is fresh, the affected cerebral hemisphere is swollen and its gyri are flattened. The mass of recent thrombus and fluid blood disrupts and distends the brain. The mass may rupture into the lateral ventricles, filling the ventricular system with blood.

      (a) Structures around the area of hemorrhage are compressed and edematous.

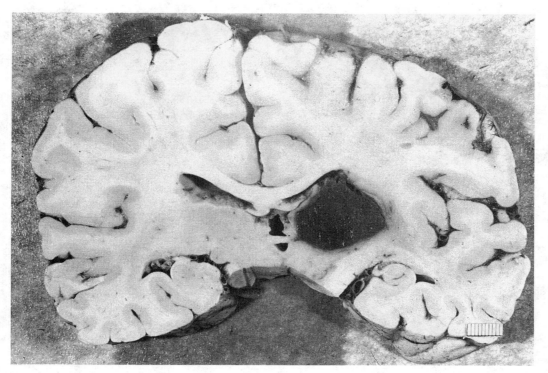

Figure 21-1. Cross section of the brain from a 70-year-old man with hypertension. A large hemorrhage is present in the area of the basal ganglia.

(b) If the patient survives, the clot shrinks and becomes chocolate-colored, and the edema disappears.

(2) Microscopic appearance

(a) In a fresh hemorrhage, masses of erythrocytes replace the destroyed tissue.

(b) Within 3 days, microglial phagocytes begin to ingest degenerating red blood cells, and within 6 to 10 days, hemosiderin begins to appear. Within 3 to 6 weeks after the initial event, the phagocytic activity clears out the central area of destruction, leaving a cystic space.

2. Subarachnoid hemorrhage is most commonly caused by trauma or by rupture of a berry aneurysm. It produces:

a. Headache, by increasing intracranial pressure

b. Nuchal rigidity, by meningeal irritation

c. Alterations in mental status

d. Hydrocephalus, by obstruction of the flow of CSF

3. Subdural hemorrhage, with rare exception, results from trauma that shears the veins or small arteries that traverse the space between the arachnoid and the dura. Most vulnerable to hemorrhage are the superior cortical veins that lead to the superior sagittal sinus (see also VI A 2).

4. Epidural hemorrhage. A skull fracture can shear the middle meningeal artery, and the resultant bleeding dissects the dura from the inner table of the skull. The expanding mass increases intracranial pressure, produces herniation, and requires prompt evacuation to save life.

B. Vascular malformations

1. AV malformation (Figure 21-2) is one of the most significant aberrations of angiogenesis. Fundamental to this lesion are congenital, low-resistance AV shunts that siphon blood from the adjacent parenchyma. In time, this tangle of abnormal vessels enlarges.

a. Distribution. AV malformation favors the regions of the cerebral hemispheres that lie within the distribution of the middle cerebral artery.

b. Clinical features include seizures, neurologic deficits, and chronic mass effects.

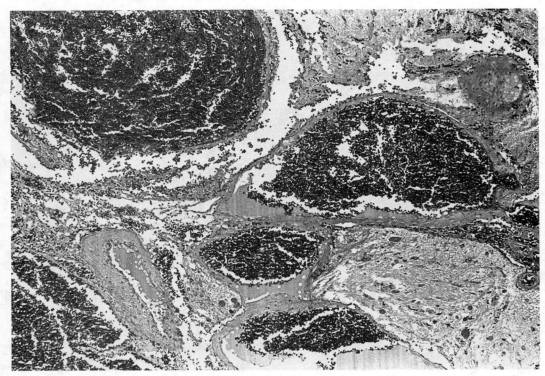

Figure 21-2. Arteriovenous malformation of the brain, showing large, blood-filled, thin-walled vessels. Brain tissue is at *lower right* (low power).

   c. Rupture of an AV malformation causes combined intraparenchymal and subarachnoid hemorrhage in two-thirds of the cases, subarachnoid hemorrhage alone in one-fourth, and intraparenchymal hemorrhage alone in the remainder.

2. Three **additional vascular malformations** are recognized entities, all of which generally are asymptomatic:

   a. Telangiectasis
   b. Venous angioma
   c. Cavernous angioma

C. Aneurysms

1. Berry aneurysms are small saccular aneurysms. They originate from a structural weakness at the branch point of a large cerebral artery in, or within several centimeters of, the circle of Willis. More than 90% of berry aneurysms occur within the carotid supply. They are multiple in about 20% of cases.

   a. Pathogenesis. The aneurysm is thought to be due to a congenital defect of the media at the bifurcation of an artery, with superimposed degeneration of the internal elastic membrane. The wall gives way under arterial pressure at such a weak point, and a berry aneurysm occurs.

   b. Rupture of a berry aneurysm is the most common cause of nontraumatic symptomatic subarachnoid hemorrhage in adults.

2. Mycotic (septic) aneurysms are infrequent. They are most common in subacute bacterial endocarditis and are due to weakening of the walls of large or, more often, small arteries by infected emboli.

   a. Mycotic aneurysms may cause single large or multiple small hemorrhages anywhere in the brain.

   b. Other consequences of septic aneurysms include the spread of infection into the subarachnoid space, which produces leptomeningitis, and extension into the parenchyma, which may cause an abscess.

3. Arteriosclerotic aneurysms are fusiform (spindle-shaped) and typically are on the internal carotid, vertebral, or basilar vessels.

D. Arterial occlusive diseases

1. Atherosclerosis appears first in the carotid artery (at the origin, bifurcation, and distal segments), the vertebral artery (at the origin and distal segments), and the basilar artery, and later in the middle, posterior, and anterior cerebral arteries, usually in that order.

   a. Pathology. Gross examination shows patches of yellow or yellowish-orange discoloration in arterial walls, often near points of branching. **Microscopic** appearance is similar to that in atherosclerosis elsewhere in the body (see Chapter 10 I B 1 d).

   b. Consequences. Atherosclerosis often leads to thrombosis.

   (1) If **thrombosis** occurs in small arteries, multiple areas of destruction in the brain may be seen as microscopic or small lesions, which appear most often in the basal ganglia, in the central white matter of the cerebrum, and in the cerebral cortex. If the thrombosis involves large arteries, encephalomalacia resulting from infarct and necrosis occurs (see II D 4).

   (2) Thrombotic stroke. As a rule, symptoms appear much more slowly than those due to cerebral hemorrhage. The clinical picture depends on the portion of the brain affected. Often, permanent hemiplegia ensues. Aphasia also may result.

2. Hypertension. About 20% of patients with systemic hypertension develop cerebral lesions, usually in the latter half of life. Most of these patients also have atherosclerosis. The arterial changes resemble those seen in the vascular system in general (see Chapter 9 IV). Changes in the brain parenchyma result from hemorrhage and ischemic necrosis.

3. Embolism. In both bacterial endocarditis and those conditions associated with thrombi in the left cardiac chambers, portions of thrombotic material travel to the cerebral circulation and produce arterial occlusions, often multiple, with areas of encephalomalacia.

4. Encephalomalacia

   a. Etiology and distribution. Encephalomalacia occurs because of atherosclerosis, arterial occlusion (thrombotic or embolic), and other causes of inadequate blood flow. Encephalomalacia is most common in the area of the cerebrum that is supplied by the middle cerebral artery.

b. **Pathophysiology.** Brain damage from vascular disorders can be separated into two processes:

(1) Vascular events lead to initial reduction and later alteration of local blood flow.

(2) Ischemia-induced chemical abnormalities cause necrosis of neurons and glial cells. Changes occur in cell signal apparatus (neurotransmitters), signal transduction (receptors), and metabolism (protein, carbohydrate, free radical formation).

c. **Pathology**

(1) **Gross appearance**

(a) When fresh, the affected area is swollen, soft, and pallid or dusky, with petechial hemorrhages peppering the area. Normal architectural markings become obscured, and there is considerable edema of surrounding brain tissue. The area becomes increasingly yellow, soft, finely cystic, and shrunken.

(b) Eventually, over a period lasting from 6 weeks to several months, a roughly rounded or stellate cystic space appears wherever tissue was destroyed.

(2) **Microscopic appearance**

(a) In the acute stage, nerve cells undergo ischemic necrosis in the gray matter, and axons swell enormously in the white matter. Marked edema is present, with greatly widened perineuronal and perivascular spaces.

(b) Many neutrophils enter the zone within the first 24 hours, then disappear in 3 to 6 days. Marginal astrocytosis begins in about 3 days and reaches its height in about 4 to 6 weeks.

5. **Other arterial occlusive conditions** may affect the CNS circulation and produce ischemic changes. They include polyarteritis nodosa (which more often affects the peripheral nervous system), thrombotic thrombocytopenic purpura, systemic lupus erythematosus, giant cell arteritis, and other, possibly allergic, vascular diseases.

E. **Thrombosis of venous sinuses and cerebral veins.** Cerebral venous disorders are much rarer than arterial disorders. They reflect either venous wall defects or coagulation abnormalities. The superior sagittal sinus and superior cerebral veins usually are affected.

1. **Clinical features.** Spontaneous thrombosis is found in poorly nourished, anemic children and in those with severe acute or chronic infections. It is rare in adults; postpartum women are the most likely victims.

2. **Pathology**

a. **Grossly,** veins are distended and firm. Hemorrhages and marked congestion of the leptomeninges and cerebrum are seen.

b. **Microscopically,** multiple pericapillary hemorrhages are seen, in association with changes due to encephalomalacia.

III. INFECTIONS OF THE CENTRAL NERVOUS SYSTEM

A. **Bacterial infections**

1. **Suppurative CNS infection** chiefly occurs secondarily to diseases of the middle ear and its related cavities, diseases of the accessory nasal sinuses, or diseases of the throat and thoracic organs. Less commonly, it follows trauma to the head, and rarely it results from the hematogenous spread of infections elsewhere.

a. **Acute suppurative meningitis (leptomeningitis)** is the most frequent pyogenic infection of the nervous system. It may occur at any age but is most common in children.

(1) **Etiology and pathogenesis.** The most frequently encountered microorganisms are meningococci, pneumococci, streptococci, and hemophilus. Staphylococci and gram-negative bacteria are seen less often. The organisms may invade the meninges directly from an infected sinus or ear, or they may "seed" the meninges in a septicemic patient.

(2) **Clinical features.** Intense headache, vomiting, increased intracranial pressure, fever, and stiff neck are found. Convulsions and motor disabilities also may be seen. The CSF is clouded and reveals increased pressure, an abnormal increase of neutrophils, increased protein, absence of sugar, and the presence of pathogenic organisms.

(3) **Pathology**

(a) **Grossly,** a varying amount of exudate is seen in the subarachnoid space, overlying the base of the brain and spinal cord.

      (b) Microscopically, the subarachnoid space contains bacteria and pus; the underlying brain and cord are edematous and moderately congested. The exudate as a rule remains confined to the leptomeninges. It contains considerable numbers of lymphocytes and large mononuclear cells. If the patient recovers, the activity of phagocytes completely clears the subarachnoid space.

    (4) Prognosis. Recovery with complete resolution is common. Permanent disabilities include localized paralysis, speech defect, or mental deficiency.

    (5) Complications. If a low-grade infection persists, trabeculae form across the subarachnoid space, followed by progressive fibrosis, with narrowing or localized obliteration of the subarachnoid space. When such changes are localized to basilar leptomeninges near the foramina, the outflow of CSF from the ventricular system is blocked, leading to **hydrocephalus**.

  b. Brain abscess can occur at any age; its incidence is 20% of that found for suppurative meningitis.

    (1) Etiology and pathogenesis

      (a) Common causative microorganisms include staphylococci, pneumococci, and streptococci. Gram-negative bacilli are rarely the cause.

      (b) Sources of brain abscess are otitis media, mastoiditis, frontal sinusitis, lung abscess, empyema, and bacterial endocarditis. These conditions may spread to cephalic structures by direct extension or as infected emboli in the bloodstream. Most multiple abscesses are embolic.

    (2) Clinical features. Symptoms and signs are those of a rapidly expanding intracranial lesion. The CSF is under increased pressure; lymphocytes and increased protein are found, but there is no change in sugar content; and no pathogenic organisms are seen (unless the abscess ruptures and meningitis ensues). The source of infection usually is evident (e.g., middle ear disease).

    (3) Pathology. Solitary abscesses are located most often in the temporal lobe or cerebellum; multiple abscesses occur most often in the cerebrum at the junction of the gray and white matter.

      (a) Grossly, an abscess appears as a cavity in the brain, which contains a thick exudate surrounded by a narrow marginal band of intensely congested tissue. The surrounding brain tissue shows marked edema, with swollen white matter.

      (b) Microscopically, the appearance is that of necrotic tissue.

    (4) Complications. If infection breaks beyond the abscess wall because of the virulence of the organism, poor resistance of the patient, or inadequate development of the abscess wall, a spreading **suppurative encephalitis** may ensue.

  c. Septic thrombosis (thrombophlebitis) develops in transverse sinuses from otitis media or mastoiditis or from localized osteomyelitis and epidural abscess. It may occur in the cavernous sinus following infections of the face, particularly of the upper lip, with retrograde thrombophlebitis of the angular and ophthalmic veins.

2. Tuberculous meningitis (leptomeningitis) is the most common form of tuberculous infection in the nervous system.

  a. Pathogenesis. The condition is secondary to infection in the mediastinal or mesenteric glands, bones, joints, lungs, or genitourinary tract. It is usually, but not always, the result of miliary dissemination.

  b. Clinical features. The onset is insidious, with 2 to 3 weeks of anorexia, loss of weight, and change of disposition. Drowsiness with occasional delirium is followed by characteristic lucid intervals. The CSF contains lymphocytes, increased protein, decreased sugar, and tubercle bacilli.

  c. Pathology

    (1) Grossly, there is a delicate, white or gray-white, lacy exudate in the leptomeninges at the base of the brain. The exudate tends to pool in all basilar cisterns, particularly those in the sylvian fissure. At the margins of this thin exudate are sharply outlined, round white nodules (tubercles).

    (2) Microscopically, the subarachnoid space is extended in places by the exudate and is filled with granulomas composed of lymphocytes and large mononuclear cells. Tubercle bacilli are present.

3. Neurosyphilis is one manifestation of **tertiary syphilis,** developing in approximately 2% of infected persons. Several forms of neurosyphilis are recognized.

  a. Meningovascular syphilis, which may occur a few years after initial infection, is characterized by syphilitic **arteritis** in association with **meningitis.** The neural parenchyma may be involved secondarily.

    (1) Clinical features. Symptoms vary greatly, depending on the predominance of spinal or cerebral meningitis. The CSF usually has a normal pressure, few cells (20 to 100, chiefly lymphocytes), and increased protein; serology is positive in 90% to 100% of affected patients.

    (2) Pathology

      (a) Grossly, a yellowish opaque exudate is found in the meninges, at times containing tiny, firm nodules.

      (b) Microscopically, there is infiltration of the subarachnoid space and pia by plasma cells and lymphocytes, followed by extension of the exudate into the perivascular spaces of the superficial parenchyma. Proliferation of fibroblasts and capillaries gives rise to syphilitic granulomas (**gummas**). Spirochetes rarely are demonstrable in the leptomeninges and blood vessel walls.

  b. Parenchymatous syphilis

    (1) Tabes dorsalis typically begins 8 to 12 years after initial infection, most often in men in the fourth and fifth decades of life. About 2% to 3% of persons with syphilis develop tabes.

      (a) Clinical features. The onset is insidious. Signs and symptoms include lightning pains constricting the chest, abdominal pains, and ataxia when walking with a wide stride. Other features are sensory loss, analgesia, loss of vibratory sense, and diminution and loss of deep tendon reflexes. "Trophic changes" (Charcot's joints, leg ulcers) of unknown etiology also occur. The spinal fluid shows increased protein and lymphocytes; serology is positive in 70% of patients.

      (b) Pathology. The posterior columns of the spinal cord are reduced in size. **Microscopic examination** in the early stages shows localized changes around the dorsal roots in the lumbar region, with granulation tissue formation as occurs in meningovascular syphilis. Spirochetes are present in these radicular leptomeningeal sheaths. Degeneration of axons and myelin sheaths in the dorsal roots also occurs.

    (2) General paresis typically begins 10 to 15 years after the initial infection, most often in men in the fourth and fifth decades of life. General paresis comprises fewer than 10% of cases of neurosyphilis.

      (a) Clinical features. Because the cerebral cortex is involved, the earliest symptoms are mental (e.g., impairment of intellectual efficiency, memory, and judgment; delusions). Until they die, patients are bedridden and incontinent. CSF serology is positive in 95% to 100% of cases, and there is an increase in protein and lymphocytes.

      (b) Pathology

        (i) Gross examination shows atrophy of cerebral gyri, most marked in the frontal lobes.

        (ii) Microscopic examination shows mild to marked leptomeningeal infiltration by lymphocytes and plasma cells. Gradual degeneration of nerve cells may result from syphilitic capillary changes and consequent anoxia.

B. Viral infections

  1. General features

    a. Pathogenesis. When viruses involve the CNS, they invade both neural and meningeal areas, producing a **meningoencephalitis.** Infection may occur via an insect bite (equine encephalitis), by the gastrointestinal route (poliomyelitis), or via the skin or mucosa (herpes); it may reach the CNS by ascending via the peripheral nerves (rabies) or by hematogenous spread.

    b. Pathology

      (1) Nervous system response to viral infection may be a neuron degeneration, with associated gliosis; a perivascular inflammatory response (chiefly in mononuclear cells) often appears.

      (2) Inclusion bodies are seen in neural and glial cells in some infections [e.g., cytomegalovirus (CMV)]. These bodies may be nuclear (herpes) or cytoplasmic (rabies). The characteristic **Negri bodies** seen in rabies are eosinophilic, oval to bullet-shaped, intracytoplasmic inclusions found only in neurons.

2. **Poliomyelitis** is caused by poliovirus, a small RNA virus that is transmitted gastrointestinally by sewage-contaminated water. The virus is neurotropic, chiefly affecting the spinal cord and brain stem.
    a. **Clinical features.** Patients may or may not manifest gastrointestinal symptoms; but within a few weeks of infection, they show lower motor neuron paralysis, usually affecting the lower limbs. The brain stem neurons may become affected, and the resultant respiratory paralysis may be fatal. Surviving patients have significant neurologic sequelae, especially affecting the legs.
    b. **Pathology.** Grossly, the spinal cord may show small hemorrhages and congestion. The anterior horn cells of the cord are affected predominantly, with an initial neutrophilic infiltration. Later, gliosis takes place.

3. **Rabies.** Rabid animals (chiefly wild animals in the United States, chiefly dogs elsewhere) secrete the RNA virus (rhabdoviridae) in the saliva and transmit it to humans by bite.
    a. **Clinical features.** In classic, untreated rabies, about 1 month after the bite the patient exhibits restlessness and hydrophobia; symptoms progress until death occurs.
    b. **Pathology.** The virus may infect neurons throughout the nervous system, destroying these cells and causing a reactive gliosis. **Negri bodies** [see III B 1 b (2)] are diagnostic of the disease. Autopsied cases have shown myocarditic lesions in addition to the neuropathologic changes.

4. **Herpes simplex encephalitis**
    a. **Clinical features.** Herpes simplex encephalitis frequently has an acute course, with fever, somnolence, and then coma. If the disease is not fatal, neurologic and mental deficiencies often result.
    b. **Pathology**
        (1) **Grossly,** the brain may show zones of necrosis and softening.
        (2) **Microscopically,** this disease is reflected by perivasculitis, neuronal destruction, and glial proliferation. Intranuclear inclusions are characteristic. Demonstration of the virus by electron microscopy (EM) or by immunohistologic methods is diagnostic.

5. **Subacute sclerosing panencephalitis (SSPE).** This progressive disorder is associated with prior **measles** infection.
    a. **Clinical features.** SSPE is a rare childhood disease characterized by involuntary muscular movements and dementia. It is fatal within 1 to 2 years and at present is unresponsive to any known treatment.
    b. **Pathology.** The brain shows multifocal areas of neuronal destruction and gliosis. Occasional intranuclear inclusions are seen.

6. **Progressive multifocal leukoencephalopathy** is a rare subacute disorder that usually occurs in adult patients with an antecedent and debilitating disease, usually a malignancy (most often lymphoma). A **papovavirus** has been confirmed as the causative agent.
    a. **Clinical features.** The symptoms of hemiparesis, intellectual impairment, blindness, and aphasia reflect the predominant cerebral involvement. The disease is progressive and, within 3 to 6 months, contributes to the death of a patient already compromised by systemic illness.
    b. **Pathology.** The basic lesion of progressive multifocal leukoencephalopathy is a well-defined focus of demyelinization associated with viral infestation. Between the area of demyelinization and the intact white matter are prominent oligodendroglia containing intranuclear inclusions.

C. **Toxoplasmosis.** Caused by the protozoan *Toxoplasma gondii,* toxoplasmosis may be acquired transplacentally or subsequently in life and may range in severity from an asymptomatic infection to a fulminating disseminated, fatal disease. The organisms enter the bloodstream and are carried to many organs, producing the most severe lesions in the CNS.

1. **Congenital toxoplasmosis**
    a. **Clinical features.** About 30% of infected infants are symptomatic at birth or shortly thereafter. Hydrocephalus is common, as are bilateral focal chorioretinitis, intracerebral calcification, convulsions, and ocular palsies. The CSF shows an increase in cells and protein. Infants born with inapparent infection may develop CNS and ocular symptoms later in life. Mothers of affected children usually appear healthy.
    b. **Pathology**
        (1) **Gross appearance.** Depressed, soft, sharply circumscribed yellowish areas are seen on

the surfaces of the cerebral hemispheres; stenosis of the aqueduct of Sylvius with internal hydrocephalus is noted in most cases.

    (2) Microscopic appearance. Sharply outlined, inflammatory, necrotizing lesions are seen in the brain tissue, with associated secondary leptomeningitis. Toxoplasmal cysts are plentiful in the lesions and destroy all neural and glial structures.

  c. Prognosis. Affected infants may die within a few days or months after birth, or they may survive with apparently arrested infection but with defects due to neural destruction (e.g., mental deficiency, chronic hydrocephalus, blindness, and seizures).

  2. Acquired toxoplasmosis. Acute, fulminating, often fatal infection occurs in immunodeficient hosts, especially patients with AIDS. A mild, predominantly lymphatic form is more common (see Chapter 8 IX A).

D. Fungal CNS infections occur in immunocompromised hosts, especially in patients with malignant lymphoma and leukemia or in those taking immunosuppressant drugs. **Cryptococcal infection** (Figure 21-3) is most common, with extraneural lesions occurring most frequently in the lungs. **Actinomycosis** and **coccidioidomycosis** also may involve the nervous system. Clinically and pathologically, fungal CNS infections resemble tuberculous meningitis.

IV. METABOLIC DISORDERS AFFECTING THE CENTRAL NERVOUS SYSTEM

A. Pernicious anemia [see also Chapter 8 I A 3 a (2) (a)]. **Vitamin B$_{12}$ deficiency** causes both a megaloblastic anemia and a neurologic disorder known as **subacute combined degeneration of the spinal cord (combined system disease),** in which both the posterior and lateral columns are affected.

  1. Clinical features. Dorsolateral degeneration of the spinal cord occurs in 30% to 50% of untreated cases of pernicious anemia. The first neurologic symptom, paresthesia in the distal parts of the extremities, is followed by unsteady gait and impaired sense of both position and vibration. Vitamin B$_{12}$ therapy arrests the degenerative process but cannot restore destroyed nerve fibers.

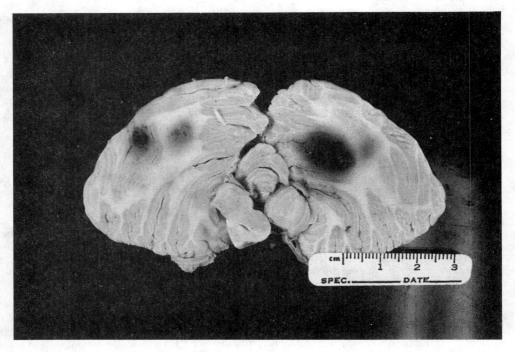

Figure 21-3. Cerebellum from a 30-year-old woman with leukemia and extensive chemotherapy-related immunosuppression. Several hemorrhagic foci can be seen. These embolic septic foci (abscesses) contain cryptococcal organisms; cryptococcal endocarditis is the presumed source.

2. Pathology
   a. Grossly, the posterior and lateral columns show gray discoloration.
   b. Microscopically, degeneration of myelin sheaths and axons characteristically is seen in the posterior columns and lateral pyramidal tracts (hence the term **dorsolateral degeneration**) and usually is most severe in the middle and upper thoracic segments of the cord.

B. Wernicke's syndrome (Wernicke's encephalopathy) is a complication of **chronic alcoholism.**

1. **Clinical features.** Symptoms develop rapidly and include severe ataxia, mental confusion, delirium, and restlessness. Severe cases are fatal.

2. **Pathology.** Lesions are strikingly localized to periventricular gray matter around the third ventricle, the aqueduct of Sylvius, and sometimes the floor of the fourth ventricle.
   a. Grossly, marked congestion of periventricular gray matter usually accompanies many petechial hemorrhages.
   b. Microscopically, capillaries are more prominent than usual, because of endothelial hypertrophy and hyperplasia. Nerve cells supplied by these vessels undergo acute ischemic necrosis.

V. CENTRAL NERVOUS SYSTEM INTOXICATIONS

A. Medicinal agents, beneficial in proper amounts, are injurious in overdoses (which may be taken by accident or with suicidal intent).

1. Some agents (e.g., phenobarbital, ether, chloroform) produce **depressed respiration** and cause death without organic neural damage.

2. Some drugs (e.g., morphine) produce **nerve cell degeneration,** especially if taken chronically.

B. Alcohol

1. **Acute ethyl alcohol intoxication** (see also Chapter 4 IV B 1). If the patient dies, the brain and leptomeninges are edematous and congested; occasionally, petechial hemorrhages are noted in cerebral white matter. Mild diffuse and degenerative changes occur in nerve cells, especially in those of the cerebellar cortex.

2. **Methyl alcohol (methanol) intoxication** (see also Chapter 4 III A). More severe degenerative changes occur in the brain stem and cerebral cortex. Petechial hemorrhages and degeneration of nerve cells occur in the retina and in optic nerve fibers. Blindness is common.

C. Carbon monoxide. Inhalation causes headache, visual disturbances, nausea, vomiting, convulsions, coma, and respiratory paralysis, with symptoms growing more severe as the concentration of gas or the length of exposure increases. **Pathologically,** in the acute stage, the brain is hyperemic and edematous, with scattered petechial hemorrhages.

D. Bacterial toxins

1. **Tetanus toxin** chiefly affects motor neurons of the spinal cord and brain stem.

2. In **botulism,** the *Clostridium botulinum* toxin affects the brain stem nuclei; death from respiratory paralysis occurs.

VI. TRAUMA TO THE HEAD AND SPINE. Vehicular accidents cause most head and spine injuries. Other causes include falls, blows on the chin, and childbirth (e.g., injury to the newborn from instrumental delivery).

A. Head injuries result in intracranial hemorrhage (epidural, subdural, subarachnoid), concussion, contusion, or laceration of the brain.

1. **Epidural hemorrhage** is the least common of traumatic hemorrhages and is due to laceration of the middle meningeal artery and vein from a fracture of the skull.
   a. Clinical features. Loss of consciousness follows the injury, often with apparent recovery and then relapse. Signs of increased intracranial pressure are noted, followed by depressed respiration and death unless the hemorrhage is promptly evacuated.

   b. **Pathology.** The hemorrhage is external to the dura, which is firmly attached to the skull and limits the spread of the hemorrhage. Many small vessels between the dura and skull are torn incidentally as the dura is dissected by the hemorrhage. The dura is pressed inward in a localized area, causing focal compression of the brain, increased intracranial pressure, and finally subtentorial herniation.

2. **Subdural hematoma.** In this condition, trauma to the head produces a tear in a meningeal vein, commonly one of the superior cerebral veins that lie relatively unprotected in the subdural space. The trauma most often is a blow to the frontal or occipital region or a birth injury.
   a. **Clinical features**
      (1) In the **acute phase,** signs and symptoms are expressions of mass effect, namely, increasing intracranial pressure and transtentorial herniation.
      (2) **Chronic subdural hematoma** may follow a seemingly insignificant head injury. After a latent period of several months, nonlocalizing and diagnostically confusing signs may appear, such as deterioration of mental capacity.
   b. **Pathology**
      (1) **Grossly,** a hematoma forms between the dura and leptomeninges. After 3 days, transparent membranes line the inner and outer surfaces of the hematoma, encapsulating it.
      (2) **Microscopically,** these inner and outer encapsulating membranes are formed by the outgrowth of fibroblasts and capillaries from the inner surface of the dura.

3. **Subarachnoid hemorrhage** (see II A 2), although common after head injuries, usually is not a major consequence but accompanies other, more serious lesions.

4. **Concussion** is characterized by widespread paralysis of functions of the brain without visible organic changes and with a strong tendency to spontaneous recovery.
   a. The **pathogenesis** of a concussion is not established, but the condition is possibly due to acceleration effects or shearing (rotational) strains on the brain.
   b. **Clinical features.** In mild cases, the patient is momentarily dazed or unconscious, with subsequent temporary impairment of higher mental functions. In severe cases, there is prolonged unconsciousness, low blood pressure, slowed pulse and respiration, and flaccid muscles. Vomiting, headache, and delirium are common upon return of consciousness. Complete recovery is usual.

5. **Contusion** is essentially a bruise on the brain consequent to a blow on the calvarium. It probably is due to stress on the vascular network, with tearing of capillaries. The lesion may be located directly beneath the area of impact or opposite it (**contrecoup**). Most contusions affect the frontal and temporal poles of the cerebrum.
   a. **Clinical features.** Unconsciousness, which may progress to coma (and to death in a severe injury), is the common clinical presentation.
   b. **Pathology**
      (1) **Grossly,** recent contusions show swollen, edematous gyri studded with petechial hemorrhages. Old contusions are sunken areas, which may be finely cystic.
      (2) **Microscopically,** fresh contusions show an edematous area of cortex and subcortical white matter containing many fresh pericapillary hemorrhages [**Duret's hemorrhages** (see VIII A 3)]. In old contusions, areas of gliosis are seen.

6. **Laceration** of the brain is caused by penetrating wounds. Symptoms depend on the site of the lesion that shows complete destruction of all neural, glial, and vascular elements in the line of the tear.

B. **Spinal injuries**

1. **Hemorrhages in the meninges** are relatively uncommon in the spinal canal but may result from the spread of a cranial subdural hemorrhage. **Epidural hemorrhages** may follow fractures of the vertebrae.

2. **Concussion of the spinal cord** is much less frequent than concussion of the brain. The patient is paralyzed below the level of the injury. Complete return of function usually occurs.

3. **Hematomyelia,** hemorrhage into the cord, can result from flexion of the spine or a severe blow to the back.
   a. **Clinical features.** Below the level of the lesion, pain and temperature perception are lost and extremities are paralyzed.

b. Pathology. The hemorrhage is seen **grossly** and **microscopically** in the spinal cord and shows a tendency to extend longitudinally in cephalad and caudad directions.

4. Compression and contusion of the spinal cord (cord crush) follows dislocation of a vertebra.
  a. Etiology. Cord crush occurs commonly in the lower cervical region following a sudden, forcible flexion of the head, as occurs in an automobile accident, or in the lower dorsal and lumbar region from a heavy blow across the lower back or a fall.
  b. Clinical features. The patient is paralyzed and loses sensation below the level of the crush. If the patient survives, permanent disability results.

5. Laceration of the spinal cord. In stab wounds, a knife usually enters obliquely, hemisecting or completely transecting the cord. Bullet wounds can partially or completely tear the cord.

C. Herniated intervertebral disk (extrusion of the nucleus pulposus) is common in men 30 to 50 years of age. The most common location is the lumbar and lumbosacral area, wherein it presents as low back pain (**sciatica**) following mild to moderate trauma to the back. Disk herniation also may occur in the cervical region. **Pathologically,** the center of the intervertebral disk (nucleus pulposus) extrudes through a tear in the annulus fibrosus; in the common location in the lower back, this herniation usually occurs at the level of L4-L5 or L5-S1.

VII. DEMYELINATING AND DEGENERATIVE CENTRAL NERVOUS SYSTEM DISEASES

A. General concepts

1. In **demyelinating disorders,** the **white matter** is primarily affected. Although myelin destruction is dominant, there is also a lesser degeneration of axons and, rarely, delayed necrosis of other neural and glial elements.

2. In the **degenerative diseases, neurons** are primarily affected, often in one or more selective functional groupings.

3. There is no general agreement on the cause of these diseases, but many are now considered to be **autoimmune in etiology.** Progressive multifocal leukoencephalopathy (see III B 6) is a demyelinating disorder caused by a virus.

B. Specific disorders

1. Multiple sclerosis (MS) affects young adults principally, with onset between the ages of 20 and 40 years.
  a. Clinical features. Symptoms are varied because of the widespread dissemination of lesions and the variability in their location, size, and number. The onset can be sudden or slow, and remissions and relapses are common. Since a few axons probably are destroyed in each lesion, and since later lesions frequently strike the same tract, a cumulative effect of axonal loss leads to eventual permanent symptoms.
  b. Pathology
    (1) Gross appearance. The basic lesion is a discrete locus of demyelination, or **"plaque,"** which produces an acute focal neurologic deficit in accord with its anatomic location. Plaques are found scattered throughout the brain and spinal cord and vary in size from a few millimeters to 5 or 6 cm (average size is 0.5 to 2 cm).
    (2) Microscopic appearance. Localized edema, congestion, and microglial proliferation are followed by perivascular astrocytosis and infiltration by lymphocytes. Astrocytosis is progressive; it becomes increasingly fibrillar and forms a scar or **sclerotic plaque.**

2. Leukodystrophies are inborn errors of metabolism in which the formation of myelin or its composition is abnormal and in which the myelin tends to break down. All syndromes in this group are familial, with infantile or childhood demise. The prototype is **Krabbe's disease,** in which myelin cerebroside is defective and accumulates in various parts of the neuraxis.

3. Amyotrophic lateral sclerosis (ALS) is a chronic disease that involves both upper and lower motor neurons of the brain stem and spinal cord. It occurs most commonly in men in the fourth to fifth decade of life.
  a. Clinical features. ALS presents as weakness and atrophy of various muscle groups, commonly the intrinsic muscles of the hand and muscles of the arm and shoulder. Fasciculations are visible through the skin. The outcome is fatal, often within 2 to 3 years, because of respiratory paralysis or intercurrent infection.

    b. **Pathology.** The motor cells in the anterior horns progressively diminish in number, with eventual total disappearance and associated degeneration of the ventral nerve roots. The disease is most severe in the cervical cord.

4. **Werdnig-Hoffmann disease (infantile spinal muscular atrophy)** is a degeneration of the lower motor neurons of the spinal cord and medulla.

    a. **Clinical features.** This disorder is the most common neuromuscular cause of profound weakness during childhood. An autosomal recessive inheritance is noted in many cases, but the etiology is obscure, and there is no effective therapy. Respiratory insufficiency and superimposed infection usually are the causes of death.

    b. **Pathology.** In the spinal cord, anterior horn cell loss is grossly apparent. The spinal and cranial lower motor neurons are markedly reduced in number. Finding numerous small, round, atrophic fibers on muscle biopsy establishes the diagnosis.

5. **Syringomyelia** is the development of an abnormal cleft or cavity (**syrinx**) in cord tissue. The cause is unknown; the condition may represent reactive astrocytosis secondary to unknown injury.

    a. **Clinical features.** Symptoms of this chronic disease usually begin in early adult life. The classic sign is "dissociated" sensory impairment, in which pain and temperature sensation are diminished or absent but touch, position, and vibratory perceptions are retained.

    b. **Pathology**

        (1) **Gross appearance.** The cavity most often is in the cervical spinal cord but may extend almost the full length of the cord. At the level of the cavity, the cord may appear distended or fusiform or may be collapsed and flattened. The syrinx is filled with colorless or amber-tinged fluid.

        (2) **Microscopic appearance.** Examination of the wall of the syrinx shows that it is composed of glial tissue. Cavity formation usually starts near the center of the cord; hence, early compression or destruction of pain fibers is found.

6. **Parkinson's disease (paralysis agitans)** affects the dopaminergic fibers of the substantia nigra and striatum.

    a. **Clinical features.** This slowly progressive disorder of unknown cause usually affects elderly men, causing tremor, rigidity, and slow, labored muscular activity. Speech is unclear, but mental processes are normal.

    b. **Pathology.** Gradual degeneration and loss of nerve cells with gliosis occur, especially in the substantia nigra. Some cells contain spherical eosinophilic cytoplasmic inclusions (**Lewy bodies**), often with peripheral clear halos.

7. **Creutzfeldt-Jakob disease** appears to be caused by a viruslike agent.

    a. **Clinical features.** This rapidly fatal dementia occurs in the fifth to sixth decade of life. Pyramidal and extrapyramidal symptoms, and sometimes abnormal reflexes and bladder dysfunction (signs of lower motor neuron dysfunction), are found.

    b. **Pathology.** Severe atrophy of the brain is grossly apparent and is manifested histologically by marked loss of nerve cells and intense astrocytosis in the cerebral cortex, caudate nucleus, and putamen.

8. **Alzheimer's disease** is a progressive dementing disorder that begins between the ages of 45 and 60. It affects over 2 million Americans and probably will increase in incidence as the population ages.

    a. **Etiology** is still unknown. Family clusters of the disease and chromosomal studies in sporadic cases suggest a **genetic predisposition**. Clinical and pathologic similarity to Down syndrome support the genetic concept. Genetic analysis has shown a linkage between chromosome 21 (Down syndrome chromosome) and the occurrence of Alzheimer's disease in several large kindreds. Theories of etiology have included slow virus infection, toxins, and trauma.

    b. **Pathology**

        (1) **Grossly,** the widespread atrophy of gyri is usually more intense in the frontal lobes.

        (2) **Microscopically,** diffuse loss of nerve cells in all cortical layers accompanies diffuse fibrillary astrocytosis and amyloid deposits. Characteristic forms of nerve cell degeneration are seen—**neurofibrillary tangles,** senile plaques—wherein intracellular neurofibrils are thickened.

        (3) Recent research into the **neural degeneration** seen in this disease has shown abnormalities (hyperphosphorylation) of tau protein, normally synthesized in gray matter. The accumulation of abnormal tau protein into tangles and plaques in Alzheimer's

brains suggests that understanding the molecular and biochemical changes in this protein may shed light on the pathogenesis of the disease.

9. **Pick's disease** is clinically similar to Alzheimer's disease; it affects women more often than men.
   a. **Etiology.** As in Alzheimer's disease, the cause is unknown.
   b. **Pathology.** In Pick's disease, atrophy involves only the frontal and temporal lobes. Neurofibrillary tangles rarely are found.

VIII. CENTRAL NERVOUS SYSTEM NEOPLASMS

A. **General considerations**

1. **Incidence and distribution.** Primary CNS tumors account for about 9% to 10% of all cancer deaths. Approximately 10% of all nervous system disorders are neoplasms.
   a. All age-groups are affected by brain tumors, but important **age differences** appear in both the distribution of tumors and the histologic types encountered.
      (1) In the child, about 70% of all brain tumors are found below the tentorium; in the adult, 70% are supratentorial.
      (2) In the child, brain tumors account for a major proportion of all neoplasms (about 20%), trailing the leukemias. In the adult, tumors of the lung, breast, gastrointestinal system, and hematopoietic system exceed neural tumors in occurrence.
      (3) In the child, the most common brain tumors are astrocytic tumors (including glioblastomas), followed by medulloblastomas, ependymomas, and craniopharyngiomas. In the adult, the astrocytic tumors are also the most prevalent but are followed by metastatic tumors and meningiomas.
   b. The distribution of CNS tumors by sex is rather consistently biased against men.

2. **Benign and malignant tendencies of CNS tumors**
   a. Neoplasms derived from virtually every cell type in the nervous system have been reported—many of them histologically malignant and some benign. In most organ systems, a clear correlation exists between the histologic classification of tumors and the clinical outcome. With brain tumors, this correlation often is obscure.
   b. The definitions of benign and malignant, thus, require special clarification for tumors of the CNS. For this purpose, brain tumors may be divided conveniently into those of glial and those of nonglial origin.
      (1) The **glial tumors** tend to grow by infiltration. This infiltrative quality and the spongelike quality of the brain make these tumors biologically malignant and makes their complete removal usually impossible.
      (2) The **nonglial tumors** generally grow by expansion and, therefore, offer the surgeon a better opportunity for total removal.
   c. An enigmatic and unique property of most brain tumors is that, regardless of their degree of histologic malignancy, they only rarely metastasize outside the CNS.

3. **Pathophysiologic effects of CNS tumors**
   a. **Direct effects**
      (1) Tumors of the brain produce symptoms directly, by interfering with local neurologic function in the tumor area; that is, by inhibiting the afferent impulses of local neurons, thereby rendering the neurons electrically unstable and liable to epileptiform discharges.
      (2) The location of tumors is of prime importance, with varying functional significance.
   b. **Secondary effects**
      (1) **Edema** is probably the most important factor in the symptoms of brain tumors and is the ultimate determinant of the level of neurologic function that can be expected in the presence of the tumor.
      (2) **Other indirect effects** of CNS tumors include the following:
         (a) **Circulatory effects** (e.g., compression of the brain or cord, with collapse of veins and capillary beds, producing edema, ischemia, degeneration of neural tissue)
         (b) **Compression, distortion, and displacement of nearby vital structures,** as a result of edema formation
         (c) **Herniations** of the brain and cerebellar tonsils
         (d) **Interference with CSF circulation,** with the added hazard of internal hydrocephalus

(e) **Papilledema** (i.e., swelling due to edema of optic nerve papillae, with engorgement of retinal veins)

(3) **Another consequence of brain swelling and herniation is the Duret's hemorrhage** in the midbrain and pons. This lesion results from rapid, unilateral brain swelling, in which pressure is unevenly transmitted to the brain stem, resulting in shearing of midline vessels and destruction of the median portions of the upper brain stem.

4. **Clinical features**
   a. Common symptoms of brain tumors are headache, nausea, and vomiting—often of the projectile type. Lethargy, seizures, paralysis, aphasia, blindness, deafness, or abnormal behavior also may be seen.
   b. Destruction of the reticular formation by herniation results in loss of consciousness, respiratory failure, and death.

B. **Specific tumors**

1. **Tumors of astrocytic origin**
   a. **Morphologic changes**
      (1) **Normal astrocytes,** in the presence of injury, generally react by forming glial fibrils and expanding their cytoplasm, becoming greatly swollen or bloated (**gemistocytic astrocytes**).
      (2) **Neoplastic astrocytes** may take on many forms, recapitulating normal cells or reactive processes and generally displaying the characteristics of normal astrocytes in that a close vascular relationship is maintained. The nucleus, however, reveals the changes that are associated with any neoplasm.
   b. **Astrocytomas** comprise about 30% of all gliomas. They occur most often in the central white matter of the cerebrum in adults and in the cerebellar hemispheres in children and young adults. The two major subtypes—**protoplasmic** and **fibrillary**—depend on which type of astrocyte predominates.
      (1) **Pathology**
         (a) **Grossly,** astrocytomas are white or gray-white, firm, poorly demarcated tumors whose margins are extremely difficult to determine. They may contain tiny cysts or large cavities filled with clear yellowish fluid.
         (b) **Microscopically,** the appearance varies from highly to sparsely cellular, and the tumors are highly fibrillar. Mitoses are rare or absent, and the architecture is uniform. Tiny cysts are due to the gradual degeneration of small numbers of astrocytes.
      (2) **Prognosis.** Astrocytomas are slow growing, occasionally becoming more malignant, with transformation into glioblastomas. Survival may range from 1 to 10 years, depending on pathologic grade.
   c. **Astrocytomas of the cerebellum** are very distinctive lesions, both clinically and pathologically.
      (1) These tumors, which may account for 30% of all posterior fossa tumors in children, occur almost exclusively in persons under age 20. Treatment consists of operative removal of the tumor.
      (2) When the tumor is adequately removed, the **prognosis** for patients with cerebellar astrocytoma is excellent; at least 90% of patients survive. Of the survivors, probably fewer than 10% suffer any continued neurologic deficit.
   d. **Glioblastoma multiforme** is a rapidly growing lesion with a variety of symptoms, reflecting rapidly increasing intracranial pressure. The tumor occurs more commonly in men and is the most common of all gliomas, comprising 40%.
      (1) **Pathology**
         (a) **Gross examination** shows a usually massive, well-demarcated, soft, multicolored, highly vascular tumor growing in the central white matter of the cerebrum. Rapid expansion of the tumor plus edema produce marked compression, distortion, and displacement of nearby structures. Not infrequently, the tumor invades the corpus callosum, crossing to the opposite hemisphere.
         (b) **Microscopic examination** shows a highly cellular, highly vascular neoplasm, which varies in appearance from area to area and shows extensive necrosis and multiple mitoses (Figure 21-4). The numerous capillaries commonly show intense endothelial hyperplasia.

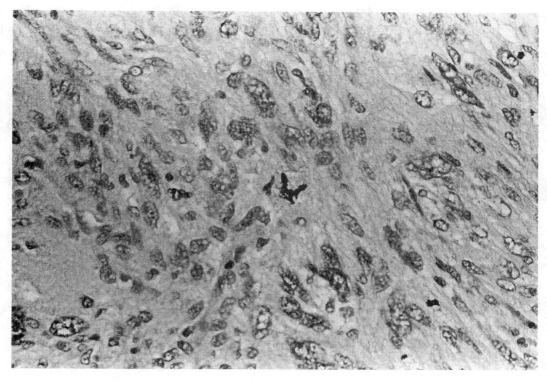

Figure 21-4. Glioblastoma multiforme with tripolar mitosis in *center* (high power).

  (c) **Molecular pathology.** Abnormalities of chromosomes 7, 9, and 10 are common in glioblastomas. Over 50% of these tumors express the oncogene c-*sis,* and 30% express c-*erb* B.

 (2) **Prognosis** is dismal, although it is somewhat better with aggressive modern radiotherapy.

e. **Oligodendrogliomas** account for 5% to 8% of all intracranial tumors. They most commonly occur in the cerebral hemispheres of adults.

 (1) **Clinically,** the outstanding feature of oligodendrogliomas is their indolent clinical course.

 (2) **Pathology**

  (a) **Grossly,** oligodendrogliomas are generally well-circumscribed tumors of the white matter, but they often break through into the cortex.

  (b) **Histologically,** the tumors are composed of small, rather uniform cells that display a honeycomb or "fried egg" appearance, with small, rounded nuclei surrounded by clear spaces (Figure 21-5). Calcification is prominent.

 (3) **Prognosis.** With operative removal (when possible), it is estimated that about half of the patients survive 5 years.

2. **Ependymomas** are derived from the cells forming the ependymal lining of the ventricles in the brain and the central canal in the spinal cord. Some 50% of ependymomas are located below the tentorium, and 40% are above it. A few are located in the spinal cord or filum terminale. The tumors occur in all age-groups, with the highest percentage occurring at about age 3 to 4. Papilledema and headache are common presentations.

 a. **Pathology.** The histologic appearance varies, but in nearly every tumor there is a typical perivascular **pseudorosette** pattern. With special staining, ependymomas may be identified precisely by the presence of **blepharoplasts** in the cytoplasm near the nucleus.

 b. **Prognosis** varies with location of the tumor. Supratentorial ependymomas carry a more guarded prognosis than those in the posterior fossa. The average survival is 4 years or more.

3. **Medulloblastomas** are clinically and pathologically malignant tumors that occur chiefly in children under age 14. The cerebellum is the major site of occurrence. From 50% to 80% of

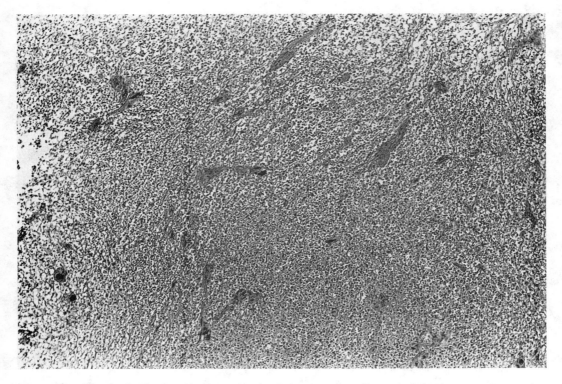

Figure 21-5. Oligodendroglioma, with clear perinuclear halos giving the cells a typical "fried-egg" appearance (low power).

the tumors arise in the midline posteriorly and have a propensity to spread along the CSF pathway. The medulloblastoma is one of the small-cell tumors of the CNS and peripheral nervous system, classified currently as **primitive neuroectodermal tumors (PNET)**.

    a. Pathology
        (1) Grossly, medulloblastomas are homogeneous, reddish-gray, finely granular, well-defined neoplasms usually arising from the roof of the fourth ventricle and extending into and filling much of this cavity.
        (2) Microscopically, they are highly cellular, uniform, relatively avascular tumors whose component cells tend to cluster.
    b. Prognosis. Most patients survive between 1 and 2 years after the first onset of symptoms.

4. Meningiomas are common tumors, accounting for 15% to 20% of all intracranial tumors in adults (usually women); however, they are uncommon in children. About 50% of meningiomas are situated near the vertex and the midline. **Spinal meningiomas** are among the most common intraspinal tumors, but are rare compared to the intracranial meningiomas.

    a. Clinical features. Symptoms may be minimal. The tumors may produce slowly evolving deficits.
    b. Pathology
        (1) Grossly, meningiomas are firm to rubbery tumors that have a white or red gritty appearance. They are usually clearly demarcated from the surrounding brain, which they push inward but do not truly invade. They can be shelled out, leaving the depressed brain beneath.
        (2) Microscopically, there is uniformity of the cells, which contain ovoid nuclei, often with intranuclear vacuoles. The cells often form whorls (Figure 21-6) and **psammoma bodies** are common.
    c. Prognosis. Meningiomas are slowly growing tumors. Because of their location, tumors may be incompletely excised. Such lesions may recur.

5. Hemangioblastomas. These tumors of blood vessel origin appear most often in the cerebellum of young adults and constitute 7% of primary posterior fossa tumors.

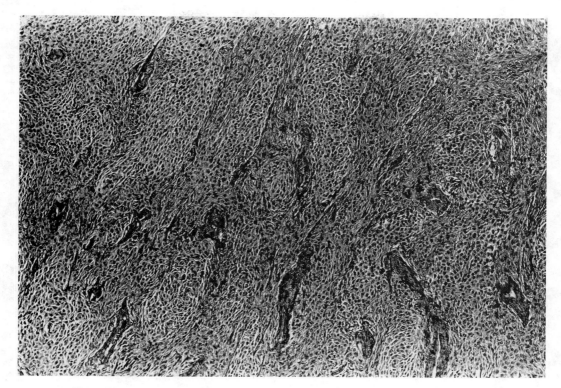

Figure 21-6. Meningioma showing characteristic wavy bundles of tumor cells (low power).

    a. Clinical features. Patients present with disorders of gait and locomotion. Occasionally, polycythemia has been reported. Analysis of the cyst fluid shows **erythropoietin**.
    b. Pathology
        (1) Grossly, the tumor is a sharply outlined, spongy, purplish-red or brown neoplasm, which may be solid or cystic. Sometimes a large cyst is present with a small mural nodule of tumor.
        (2) Microscopically, the tumor varies from an almost purely vascular type with capillaries or large cavernous channels, to a highly cellular tumor in which the many capillaries are overshadowed by large polygonal cells containing lipids.
    c. Prognosis. Solitary hemangioblastomas can be easily shelled out, and the patient can enjoy an excellent prognosis.
    d. Von Hippel-Lindau disease is a rare familial disorder in which multiple hemangioblastomas of the CNS and retina are associated with malformations, tumors of other organs [notably the kidney (renal cell carcinoma) and adrenal gland (pheochromocytoma)], and cysts of the pancreas, liver, and kidney.

6. Neurilemmomas (schwannomas) are tumors of **nerve sheath origin**. They are common, accounting for 8% to 10% of all intracranial tumors, and occur mostly in middle-aged adults. The most common intracranial schwannoma affects the eighth cranial nerve (**acoustic neuroma**).
    a. Clinical features. Patients present with hearing loss, disequilibrium (causing dizziness and ataxia), and headache. The tumors often are misdiagnosed as sensorineural deafness and, thus, are missed entirely.
    b. Pathology
        (1) Gross appearance. Schwannomas occur in conjunction with a nerve but grow external to it in most cases. The tumors may appear spherical or oblong and, on cut section, are either homogeneous or variegated. They are granular or cystic in consistency.
        (2) Microscopic appearance is described in Chapter 25 III B 5.
    c. Prognosis. Treatment is resection of as much of the tumor as possible. If total resection is not accomplished, the tumor often recurs. Overall, the prognosis is good.

7. **Craniopharyngiomas** chiefly affect children between age 4 and 16. These tumors classically are calcified suprasellar lesions that produce visual disturbances and hypothalamic syndromes.
   a. **Pathology**
      (1) **Gross appearance.** The tumors usually are several centimeters in size, are multiloculated, and may be encapsulated by the surrounding brain into which they push. The cysts of the tumors contain a "machine-oil" material in which cholesterol crystals are suspended. Solid portions of the tumors are granular or crumbly.
      (2) **Microscopic appearance.** The tumors are variegated and usually are multicystic. The solid regions contain foreign-body reactions, fibrous tissue, mineralization, and even bone formation in reaction to the degeneration products of the tumors. The tumor cells themselves may be epithelial in appearance or may resemble tooth bud or squamous epithelium. Some resemble jaw tumors (**ameloblastomas**).
   b. **Prognosis.** The treatment is total removal. If any tumor is left, recurrence is the rule. Survival for many years is common.

8. **Chordomas** are slow-growing, persistent tumors. They affect men more often than women, and their occurrence peaks during the third and fourth decades of life. About 60% occur in the sacrococcygeal region, and about 30% occur in the region of the clivus at the base of the skull. The tumors aggressively invade bone; and at the base of the brain, they infiltrate the basal structures of the skull.
   a. **Pathology**
      (1) **Grossly,** the tumors are gelatinous, gray-white, friable, and lobulated.
      (2) **Microscopically,** they are composed of clear cells in an amphophilic matrix. The large, water-clear, **physaliphorous cells** are characteristic, but sometimes confused with cartilaginous tumors, metastatic renal cell cancer, or liposarcomas. The tumors are thought to arise in notochordal remnants.
   b. **Prognosis.** Most patients die of locally aggressive disease after a prolonged course.

9. **Tumors of the pineal body.** The pineal body gives rise to a series of tumors, most of which are **teratoid** in character and identical to germ cell tumors of the ovary and testis. Characteristically, they affect younger men, generally under age 20.
   a. **Clinical features.** Pineal tumors present with signs of increased intracranial pressue due to obstruction of the aqueduct or posterior third ventricle.
   b. **Pathology**
      (1) **Grossly,** the tumors may vary in their cellular composition, appearing variegated in color and consistency, with cyst formation common.
      (2) **Microscopically,** pineal teratomas typically resemble teratomas that arise in the gonads (see Chapter 17 I E 1 d and Chapter 18 V B 2).
   c. **Prognosis.** Patients with the **pure seminoma type** of pineal tumors have the best prognosis (with an average patient survival of 5 to 10 years), because of their radiosensitivity. **Other pineal tumor types** show poorer patient survival rates in direct correspondence to their poorer response to radiation therapy and the difficulty of operative removal.

10. **Lymphomas of the brain (microgliomatosis).** Primary neoplasms of the reticuloendothelial system in the brain are uncommon and occur most often during the sixth and seventh decades of life or in persons who are immunocompromised (e.g., renal transplant recipients, patients with AIDS). In immunocompromised patients, lymphomas are the most common primary brain neoplasm.
   a. **Clinical features.** The tumors present in a subtle fashion as disorders of higher neural functioning and mentation, with headache and seizures. The average duration of symptoms prior to diagnosis is a few months.
   b. **Pathology**
      (1) **Grossly,** the tumors are seen most often in the cerebrum and usually are multifocal in character. They appear to arise in the perivascular spaces of many vessels and in some cases resemble encephalitis rather than tumors.
      (2) **Microscopically,** lymphomas of the brain may resemble the classic forms of lymphomas elsewhere. Most mark as B-cell neoplasms.
   c. **Prognosis.** The treatment is irradiation and chemotherapy. Survival for 1 to 2 years is common, but apparent total cures have been seen. Prompt, often dramatic, response to radiation therapy is characteristic of the lesion.

11. **Metastatic tumors.** Probably between 20% and 25% of all brain tumors represent metastatic lesions. Metastasis to the brain usually is an intravascular process, but direct invasion and diffuse spread by a paracranial tumor also may occur.
    a. **Common sources of metastatic CNS tumors**
       (1) The tumor most commonly producing metastases in the CNS is **lung carcinoma;** 40% to 50% of patients who die from this disease show brain involvement. The **leukemias** are also tumors that commonly spread to the brain, as are carcinomas of the large intestine, the kidney, and the breast.
       (2) Less common tumors that have a high incidence of brain metastases include malignant melanoma (nearly 50% of patients have brain lesions), follicular thyroid carcinoma, and the sarcomas. Some tumors, most notably carcinoma of the breast, metastasize to the dura mater and skull.
    b. **Clinical features.** Signs and symptoms of metastatic tumors of the brain are varied, but generally are those typical of any brain tumor.
    c. **Pathology**
       (1) **Grossly,** most metastatic tumors are at the junction of the gray and white matter, where the circulation is slower and the number of vessels is diminished.
       (2) **Microscopically,** metastatic tumors generally display an intimate relationship with vessels, are discrete from the surrounding brain, and show the typical characteristics of the primary tumor.

IX. DISORDERS OF THE PERIPHERAL NERVOUS SYSTEM

A. **Peripheral neuropathy**

1. **General considerations**
   a. **Mononeuropathy** indicates a focal pathologic process affecting just one nerve (or only a few). **Polyneuropathy** and **polyneuritis** indicate widespread degeneration of the peripheral nerves.
   b. **Predisposing causes** are extremely varied.
      (1) Neuropathy may be associated with a chronic focal **infection** or may complicate almost any acute infectious disease (e.g., typhoid fever, pneumonia, malaria, measles). **Guillain-Barré** syndrome is believed to result from an immunologic reaction following infection (sensitized lymphocytes attack and destroy myelin).
      (2) It may result from **poisoning** by heavy metals (e.g., lead, arsenic, mercury, thallium), alcohol, or other chemicals (e.g., carbon tetrachloride).
      (3) It may occur in **metabolic and deficiency disorders** (e.g., diabetes mellitus, hematoporphyrinuria, beriberi, pellagra) or may be associated with pregnancy, prolonged vomiting, or diarrhea.
      (4) **Familial peripheral neuropathies** are rare. **Charcot-Marie-Tooth disease** is the prototype. The neuropathy chiefly involves the lower extremities.
   c. **Site.** Any combination of peripheral nerves, including the cranial nerves, may be affected by multiple neuropathies. Nerves supplying the extremities, especially the distal parts, are involved most often.
   d. **Pathology**
      (1) **Grossly,** abnormalities are not seen in multiple neuropathies.
      (2) **Microscopically,** the myelin sheaths are first swollen, then fragmented, forming droplets and globules that lie in groups along the course of degenerating fibers (**wallerian degeneration**). They stain progressively poorly and then disappear. Axons also become swollen and fragmented, then disappear.

2. **Traumatic neuropathy**
   a. **Mechanism of injury.** Damage to peripheral nerves may occur by the following means:
      (1) **Compression** by a neoplasm, a callus, an aneurysm, prolonged pressure against a hard surface, necrosis, or bandages
      (2) **Tension or stretching** by abnormal movements (e.g., overextension of a limb) or by bone fracture, with wide separation of fragments
      (3) **Severance** by knife, bullet, or jagged edge of fractured bone
   b. Peripheral nerves, unlike CNS neurons, are capable of **regeneration**. After injury, degeneration and regeneration of affected peripheral nerves proceed concomitantly. Regeneration is affected by the nerve involved, by the degree of separation of the severed nerve ends, by the state of the blood supply, and by any complicating infections.

   3. **Neuropathy of vascular disorders**
      a. **Vasculitis,** such as polyarteritis, can produce clinical neuropathy by what is presumed is-chemic injury to specific nerves or nerve groups.
      b. **Diabetic neuropathies** are presumed due to focal ischemic changes in small vessels, such as microangiopathy.

   4. **Intoxications**
      a. **Arsenic poisoning** leads to a polyneuropathy that begins about 1 to 2 months after acute exposure or may occur later in cases of low-grade chronic ingestion. Symptoms include numbness, tingling, pain, and weakness, especially of the legs.
      b. **Lead poisoning** produces a neuropathy that is chiefly motor, with a predilection for the wrist, fingers, and arms.
      c. **Alcohol intoxication** results in a neuropathy that is usually characterized by a severe sen-sory loss with sparing of the motor nerves.

B. Infiltrative disorders. The prototype is **amyloidosis,** in which amyloid is deposited within nerves, leading to focal degeneration.

C. Neoplasms. These growths include benign **schwannomas** and **neurofibromas,** their **malignant counterparts,** and **von Recklinghausen's disease (neurofibromatosis)** [see Chapter 25 III B 5 and III D 3 c]. In neurofibromatosis, multiple neoplasms and hamartomas affect other organ systems as well as peripheral nerves, and malignant transformation of neurofibromas may occur.

X. NEUROMUSCULAR AND MOTOR UNIT DISORDERS

A. Muscular dystrophies are hereditary progressive neuromuscular disorders. **Duchenne (pseudo-hypertrophic) muscular dystrophy** is the prototype. This X-linked recessive disorder affects chil-dren, chiefly boys.

   1. **Clinical features.** Duchenne muscular dystrophy becomes evident through weakness and fall-ing when the child begins to walk.
      a. Early on, the pelvic girdle is the muscle group mainly involved; therefore, the legs are weak and the children tend to use their arms and shoulders. As the disease progresses, all muscles are involved.
      b. The diagnosis is confirmed by the marked elevation of muscle enzymes, especially creatine kinase.

   2. **Pathology**
      a. **Grossly,** the muscles appear atrophic and yellowish.
      b. **Microscopically,** variation in fiber size reflects some degenerated and some hypertrophied fibers. In older patients, muscle tissue is replaced by fat.

   3. **Prognosis.** Most children die before age 20, often of pneumonia associated with respiratory muscle weakness.

B. Polymyositis (see also Chapter 6 IV E) is a diffuse inflammatory disease of unknown origin and affects mostly women.

   1. **Clinical features.** Polymyositis causes symmetrical muscle weakness (more marked in prox-imal muscle groups—shoulder and pelvic girdles) and pain.
      a. Some patients show an associated inflammatory skin lesion (**dermatomyositis**).
      b. In 15% to 50% of affected adults, an associated visceral malignancy (for the most part, carcinoma of the lung, breast, or colon) is present or develops shortly after recognition of the myositis.

   2. **Pathology.** Muscle biopsy shows variation in fiber size and muscle degeneration, with vac-uolation and necrosis. An inflammatory infiltrate is seen. Muscle enzymes are elevated.

   3. **Prognosis.** In cases not associated with malignancy, the course and prognosis are variable. Children fare better than adults.

C. Myasthenia gravis is a common disorder that usually affects women in the third or fourth decade of life.

1. **Pathogenesis.** As many as 80% of myasthenic patients have antibodies directed against neuromuscular acetylcholine receptors. Immunoglobulin G (IgG) and complement on the muscle receptor sites probably interfere with neural transmission.

2. **Clinical features.** Myasthenia gravis presents as weakness relieved by rest and worsened by exercise. Often cranial and extraocular muscles are involved. The course of the disease fluctuates, with partial remissions followed by relapse and progression.
   a. Electromyographic (EMG) studies characteristically show decremental responses to repeated nerve stimulation.
   b. Associated abnormalities are common; 75% to 80% of patients have thymic hyperplasia, and 10% to 15% have a **thymoma**.

3. **Pathology.** In the muscle, the characteristic findings are **lymphorrhages** (lymphocytic infiltrates) around degenerating myofibers. EM shows abnormal myoneural junctions with widened clefts.

4. **Prognosis**
   a. Death, usually due to intercurrent infection (pneumonia associated with respiratory muscle weakness), occurs in most cases after several years.
   b. In some patients, especially those with thymoma, complete resection of the thymic lesion results in remission of the myasthenia. Removal of a nontumoral hyperplastic thymus as therapy for myasthenia remains controversial; only young women seem to benefit from this therapy.

STUDY QUESTIONS

Directions: Each of the numbered items or incomplete statements in this section is followed by answers or by completions of the statement. Select the **one** lettered answer or completion that is **best** in each case.

1. In an animal or a patient with rabies infection, the main histologic characteristic in the brain would be

(A) Lewy bodies
(B) neurofibrillary tangles
(C) Negri bodies
(D) Duret bodies
(E) amyloid plaques

2. Astrocytomas of the cerebellum are characterized by

(A) multiple recurrences
(B) poor survival rate
(C) long-term continued neurologic deficit following therapy
(D) occurrence in childhood and adolescence
(E) transformation of glioblastoma

3. A 27-year-old woman presents with a sudden onset of right-sided blindness and weakness in her left leg. There is no history of trauma; however, she experienced a similar episode 8 months ago and was diagnosed as having aseptic meningitis. The most probable diagnosis is

(A) meningeal carcinomatosis
(B) multiple sclerosis (MS)
(C) pernicious anemia
(D) meningioma of the falx
(E) tabes dorsalis

4. A 39-year-old man complains that he has noticed a progressive hearing loss over a 2-year period. Except for occasional headaches, he has no other complaints. Evaluation discloses severe sensorineural hearing loss on the left side. X-rays show a 1.5-cm mass at the left cerebellopontine angle. The mass is most likely to be a

(A) meningioma
(B) tuberculous abscess
(C) glioblastoma
(D) schwannoma
(E) metastatic tumor from the lung

5. A 31-year-old man presents with difficulty in locomotion and an elevated red blood cell count (polycythemia). Family history reveals the presence of kidney and brain tumors in several family members. Computed tomography (CT) of the brain shows a vascular lesion in the cerebellum of this patient. The most likely diagnosis is

(A) astrocytoma
(B) medulloblastoma
(C) hemangioblastoma
(D) ependymoma
(E) glioblastoma multiforme

6. A 28-year-old woman presents with progressive generalized weakness and a recent onset of diplopia. Physical examination discloses weakness of the eyelids and extraocular muscles as well as generalized muscle weakness that is worsened with exercise. The most likely diagnosis is

(A) systemic lupus erythematosus (SLE)
(B) myasthenia gravis
(C) Hodgkin's disease
(D) Duchenne muscular dystrophy
(E) polymyositis

7. Congenital malformations of the central nervous system (CNS) may result from all of the following EXCEPT

(A) maternal irradiation
(B) in utero viral infections
(C) maternal vitamin deficiency
(D) maternal anoxia
(E) birth trauma

8. All of the following statements concerning Alzheimer's disease are true EXCEPT

(A) atrophic gyri and enlarged sulci are seen
(B) cerebellar atrophy is prominent
(C) neurofibrillary tangles are characteristic
(D) the disease course is prolonged and progressive
(E) it occurs in the fifth and sixth decades of life

1-C   4-D   7-E
2-D   5-C   8-B
3-B   6-B

9. Chordomas are nervous system neoplasms that have all of the following characteristics EXCEPT

(A) occurrence in childhood
(B) location in the sacrococcygeal region
(C) slow growth
(D) prolonged clinical course
(E) late metastasis

Directions: The group of items in this section consists of lettered options followed by a set of numbered items. For each item, select the **one** lettered option that is most closely associated with it. Each lettered option may be selected once, more than once, or not at all.

Questions 10–14

Match each of the following disorders of the nervous system with the neural component that is dominantly affected.

(A) Peripheral sensory neurons
(B) Basal ganglia
(C) Substantia nigra
(D) Cerebral cortex
(E) Anterior horn cells of the spinal cord

10. Huntington's disease

11. Charcot-Marie-Tooth disease

12. Amyotrophic lateral sclerosis (ALS)

13. Parkinson's disease

14. Pick's disease

9-A   12-E
10-B   13-C
11-A   14-D

ANSWERS AND EXPLANATIONS

1. The answer is C *[III B 1 b (2), 3 b].*
Negri bodies are eosinophilic ovoid or bullet-shaped intracytoplasmic inclusions characteristically seen in neurons infected with the rabies virus. Lewy bodies are eosinophilic cytoplasmic inclusions surrounded by a clear halo; they are found in neurons of patients with Parkinson's disease. Neurofibrillary tangles and amyloid plaques are seen in degenerative disorders, especially Alzheimer's disease. Duret bodies do not exist; Duret's hemorrhages are found in the midbrain and pons as a result of brain swelling and herniation.

2. The answer is D *[VIII B 1 c].*
Astrocytomas of the cerebellum are clinically and pathologically distinctive lesions in that they occur almost exclusively in patients under age 20. In addition, the prognosis for these patients is excellent because the location of the lesion allows for complete operative removal of the tumor. Prolonged neurologic deficit is rare, with only about 10% of patients experiencing this complication. Transformation to highly malignant glioblastoma is virtually unknown.

3. The answer is B *[VII B 1].*
Multiple sclerosis (MS) is a strong possibility in a young patient with neurologic signs that remit and recur. Meningeal carcinomatosis is unlikely in this age-group and in a patient with no known primary site. Pernicious anemia and tabes dorsalis would not remit and recur. Meningioma would not remit.

4. The answer is D *[VIII B 6 a].*
The sensorineural hearing loss, occasional headaches, and intracranial mass in this man are classic findings in cases of eighth cranial nerve schwannoma (acoustic neuroma). Although a meningioma may occur at the cerebellopontine angle, it is unusual. The hearing loss symptoms point toward a tumor of cranial nerve VIII. All other possibilities are ruled out by the 2-year history in this case.

5. The answer is C *[VIII B 5].*
The most likely diagnosis in this young patient with a cerebellar tumor and polycythemia is hemangioblastoma. The positive family history of kidney and brain tumors is a great clue to the diagnosis of hemangioblastoma, since this feature is characteristic of von Hippel-Lindau disease. Glioblastoma multiforme is a tumor of the cerebrum; it rarely occurs in the cerebellum. Ependymoma also is not a tumor of the cerebellum. Although astrocytoma could occur in the cerebellum, it is an unusual tumor in this age-group and typically would not be associated with the clinical and historical features noted in this case. Medulloblastoma also is unlikely in a patient of this age; it typically is a tumor of children younger than age 14.

6. The answer is B *[X C].*
A clinical presentation of generalized muscle weakness with extraocular involvement in a young woman suggests the diagnosis of myasthenia gravis. Although systemic lupus erythematosus (SLE) and Hodgkin's disease also occur in women of this age-group, neurologic symptoms are somewhat rare and not so well defined in these diseases. Muscular dystrophy chiefly affects boys and becomes apparent in the toddler stage. Polymyositis usually affects specific muscle groups and is not characterized by generalized weakness.

7. The answer is E *[I A].*
Irradiation of the pregnant mother, viral infections in utero, maternal vitamin deficiency, and maternal anoxia all are conditions that have been associated with central nervous system (CNS) malformations in both humans and animals. In the United States, irradiation and viral infections account for most instances in which cause is known or suspected. Trauma at birth may lead to neurologic defects, but it is not associated with congenital malformation.

8. The answer is B *[VII B 8].*
The cerebral cortex, especially the frontal lobes, is involved most prominently in Alzheimer's disease; cerebellar disease does not occur or is minor in extent. Alzheimer's disease has a prolonged and progressive course that typically begins in the fifth or sixth decade of life. The gross pathologic features include widespread atrophy of the gyri and enlarged sulci; microscopically, the features are diffuse fibrillary astrocytosis and a characteristic form of nerve cell degeneration called neurofibrillary tangles.

9. The answer is A *[VIII B 8].*

Chordomas are slow-growing, persistent tumors that affect adults (men more often than women). About 60% of these tumors occur in the sacrococcygeal area. The tumors grow slowly and have a prolonged course, with late dissemination.

10–14. The answers are: 10-B *[I F 1],* **11-A** *[IX A 1 b (4)],* **12-E** *[VII B 3],* **13-C** *[VII B 6],* **14-D** *[VII B 9].*

Huntington's disease, which consists of abnormal, involuntary movements (chorea) and mental deterioration, affects the basal ganglia. Charcot-Marie-Tooth disease involves the peripheral sensory nerves, which show degenerated axons, loss of myelin, and fibrosis. Atrophy of the anterior horns of the spinal cord (especially of the cervical and lumbar areas) is associated with massive loss of neurons and gliosis and is characteristic of amyotrophic lateral sclerosis (ALS). Clinically, the features are corresponding muscle weakness and spasticity. Loss of pigmented nuclei of the brain stem is characteristic of Parkinson's disease; usually, this loss includes depigmentation of the substantia nigra. Pick's disease is a presenile dementia characterized by degeneration (loss of neurons) of the frontal and temporal lobes of the cerebral cortex.

22
Head and Neck

Maria J. Merino
Virginia A. LiVolsi

I. MOUTH

A. Normal structure. The mouth is lined by stratified squamous epithelium and underlying fibro-connective tissue in which blood vessels and nerves are found.

B. Congenital abnormalities

1. **Cleft lip** is due to failure of the globular processes to unite with the maxilla. It usually affects the upper lip.

2. **Cleft palate** is caused by premature closure of the coronal or lambdoid sutures and may involve the soft, the hard, or both palates. It usually is associated with cleft lip; and in such cases the nasal cavities communicate with the oral area, interfering with feeding.

3. **Fordyce's disease,** a benign asymptomatic condition, is characterized by the presence of painless yellow to white granules in the mucosa of the cheeks, lips, and gingivae. The plaques consist of displaced ectopic sebaceous glands.

C. Inflammatory disorders. Inflammation of the oral mucosa is called **stomatitis,** and the term **gingivostomatitis** is used when the inflammation also involves the gums. These conditions often are the consequence of ill-fitting dentures or poor dental hygiene.

1. **Herpetic gingivostomatitis** is caused by herpes simplex virus (HSV) type 1.
   a. It is characterized by the development of vesicular lesions that fuse and rupture, forming small ulcers (Figure 22-1).
   b. Most often affected are infants and children, who commonly present with soreness of the oral cavity, malaise, and fever. The disease resolves within 7 to 12 days.

2. **Monilial (candidal) stomatitis** is caused by *Candida albicans* and occurs predominantly in children with neglected oral hygiene and in adults who have debilitating diseases or who are receiving immunosuppressive therapy.
   a. The lesions appear as white elevated patches, which are scattered over the oral mucosa, tongue, palate, and pharynx. Confluence of these lesions may lead to the formation of extensive membranes consisting of a mixture of necrotic epithelium, fungal organisms, and acute inflammatory cells.
   b. If the disease advances, systemic involvement of organs may occur.

3. **Aphthous stomatitis** is a painful condition with an unknown etiology.
   a. It is characterized by yellow-white ulcers of different sizes. Histologically, the epithelium is preserved, but fibrinous exudate is present in varying amounts beneath it.
   b. The duration of the ulcers varies from 7 to 10 days, but chronic conditions may last years.

4. **Syphilis** in any stage can involve the oral mucosa.
   a. The primary stage is characterized by **chancre;** the second stage, by patches in the oral mucosa and macules on the tongue; and the third stage, by **gummas** in the hard or soft palate and by glossitis.
   b. **Microscopically,** marked lymphoplasmacytic infiltration is present, most prominently around the small and medium-sized vessels.

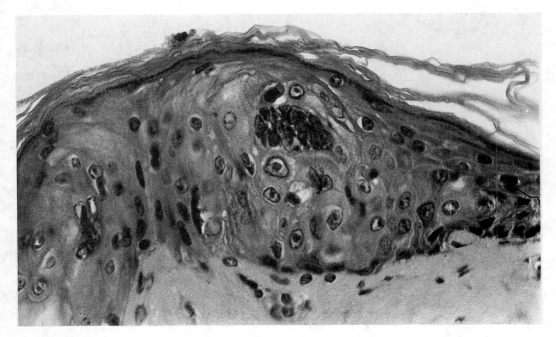

Figure 22-1. Herpetic stomatitis, showing multinuclear inclusion cells characteristic of herpes (high power).

D. Benign tumors and tumorlike conditions

1. **Gingival hyperplasia** occurs predominantly in patients receiving phenytoin. The gingiva appears as a pink, lobulated mass because collagenous tissue proliferates and new blood vessels form. The hyperplasia usually recedes after the drug is discontinued. The tongue may be similarly affected.

2. A **ranula** is a unilateral cyst on the floor of the mouth near the frenulum. It varies in size and is believed to be either a retention cyst that results from mechanical interference with secretions of the sublingual glands or a remnant of a branchial cleft cyst.

3. A **mucocele** is a cyst that occurs predominantly on the lips. It is characterized by pools of mucus and inflammatory cells within the minor salivary glands.

4. An **epulis** is a tumorlike mass that appears in the gingiva as a sessile or pedunculated, rubbery, red–blue or pink mass. It is situated on the outer surface of the gum and involves the mandible more often than the maxilla. **Histologically,** it consists of a fibrous stroma in which numerous multinucleate giant cells are seen admixed with chronic inflammatory cells.

5. A **fibroma** occurs predominantly on the inner surface of the cheek and lips. It usually follows irritation from dentures or other trauma to the area. **Histologically,** this exophytic type of soft tissue proliferation, with chronic inflammatory cells, is covered by squamous mucosa that may be either thickened or atrophic.

6. A **granular cell tumor** (see Chapter 25 III B 5 c) is one of the most common benign tumors affecting the tongue. Hyperplasia of the squamous mucosa overlying the lesion may simulate cancer.

E. Leukoplakia.

This lesion of the mucous membranes is regarded by some authorities as a precancerous condition. Chronic irritation and trauma to the area are believed to be local etiologic factors.

1. **Clinical features.** Leukoplakia is more common in men than in women. The lesion consists of one or several white patches, not less than 5 mm in diameter, with raised, ill-defined borders.

2. **Histologically,** the condition shows hyperkeratosis, parakeratosis, thickening of the stratified squamous mucosa, and varying degrees of cellular atypia, especially in the basal layer. Evidence of inflammation may be present in the underlying connective tissue.

F. Squamous cell carcinoma of the mouth. Cancer of the mouth is an important clinical problem, constituting about 5% to 10% of all malignant tumors. The lips, larynx, and tongue are the sites most often involved. The most common malignant lesion of the oral mucosa is squamous cell carcinoma (SCC).

1. **Etiology**
   a. Cancer of the tongue and larynx occurs often in smokers, especially in those who smoke and drink heavily.
   b. Tobacco chewers have a high incidence of buccal mucosal tumors, especially at the site where tobacco is held in the mouth.
   c. Carcinoma of the lips affects pipe smokers and persons chronically exposed to sunlight.

2. **Clinical features.** The lesion starts as a small indurated plaque, nodule, or ulcer, which may increase in size and project as a large cauliflower-like mass that interferes with speech and chewing and destroys the adjacent tissues.

3. **Pathology**
   a. **Carcinoma in situ** is considered to be a precursor of invasive cancer and may be found at the margins of an obvious cancer. **Histologically,** it is characterized by immaturity and disorganization of the squamous epithelium, with pleomorphism and atypia of individual cells. Mitoses are present. The lesion is limited by an intact basement membrane.
   b. **Infiltrating carcinoma** usually is well differentiated, exhibits abundant keratin formation, and invades adjacent tissues (Figures 22-2 and 22-3).

4. **Prognosis.** These tumors frequently metastasize by lymphatics to the neck lymph nodes. Prognosis depends on several factors, such as degree of differentiation, size of the primary tumor, depth of invasion, and spread of metastases. Multifocal tumors are commonly associated with a poor prognosis.

5. **Treatment** usually depends on the site and size of the tumor and its surgical accessibility. If surgical resection is possible, a radical lymph node dissection is often performed, followed by radiation of the involved area.

II. NASOPHARYNX

A. Normal structure. The pharynx is encircled by aggregations of lymphoid tissue, which form the **tonsillar ring of Waldeyer** (the nasopharyngeal, tubal, palatine, and lingual tonsils). These lymphoid aggregates are covered by either pseudostratified columnar epithelium or stratified squamous epithelium.

B. Inflammatory disorders

1. **Tonsillitis.** With either acute or chronic inflammation, the tonsils appear enlarged and red. The causative agents most commonly are β-hemolytic streptococci (e.g., *Streptococcus pyogenes*) and pneumococci, but tonsillitis also may result from viruses and other organisms. **Histologically,** the crypts of squamous epithelia contain numerous neutrophils and desquamated epithelial cells.

2. **Pharyngitis.** Infections of the oropharynx are commonly caused by viruses or bacteria, such as streptococci and, less frequently, staphylococci. Characteristics are intense infiltration by inflammatory cells, edema, and hyperplasia of tissues. With antibiotics, the process resolves in a few days.

C. Benign tumors

1. **Nasal polyp** is a nonspecific proliferation of edematous stroma and nasal mucosa found in patients with clinical histories of allergies. It is a very common condition.

2. **Angiofibroma** is an infrequent tumor that may have an endocrine pathogenesis.
   a. **Clinical features.** The characteristic symptoms are nasal obstruction, epistaxis, and nasal discharge. Patients usually are males between age 12 and 25.
   b. **Pathology**
      (1) **Macroscopically,** the lesion is a firm, rubbery, gray or purple–red tumor that usually has a broad attachment to the wall of the nasopharynx. The surface may become ulcerated.

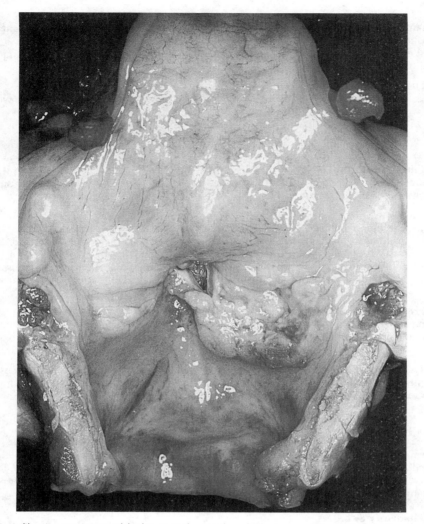

Figure 22-2. Infiltrating carcinoma of the larynx in the vocal cord. The tumor protrudes into the lumen of the larynx.

      (2) Microscopically, the tumor consists of vascular fibrous connective tissue intermingled with spindle-shaped cells and chronic inflammatory cells, such as lymphocytes and plasma cells. The vessels are small to medium-sized malformed arteries with incomplete elastic laminae. The vascularity is so pronounced that the tumor may be confused with a hemangioma.

   c. Treatment. Angiofibroma has a tendency to remit spontaneously. Removal of the lesion is difficult and dangerous because of potential severe hemorrhage, which may be difficult to control. As an androgen-dependent tumor, it may respond to hormone therapy.

D. Lymphoepithelioma is also known as nasopharyngeal carcinoma. This describes a poorly differentiated carcinoma that can appear at any site in the upper respiratory tract but most frequently is found in the lateral wall of the nasopharynx, around the ostium of the eustachian tube.

   1. Clinical features. Lymphoepithelioma occurs in young adults, often of Asian lineage. The patient usually presents with nasal obstruction, bleeding, middle ear discomfort, cranial nerve palsies, or enlarged lymph nodes in the neck. Association with Epstein-Barr virus (EBV) infection has been noted for many patients.

   2. Pathology. Lymphoid elements are admixed with malignant epithelial cells identical to those of a poorly differentiated SCC. The lymphoid cells are not considered neoplastic. Only the epithelial component is present in metastases.

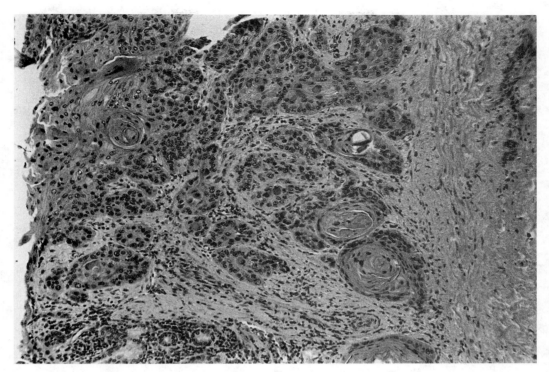

Figure 22-3. Infiltrating well-differentiated squamous cell carcinoma (SCC) of the larynx, exhibiting keratin formation (high power).

      3. Prognosis and treatment. The tumor grows rapidly and tends to metastasize early. The treatment of choice is radiotherapy, as surgical control is virtually impossible.

III. LARYNX. Hoarseness is the most common symptom of any laryngeal disease.

   A. Laryngitis usually occurs as part of any inflammatory process in the respiratory tract. It calls for special attention when it occurs in infants or children, because significant edema in the young can cause laryngeal obstruction and difficulty in breathing.

   B. Benign laryngeal tumors

      1. Laryngeal polyps are sessile or pedunculated nodules that occur predominantly in the vocal cords. They are most common in adult men, often those who are speakers or singers, and generally cause hoarseness.

         a. Pathology. A laryngeal polyp consists of a proliferative stroma covered by benign squamous epithelium. The stroma may be very vascular and may exhibit varying degrees of chronic inflammation.

         b. Treatment. These benign lesions are best treated by surgical excision.

      2. Papillomatosis is probably of viral origin and has been related to human papillomavirus (HPV). The lesion can occur at any age, including childhood.

         a. Pathology. Papillomatosis is a true neoplasm, composed of friable nodules or excrescences located on the true vocal cords. **Histologically,** a central core of fibrous tissue is covered by hyperplastic squamous epithelium.

         b. Prognosis. This tumor is believed to predispose to carcinoma, although malignant transformation is rare in children.

   C. Laryngeal carcinoma

      1. Squamous cell carcinoma (SCC) [see Figures 22-2 and 22-3] is the most common epithelial tumor of the larynx. As in the oral cavity, it occurs as **carcinoma in situ** or as an **invasive carcinoma.** Prognosis is directly related to the extent (i.e., stage) of the tumor.

2. **Verrucous carcinoma** appears grossly as a large, fungating papillary growth. **Histologically,** it is a very well-differentiated squamous cell tumor and, therefore, may be difficult to diagnose in biopsy material. Resection is the treatment of choice; radiotherapy is not used because it may alter the biologic behavior of the tumor so that it becomes a highly aggressive neoplasm.

IV. JAW

A. **Osteomyelitis of the jaw** can occur in both acute and chronic forms. The chronic form usually is secondary to a dental or periodontal infection. In both forms, the radiologic and pathologic features are identical to those seen with osteomyelitis in any other bone (see Chapter 23 I F).

B. **Cysts of the maxilla and mandible** may arise as a result of a defect in tooth development (**odontogenic**), or their appearance may be secondary to inflammation of the dental pulp (**nonodontogenic**).

1. **Odontogenic cysts**
   a. A **radicular (periapical) cyst** arising in an epithelial dental granuloma is the result of inflammation and necrosis of the dental pulp. The cyst is attached to the roots of the tooth and may become very large. As a rule, it is lined by squamous epithelium; rarely, the lining is columnar epithelium. Periapical cyst is the most common cyst of the jaw.
   b. A **follicular (dentigerous) cyst** commonly occurs in the maxilla, where it is derived from misplaced tooth epithelial buds. The cyst is lined by stratified squamous epithelium and contains serous or mucoid material. Secondary infection may occur. The treatment of choice is curettage of the lesion, and recurrences are unusual.
   c. An **eruption cyst** is a small dentigerous cyst occurring on teeth that have already erupted and causing the gingiva to swell. It is lined by stratified squamous epithelium.
   d. A **primordial cyst** usually has no special relationship with the teeth, although it may appear in the area of a missing tooth. It is lined by stratified squamous epithelium, and the lumen is filled with keratinocytes.
   e. An **odontogenic keratocyst,** constituting about 5% of dental cysts, presents **radiologically** as a radiolucency in the jaw. **Histologically,** the cyst is lined by keratinizing squamous epithelium. Keratocysts recur in as many as 60% of cases.

2. **Nonodontogenic cysts**
   a. A **nasopalatine cyst** is found in the midline of the maxilla behind the central incisors, superior to the incisive papilla. The cyst wall contains numerous mucous glands, nerves, and vessels. The epithelial lining may be squamous, transitional, or cylindrical.
   b. A **globulomaxillary cyst** is located beneath the maxillary lateral incisor and cuspid. It is only symptomatic if infected. It is lined by stratified squamous cuboidal epithelium.
   c. A **nasolabial cyst** may develop from epithelial remnants at the site of fusion of the facial processes. It is situated on the alveolar process near the base of a nostril. The lining of the cyst is similar to that of nasopalatine and globulomaxillary cysts.

C. **Tumors of the jaw**

1. **Adamantinoma (ameloblastoma)** is a true neoplasm resembling the morphology of a developing tooth. The lesion occurs most commonly in the mandible. Its origin has not been definitely established.
   a. **Clinical features and diagnosis.** There is a slight predilection for women age 30 to 50. The lesion presents as a painless swelling, which may ulcerate and cause limitation of function in later stages. Radiologically, the lesion appears as a unilocular or multilocular radiolucency with well-defined margins. An embedded tooth may be present.
   b. **Pathology.** An adamantinoma consists of epithelial strands that vary in size and resemble the enamel of a tooth. The peripheral layer of cells shows centrally placed nuclei, with pink cytoplasm facing the surrounding stroma. Toward the center of the epithelial strands, the cells undergo hydropic degeneration, giving rise to cyst formation. The older the lesion, the greater the cystic development.
   c. **Prognosis and treatment**
      (1) The tumor is locally aggressive and destroys bone and adjacent structures by expanding. Metastases to lungs and lymph nodes have been described, but it is not clear whether these represent other types of tumors.
      (2) The tumor is very radioresistant. The usual therapy is curettage or resection of the lesion, but recurrence is common.

2. Odontoma is a hamartoma arising from tissues involved in tooth formation.
   a. Clinical features and diagnosis. The lesion often is diagnosed in the second decade of life, predominantly in women. It presents as an asymptomatic mass in the premolar or molar area of the mandible. Expansion into the jaws is very unusual. Radiology shows a radiolucent lesion with varying degrees of radiodensity.
   b. Pathology. The lesion consists of varying proportions of dentin, enamel, cementum, and pulp tissue. If the tissues show a random arrangement, the lesion is called **complex odontoma**. If the tissues follow normal formation patterns, the lesion is called **compound odontoma**.
   c. Prognosis and treatment. Therapy is simple curettage, and recurrences are rare.

3. Cementoma is a tumor in which soft tissues have been partly or entirely replaced by cementum-like structures, cementicles. The mandible is affected more often than the maxilla.
   a. Clinical features and diagnosis. Cementomas can be single or multiple and occur predominantly in women. The tumor almost always appears around the root of a premolar or molar and sometimes is fused to the tooth. Radiologically, a central radiopaque mass is present, surrounded by a uniform radiolucent shell.
   b. Pathology. Histologically, irregular osteoid formation and large hyperchromatic osteoblasts are seen within a background of proliferative fibrovascular tissue.
   c. Prognosis and treatment. Cementomas have the capacity to recur and invade locally. Although their malignant potential is low, rare cases of metastasis to the lungs have been reported. Treatment is aimed at complete removal of the lesion.

4. Other tumors
   a. The jaw may be affected by benign and malignant tumors similar to those occurring in the long bones. Of these, the most common are osteoid osteomas, giant cell tumors, fibrous dysplasia, Paget's disease, ossifying fibromas, and osteosarcomas.
   b. Secondary involvement of the mandible is common after SCCs of the buccal and oral mucosae. Tumors such as those of the breast and lung can also metastasize to the mandible and simulate primary neoplasms.

V. SALIVARY GLANDS

A. Normal structure

1. Types. The salivary glands are of two types.
   a. The **major salivary glands** are large and bilateral. These include:
      (1) The **parotid glands,** located at the angle of the jaw and sides of the face
      (2) The **submaxillary glands,** located under the jaw
      (3) The **sublingual glands,** located under the tongue
   b. The **minor salivary glands** are small and are present throughout the oral cavity, pharynx, nasopharynx, nose, paranasal sinuses, and larynx.

2. Acini. All of the salivary glands contain both mucous and serous acini, with the exception of the parotid glands (which are exclusively serous) and the sublingual glands (which are exclusively mucous).

B. Sialadenosis is asymptomatic enlargement of salivary glands unrelated to inflammation, salivary stones, or tumors. It occurs most frequently in the parotid glands, causing "chipmunk facies."

1. Pathogenesis. A number of **associated conditions** may lead to sialadenosis, including:
   a. Nutritional deficiencies, especially the protein malnutrition seen in alcoholics
   b. Ingestion of substances containing iodides, lead, or mercury
   c. Hormonal imbalances, especially those that occur in hypothyroidism, diabetes mellitus, and pregnancy

2. Diagnosis is suggested by the patient's history and may be confirmed by chemical diagnosis of the saliva or by biopsy.

C. Sialolithiasis. Stones are found in the large ducts of the major salivary glands, with 80% occurring in the submandibular, fewer than 20% in the parotid, and about 1% to 2% in the sublingual glands.

1. Etiology. The cause is unknown, but sialolithiasis probably reflects subtle abnormalities of salivary secretion—perhaps from local electrolyte imbalance and local dehydration—leading to precipitation of insoluble calcium salts.

2. Clinical features and diagnosis. Most stones occur in adults. Salivation can produce acute pain, and the gland swells after ingestion of spicy or tart food. Physical examination typically shows a palpable mass at the affected site. Sialography, with introduction of a radiopaque medium into major salivary ducts, is diagnostically useful.

3. Treatment. Most stones can be removed manually under local anesthesia, but some may require surgical excision of the entire submandibular gland or parotid lobectomy (e.g., because of location). Adequate hydration and, perhaps, a change in diet may help to prevent recurrences.

D. Parotitis

1. Acute suppurative parotitis occurs in the very young or the elderly. The organism that is cultured most frequently is *Staphylococcus aureus.* Acute parotid inflammation and swelling also occur in **mumps;** suppuration does not occur.
  a. Predisposing factors are debilitation and dehydration. About 50% of patients have major systemic infections, and 25% have malignancies and usually are undergoing chemotherapy.
  b. Treatment consists of appropriate antibiotic therapy. Surgical drainage occasionally is required. A mortality rate of about 20% reflects the seriousness of the underlying illness rather than of the parotitis per se.

2. Chronic recurrent parotitis can occur in the presence or absence of stones. It is characterized by recurring pain, decreased salivary secretion, and increased salivary sodium concentration. Sialography demonstrates parotid duct irregularities due to stenosis and dilation.

3. Submaxillary gland inflammation, in contrast to that of the parotid, is invariably due to stones.

E. Mikulicz's disease and Mikulicz's syndrome

1. Many conditions have been listed in the wastebasket diagnosis of **Mikulicz's disease,** including lymphoma, tuberculosis, sarcoidosis, and salivary gland enlargement due to nutritional deficiencies. Mikulicz described one patient with bilateral lacrimal, submandibular, and parotid gland swelling that histologically resembled severe chronic inflammation, with atrophy of these glands. It is now believed that this patient had Sjögren's syndrome.

2. Mikulicz's syndrome refers to bilateral swelling of the lacrimal, submandibular, and parotid glands due to known causes such as sarcoidosis and tuberculosis.

3. Because of overuse and confusion surrounding these terms, it is better to define the specific lesion rather than to employ the eponym.

F. Sjögren's syndrome is a systemic condition, with both inflammatory and neoplastic characteristics. Women, frequently postmenopausal, are afflicted more commonly than men, in a ratio of 9:1. Although Sjögren's syndrome is a benign disease in the majority of cases, it is now known that some patients have a predisposition to develop malignant lymphoma.

1. Clinical features
  a. The triad of **xerostomia** (dry mouth), **xerophthalmia** (dry eyes), and **arthritis** is classic, although these symptoms may not always appear in one patient.
    (1) The xerostomia and xerophthalmia are due to a marked decrease in the secretion of the salivary and lacrimal glands; the combination of dry mouth and dry eyes often is referred to as the **sicca syndrome**.
    (2) Swelling of the salivary and lacrimal glands may or may not occur, and it may be unilateral.
    (3) Rheumatoid arthritis is seen in more than half of the patients; others may have another collagen vascular disease, such as systemic lupus erythematosus (SLE), polyarteritis, scleroderma, or polymyositis.
  b. Autoantibodies to normal salivary duct epithelium have been demonstrated in the serum of patients with Sjögren's syndrome—by immunofluorescent techniques.

2. Pathology
  a. Histologically, the salivary glands in patients with Sjögren's syndrome show atrophy of acinar tissue, with fibrosis of inter- and intralobular tissue and lymphoplasmacytic infiltration. The histologic findings in Mikulicz's syndrome are similar. A histologically similar lesion isolated to one salivary gland and presenting as a mass is termed **lymphoepithelial lesion of Godwin**.

b. The diagnosis of Sjögren's syndrome is confirmed by the presence of **epimyoepithelial islands,** the result of altered (metaplastic) ducts that become suspended in lymphoid tissue.

   (1) These islands are most valuable in distinguishing the lesion from lymphoma, a misdiagnosis often made because of marked lymphoid infiltration of the salivary glands.

   (2) The distinctive epimyoepithelial islands found in Sjögren's syndrome are not present in diseases of the minor salivary glands; only atrophy and lymphocytic infiltration are seen.

3. Diagnosis

   a. The diagnosis is clinically obvious in classic cases of Sjögren's syndrome.

   b. In other cases, needle biopsy can be informative. Since characteristic microscopic changes are present throughout the salivary and lacrimal systems, a minor salivary gland can be biopsied under local anesthesia. This simple and reliable office procedure avoids the risk of injury to the facial nerve.

G. Tumors of the salivary glands

   1. General considerations. A wide diversity of neoplasms can arise in salivary tissue. Almost all salivary tissue tumors are now believed to be epithelial, either acinar or ductal cell in origin.

   a. Location. Most tumors of the salivary glands (about 80%) occur in the parotid gland; the next most common site is the submandibular gland, followed by the salivary glands of the palate.

   b. Clinical features

   (1) A **benign tumor** usually presents as a painless lump that gradually increases in size.

   (2) A **malignant lesion** is suggested by the presence of pain, functional disturbances (e.g., seventh cranial nerve weakness), or ulceration (in minor glands). The course of a malignant tumor depends on the histologic type. The tumor may be painful as a result of rapid growth; and by invasion or spread, it may produce diverse problems, some potentially fatal. As an example, patients may die from the local disabling effects of the tumor.

   (a) The tumor may produce nerve palsy through invasion of nerves and may spread to the base of the brain. It may extend to the skin or bones.

   (b) The tumor may grow to the floor of the mouth, into the tongue or pharynx; dysphagia may result, and aspiration may occur.

   (c) It may invade the jugular vein or carotid artery, leading to exsanguination.

   c. Treatment. Surgery is the primary therapy for all salivary gland tumors.

   (1) Benign neoplasms are best treated by lobectomy when in the parotid gland, total excision when in the submandibular or sublingual gland, and wide excision when in a minor salivary gland. Recurrence is common after inadequate resection.

   (2) Treatment of **malignant neoplasms** is determined by the grade, type, and extent of the lesion.

   (a) High-grade, aggressive tumors may require radical excision, including sacrifice of the seventh cranial nerve, and radical neck dissection. Wide excision usually suffices in low-grade, slowly growing cancers. "Shelling-out" procedures are to be condemned.

   (b) Radiation therapy postoperatively may be of secondary value to control microscopic residues or may be of use to palliate unresectable local disease. The value of adjuvant chemotherapy requires additional study.

2. Benign tumors

   a. Benign mixed tumors (BMTs; pleomorphic adenomas) comprise 80% to 85% of all salivary gland tumors. The tumor usually is found in the superficial lobe of the parotid gland; occasionally, it may lie on or near the seventh cranial nerve.

   (1) Clinical features. A BMT appears as an asymptomatic, slowly enlarging mass. Although it can reach an enormous size in the parotid, it does not invade the facial nerve or infiltrate the skin. Adults of all ages may be affected.

   (2) Pathology

   (a) Grossly, a pleomorphic adenoma is well circumscribed (Figure 22-4) and, at times, encapsulated. Often, small outpouchings or satellite nodules are present; hence, a high rate of recurrence follows enucleation or shelling out of the tumor, because satellites remain.

   (b) Microscopically, a BMT appears as shown in Figure 22-5. The cartilaginous material in the tumor has been identified as mucins of epithelial origin. It is suggested

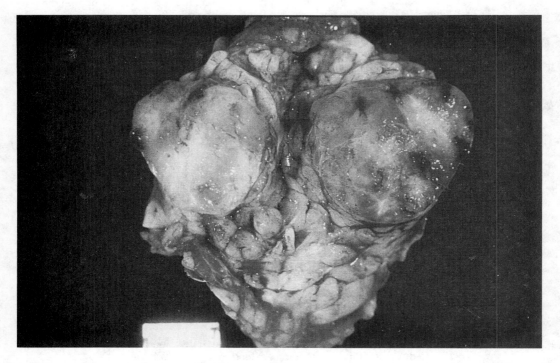

Figure 22-4. Circumscribed nodule in the parotid gland, with the cartilaginous appearance characteristic of a benign mixed tumor (BMT).

that myoepithelial cells undergoing metaplastic change have the capacity to act as facultative chondrocytes, elaborating a matrix of mesenchymal components similar to hyaline cartilage.

    (3) Prognosis. BMT may be seeded in the operative site if the tumor is incised. The patient eventually may present with multiple nodules in the scar, which may grow locally and expand. This tumor is a recurrent BMT, not a malignancy.

  b. Papillary cystadenoma lymphomatosum (Warthin's tumor) constitutes about 10% of benign salivary tumors. It is found almost exclusively in the parotid gland, frequently in the tail, and occasionally separate from the main body of the gland. About 10% are bilateral. The tumor occurs 8 to 10 times more often in men than in women; older age-groups primarily are affected.

    (1) Diagnosis. Warthin's tumor, alone among salivary neoplasms, concentrates technetium 99m, which make its identification possible preoperatively.

    (2) Pathology. Grossly, the lesion is soft, almost fluctuant, brown, and cystic in some areas. Its histologic appearance is that of tall eosinophilic cells in lymphoid stroma.

    (3) Prognosis. The tumor frequently is multicentric in origin, accounting for its tendency to recur after local excision. Very rarely, malignant lymphoma or undifferentiated carcinoma arises in a Warthin's tumor.

3. Malignant tumors

  a. Mucoepidermoid carcinomas are the most common, constituting about one-third of malignant salivary gland tumors. Some 60% to 70% occur in the parotid glands, 15% to 20% in the minor salivary glands, and 10% in the submaxillary glands. The tumor often may be seen in the hard or soft palate.

    (1) Pathology. Circumscribed but nonencapsulated, the tumor contains mucus-secreting and epidermoid cells and an intermediate type of basal or non–mucus-secreting cell. Low-grade, well-differentiated tumors, intermediate-grade lesions, and high-grade aggressive cancers are seen.

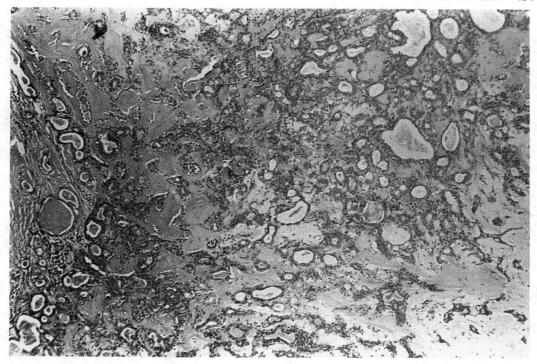

Figure 22-5. Benign mixed tumor (BMT), with fibrous and myxoid stroma and epithelial structures (tubules and glands) [low power].

    (2) Prognosis depends directly on the grade of the tumor. Most patients have an excellent prognosis, with the 5-year survival rate approaching 90%. However, in approximately 10% of patients, the tumor takes a highly malignant course.
        (a) Two-thirds of patients with high-grade tumors develop regional node metastases, and one-third have distant metastases over a 5-year period. Death often is due to uncontrolled local and distant metastases.
        (b) The low-grade tumors have a clinical course approaching that of benign mixed tumors.
  b. Malignant mixed tumors (MMTs) comprise about 10% to 15% of salivary gland cancers. The tumor most often involves the parotid glands, less often the submaxillary glands, and rarely the minor salivary glands. It occurs twice as frequently in women as in men.
    (1) Clinical features. Patients usually have a typical clinical history of an untreated salivary gland tumor that has been present for many years, with recent rapid enlargement. On average, patients with MMTs are 10 to 20 years older than those with BMTs. Pain and facial nerve paralysis are often seen.
    (2) Pathology. The finding of a BMT associated with an obvious carcinoma supports the diagnosis of an MMT.
        (a) An MMT (or carcinoma, e.g., mixed tumor) consists of carcinomas of the single-cell type, such as epidermoid, adeno-, and spindle-cell carcinomas. One of these carcinomas appears to become malignant, overgrowing and infiltrating the benign tumor.
        (b) Recurrences and metastases from an MMT do not show the pleomorphic spectrum of a BMT.
    (3) Prognosis. Patients with extensive tumors or those previously treated have a poor prognosis. Local recurrence, nodal metastases, and widespread bone and visceral metastases are common.
  c. Adenoid cystic carcinomas (cylindromas) occur in all salivary glands but are most common in the submaxillary and minor salivary glands. They are the most frequently encountered neoplasms of the minor salivary glands, accounting for 16% to 25% of all tumors of these glands and over 50% of malignant tumors of these glands.
    (1) Clinical features. Local pain is a prominent feature in half of the patients. Facial paralysis is an ominous sign.

(2) Pathology

   (a) The term cylindroma conveys the structural pattern of the tumors—the enclosure of mucin or hyaline cylinders within epithelial islands. Often, the small, darkly stained cells appear as anastomosing cords lying in a mucoid or hyaline stroma. The neoplasm is not encapsulated.

   (b) The most striking characteristic is the tumor's **affinity for nerves,** with growth into and within the perineural spaces. The tumor may extend along nerves to the base of the brain. Hence, at the time of resection, the nerves must be carefully examined by frozen section to detect perineural invasion at the resection margins. A solid histologic pattern of a larger cell type with areas of necrosis portends a rapid, fulminant clinical course.

(3) Prognosis. The lesion is deceptively slow growing but has a relentless clinical course.

   (a) Because the tumor may infiltrate insidiously at margins and resection often is inadequate, recurrence is common and the ultimate prognosis is poor. Thus, although the cure rate at 5 years is approximately 75%, it drops to 15% to 20% when patients are followed for 10 to 20 years.

   (b) In the late stage, metastases to lungs, bones, and viscera are common. Silent lung metastases are not unusual and should not deter the surgeon from trying to control local disease. Radiotherapy is a useful adjunct in controlling a locally persistent or recurrent malignant tumor.

d. Acinic cell carcinomas usually arise in the parotid glands. Only 5% occur in the submaxillary glands, and rarely have these tumors been reported in minor salivary glands. About 70% are found in women.

   (1) Clinical features. An acinic cell carcinoma mimics a mixed tumor.

   (2) Pathology. This grossly circumscribed but microscopically invasive tumor resembles the cellular lining of the acini of the parotid gland, being composed of basophilic cells with granular cytoplasm. Cyst formation is common.

   (3) Prognosis. Acinic cell carcinoma is a low-grade carcinoma, recurring locally and rarely producing distant metastases. Regional nodes are involved infrequently. The 5-year cure rate is 90%; however, the cure rate becomes poorer as follow-up periods grow longer.

e. Other malignant tumors, not easily classifiable into the preceding groups, do occur but are rare.

   (1) SCCs originating primarily in salivary tissue have been recorded, but these might be part of high-grade mucoepidermoid tumors, or they might be carcinomas arising in a BMT which is not identified or has been destroyed by the malignancy.

   (2) Malignant lymphomas may appear initially as intraparotid masses, since nodes occur in the parotid gland.

   (3) Metastatic tumors of the intraparotid nodes may mimic primary salivary gland cancers. These usually are melanomas of head or eye origin or SCCs from the head or neck.

   (4) Polymorphous low-grade adenocarcinoma is a recently recognized carcinoma of minor salivary glands, predominantly involving the palate. It shares microscopic features with the mixed tumor and adenoid cystic carcinoma. Its course is biologically indolent; and although it may recur locally, death from this tumor is almost unknown.

STUDY QUESTIONS

Directions: Each of the numbered items or incomplete statements in this section is followed by answers or by completions of the statement. Select the **one** lettered answer or completion that is **best** in each case.

1. During a routine preschool physical examination, a 5-year-old child is discovered to have elevated, partially confluent white patches on the hard palate. These lesions

(A) probably represent leukoplakia and should be biopsied
(B) will probably reveal blastomycosis yeast forms on a potassium hydroxide (KOH) preparation
(C) may signal an underlying immunodeficiency
(D) represent Fordyce's disease

2. Epstein-Barr virus (EBV) infection is associated with

(A) herpetic stomatitis
(B) aphthous stomatitis
(C) papillomatosis
(D) osteomyelitis
(E) lymphoepithelioma

3. Patients undergoing long-term phenytoin therapy may develop which complication?

(A) Leukoplakia
(B) Moniliasis
(C) Dental caries
(D) Gingival hyperplasia
(E) Squamous cell carcinoma (SCC)

4. A 70-year-old man with a history of recurrent "cold sores" and cigar smoking presents with a raised nonhealing ulcer of the inner lower lip. A biopsy reveals infiltrating squamous cell carcinoma (SCC). Which statement is true?

(A) Areas of leukoplakia at sites distant from the ulcer need not be biopsied
(B) Radical lymph node dissection is not indicated because of the history of herpes infection
(C) Radiation therapy is more effective than chemotherapy in control of local spread
(D) The lymphoid tissue of Waldeyer's ring is a frequent site of metastases

5. A 55-year-old woman presents with a history of bilateral eye irritation and dry mouth. A biopsy of a minor salivary gland reveals metaplastic secretory ducts surrounded by lymphocytes. The most likely diagnosis is

(A) malignant lymphoma
(B) Sjögren's syndrome
(C) sarcoidosis
(D) sialadenosis

6. Which of the following is a characteristic of laryngeal polyps?

(A) Occurrence at any age
(B) Viral etiology
(C) Multifocality
(D) Malignant transformation
(E) Occurrence in singers

7. Adenoid cystic carcinoma is a tumor of the salivary glands that is characterized by

(A) frequent involvement of the parotid glands
(B) nerve invasion in the area of the tumor
(C) grossly cystic appearance
(D) short survival in affected patients
(E) circumscribed growth pattern

8. Angiofibroma of the nasopharynx is characterized by

(A) frequent occurrence in young females
(B) occurrence in cigarette smokers
(C) association with human papillomavirus (HPV)
(D) capacity to undergo malignant transformation
(E) presence of steroid receptors

9. Risk factors for acute suppurative sialadenitis include all of the following EXCEPT

(A) dehydration
(B) stones
(C) stenosis of the duct system
(D) mumps
(E) debilitation

1-C	4-C	7-B
2-E	5-B	8-E
3-D	6-E	9-D

10. Lymphoepithelioma is a malignant neoplasm of the nasopharynx characterized by all of the following EXCEPT

(A) high incidence in young Asians
(B) rapid growth
(C) lymphoid and epithelial elements
(D) high rate of cure with surgical resection
(E) some association with Epstein-Barr virus (EBV) infection

11. Characteristics of Sjögren's syndrome include all of the following EXCEPT

(A) swelling of the lacrimal and salivary glands
(B) formation of epimyoepithelial islands
(C) association with rheumatoid arthritis
(D) metastasis to regional lymph nodes
(E) development of malignant lymphoma

12. All of the following statements regarding benign mixed tumor (BMT) of the salivary glands are true EXCEPT

(A) it most commonly occurs in the parotid
(B) it is a rapidly growing asymptomatic mass
(C) it does not invade skin or nerves
(D) it is the most common salivary gland neoplasm

13. All of the following statements concerning sialolithiasis are true EXCEPT

(A) it occurs most often in adults
(B) it presents clinically as a painful swelling
(C) it can be treated with antibiotics
(D) it occurs most frequently in the submandibular gland

10-D   13-C
11-D
12-B

ANSWERS AND EXPLANATIONS

1. The answer is C *[I C 2].*
The most common cause of elevated white oral plaques in children is candidal stomatitis. Although this inflammation may occur in otherwise healthy children, *Candida* infection often occurs in immunosuppressed individuals,. Leukoplakia is a dysplastic epithelial process found in adults. Blastomycosis infection is rare and does not present as oral plaques. Fordyce's disease is characterized by discrete small granules of the cheeks, lips, and gingivae.

2. The answer is E *[II D].*
The Epstein-Barr virus (EBV) genome has been found in the majority of cases of lymphoepithelioma tumors so studied. Herpes simplex virus (HSV) is the cause of herpetic stomatitis. Human papillomavirus (HPV) is associated with papillomatosis. Osteomyelitis is usually caused by bacteria. Aphthous stomatitis does not have an infectious etiology.

3. The answer is D *[I D 1].*
Gingival hyperplasia can occur in patients receiving long-term phenytoin therapy. Lobulated masses of gingival tissue enlarge because collagen proliferates and new vessels form. The hyperplasia usually recedes following discontinuation of the drug therapy.

4. The answer is C *[I F].*
Following surgical excision and radical lymph node dissection, radiation therapy is used because chemotherapy has not been effective in controlling squamous cell carcinoma (SCC). Multifocality of SCC is common, and any clinically suspicious areas should be biopsied. Although Waldeyer's ring may be directly invaded by cancer, the usual spread of metastases is to regional lymph nodes.

5. The answer is B *[V F].*
The histologic features described and the history provided are typical of Sjögren's syndrome. Although malignant lymphoma may arise in the syndrome, it is rare and is usually heralded by a suddenly enlarging gland and lymphadenopathy. The histologic features of sarcoidosis (noncaseating granulomas) are not present. Sialadenosis is not an inflammatory condition.

6. The answer is E *[III B 1 a].*
A laryngeal polyp is a localized proliferation on the vocal cord and consists of proliferative fibrous and vascular tissue. No relationship to viral causation has been documented. It has been found most commonly in adult men who use their voices in occupations such as singers and announcers. The lesion is not believed to predispose to carcinoma.

7. The answer is B *[V G 3 c].*
An adenoid cystic carcinoma (also known as cylindromatous carcinoma) can be found in any salivary gland but occurs most frequently in the submandibular and minor salivary glands. The most striking histologic feature of this tumor is its propensity for nerve invasion—and its subsequent growth in the perineural spaces. The tumor grows slowly but relentlessly; the 5-year survival rate is nearly 75%, but the 10- to 15-year survival rate is only 15% to 20%. The term adenoid cystic refers to the histopathologic appearance but not to a grossly cystic appearance; the tumor always grows in an infiltrative pattern and is not circumscribed.

8. The answer is E *[II C 2].*
Angiofibroma of the nasopharynx is an uncommon benign tumor that occurs in young males between age 12 and 25. This lesion consists of vascular fibrous tissue intermingled with spindle cells and chronic inflammatory cells. It is extremely vascular and presents with epistaxis. Angiofibroma is postulated to have a hormonal dependence and contains steroid hormone receptors. It commonly regresses spontaneously.

9. The answer is D *[V D 1, 3].*
Suppuration and acute sialadenitis imply the presence of an infecting organism that is a bacterium. In the setting of dehydration, debilitation, or duct obstruction (due to either stenosis or stones), the acute inflammation usually is accompanied by bacterial infection, often with *Staphylococcus aureus*. Although acute parotitis occurs in mumps, there is no suppuration or abscess formation in this disease. Although stones are less common in the parotid gland as compared with the submaxillary or submandibular gland, they do, in fact, occur with acute suppurative parotitis.

10. The answer is D *[II D]*.
Lymphoepithelioma is a highly malignant tumor of the upper respiratory tract; it occurs in young adults, particularly those of Asian heritage. A link to Epstein-Barr virus (EBV) infection has been noted. The tumor consists of both malignant epithelial cells and nonneoplastic lymphoid cells, which probably represent an immune response to the malignant epithelial component. Radiotherapy is the treatment of choice since the epithelial component grows rapidly and tends to metastasize early. Surgical control is virtually impossible.

11. The answer is D *[V F]*.
Characteristics of Sjögren's syndrome include enlargement of lacrimal and salivary glands; histologic evidence of lymphoplasmacytic infiltration, acinar tissue atrophy, and ductal destruction; and formation of epimyoepithelial islands. The disorder frequently is associated with rheumatoid arthritis. Some patients with Sjögren's syndrome appear to be at increased risk for development of lymphoma. Sjögren's syndrome itself is not a malignant condition; hence, metastases to regional lymph nodes would not occur.

12. The answer is B *[V G 2 a]*.
Benign mixed tumors (BMTs) of the salivary glands (also called pleomorphic adenomas) comprise 80% to 85% of all salivary gland tumors. The most common location for these tumors is the parotid gland. The tumors usually occur in patients between age 20 and 40. The histology of pleomorphic adenomas is dominated by epithelial and myoepithelial cells in a matrix of myxomatous tissue, which sometimes contains islands of cartilage and bone.

13. The answer is C *[V C 2]*.
Sialolithiasis (stone formation within the salivary gland ducts) occurs most often in adults and usually affects the submandibular gland. Nearly 80% of cases involve this gland, about 18% to 20% involve the parotid, and only 1% to 2% occur in the sublingual gland. In most cases, surgical removal of the stone is curative. Antibiotics would not be helpful unless secondary infection occurs. The stones produce pain and swelling in the affected gland.

23

Bones and Joints

Maria J. Merino

I. BONES

A. Normal histology and development

1. Bone tissue consists of several **layers**.
   a. The **cortex,** a dense outer layer, is covered by connective tissue called the **periosteum**. The cortex is essential for mechanical function, and it is less sensitive to metabolic disorders than the medulla.
   b. The **medulla,** an inner network of thin trabeculae, lies within the marrow cavity.
   c. The inner surface of the cortex and the outer surface of the medulla are lined by the **endosteum**.

2. Bone consists of three **types of cells**.
   a. **Osteoblasts** are mononuclear cells with basophilic cytoplasm due to abundant endoplasmic reticulum. The cytoplasmic borders of the cells are blurred; however, narrow spaces do exist between them. Osteoblasts are actively engaged in synthesizing collagen and ground substance and in transporting minerals for the calcification of the organic matrix. The origin of osteoblasts is unknown and remains controversial.
   b. **Osteocytes** are osteoblasts that become embedded and incorporated into an osteoid matrix. They communicate with the overlying osteoblasts by canaliculi through which cell processes extend, and they are able to form and to resorb bone.
   c. **Osteoclasts** are large cells and are usually multinucleate (with 5 to 10 nuclei). In the presence of parathyroid hormone, osteoclasts cause bone resorption by first releasing phosphorus and calcium from the bone and then digesting the bone matrix, creating **resorption (Howship's) lacunae,** which are spaces or pits along bone surfaces.

3. **Bone development** occurs by means of two phenomena.
   a. **Long bones** develop by **endochondral ossification**. The cartilaginous surface is replaced by bone, and the cartilage is left serving as the epiphyseal plate and articular surface.
   b. **Flat bones** develop by **intramembranous ossification**. The mesenchymal cells differentiate directly into bone; there is no cartilaginous phase.

4. Three major **hormones** control calcium and phosphate metabolism: **parathyroid hormone** (parathormone, PTH), **calcitonin,** and the **metabolites of vitamin D,** 25-hydroxyvitamin D_3 and 1,25-dihydroxyvitamin D_3 [1,25-$(OH)_2D_3$].

B. Congenital bone disorders

1. **Osteogenesis imperfecta** is a hereditary disorder of connective tissue that is manifested clinically by a predisposition to multiple bone fractures.
   a. In **osteogenesis imperfecta congenita,** the fetus develops multiple fractures; and, thus, the infant is born with crippling deformities. Few patients are capable of reproduction; hence, the genetic pattern remains uncertain.
   b. **Osteogenesis imperfecta tarda** is usually transmitted as an autosomal dominant trait. It appears after the perinatal period, with bowing of the extremities, blue sclerae, and other manifestations of defects in collagen synthesis. Fractures usually heal normally. The bones show marked osteopenia with a porous cortex because osteoblasts do not synthesize the normal amount of bone matrix. The disease is less severe after puberty.

2. **Osteopetrosis** is a hereditary disorder characterized by abnormally dense bone.
    a. **Clinical features.** There are two forms.
        (1) The **benign form** is autosomal dominant. Patients may have multiple fractures. Diagnosis of the disease often is not made until the second or third decade of life. Osteomyelitis is a common complication.
        (2) The **malignant form** is recessive. Patients may show slow growth, mental retardation, and deafness. Affected children usually die before the second decade of life because they are susceptible to anemia and secondary infections.
    b. **Pathology.** The condition involves an extreme reduction in the size of the medullary cavities and an increased density and widening of all cortical bones except the membranous bones, such as the cranium. The ends of the long bones appear club-shaped with alternating zones of radiolucency and radiopacity, depending on the progression of the disease. A large number of osteoclasts are present but are incapable of resorbing bone because they cannot release acid phosphatase.

C. **Metabolic bone diseases: disorders of remodeling (formation and resorption)**

1. **Osteopenia** and **osteoporosis** are characterized by a decrease in bone mass. The decrease is in the amount of osseous tissue per unit of bone volume. It has been suggested that the term **osteoporosis** be reserved for those cases in which **osteopenia** causes clinical symptoms.

2. **Pathophysiology**
    a. **Senile osteopenia.** With increasing age comes a continuous loss of bone at both the trabecular and cortical layers, which become thinner by internal resorption.
    b. **Steroid-induced osteopenia.** The catabolic effect of corticosteroids may affect trabecular bone, producing a decrease in bone formation. Steroids also decrease intestinal absorption and renal resorption of calcium, so that less calcium reaches the bone.

3. **Clinical features**
    a. **Postmenopausal osteoporosis.** This form of osteopenia is most common in women, especially after the fifth decade of life.
        (1) The decrease in bone volume is due not only to a disorder in remodeling but also to a decreased amount of bone deposited by osteoblasts. Compression of vertebral bodies and fractures are common consequences.
        (2) No effective treatment has been found; but calcium supplements, exercise, and (in some cases) estrogen therapy help to reduce the risk.
    b. **Immobilization osteoporosis.** Confinement to bed for periods longer than 6 months can result in a loss of 30% of initial bone volume. The lack of exercise probably leads to an increase in bone resorption and a decrease in bone formation.

4. **Pathology.** The entire skeleton may show low density, with conspicuous sparsity and thinning of the spongy trabeculae of the affected bone, resulting from an imbalance between resorption and formation in the remodeling sequence.

D. **Hormonal disorders affecting bone**

1. **Primary hyperparathyroidism**
    a. **Pathogenesis.** In bone, PTH stimulates the active phase of the remodeling sequence. Thus, when blood levels of PTH are elevated because of parathyroid hyperplasia or adenoma, bone is affected.
    b. **Clinical features.** Primary hyperparathyroidism predominantly affects women age 30 to 50.
        (1) The clinical symptoms are those of hypercalcemia (see Chapter 20 IV B 1). Patients may present with bone pain, which is more severe in the lower extremities. Pathologic fractures and bone deformities may be seen.
        (2) Serum calcium levels are elevated above 11.5 mg/dl, and phosphorus levels are reduced to less than 2 mg/dl.
    c. **Pathology**
        (1) **Histologically,** the bone tissue shows an increased number of osteoclasts, which resorb the walls of the haversian canals of cortical bone and the surfaces of spongy trabeculae, and the bone is replaced with fibrous tissue.
        (2) Occasionally, proliferation of osteoclasts that contain hemosiderin pigment is very prominent within the fibrous stroma. The lesions, called **brown tumors,** can occur in any bone but are most common in the jaw.
    d. **Treatment** consists of removal of the parathyroid lesion (see Chapter 20 IV C 3).

2. Secondary hyperparathyroidism. In renal failure and other conditions causing hypocalcemia or hyperphosphatemia, there is a compensatory increase in the secretion of PTH. The histologic appearance of bone is the same as in primary hyperparathyroidism but with more severe marrow fibrosis.

3. Hypoparathyroidism often is the result of accidental surgical removal of the parathyroid glands, although idiopathic hypoparathyroidism can occur.
   a. Clinical features. The signs and symptoms are dominated by hypocalcemia, with soft tissue calcification and ossification, abnormal dentition, and otosclerosis.
   b. Pathology. Histologically, bone shows a markedly decreased turnover rate, with active osteoblasts and a lack of osteoclasts.
   c. Treatment is the administration of synthetic PTH or vitamin D.

E. Nutritional disorders affecting bone

1. Vitamin D deficiency affects bone, causing **rickets** in children and **osteomalacia** in adults.
   a. Clinical features
      (1) If vitamin D deficiency occurs in children before epiphyseal closure, the disorder known as **rickets** results, with bone deformities and pain. Symptoms may include a **rachitic rosary** (swelling at the osteochondral junctions of the ribs), bowing of the legs, fractures, and pelvic disorders.
      (2) In adults, the corresponding deficiency disorder is **osteomalacia;** diagnosis can be made on bone biopsy only, because bone growth has already been completed.
   b. Pathology. Histologically, uncalcified osteoid cartilage increases and calcified bone decreases.
   c. Treatment. The disease responds to the administration of vitamin D.

2. Vitamin C deficiency causes increased capillary fragility, which results in hemorrhages in the periosteum as well as in the gums and skin. **Histologically,** the trabecular bone mass decreases, and osteoblasts are abnormal.

3. Vitamin A disorders
   a. Hypervitaminosis A causes abundant mineralization of the periosteum and abnormal bone formation. In children, the premature epiphyseal closure results in permanent skeletal deformities.
   b. Vitamin A deficiency, besides its effects on vision, also causes bone changes. Remodeling ceases, and osteoclastic activity disappears. The bones are short and thick, with a predominance of new cancellous periosteum.

F. Infectious bone disease: osteomyelitis. Osteomyelitis is inflammation of the medullary and cortical portions of bone, including the periosteum. In children, the long bones are most often affected; in adults, the vertebrae.

1. Pathogenesis
   a. The causative organism is most often *Staphylococcus aureus;* occasionally, other bacteria or fungi are the cause.
   b. The bone infection is a result of:
      (1) Most commonly, the hematogenous spread of bacteria from a distant focus of sepsis
      (2) Invasion of bone from adjacent septic arthritis or soft tissue abscesses
      (3) Penetrating trauma
      (4) Complications of fractures
      (5) Complications of surgery
   c. At increased risk for developing osteomyelitis are persons with sickle cell disease, hemodialysis patients, patients with bone or joint prostheses, and intravenous drug abusers.
   d. As bone is altered or destroyed by inflammation, repair and remodeling take place, with new bone formation. Occasionally, inflammation may persist in regions of relative avascularity, where it is impossible to achieve high tissue levels of antibiotics.

2. Types
   a. Pyogenic osteomyelitis most commonly affects children and young adults and involves the femur, tibia, humerus, and radius. Often no source of infection is obvious, but the usual causative organism is *S. aureus.*
   b. Chronic osteomyelitis may develop when the acute process is not properly treated; flare-ups of osteomyelitis may occur at intervals of months or years.

    c. Tuberculous osteomyelitis affects both children and adults and occurs by hematogenous spread of tuberculous organisms to bone; however, the primary focus of the disease may be difficult to find. Spinal involvement (**Pott's disease**) produces destruction and collapse of vertebral bodies. Hips, knees, ankles, and hands often are affected as well. Progressive destruction with little ossification is the rule, and there may be marked epiphyseal involvement.

  3. Clinical features. Fever, local pain, marked leukocytosis, and an elevated sedimentation rate often occur. X-rays may be normal until bone resorption takes place, or the medullary cavity may show increased density.

  4. Pathology. The pathologic appearance of osteomyelitis is variable, depending on the causative organism, host factors, and therapy.

    a. Suppurative inflammation is initiated in the marrow cavities, haversian canals, or subperiosteal spaces. Fibrosis, granulation tissue formation, lymphocytes, plasma cells, and macrophages are seen. Repair follows the initial acute phase.

    b. The structural integrity of the bone depends on the degree of new bone formation and bone remodeling.

  5. Treatment consists of surgical debridement and administration of antibiotics.

G. Idiopathic bone disorders

  1. Paget's disease of the bone (osteitis deformans) affects 3% to 4% of the population over age 40, most commonly men. Characteristically, chronic focal lysis of bone tissue occurs, and a soft, fibrotic matrix replaces the tissue. The disease is usually, although not always, polyostotic, with a predilection for the skull, pelvis, tibia, and femur.

    a. Clinical features

      (1) The initial symptoms may be bone pain, fractures, and deformities. Deafness is common when the skull is affected. Height distortion may occur as a result of vertebral compression. The serum alkaline phosphatase level is markedly elevated, and radiologic findings of bone lysis and reformation are characteristic.

      (2) Occasionally, Paget's disease of bone may be associated with a malignant neoplasm, such as an osteosarcoma.

    b. Pathology

      (1) Marked medullary fibrosis is present, and numerous osteoclasts appear abnormal because of an increased number of nuclei. Lytic and formative phases rapidly succeed one another, leading to local increase in bone mass and disorganization of the normal trabecular pattern.

      (2) The high turnover of bone is characterized by the presence of numerous osteoclasts and osteoblasts, an increased calcification rate, and accumulation of woven bone. This turnover leads to a typical **"mosaic" pattern,** so termed because a cementlike material forms narrow boundaries between the original bone and the activity remodeling foci.

    c. Treatment consists of administration of calcitonin or one of the diphosphonates, both of which decrease the resorption and, therefore, the high turnover rate.

  2. Avascular necrosis predominantly affects the head of the femur in men. It is often associated with alcoholism, corticosteroid therapy, hyperuricemia, Gaucher's disease, systemic lupus erythematosus (SLE), and trauma. Radiologically, reparative foci are seen, replacing necrotic bone.

  3. Legg-Calvé-Perthes disease is a childhood disorder of the head of the femur and is similar to avascular necrosis of adulthood. The typical age at onset is 5 to 9 years, and the earliest manifestations are an intermittent limp and pain.

H. Cystic and neoplastic bone lesions (Table 23-1)

  1. Cystic lesions

    a. Solitary (unicameral) bone cysts are benign lesions of unknown etiology that occur predominantly in the distal end of the long bones (humerus and femur) of young males.

      (1) Clinical features. The most common symptoms are pain in the affected areas and swelling of the soft tissues; in occasional patients, fractures occur. Radiologically, a cyst with a smooth thin cortex is seen in close proximity to the epiphysis.

      (2) Pathology

        (a) Grossly, the cyst has ridges dividing the cavity, giving it a multiloculated appearance. The cavity is filled with clear or bloody fluid.

Table 23-1. Bone Tumors

	Cystic	Chondroblastic	Osteoblastic	Other
Benign	Solitary bone cyst Aneurysmal bone cyst	Chondroma Osteochondroma Chondroblastoma Chondromyxoid fibroma	Osteoma Osteoid osteoma Osteoblastoma	Fibrous dysplasia
Malignant	. . .	Chondrosarcoma	Osteosarcoma	Giant cell tumor of bone Plasma cell myeloma Ewing's sarcoma Malignant lymphoma Metastatic tumors

   (b) **Microscopically,** specific features are lacking, but strands of fibrous tissue may be present, with occasional osteoid and granular tissue formation.
   (3) **Treatment and prognosis.** Curettage followed by the insertion of bone chips is successful. Recurrences are very rare.
  b. **Aneurysmal bone cysts** occur in the metaphysis of the long bones and in the vertebrae; they are seen most frequently in females in the second and third decades of life.
   (1) **Clinical features.** Swelling, pain, and tenderness of the affected area are the most common symptoms. Radiologically, a circumscribed zone of rarefaction is visible, with extension into the soft tissues.
   (2) **Pathology**
      (a) **Grossly,** the lesion varies in size from a few centimeters to 20 cm. The bone is greatly distorted and has an irregular outline. On cut surface, it has a spongy appearance, with cystic spaces of various sizes. The spaces contain blood and are in different stages of organization.
      (b) **Microscopically,** the essential feature is the presence of cavernous spaces with walls that lack normal endothelial linings. Solid areas of fibrous tissue contain osteoid and mature bone, and giant cells may be present. The histologic differential diagnosis includes giant cell tumor of the bone and telangiectatic osteosarcoma.
   (3) **Treatment and prognosis.** The most successful treatment is removal of the entire lesion—or as much of it as possible—followed by the insertion of bone chips. Recurrences may appear in up to 21% of cases.

 2. **Benign disorders**
  a. **Fibrous dysplasia.** This poorly understood condition can affect any bone; but the ribs, femur, tibia, and maxilla are most commonly involved. The disorder is usually monostotic; but in 20% of cases, lesions are polyostotic. At that point, they become a component of **Albright's syndrome,** as are precocious puberty and cutaneous pigmentation.
   (1) **Clinical features.** Symptomatology varies from vaginal bleeding and other endocrinologic symptoms in the infant with Albright's syndrome to bone pain in the elderly. Repeated fractures may lead to bone deformities. X-rays usually demonstrate well-defined zones of rarefaction surrounded by narrow rims of sclerotic bone.
   (2) **Pathology. Histologically,** the major feature is the proliferation of fibroblasts, which produce a dense collagenous matrix. There is no evidence that the woven immature bone ever grows into trabecular lamellar bone. In some areas of the lesion, poorly oriented trabeculae of semicalcified bone are present. Fibrosis with osteoid, giant cells, macrophages, and islands of cartilage are seen.
   (3) **Treatment and prognosis.** A monostotic lesion is treated by either curettage or local resection. Polyostotic lesions are treated conservatively because they commonly stop growing after puberty.
  b. **Chondroma (endochondroma),** a benign cartilaginous lesion, can be solitary or multiple and usually affects the small bones of the hands and feet. Patients frequently are in the second to fifth decades of life.
   (1) **Two syndromes** have multiple chondromas as components. In both of these syndromes, a relatively high risk of malignant transformation accompanies the development of chondrosarcomas.

(a) Ollier's disease (enchondromatosis) is a rare, nonhereditary disorder in which multiple chondromas are present in the metaphysis and diaphysis of various bones.

(b) Maffucci's syndrome is a congenital disease characterized by dyschondroplasia and multiple hemangiomas in the skin and viscera.

(2) Clinical features. Lesions are usually asymptomatic. X-rays show a localized, radiolucent cystic defect with distortion of the bony contour. Central areas of calcification may be present.

(3) Pathology. This neoplasm is thought to originate from heterotropic cartilaginous cell nests in the medullary cavities of bones.

(a) Grossly, the lesion appears as a confluent mass of bluish hyaline cartilage with a lobular configuration.

(b) Microscopically, the cartilage appears moderately cellular, with occasional binucleate cells. Mitoses are absent.

(4) Treatment is curettage of the lesion.

c. Osteochondroma is the most common benign tumor of bone affecting patients under age 21. The lesions may be single or multiple and predominantly involve the metaphysis of long bones.

(1) Clinical features. Symptoms are usually pain and compression of adjacent structures by large tumor masses.

(2) Pathology

(a) Grossly, the tumor may range in size from 1 to several centimeters and appears as a stalked protuberance, with a lobulated surface jutting from the affected bone. The periosteum of the adjacent bone covers the lesion.

(b) Microscopically, the cartilaginous cells appear lined up, mimicking the orientation of cartilaginous cells in a normal epiphysis. No mitoses are present.

(3) Treatment and prognosis. Resection of the lesion usually is curative.

d. Chondroblastoma is a rare cartilaginous tumor that almost always involves the epiphyseal portion of the long bones. The tumor predominantly affects males in the second decade of life.

(1) Clinical features. Patients present with local pain, stiffness, and limitation of motion. X-rays show a central area of bone destruction delineated from the surrounding normal bone by a thin margin of increased bone density.

(2) Pathology

(a) Grossly, the tumor is round or oval in shape, with areas of cystic degeneration and hemorrhage.

(b) Microscopically, proliferation of chondroblasts is intermixed with varying amounts of fibrous stroma and chondroid material. Multinucleate giant cells and calcifications are present. Mitoses are virtually absent.

(3) Treatment and prognosis. A conservative approach, such as curettage or local excision, is best. Although chondroblastomas are considered to be benign, metastasis to the lungs has been reported.

e. Chondromyxoid fibroma is most commonly located in the metaphysis of long bones but occasionally can involve the epiphysis. It primarily affects males in the first and second decades of life.

(1) Clinical features. Pain is the most common symptom. The lesion appears in x-rays as a sharply outlined mass with a rim of sclerotic bone.

(2) Pathology

(a) Grossly, the tumor is a well-circumscribed, solid mass with a cartilaginous appearance. The cortex of the bone is expanded by the tumor, which is limited by the periosteum.

(b) Microscopically, a variety of fibrous, myxomatous, and chondroid elements are seen together with multinucleate giant cells and macrophages that contain hemosiderin. When the tumor forms lobules, a condensation of nuclei occurs beneath the rim of the compressed adjacent tissue.

(3) Treatment and prognosis. Cure can be obtained by complete excision of the lesion, including a rim of normal bone. The incidence of local recurrence is about 20%.

f. Osteoma. This benign tumor almost exclusively involves the skull and facial bones; the frontal sinus is the most common location. Males are affected more often than females, and the lesion can occur at any age. Although osteoma is predominantly a solitary lesion, multiple osteomas can occur in association with intestinal polyposis and soft tissue tumors (**Gardner's syndrome**).

   (1) **Clinical features.** The lesion is asymptomatic unless it interferes with drainage from the paranasal sinus.
   (2) **Pathology.** The tumor of normal dense and mature bone originates from the periosteum. There is little evidence of osteoblastic activity.
   (3) **Treatment.** Resection of the lesion usually is curative.

   g. **Osteoid osteoma** is common in young persons, mostly males.
   (1) **Clinical features.** Patients present with increasing pain that tends to be more severe at night and is relieved by aspirin. X-rays show the lesion as a central radiolucent area (the **nidus**) surrounded by dense sclerotic bone.
   (2) **Pathology**
      (a) **Grossly,** an osteoid osteoma appears as a small round or oval mass containing a central red-brown, friable area (the **nidus**). Frequently, the nidus becomes dislodged from the surrounding sclerotic bone.
      (b) **Microscopically,** the nidus appears as a maze of irregular bone trabeculae, fibrous tissue, and vessels. The center of the nidus is rich in osteoblasts, calcification, and multinucleate giant cells.
   (3) **Treatment and prognosis.** The entire nidus and a rim of sclerotic bone must be excised in order to avoid recurrences of the lesion or persistence of the symptoms.

   h. **Osteoblastoma** predominantly affects the vertebrae and long bones of young males in the first three decades of life.
   (1) **Clinical features.** Symptoms are rarely present. X-rays demonstrate a well-circumscribed lesion surrounded by a zone of sclerotic bone and thickened periosteum. Some tumors may appear as obstructive and expansile masses.
   (2) **Pathology**
      (a) **Grossly,** the lesions vary in size from a few to several centimeters.
      (b) **Microscopically,** osteoblasts proliferate and osteoid production increases. Osteoclasts and multinucleate giant cells may be very numerous, especially in areas of blood extravasation.
   (3) The **treatment** of choice is removal of the entire lesion by curettage.

3. **Malignant tumors**
   a. **Osteosarcoma (osteogenic sarcoma)** is a highly malignant bone tumor characterized by the production of osteoid and bone. Most osteosarcomas arise in the metaphyseal end of long bones (predominantly the femur, humerus, and tibia), but they can involve any bone, including the small bones of the hands, feet, and face.
   (1) **Incidence.** Osteosarcoma is the most common primary malignant tumor of bone (next to multiple myeloma), accounting for approximately 16% of all bone malignancies. The disease predominantly affects young males between age 10 and 20.
   (2) **Etiology.** The etiology is unknown; however, two factors that predispose to the development of osteosarcoma are radiation and preexisting bone disorders, such as Paget's disease. The suspected roles of trauma and viral disease are not clearly established.
   (3) **Clinical features**
      (a) In general, the presenting symptoms are pain and swelling of the affected region; large tumor masses may cause limitation of motion of the nearby joints. Patients with rapidly growing tumors may experience weight loss and secondary anemia.
      (b) Radiologically, there is evidence of bone destruction with penetration of the cortex, subperiosteal elevation (**Codman's triangle**), and infiltration of adjacent soft tissues.
   (4) **Pathology**
      (a) **Gross appearance.** The tumor appears as a large necrotic and hemorrhagic mass (Figure 23-1). The lesion usually ends in the epiphyseal cartilage and rarely extends into the nearby joint space.
      (b) **Microscopic appearance**
         (i) Three **types** of osteosarcomas have been differentiated according to their predominant histologic patterns: **osteoblastic, fibroblastic,** and **chondroblastic**.
         (ii) The hallmark of the tumor is the presence of a malignant stroma that contains osteoid and bone (Figure 23-2). The stroma shows bizarre pleomorphic cells, with hyperchromatic, irregular nuclei and abundant mitoses. Multinucleate

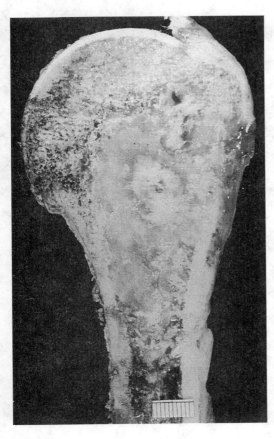

Figure 23-1. Section of a femoral head with osteosarcoma. The necrosis and hemorrhage involve the medullary cavity and extend into the cortical bone.

giant cells are seen most often near zones of necrosis and calcification. Malignant cartilage may be present in small foci or as a large proportion of the tumor.

    (5) Treatment and prognosis

        (a) Surgical amputation of the affected limb is the best treatment for avoiding early dissemination of the tumor. Adjunctive chemotherapy has improved results and lengthened survival times; radiation therapy has proven ineffective.

        (b) Osteosarcoma is a highly malignant tumor, with a 5-year survival rate of 5% to 20%; the lower percentage generally prevails. Death usually occurs by hematogenous dissemination of the disease to the lungs and liver and to other bones.

  b. Chondrosarcoma is a malignant cartilaginous tumor. The most common locations are the spine, pelvic bones, and upper ends of the femur and humerus. The tumor may arise de novo (**primary chondrosarcoma**) or originate from a preexisting benign cartilaginous lesion (**secondary chondrosarcoma**).

    (1) Incidence. Chondrosarcomas comprise between 7% and 15% of all bone neoplasms. The tumor occurs in patients between age 30 and 60 and in men three times more often than in women.

    (2) Clinical features

        (a) Local swelling and pain are the most common symptoms. A history of a mass that has been present for months or years can be obtained in many cases.

        (b) Radiologically, the affected area shows cortical bone destruction, with occasional medullary involvement and mottled densities produced by calcification and ossification.

    (3) Pathology

        (a) Grossly, a chondrosarcoma appears as a lobulated white or gray mass that contains mucoid material and foci of calcification (Figure 23-3).

        (b) Microscopically, there are islands of immature or poorly developed cartilage in which anaplastic cells with two or more nuclei are present within the lacunar space.

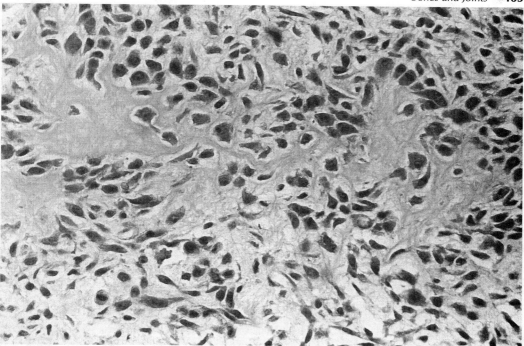

Figure 23-2. Osteosarcoma, showing malignant stroma and osteoid formation (high power).

- **(4) Treatment and prognosis**
    - **(a)** Total resection of the tumor is the treatment of choice, but the location of the tumor may make this procedure difficult to accomplish.
    - **(b)** The neoplasm is slow growing and can remain locally aggressive for years, with a high tendency to recur and implant in soft tissues. Hematogenous dissemination to the lungs, liver, and kidneys takes place over the years, with eventual death of the patient. The 10-year survival rate ranges from 50% to 60%.
- **c. Giant cell tumor of bone (osteoclastoma)** is an uncommon malignant tumor characterized by multinucleate giant cells. It occurs predominantly in women over age 19 and peaks in the third decade of life. The lesion almost always is localized in the distal portion of the long bones (femur or humerus), and 50% of these tumors occur in the area of the knee. Occasionally, the tumor involves the skull, pelvis, or small bones of the hands and feet.
    - **(1) Clinical features.** Patients present with pain, tenderness, functional disability, and large bulky masses. X-rays show an expanding zone of radiolucency, with no reactive sclerosis in the surrounding margins.
    - **(2) Pathology.** The tumor is believed to originate from the mesenchymal cells of connective tissue.
        - **(a) Grossly,** the tumor characteristically appears as multiple hemorrhagic cystic cavities that destroy the adjacent bone and are enclosed by a thin shell of new bone formation.
        - **(b) Microscopically,** a vascularized stroma composed of spindle cells that contain multinucleate giant cells intermixes with areas of hemorrhage, inflammation, and hemosiderin deposits. Mitoses are present.
    - **(3) Treatment and prognosis**
        - **(a)** Adequate removal of the lesion by complete resection or curettage is the treatment of choice.
        - **(b)** The behavior of giant cell tumors is not predictable from the histologic appearance because well-differentiated, benign-appearing tumors have been known to metastasize. In general, about one-third of the tumors will behave in a benign fashion, one-third will recur, and one-third will be frankly malignant.
        - **(c)** Metastatic spread can occur to any organ, but the lungs are most commonly involved.

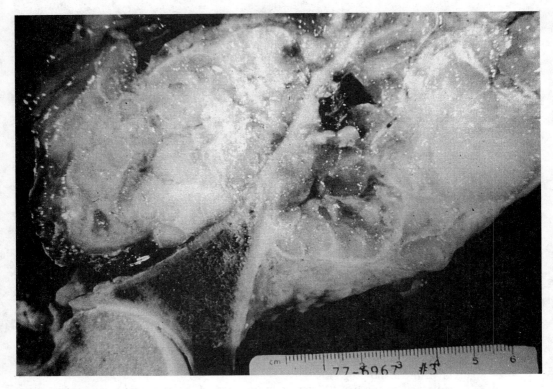

Figure 23-3. Chondrosarcoma of the ischium, with characteristic white-gray lobulated appearance.

    d. Multiple myeloma (plasma cell myeloma) [see also Chapter 8 VII A] is the most common primary tumor affecting the bones, even though it is a plasma cell neoplasm and, thus, not a true primary bone neoplasm. This multicentric disease involves several sites at the time of diagnosis. The etiology remains unknown, but observations suggest that chronic inflammation (e.g., from infection) may play an important role.

      (1) Clinical features. In bone, multiple myeloma may cause pain in areas such as the back, thorax, and head, where occasionally a tumor mass may be palpated. Multiple destructive ("punched-out") lesions are seen radiologically.

      (2) Pathology. Histologically, the tumor consists of masses of mature plasma cells with varying degrees of atypia and anaplasia (see Chapter 8, Figure 8-9). Binucleate forms and mitoses can be present.

    e. Ewing's sarcoma is a rare primary malignant tumor. It originates in the medullary cavities of the long bones predominantly, although any bone can be involved.

      (1) Incidence. Ewing's sarcoma accounts for fewer than 2% of all bone malignancies. It is found most commonly in young males between age 10 and 30.

      (2) Clinical features

        (a) Pain is the most common symptom, but other features may be a palpable mass, tenderness, and compromised function of the involved area.

        (b) A destructive lesion is seen radiologically. As the tumor breaks through the cortex, it gradually elevates the periosteum. The multiple layers of subperiosteal reactive new bone produced give the lesion its characteristic "onion-skin" appearance.

      (3) Pathology. The tumor is believed to originate from undifferentiated mesenchymal cells of the medullary cavity.

        (a) Grossly, the extent of the lesion is often greater than is appreciated on x-rays. The affected bone characteristically shows destruction of the medullary cavity by hemorrhage and necrosis, which can permeate the cortex and extend into adjacent soft tissues.

(b) Microscopically, the tumor consists of undifferentiated small round cells arranged in sheets or cords. The cells are larger than lymphocytes and have prominent nuclei and scanty cytoplasm. The tumor has a rich vascular background, and fibrous tissue is visible.

(4) Treatment and prognosis. The treatment consists of amputation of the affected limb, if possible. Newer chemotherapeutic agents have been used with relative success. However, the disease is highly aggressive and malignant, with 5-year survival rates that range from 0% to 12%. Metastases occur through hematogenous dissemination and can involve any organ.

f. Lymphoma. Primary malignant lymphoma of the bone is quite rare and generally arises in the diaphyseal area of the long bones. The histology is similar to that of diffuse histiocytic lymphomas of the lymph nodes.

g. Metastatic tumors to bones are the most common form of malignancy in adult bones. The primary tumors most frequently are carcinomas of the prostate, breast, thyroid, and kidney; other tumors metastasizing to bone include those of the lung, stomach, and bowel.

II. JOINTS

A. Anatomy and histology. A **diarthrosis,** or **synovial joint,** allows bodily movement. The synovial joint consists of two molded bone ends connected through the joint **capsule,** which is formed by dense fibroconnective tissue. The bone and cartilaginous surfaces are covered by a thin membrane, the **synovium,** which can produce a clear (synovial) fluid that acts as a lubricant. All of the elements that form joints are of mesenchymal derivation.

B. Inflammatory disorders

1. Infectious arthritis

a. Bacterial (pyogenic, septic) arthritis is an acute inflammatory process. Any joint may be involved, but the most frequently affected are the knee, hip, ankle, and wrist. The arthritis usually is monarticular, particularly in children, although polyarticular septic arthritis can occur.

(1) Etiology

(a) Gonococci, staphylococci, streptococci, and pneumococci are the most common organisms involved. In young children, *Haemophilus influenzae* and gram-negative rods are often the causative organisms.

(b) Bacterial arthritis is acquired through hematogenous spread from a primary septic focus, such as pneumonia, otitis media, endocarditis, or any site of gonorrheal infection.

(2) Clinical features

(a) In general, bacterial arthritis is most common in persons between age 20 and 40 because this age-group is most susceptible to the causative infections.

(b) Affected patients present with acute pain, swelling, tenderness, and redness of the involved joint, with associated systemic symptoms such as fever and malaise. There may be limitation of joint motion.

(c) Radiologically, the early phase of the disease shows prominent accumulation of fluid. In the later stages, there is evidence of destruction of the articular surfaces.

(3) Pathology. Findings depend largely on the nature of the causative organism and the stage of the disease process.

(a) In the early stages, congestion and edema of the synovial membranes involve collection of fluid in the joint space.

(b) As the process progresses, an intense purulent inflammatory exudate accompanies areas of necrosis in the synovium and articular cartilage.

(c) If the disease is controlled in an early phase, the process resolves without sequelae; if not, fibrosis and calcification of the joint occur, resulting in ankylosis.

(4) Treatment. Antibiotics are administered.

b. Tuberculous arthritis is a chronic inflammatory process. This type of arthritis occurs predominantly in children and is a complication of pulmonary or miliary tuberculosis. The spine is the most common location.

(1) Clinical features. The clinical manifestations are the same as those of infectious arthritis, but they present late in the course of the disease after joint destruction has already occurred.

    (2) Pathology
        (a) Tuberculous arthritis is characterized by the presence of confluent tubercles and necrotizing granulation tissue. The joint space may be filled with thick, purulent material, and acid-fast bacilli may be identified in cultures.
        (b) Destruction and obliteration of the joint space are common. Erosion of articular cartilage and bone leads to ankylosis.
    (3) Treatment. Antituberculous drugs are administered.

  2. Rheumatoid arthritis is an inflammatory disease of the joints that affects approximately 4% of the American population. It is three times more common in women than in men, and it usually starts during the fourth or fifth decade of life.
    a. Etiology. The etiology is unknown, but two sources are suspected—infection and an autoimmune response.
    b. Clinical features. Rheumatoid arthritis is a systemic disease that may involve a variety of organs, and the initial symptoms (e.g., fatigue, fever, malaise) may not relate to joint involvement.
      (1) Features of joint involvement
        (a) Rheumatoid arthritis usually involves the interphalangeal joints of the fingers and the metacarpophalangeal joints of the hands and the feet in a bilaterally symmetrical fashion. Eventually, any joint may be involved.
        (b) Affected joints show morning stiffness, pain on movement, sensitivity to pressure, swelling, redness, and warmth. In later stages, ankylosis is permanent.
        (c) In late stages of the disease, the joints may be contracted into various deforming and incapacitating positions. The hands show ulnar deviation of the fingers and dislocation of the interphalangeal joints. The wrists become fixed, with ankylosis of the elbows in flexion.
      (2) Systemic involvement. Since the disease process may involve other mesodermal surfaces, patients may develop pericarditis, pleuritis, and cardiac problems. About 15% of patients develop systemic amyloidosis.
      (3) Laboratory findings
        (a) Hypergammaglobulinemia is characteristic. The serum contains an antibody against immunoglobulin G—**rheumatoid factor (RF)**. The serum titers depend on the severity of the disease.
        (b) Typically, in advanced stages, x-rays show erosion of the juxtaarticular surfaces.
    c. Pathology
      (1) The inflammatory process causes diffuse thickening and hyperplasia of the synovium. Eventually, a vascularized mass called a **pannus** replaces the synovium. The pannus consists of lymphocytes and plasma cells surrounding areas of necrosis with palisading fibroblasts.
      (2) The pannus and the inflammatory component wear away the articular surfaces and erode the bone, leading to hemorrhage and granulation tissue formation, which diminish the synovial spaces.
      (3) Fibrosis is the end result of the disease.
    d. Treatment and prognosis. Aspirin and corticosteroids are used in treatment. Recurrences and exacerbations of the disease are common.

C. Degenerative and metabolic diseases

  1. Osteoarthritis is the most common noninflammatory degenerative disease affecting the movable joints. This progressive disease of the fifth decade of life and beyond afflicts approximately one-fifth of the American population.
    a. Etiology
      (1) Of the factors involved in the development of osteoarthritis, the wear and tear of aging is probably the most important.
      (2) Other factors include:
        (a) Obesity
        (b) Previous injury to the joint (particularly infections and trauma)
        (c) Excessive use (e.g., through athletics) of the joint
        (d) Synovial diseases
    b. Clinical features
      (1) The joints most frequently involved are the hips, the knees, the distal joints of the fingers, and the vertebral joints. Osteoarthritis may be monarticular or polyarticular.

(2) The disease begins insidiously; the affected joint shows decreased mobility. As the disease progresses, there may be pain, crepitation, and effusion, but there is no clinical evidence of inflammation.

(3) Nodules occasionally are noted at the base of the terminal phalanges of the fingers (**Heberden's nodes**).

(4) Radiologically, there is evidence of erosion of articular surfaces and the underlying bone, with a decrease in size of the articular spaces.

  c. Pathology

    (1) Gross appearance

      (a) The initial changes are in the articular cartilage. The amount of cartilage gradually shrinks, and articulation takes place over a smaller than normal surface area. Therefore, the articular surfaces erode and appear chipped, pitted, and shredded. Macroscopic pieces of cartilage (**"joint mice"**) may flake into the joint space.

      (b) Perichondrial soft tissues proliferate, and this change may give rise to cartilaginous formation and ossification. This condition produces "lipping" of the bone ends, which is responsible for loss of joint motion and deformities.

    (2) Microscopic appearance. Histologically, the synovial tissues are thickened, but show little evidence of inflammation.

  d. Treatment. There is no adequate treatment for this chronic disease, but supportive measures include exercise, aspirin, and occasionally corticosteroids.

2. Gout is rare, accounting for 2% to 5% of articular diseases. The majority of patients are middle-aged or elderly men.

  a. Pathogenesis. Gout has its origin in an inborn error in purine metabolism. The result is an abnormally high serum level of uric acid, with consequent formation of urate deposits (tophi) in the joints. The disease is inherited as an autosomal recessive trait.

  b. Clinical features

    (1) Gout typically begins as an acute attack of arthritis in the metatarsophalangeal joint of a great toe; that joint becomes tender and swollen. Occasionally, the first attack occurs in a different joint, such as another foot joint, the knee, or a finger joint. Attacks usually occur first at night and may last several days.

    (2) Serum levels of uric acid are elevated to more than 6 mg/dl.

    (3) Deposition of urates can also occur in the kidney, causing urolithiasis and other renal disease.

  c. Pathology. Microscopically, evidence of deposits of urates (**tophi**) may be seen anywhere in or around the joints. The tophi appear as a collection of filamentous urate crystals when fixed in absolute alcohol. Many of the individual agglomerations of urates have roundish contours and are surrounded by foreign-body giant cells.

  d. Treatment. Colchicine is used to reduce swelling and pain. Prophylaxis with probenecid (a uricosuric) and allopurinol (a purine antimetabolite) has replaced the traditional purine-free diet.

D. Malignant neoplasms

1. Synovial sarcoma (see Chapter 25 III D 4 b) occurs in the extremities in close proximity to large joints. The areas around the knee, foot, and ankle are most frequently involved.

  a. Histologically, the tumor typically has a biphasic appearance because it consists of two cell types found in close association: epithelial (pseudoglandular) cells that resemble those seen in carcinomas and cells that resemble spindle-cell fibrosarcomas. Calcifications are common.

  b. In a few cases, the tumor lacks the epithelial pseudoglandular component and shows only the sarcomatous stroma. These tumors are designated as **monophasic synovial sarcomas**.

2. Epithelioid sarcoma is a malignant tumor that predominantly involves areas of the hand, finger, and forearm. The tumor is frequently misdiagnosed as benign granulomatous disease (e.g., a rheumatoid nodule) because its **histologic appearance** shows granulomatous features, with large histiocytic or epithelioid cells surrounding zones of necrosis.

STUDY QUESTIONS

Directions: Each of the numbered items or incomplete statements in this section is followed by answers or by completions of the statement. Select the **one** lettered answer or completion that is **best** in each case.

1. Osteomalacia is characterized by which mechanism?

(A) Pronounced mineralization of the periosteum
(B) Increased deposition of uncalcified osteoid
(C) Abnormal osteoblastic activity
(D) Increased capillary fragility
(E) Abnormal crystalline structure of the bone

2. The most common benign bone tumor affecting persons under 21 is

(A) chondromyxoid fibroma
(B) osteochondroma
(C) giant cell tumor
(D) aneurysmal bone cyst
(E) osteogenic sarcoma

3. Which bone disorder tends to occur in the femoral epiphyses of young women?

(A) Chondroblastoma
(B) Benign bone cyst
(C) Giant cell tumor
(D) Fibrous dysplasia
(E) Osteosarcoma

4. What is the most common degenerative disease affecting the joints?

(A) Rheumatoid arthritis
(B) Osteoarthritis
(C) Gouty arthritis
(D) Villonodular synovitis
(E) Migratory polyarthritis

5. The pathologic process present in Paget's disease is

(A) loss of cortical bone because of unopposed osteoclastic activity
(B) normal osteoid production with decreased calcification
(C) abnormal remodeling of bone, with increased numbers of osteoclasts and osteoblasts
(D) malignant proliferation of osteoblasts
(E) reactivation of closed epiphyseal junctions

6. Septic bacterial arthritis is similar to gouty arthritis in that

(A) affected joints are warm, swollen, and painful
(B) crystals are often found in joint fluid
(C) elderly men are most commonly affected
(D) antibiotics are the treatment of choice
(E) there is an elevation of serum rheumatoid factor

7. An 18-year-old woman presents with distal arm pain and swelling. Radiographs reveal an expansile cystic lesion of the distal radius. A biopsy reveals fibrosis, mature bone formation, and scattered osteoclast-like giant cells. The most likely diagnosis is

(A) brown tumor
(B) tuberculous osteomyelitis
(C) aneurysmal bone cyst
(D) Ewing's sarcoma
(E) osteochondroma

8. A 40-year-old woman complains of a low-grade fever, malaise, and stiffness in her joints each morning. What is the most likely diagnosis?

(A) Metastatic carcinoma
(B) Osteoarthritis
(C) Rheumatoid arthritis
(D) Gout
(E) Villonodular synovitis

9. A 40-year-old man presents with a single inflamed metatarsophalangeal joint. Examination of joint fluid reveals urate crystals. Which statement is true of this disorder?

(A) It is characterized by pannus formation
(B) It is accompanied by hypergammaglobulinemia
(C) It afflicts about one-fifth of the American population
(D) It is associated with Heberden's nodes
(E) It is inherited in an autosomal recessive manner

1-B	4-B	7-C
2-B	5-C	8-C
3-C	6-A	9-E

10. A decrease in bone mineral mass can be seen
in all of the following people EXCEPT

(A) the elderly
(B) patients with hypoparathyroidism
(C) postmenopausal women
(D) patients on chronic steroid therapy
(E) people with vitamin D deficiency

ANSWERS AND EXPLANATIONS

1. The answer is B *[I E 1].*
Osteomalacia (the adult counterpart of rickets) is caused by vitamin D deficiency, the effect of which is an increase in the uncalcified osteoid matrix and cartilage, and a decrease in the amount of calcified bone. The disease responds to the administration of vitamin D.

2. The answer is B *[I H 2 c].*
Osteochondroma (also referred to as osteocartilaginous exostosis) is a benign new-bone growth that often protrudes from the outer contour of bones and is capped by growing cartilage. The multifocal and clearly hereditary form of this lesion is known as hereditary multiple cartilaginous exostosis. Whether the lesions are multiple or isolated, nearly 80% are noted prior to age 21.

3. The answer is C *[I H 3 c].*
Giant cell tumor (osteoclastoma) is a rare bone tumor that is characterized by the presence of multinucleate giant cells, which some authorities believe are osteoclasts. This tumor most frequently occurs in women between age 20 and 30. The lesion usually is found in the distal portion of long bones, such as the femur or humerus.

4. The answer is B *[II C 1].*
Osteoarthritis is the most common form of arthritis. Unlike rheumatoid arthritis, which affects the synovial membranes, osteoarthritis destroys articular cartilage. Osteoarthritis may be monarticular or polyarticular, but typically it affects the joints of the spine and the extremities.

5. The answer is C *[I G 1].*
Paget's disease is characterized by increased bone remodeling, with increased activity of both osteoclasts and osteoblasts accompanying disorganized new bone formation. Activated osteoclasts are seen in hyperparathyroidism; decreased calcification of osteoid is seen in osteomalacia; malignant osteoblasts are seen in osteosarcoma; and reactivation of closed epiphyseal junctions is never observed in any disease process.

6. The answer is A *[II B 1, C 2].*
Both septic bacterial arthritis and gouty arthritis can present as acute inflammatory arthritis with similar clinical presentations. Bacterial arthritis can occur in either sex at any age but is more common in a younger age group than gouty arthritis. Crystals are not found in joint fluid in cases of bacterial arthritis, unless, of course, bacterial infection is superimposed on crystal arthropathy. Antibiotics are used in infectious, but not in noninfectious, arthritis. Rheumatoid factor is present in patients with rheumatoid arthritis and is not elevated in patients with bacterial or gouty arthritis.

7. The answer is C *[I H 1 b].*
Of the choices given, only aneurysmal bone cyst presents as an expansile cystic lesion. Although brown tumors have some histologic similarities (fibrosis and giant cells), these tumors occur predominantly in the jaw, in patients with hyperparathyroidism, and they are not cystic. Tuberculous osteomyelitis would present as a lytic, not a cystic lesion, and the histology would reveal a granulomatous process with inflammatory giant cells. Ewing's sarcoma and osteochondroma do not present as cystic lesions.

8. The answer is C *[II B 2].*
Rheumatoid arthritis is a systemic inflammatory disease affecting the joints. It produces symptoms such as fever, malaise, anemia, and leukocytosis, along with joint stiffness and soft tissue swelling around the affected joints. Other complications may occur, including pericarditis, pleuritis, and cardiovascular conditions.

9. The answer is E *[II C 2].*
Gout is an inflammatory arthropathy caused by crystalline urate deposits in joint spaces. This disorder is secondary to an inborn error of purine metabolism, which is inherited in an autosomal recessive manner. Gout is relatively rare, affecting only 2.5% of the population. Pannus formation and hypergammaglobulinemia are found in rheumatoid arthritis. Heberden's nodes—firm periarticular nodules of the distal phalanges—are associated with osteoarthritis.

10. The answer is B *[I C, E 1]*.
Hyperparathyroidism, not hypoparathyroidism, produces progressive calcium waste and demineralization of bone. Osteopenia is characterized by decreased bone mineral mass, which occurs with increasing age. Postmenopausal women are also at increased risk for osteoporosis, which is characterized by rarefaction of bone structure. The catabolic effects of steroid therapy also can decrease trabecular bone formation and alter calcium metabolism. Vitamin D deficiency causes a decrease in calcified bone.

24
Skin
Maria J. Merino

I. GENERAL CONCEPTS

A. Normal anatomy and histology. The normal structure of the skin is shown in Figure 24-1.

B. Types of histopathologic changes

1. **Epidermis.** The epidermis is an avascular structure of ectodermal origin. Common **histopathologic changes** include the following.
   a. **Hyperkeratosis** is thickening of the stratum corneum, as occurs in the common wart.
   b. **Acanthosis** is thickening of the stratum spinosum (prickle cell layer) that results from chronic external irritation, as in the formation of a callus.
   c. **Parakeratosis** is the retention of the keratocyte nuclei in the stratum corneum, as occurs in psoriasis vulgaris. Parakeratosis appears under conditions of rapid keratin formation, with no time for normal resorption of the keratinocyte nuclei.
   d. **Spongiosis** is intercellular edema of the epidermis, as is seen in acute inflammatory disorders, such as contact dermatitis from poison ivy.

2. **Dermis.** The dermis is a dense connective tissue structure of mesodermal origin. It provides the blood supply of the skin. The dermis is subject to the following **changes**.
   a. With **age,** elastic tissue and mucopolysaccharide content decrease, resulting in a thinner dermis. The subcutaneous fat also atrophies.
   b. With **chronic light exposure,** the elastic collagen fibers of the dermis degenerate, giving the clinical appearance of severe wrinkling.
   c. Extreme **stretching** of the skin leads to rupture and loss of elastic tissue, as seen during pregnancy in the striae gravidarum.
   d. In **wound repair,** a scar is formed when new collagen fibrils are deposited parallel to the surface of the skin. In **keloidal wound repair,** seen predominantly in blacks, a neoplastic proliferation of collagen occurs.

3. **Hair loss**
   a. **Male-pattern alopecia (balding)** is a common abnormality seen in 80% of white men in approximately the sixth decade of life. It is induced by androgens; the active moiety is thought to be 5-dihydroxytestosterone. This irreversible process is not found in men castrated before puberty, but it may be induced in a castrate by the administration of androgens.
   b. **Excessive hair loss** may be secondary to other conditions, such as extreme stress (e.g., after a myocardial infarction) or administration of a toxic drug (e.g., chemotherapy for a neoplasm).

C. Types and distribution of lesions

1. **Types**
   a. **Macules** are circumscribed flat areas of skin distinguishable by color (e.g., freckles).
   b. **Papules** are solid elevated skin lesions that are usually less than 1 cm in diameter. They can arise in the dermis, epidermis, or both (e.g., the lesions of seborrheic keratosis).
   c. **Nodules** are palpable, solid, round, or ellipsoid lesions in the deep skin or subcutaneous tissues. Nodules are larger and situated deeper than papules (e.g., the nodules of rheumatoid arthritis).
   d. **Wheals** are rounded or flat-topped elevations of skin. They are short-lived and result from edema of the upper dermis. They follow the release of mast cell products into the tissue (e.g., mosquito bites).

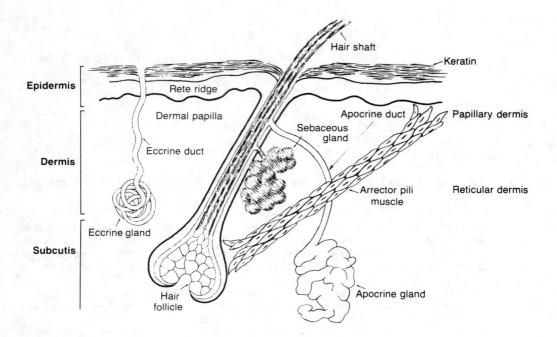

Figure 24-1. The skin and its adnexa.

    e. Vesicles are elevated lesions that contain fluid. When they are larger than 0.5 cm, they are referred to as **bullae** or **blisters** (e.g., the blisters of second-degree burns).

    f. Cysts are walled cavities that contain fluid, keratin, or mucin. They fluctuate on palpation (e.g., keratin cysts).

    g. Ulcers are craters that involve the dermis and epidermis, with loss of the surface epithelium due to sloughing of necrotic tissue. They can be the result of trauma, circulatory disorders, tumors, and infections (e.g., decubitus ulcers).

2. Distribution

    a. Localized lesions need not be solitary. They can be unilateral or bilateral and symmetric or asymmetric. They can occur in sun-exposed areas, intertriginous areas, or areas of trauma; or they can follow a dermatomal pattern.

    b. Generalized lesions are widespread throughout the skin.

    c. Universal lesions involve the entire integument: the skin, hair, and nails.

II. COMMON SKIN DISEASES

    A. Acne vulgaris is an inflammatory reaction of the pilosebaceous apparatus.

    1. Etiologically, a genetic component is apparent. Diet, inadequate cleansing, stress, and weather all have been implicated in the exacerbation of acne. About 60% to 70% of affected women present with a flare-up of the disease before menstruation.

    2. Clinical features

        a. Acne occurs equally in both sexes and predominates between age 14 and 19. It primarily affects the face, neck, and upper trunk areas, which are rich in sebaceous follicles.

        b. The initial lesions are **comedones,** commonly called "blackheads" and "whiteheads." The complicated lesions include papules, pustules, nodules, and cysts, which result ultimately in scars.

    3. Pathology and pathogenesis

        a. The current pathogenetic concept is that, in adolescence, two important changes occur: Sebaceous glands become hyperplastic, and the shedding of keratin from the outer follicle becomes sluggish. A keratinous plug forms in the outer hair follicle, and sebaceous material accumulates below it. As the proximal follicle accumulates debris, it becomes distended and eventually ruptures into the surrounding dermis, stimulating an intense acute inflammatory reaction.

    b. The anaerobic bacterium *Corynebacterium acnes* is involved in the development of the complicated acne lesions; however, its role is unclear.

   4. Treatment. Acne is treated, often successfully, with tetracyclines and vitamin A derivatives.

B. Acne rosacea is a dermatitis that affects the center and sides of the face where hair follicles and sebaceous glands are present. In one form, known as **rhinophyma,** which is seen predominantly in men, diffuse sebaceous hyperplasia of the nasal skin leads to a bulbous nose. **Histologically,** the lesion of acne rosacea is characterized by edema, telangiectasia, and inflammation in the dermis around hair follicles and capillaries. Granulomas composed of epithelioid giant cells of macrophagic origin are frequently found in the dermis.

C. Miliaria (heat rash, prickly heat) is a disease of the eccrine (sweat) apparatus. The two major types are **miliaria crystallina** and **miliaria rubra.** Both types occur following excessive sweating in parts of the body where obstruction of the intraepidermal sweat ducts is likely to occur. Both types result from pore occlusion caused by a horn plug swollen through excessive hydration. In certain cases, such as **diaper rash,** urine acts as an irritant.

   1. Pathology. In **miliaria crystallina,** vesicles form within or beneath the horny layer as a result of a ruptured sweat duct. In **miliaria rubra,** spongiotic vesicles are found in the stratum malpighii. A chronic inflammatory infiltrate is seen around and within the vesicles as well as in the adjacent dermis.

   2. Treatment. The best treatment is removal of the cause of the plugging and reduction of the warmth that stimulates the excessive perspiration.

D. Psoriasis is a disease affecting 1% to 2% of individuals of European lineage. Men in the third decade of life are affected more often than women. The disease is thought to be genetically determined and probably represents an autosomal dominant trait with incomplete penetration.

   1. Clinical features. Psoriasis is a chronic, recurrent skin disorder that can range in severity from a few mild lesions to severe exfoliation. Arthritis often occurs in severe cases. The scaly, elevated, whitish **plaques** appear predominantly on the surfaces of extensor areas, such as the elbows and knees.

   2. Pathology
     a. The psoriatic plaque is associated with rapidly dividing epidermal cells. Normally, epidermal cells take 28 days to ascend from the basal layer to the skin surface. In the psoriatic patient, they take 3 to 4 days, and two to three layers of dividing cells are often present in the epidermis.
     b. Typically, the epidermis shows marked acanthosis and elongation of the rete ridges. The dermis is so richly vascularized that bleeding easily occurs (**Auspitz sign**).
     c. A regular feature of psoriasis is the outward migration of neutrophils into the epidermis, which leads to the formation of abscesses (**Munro abscesses**). A serine protease, released by the outer epidermal keratinocytes of the psoriatic plaque, cleaves complement, which then serves as the chemotactic agent for the neutrophils. Why and how this serum protease is activated are unclear.

E. Seborrheic dermatitis is an erythematous lesion of unknown etiology. The most common and mildest form of the disease is called **dandruff.** Generalized seborrheic dermatitis in infants is often referred to as **Leiner's disease.**

   1. Clinical features. Seborrheic dermatitis may be generalized or may affect focal areas (e.g., scalp, eyebrows, face, and ears). The lesions appear as sharply demarcated brown-red areas covered with fine yellowish scales. Oozing may be present, but no vesiculation is found.

   2. Pathology. The histologic picture is not diagnostic. The horny layer shows focal areas of parakeratosis, occasionally containing a few pyknotic leukocytes. Moderate epidermal acanthosis, elongation of the rete ridges, and spongiosis appear. The dermis shows a mild chronic inflammatory infiltrate.

F. Contact dermatitis is caused by contact of the skin with an agent that acts either as a specific allergic sensitizer or as a primary irritant. The disease may be acute, subacute, or chronic. In the acute and subacute forms, diffuse erythema, edema, oozing, and crusting predominate. In the chronic form, erythema, scaling, and lichenification prevail.

1. **Acute contact dermatitis,** particularly if a specific allergic sensitizer is the cause, is characterized by the presence of vesicles or bullae, separated from one another by thin fibrous septa. The vesicles and bullae contain lymphocytes, eosinophils, neutrophils, and disintegrated epidermal cells. The epidermis shows extensive edema. The upper dermis shows vascular dilatation, edema, and inflammation.

2. **Subacute contact dermatitis** is characterized by spongiosis and the presence of small vesicles. Chronic inflammatory cells are abundant. Moderate epidermal acanthosis with varying degrees of parakeratosis appears.

3. **Chronic contact dermatitis** shows slight intercellular edema of the epidermis with acanthosis and elongation of the rete ridges. The dermis contains varying amounts of chronic inflammatory cells.

III. DISORDERS OF KERATIN PRODUCTION

A. Cutaneous horn is a small (about 1 cm) hornlike, gray-brown projection of keratin, which can arise on almost any papillary lesion, including carcinoma. **Histologically,** the horn consists of a thickened stratum corneum with focal areas of parakeratosis.

B. Warts

1. **Verruca vulgaris (common wart)** is a circumscribed, firm, elevated growth. The fingers are the most common sites of verruca vulgaris, but the lesions may occur anywhere on the skin and on the oral mucosa and genitalia.
   a. **Etiology.** The lesion is caused by human papillomavirus (HPV), which commonly can be found in the nuclei of the vacuolated cells present in the granular layer and stratum malpighii.
   b. **Pathology. Histologically,** verruca vulgaris shows acanthosis, papillomatosis, and hyperkeratosis, with areas of columnar parakeratosis. The granular layer shows vacuolar changes, with clearing of the cytoplasm and wrinkled nuclei. The basal layer of the epidermis is intact. Intracytoplasmic inclusions are seen in about 25% of the cases. The dermis is unremarkable.
   c. **Treatment.** Excision and cryosurgery of the lesion are the treatments of choice. Common warts, however, can resolve spontaneously.

2. **Verruca plana** is a slightly raised or flat wart that often occurs on the face and can be multiple.

3. **Verruca plantaris (plantar wart)** is located on the sole of the foot.

4. **Molluscum contagiosum** is characterized by small (2 mm to 4 mm) papules that have a dome-shaped appearance and may be multiple. **Histologically,** invagination of the epidermis is visible, and the epidermal cells contain large intracytoplasmic inclusion bodies. This wart is caused by a poxvirus infection.

5. **Condyloma acuminatum** is a lesion consisting of white soft verrucous nodules that often fuse and form large cauliflower-like masses around the anal and genital regions. It is caused by HPV and may be transmitted sexually.
   a. **Pathology.** The surface of the condyloma is papillomatous, wavy, and covered by a slightly thickened parakeratotic layer. **Histologically,** there is marked acanthosis of the epidermis, and vacuolated epithelial cells with clear cytoplasm and hyperchromatic nuclei (**koilocytes**) are present. The dermis may contain some chronic inflammatory cells and shows increased vascularity.
   b. **Treatment** is resection of the lesion.

C. Seborrheic keratosis (verruca senilis, basal cell papilloma) is a lesion that arises on the trunk, face, and arms of elderly people. Lesions are often seen in large numbers, but single lesions may occur.

1. **Clinical features.** Presenting as brownish, slightly raised, circumscribed, and verrucous, the lesion varies in size from a few millimeters to several centimeters.

2. **Pathology. Histologically,** hyperkeratosis, acanthosis, and papillomatosis are present. Melanin may be present in varying amounts in the epidermis. Interspersed among the epithelial cells are cystic inclusions of horny material. The border of the lesion is sharply demarcated, and the dermis is unremarkable, although chronic inflammatory cells may be present.

3. **Treatment.** This lesion is not malignant, and surgical resection is sufficient.

D. **Actinic (solar) keratosis** presents as scaly erythematous patches and plaques that occur on the face, the dorsum of the hands, and the forearms of the individuals in or past middle age. Prolonged exposure to sunlight is the essential predisposing factor. Usually the lesion measures less than 1 cm in diameter.

1. **Pathology.** The presentation is that of a dry scale, firmly adherent to an erythematous base. **Histologically,** hyperkeratosis, acanthosis, and papillomatosis are present. The epidermal cells are dysplastic, are arranged in a disorderly fashion, and have hyperchromatic nuclei. Mitoses are commonly found. The upper portion of the dermis shows basophilic degeneration of the collagen (**solar elastosis**) and dense chronic inflammatory lymphocytic infiltration.

2. **Treatment.** Although this process is not considered malignant per se, most pathologists regard it as precancerous because of its progression to squamous cell carcinoma (SCC). Treatment consists of wide excision, but smaller lesions can be frozen or excised.

E. **Ichthyosis (fish skin)** is an inherited, lifelong, dry scaly skin condition caused by overproduction of keratin and decreased keratin desquamation; the underlying molecular defect that causes the disease is unknown. It appears that the keratin itself is faulty, since the keratin layer does not shed normally, probably because of a delay in the dissolution of the desmosomal disks in the horny layer. Affected patients have increased water loss.

IV. BULLOUS DISEASES

A. **General considerations.** This group of diseases is characterized by the presence of blisters, vesicles, or bullae.

1. The lesions can be formed by the destruction of either individual cells or intracellular connections. When trauma results in rupture of keratinocytes within the epidermis, the ensuing fluid accumulation forms a blister. A blister may also result from suction, which separates the epidermis from its dermal junction.

2. Many bullous diseases, although rare, are important because they can be life-threatening.

B. **Herpes simplex** is a viral infection that characteristically leads to necrosis of the epidermal cells, resulting in blister formation.

1. **Herpes labialis (cold sore)** appears often on the edges of the lips or nostrils. A prodromal burning sensation and hyperesthesia occur. When there is accompanying fever, the condition is referred to as **herpes febrilis,** or **fever blisters.** The vesicles may develop in association with trauma, sun exposure, menstruation, or stress. Healing may take place spontaneously within 1 to 2 weeks, although the condition may become chronic with frequent recurrences.

2. **Herpes genitalis** presents in the same way, but the sores are on the genitals.

C. **Bullous pemphigoid.** This disease occurs in elderly people (80% of patients are over age 60) and is thought to be an autoimmune disorder.

1. **Clinical features.** Patients may look sick because of their multiple bullae, but they usually do not feel ill. Each lesion starts as an erythema, which then evolves into a tense bulla. The blisters do not rupture easily.

2. **Pathology**
   a. **Histologically,** multiple blisters occur, with separation of the entire epidermis at the dermoepidermal junction, which results in a blister covered entirely by epidermis. There is no acantholysis; therefore, the blister contains only inflammatory cells, predominantly eosinophils and fibrin.
   b. Immunofluorescence studies show deposits of immunoglobulin G (IgG) and complement in the basement membrane.

D. Pemphigus is also an autoimmune disease; it is potentially more serious than bullous pemphigoid. It affects patients between age 50 and 70.

1. **Clinical features.** Patients present with blisters in the skin and occasionally in the mucous membranes. The roof of the blister is quite thin and ruptures easily (in contrast to bullous pemphigoid, in which blisters are not easily ruptured). In time, the patient develops large weeping wounds over the body. These wounds encourage fluid loss and infection.

2. **Pathology. Histologically,** pemphigus is characterized by immunoglobulin and complement deposits in the epidermal intercellular space, which lead to dissolution of the epidermis and the formation of intraepidermal blisters. The separation of the cells occurs above the basal layer, leaving an intact row of basal cells. The blister contains many acantholytic keratinocytes.

E. Pemphigus vulgaris occurs mainly in individuals between age 40 and 60, 60% of whom are Jewish. A mouth lesion is the presenting sign in 50% of patients. The etiology appears to be immunologic in that the patient has antibodies circulating to the epidermis.

F. Dermatitis herpetiformis is a chronic, recurrent, pruritic disease.

1. **Clinical features.** Groups of small papules and excoriated vesicles appear symmetrically. The extensor surfaces of the extremities, the shoulders, and the buttocks are commonly affected; the oral mucosa is not. When the disease occurs during pregnancy, it is called **herpes gestationis,** and it usually disappears after termination of the pregnancy.

2. **Pathology.** The typical histologic feature is the presence of neutrophils and eosinophils at the tips of the papillae and in the subepidermal vesicles or bullae (Figure 24-2). Immunofluorescence shows granular deposits of IgA in the dermal papillae.

3. **Treatment.** As a rule, the eruption responds well to sulfapyridine and the sulfones.

G. Erythema multiforme (Stevens-Johnson syndrome). This acute, self-limited dermatosis is believed to be an allergic sensitivity reaction; it has a tendency to recur.

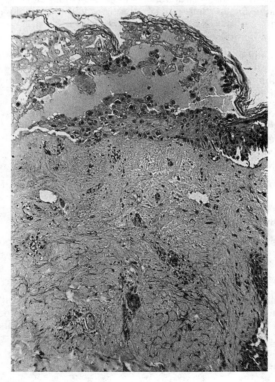

Figure 24-2. Dermatitis herpetiformis. Notice the epidermal vesicles filled with fibrin, neutrophils, and degenerating epidermal cells (low power).

1. **Clinical features.** The lesions may be multiple and widespread or focally localized, and they present as macules, papules, vesicles, or bullae. Commonly seen is the so-called **iris lesion,** a papule with peripheral extension and central cleaving. Severe cases may start abruptly with high fever, prostration, and extensive bullous eruption of the skin and mucous membranes. In cases of toxic epidermal necrolysis, the mortality rate of patients can be 5%.

2. **Pathology. Histologically,** no specific features are present. When bullae form, they are localized in the subepidermis and contain fibrin as well as eosinophils, lymphocytes, and neutrophils. The dermis contains an inflammatory infiltrate, which varies in severity, as do the clinical manifestations.

H. **Epidermolysis bullosa.** This congenital disease may be inherited as an autosomal recessive condition. It is rare, occurring in 1 in 300,000 births. Affected patients lack anchoring fibrils and have blisters over areas subject to trauma, such as the abdomen, knees, elbows, hands, and feet. The bullae heal readily, but often the resultant scarring is immobilizing.

I. **Impetigo** is an infectious disease of childhood caused by staphylococcal or streptococcal infections of the outer epidermis. It begins with the development of erythematous macules and progresses to thin-walled, pus-filled vesicles.

1. The intraepidermal or subcorneal pustule develops secondary to the bacteria-induced inflammatory reaction, apparently because of cell lysis and necrosis. There is also a neutrophilic dermal infiltrate, with overlying spongiosis.

2. When impetigo is produced by streptococci, it may be the source of glomerulonephritis.

V. INFECTIONS

A. Bacterial infections

1. **Hidradenitis suppurativa** is a chronic infection caused by staphylococci or streptococci, which enter via the hair follicles and spread to the apocrine sweat glands. The lesion begins as a red subcutaneous nodule in the axilla or anogenital region. Eventually, the nodules coalesce to form cordlike, elevated bands; suppuration and tenderness precede drainage of the purulent material. Diffuse scarring is the end result of the disease.

2. **Leprosy** is a slowly developing disease caused by *Mycobacterium leprae.* Although it manifests first in the skin and peripheral nerves, the bacterium also may be found in parenchymal organs. Typically, the patient has hypoesthesias and hypopigmented papules over the skin of the face, ears, neck, and trunk. The disease takes several forms; the one that develops depends in part on host resistance to the infecting organism.
   a. In the **lepromatous form,** host defense is inadequate, and bacterial multiplication is uncontrolled. The dermis shows diffuse infiltration by foamy histiocytes that are full of organisms.
   b. In the **tuberculoid form,** the host strongly resists the infection. Certain epithelioid granulomas contain no organisms.

3. **Tuberculosis of the skin (lupus vulgaris)**
   a. **Clinical features.** The lesions are found most commonly on the face and consist of well-demarcated, red-brown patches. Superficial ulceration occurs occasionally.
   b. **Pathology. Histologically,** tubercles composed of epithelioid and giant cells are present. Caseation and other forms of necrosis are almost always absent. The upper portion of the dermis may show extensive inflammation, but occasionally the infiltrate can extend into the subcutis, destroying the cutaneous appendages. The acid-fast bacilli may be difficult to demonstrate by special staining methods.

B. Fungal infections

1. **Moniliasis (candidiasis).** *Candida albicans* is more than a cutaneous pathogen that often affects mucosal surfaces; it can also cause systemic disease, particularly in immunosuppressed patients.
   a. **Clinical features.** In the **skin,** the primary lesion of moniliasis is a subcorneal pustule. In **mucocutaneous areas,** the lesions appear as confluent white patches with erythematous borders; adjacent tissues are inflamed.

  b. **Pathology.** The organism is present in the stratum corneum, but occasionally it can infiltrate adjacent tissues. It consists of branching mycelia (2 μ to 4 μ in diameter) and ovoid spores.

2. **Tinea (dermatophytosis, ringworm)** is the most important type of superficial fungal infection. The designation varies according to the area of the body that is affected. The fungi can be demonstrated histologically.

  a. **Tinea of the feet (tinea pedis, athlete's foot) and hands** is caused by *Trichophyton mentagrophytes* or *Trichophyton rubrum*. The lesion presents with maceration between and underneath the toes, erythematous scaling, and vesicular eruption on the soles and the palms.

  b. **Tinea cruris,** common in men, is caused by *T. rubrum,* which produces erythematous areas on the scrotum and inner surfaces of the thighs.

  c. **Tinea capitis** occurs predominantly in children and affects the hair (which tends to break off) and the scalp. It is caused by *Trichophyton tonsurans* or, less often, by *Microsporum audouinii*.

  d. **Tinea barbae** is characterized by inflammation of the bearded regions of the face and neck and is produced by *T. mentagrophytes*.

  e. **Tinea versicolor** is caused by *Pityrosporum orbiculare (Malassezia furfur),* which, like *Candida,* is a yeast. The infection is noninflammatory and affects predominantly the trunk, producing areas of brown discoloration, with fine, branlike scales.

3. **Other fungal diseases,** such as sporotrichosis, mycetoma, coccidioidomycosis, and nocardiosis, may affect the skin and be the entrance for systemic infections.

VI. NONMALIGNANT PIGMENTED LESIONS

A. **Freckles** are benign, circumscribed areas of hyperpigmentation. They vary from light to dark brown and usually become darker after sun exposure. Increased numbers of flat brown spots may be seen in certain clinical syndromes, such as Peutz-Jeghers syndrome. **Histologically,** the freckle's increased pigmentation is in the basal layer of the epidermis.

B. **Lentigo maligna**

1. **Clinical features.** This pigmented lesion occurs on the sun-exposed skin of elderly patients, predominantly on the face and neck. The lesion shows dark pigmented areas with whitish hypopigmented borders that represent foci of melanocytic regression.

2. **Pathology. Histologically,** an increased number of melanocytes are clustered in groups, some of them showing varying degrees of atypia. This lesion is considered to be a precursor of lentigo maligna melanoma.

C. **Nevocytic nevus (the common mole)** is a benign neoplasm composed of nevus cells and melanocytes. The lesion may appear flat, papillomatous, or pedunculated, and it may show marked hyperpigmentation and hairs. **Histologically,** three **types** are recognized.

1. **Intraepidermal nevus.** The upper dermis shows nests and cords of nevus cells in contact with the epidermis; some of these cells contain varying amounts of melanin. In the lower dermis, the nevus cells are scattered and embedded in collagenous tissue. Occasionally, these cells fuse and form multinucleate giant cells; this fusion occurs more commonly with mature nevi. The epidermis may show changes, such as papillomatosis and hyperkeratosis (Figure 24-3), or it may appear normal.

2. **Junction nevus.** The nevus cells, which contain melanin, are arranged in nests in the lower epidermis. They can occur in the upper dermis, but only to a minimal extent and always in conjunction with the epidermis. The dermis is unremarkable, but incontinent pigment may be present.

3. **Compound nevus.** This lesion possesses features of the other two types. Although nevus cells are present in both the dermis and epidermis, they may predominate in the dermis. When the lower one-third of the dermis is involved and the pilar units are surrounded by nevi cells, the lesion is probably congenital.

D. **Blue nevus**

1. **Clinical features.** This small, round or oval, well-circumscribed, soft nodule is blue to black in color. It commonly occurs on the buttocks, face, and arms, but it can be seen anywhere on the body.

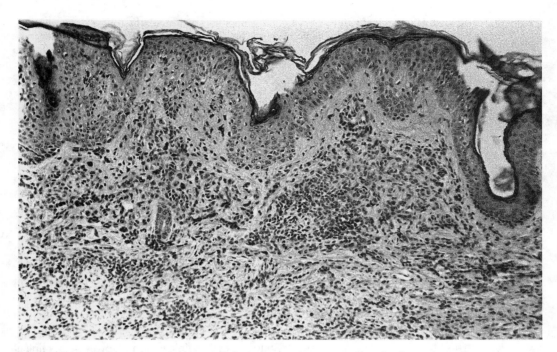

Figure 24-3. An intradermal nevus. Nevus cells lie in the dermis in nests and cords. The epidermis here is unremarkable (high power).

2. **Pathology. Histologically,** the lesion involves all of the dermis containing fibroblastic, spindle-shaped, pigmented cells. In addition, melanophages are grouped in irregular bundles extending into the subcutaneous layer. The adjacent dermis shows fibrosis, and the overlying epidermis is normal. The blue color is due to the presence of deeply located melanin.

E. Spitz nevus (spindle and epithelioid cell nevus)

1. **Clinical features.** This type of nevus occurs primarily in children and presents clinically as a solitary reddish-brown nodule.

2. **Pathology. Histologically,** the hallmark of the Spitz nevus is the proliferation of melanocytic nevus cells that look like spindle cells or epithelioid cells. The nevus cells are found at the dermoepidermal junction and throughout the dermis. Eosinophilic inclusions, called **kamino bodies,** are found in the epidermis. Mitoses are rare.

3. **Treatment.** Resection of the lesion is curative.

VII. TUMORS OF THE DERMIS

A. Granuloma pyogenicum

1. **Clinical features.** This predominantly benign, single lesion consists of a dull red, soft, raised nodule. The surface may be smooth but often shows superficial ulceration and crusting. Bleeding occurs easily when the lesion is traumatized. As a rule, the epidermis has an inward growth at the base of the lesion, causing slight pedunculation.

2. **Pathology. Histologically,** the lesion is circumscribed and is covered by a flattened epidermis. The dermis contains numerous newly formed capillaries with prominent endothelial cells. The stroma is edematous and is usually free of inflammatory infiltration.

3. **Treatment** is resection of the lesion.

B. Dermatofibroma

1. **Clinical features.** This lesion is an indolent nodule that occurs predominantly on the extremities in adults. It is usually only a few millimeters in diameter and varies from red to yellow in color.

2. Pathology. Histologically, the dermal collagen appears as irregularly arranged, intertwining and anastomosing bands mixed with scattered small capillaries. It forms nodules that merge gradually with the surrounding normal collagen. Occasionally, multinucleate giant cells and foamy macrophages are present. The overlying epidermis frequently shows marked acanthosis, predominantly in the center of the lesion (Figure 24-4).

3. Treatment is resection of the lesion.

C. Dermatofibrosarcoma protuberans

1. Clinical features. This slow-growing, protuberant tumor originates in the dermis and may become quite large. Initially, it presents as an indurated plaque from which multiple red or blue nodules arise.

2. Pathology. Histologically, the tumor consists of fibroblasts arranged in irregular strands and whorls, producing a characteristic **storiform pattern**. The fibroblasts may be atypical to varying degrees, and mitoses may be present. The tumor cells penetrate the subcutaneous fat and occasionally may infiltrate the fascia and underlying muscle. The epidermis may show atrophy or ulceration, but it does not show acanthosis.

3. Treatment and prognosis. The tumor tends to recur and may be difficult to control. Complete surgical excision of the lesion is necessary to avoid recurrences. Rarely, metastases to other organs have occurred after numerous local recurrences and the development of a malignant clone.

D. Kaposi's sarcoma

1. General features
   a. This truly unusual "sarcoma" occurs in four specific clinical forms. However, all clinical types may be related to some form of immune deficiency, and some authors have questioned the neoplastic nature of this disorder (thus, the quotation marks on "sarcoma"). The tumor is notable (and unusual) for its multicentricity, its symmetry, and its occasional spontaneous regression (although usually only some lesions regress).
   b. The cell of origin appears to be an immature pluripotential endothelial cell (either blood vascular or lymphatic).

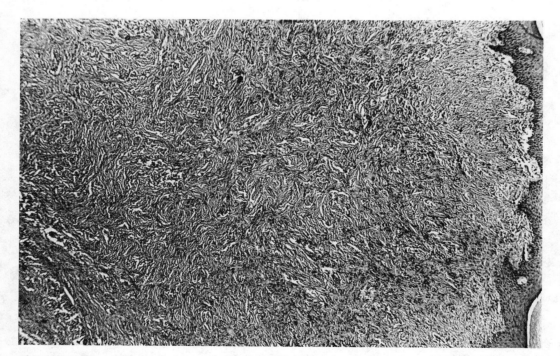

Figure 24-4. Dermatofibroma. An increased amount of dermal collagen is arranged in an irregular fashion (low power).

2. Clinical forms
  a. Classic. This relatively indolent type affects elderly patients of Mediterranean descent, particularly Eastern European Jews; over 90% of patients are men.
    (1) Small bluish nodules and plaques occur bilaterally on the feet and legs or on the hands. Classic Kaposi's sarcoma is typified as mainly cutaneous and nonvisceral in comparison to the Kaposi's sarcoma associated with AIDS. However, dissemination has been found more often in classic cases than physicians previously appreciated: Older autopsy series show a high percentage of cases with visceral disease, although this condition was clinically silent (i.e., showed no signs or symptoms).
    (2) In 10% of classic cases, Kaposi's sarcoma is associated with a malignancy, particularly lymphoma and leukemia. Kaposi's sarcoma may occur before or after such a malignancy.
    (3) The **prognosis** is very good, with the average patient surviving 8 to 13 years on low-level chemotherapy.
  b. African. As an **endemic** disease in Africa's "malaria belt," Kaposi's sarcoma affects young patients and women as often as men. Unusual forms occur: an aggressive **lymphadenopathic variety** found in young people and a **fungating form** that produces large tumors. In the 1980s, the form seen in AIDS has also occurred in this locale.
  c. Immunosuppression-related. Rarely, patients on immunosuppressive therapy for renal transplantation or for inflammatory bowel disease (IBD) acquire this tumor. If all immunosuppressive therapy is stopped, the tumor commonly regresses.
  d. AIDS-associated. This **epidemic** type has been seen in all subgroups of patients with AIDS but is particularly common in the homosexual subgroup. The tumor is *not* a direct result of viral DNA integration.
    (1) Initially, a maculopapular eruption appears on the skin or mucosa. This eruption disseminates widely and often involves the viscera and lymph nodes. In some patients, only mucosal, visceral, or lymph node sites are involved.
    (2) A uniformly poor outcome is seen in AIDS cases, but this situation is largely due to the many infectious complications that these patients incur. The **prognosis of Kaposi's sarcoma itself** is more related to the AIDS patient's immune status than to the tumor border or disease sites.
      (a) Those unusual patients with Kaposi's sarcoma and a good immune status survive for long periods (3 or more years). Rarely, patients die of directly related complications, such as pulmonary or gastrointestinal hemorrhage.
      (b) Patients with Kaposi's sarcoma and poor immune status tend to die quickly of opportunistic infections.
      (c) Total spontaneous regression of the tumor has occurred in about 4% of AIDS cases.
    (3) **Therapy** with alpha-interferon has resulted in a high proportion of complete responses, mainly in the patients with better immune status and without opportunistic infection.

3. Pathology
  a. The **distribution** within involved organs **in disseminated cases** is predictable and unlike that of usual metastases, in that distribution in disseminated cases involves capsular and sinusoidal regions of lymph nodes, mucosa and submucosa of the gastrointestinal tract, and perivascular septa in the lungs. Perhaps this difference reflects an association with lymphatics.
  b. Histologically, all forms of Kaposi's sarcoma are similar. Relatively bland spindle-shaped cells (most of which are endothelial) grow in elongated sheets. Capillaries proliferate, but may be inconspicuous because they are intermingled with a stroma composed of the spindle-shaped cells. Diagnostically, the finding of slitlike spaces, extravasated red blood cells, and hemosiderin is important (Figure 24-5).

4. Recent concepts
  a. Kaposi's sarcoma is unlike other sarcomas because of the presence of multiple simultaneous lesions in crops, its epidemic occurrence, and the phenomenon of regression. For these reasons, some pathologists have begun to refer to it as Kaposi's disease.
  b. Culture studies have shown cell dependence on various growth factors, like more normal cells. Kaposi's sarcoma may result from such factors being produced by the immune system, and, thus, may explain its epidemic occurrence with AIDS.
  c. Bacillary angiomatosis is a cutaneous vascular proliferation that clinically and histologically resembles Kaposi's sarcoma and other benign vascular lesions such as hemangiomas

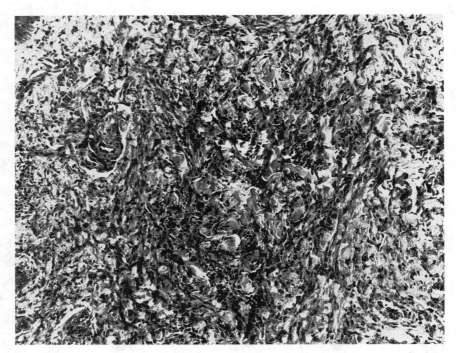

Figure 24-5. Kaposi's sarcoma involving the dermis with proliferation of vascular spaces and spindle cells that destroy the normal skin structures. Extravasated red blood cells are characteristic.

and pyogenic granuloma. This vascular proliferation frequently occurs in patients with human immunodeficiency virus (HIV) infection. The lesion—caused by bacilli and best identified by **Warthin-Starry stains**—responds well to treatment with antibiotics.

E. Angiosarcoma (hemangiosarcoma) [Figure 24-6]

1. **Clinical features.** Angiosarcoma typically occurs in the face and scalp of elderly people, with men more commonly affected than women. The lesions initially present as bright red, blue, or purple plaquelike and multinodular tumors of cystic or spongy consistency. Rarely, angiosarcomas arise in soft tissues (see Chapter 25 III D 4 f).

2. **Pathology. Histologically,** a proliferation of freely anastomosing vascular channels infiltrates and dissects the collagen in the dermis. The endothelial cells show prominent hyperchromatic nuclei, with occasional tufts protruding into the lumen. Patchy lymphoid infiltrates are present.

3. **Treatment and prognosis.** Complete surgical resection of the lesion is the treatment of choice. Radiation, chemotherapy, or both, are used as forms of adjuvant therapy. Recurrences are common, and metastases can occur in up to 40% of patients.

F. Mycosis fungoides (cutaneous lymphoma)

1. **General features.** Mycosis fungoides is a cutaneous lymphoproliferative disorder that pursues an indolent but progressive course, frequently spanning many years. Prolonged localization of this lymphoma in the skin suggests that it arises from immunocompetent T cells specialized to provide cutaneous immunity.

2. **Clinical features.** The disease may present as a diffuse, generalized erythema or as elevated plaques consisting of irregularly shaped, raised, brown-red lesions, which often undergo ulceration.

3. **Pathology**
   a. **Histologically,** skin biopsies show extensive lymphocytic infiltration of the dermis and, to a lesser extent, of the epidermis. The neoplastic cells are intermediate to large in size, and their nuclei have a characteristic lobulated cerebriform pattern. An almost pathognomonic

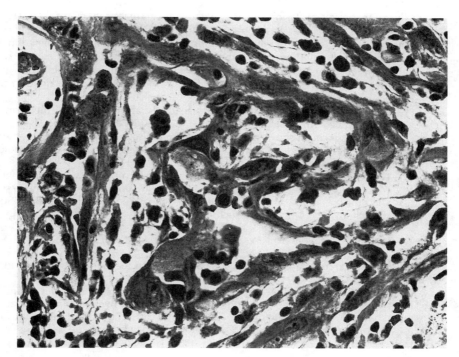

Figure 24-6. Angiosarcoma, showing prominent hyperchromatic nuclei of endothelial cells (high power).

finding is the presence in the epidermis of **Pautrier's microabscesses** (small groups of mononuclear cells surrounded by halolike clear spaces).

b. When dissemination occurs to the lymph nodes, they show involvement of the T-cell areas by foci of neoplastic cells.

4. Prognosis. In the cutaneous tumor stage, ulceration of the lesion may precede sepsis and death, but the usual course is eventual dissemination, leading to involvement of the lymph nodes, viscera, and bone marrow. The mortality rate is about 70% within 6 years.

G. Sézary syndrome is characterized by generalized pruritic erythroderma, peripheral lymphadenopathy, and the presence of Sézary cells in the peripheral blood. The course of the disease is similar to that of a malignant lymphoma.

VIII. CYSTS AND TUMORS OF THE EPIDERMIS

A. Inclusion cyst (sebaceous cyst) is a benign cystic lesion in the epidermis. This slow-growing, elevated, firm intracutaneous or subcutaneous "tumor" can occur at any site on the body.

1. Histologically, the cyst is lined by epidermis, with all layers present, and is filled with keratin, often arranged in laminated layers. Rupture of the cyst is common, and its contents incite a florid foreign-body giant cell reaction in the surrounding tissues.

2. Treatment is surgical excision of the lesion.

B. Carcinoma. Besides the carcinomas of epidermal origin discussed here, carcinomas may **metastasize to the skin,** either directly from underlying tumors or via lymphatics or the bloodstream. Cutaneous metastases from primary sites, such as the kidneys, breast, and lungs, are not uncommon.

1. Basal cell carcinoma. Derived from the basal cells of the epidermis, this tumor occurs predominantly on the hair-bearing surfaces in the adult. The face and scalp areas are the regions most commonly affected; mucous membranes, the palms, and the soles are never involved. The tumor grows by direct extension and infiltration of adjacent structures, but it very rarely metastasizes.

    a. **Clinical features.** This lesion can arise without apparent reason, but prolonged sun exposure or large doses of x-ray radiation are important predisposing factors. Basal cell carcinoma can occur as single or multiple lesions, which measure a few centimeters in diameter and have raised, rolled borders, with a central area of depression that may be ulcerated.

    b. **Pathology. Histologically,** the tumor consists of characteristic basal cells, that is, cells with large oval or elongated nuclei and little cytoplasm. The nuclei are very uniform and show no anaplasia.

      (1) The basal cells form masses of various sizes and shapes that infiltrate the dermis (Figure 24-7). Some of these masses may show contact with the epidermis. The periphery of these masses often shows an arrangement of palisade cells; the nuclei of the cells inside are disorganized. Occasionally, pigmentation, calcification, or mucinoid degeneration is present.

      (2) The connective tissue adjacent to the tumor shows proliferative changes, with an increased number of young fibroblasts. Chronic inflammatory cells may be seen.

      (3) Since the basal cell has a pluripotential capacity, it can differentiate toward squamous epithelium, hair, or adnexal structures; this accounts for the different patterns of basal cell carcinomas.

    c. **Treatment** by complete excision of the lesion is curative.

  2. Squamous cell carcinoma (SCC) can occur anywhere on the skin or on the mucous membranes.

    a. **Clinical features.** This lesion commonly arises on sun-damaged skin, but it can also arise in association with ulcers, scars, and foci of chronic osteomyelitis. Men are affected more often than women, in a ratio of 2:1. The lesion consists of a shallow ulcer surrounded by a wide, elevated, and indurated border. The ulcer may be covered by a crust with a red granular base. Occasionally, a raised, verrucous lesion occurs without evidence of ulceration.

    b. **Pathology. Histologically,** the tumor consists of irregular masses of epidermal cells, which proliferate and invade the dermis. The squamous cells may show different degrees of anaplasia as well as pleomorphism, with prominent hyperchromatic nuclei. Intercellular bridges are absent. Individual cells may undergo keratinization and pearl fomation (i.e., dense keratin formation in the cytoplasm of the cell), and mitoses are present. The dermis surrounding the invasive tumor shows a prominent chronic inflammatory reaction.

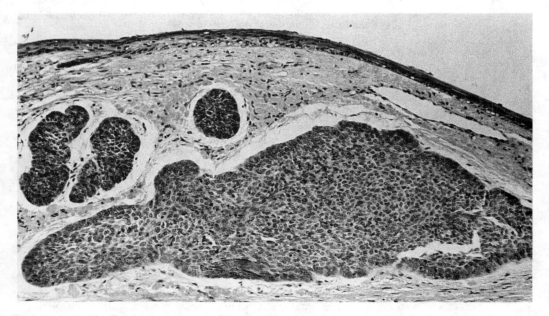

Figure 24-7. Basal cell carcinoma. Masses of varying sizes and shapes consist of basal cells. The periphery of the masses shows a palisade arrangement (high power).

   c. Prognosis depends largely on the site of the lesion. Carcinomas that arise in mucous membranes have a high rate of metastasis if not properly treated, and the regional lymph nodes are the first sites to be invaded. Tumors that originate in sun-exposed areas have a low rate of metastasis.

   d. Treatment is surgical excision of the tumor.

C. Malignant melanoma, the most malignant of the cutaneous neoplasms, arises from the epidermal melanocytes. It may arise de novo or in a preexisting nevus. Malignant melanoma is rare before puberty, but fatal cases have been reported in children.

  1. Types. The four types of malignant melanoma are **superficial spreading, nodular, lentigo maligna,** and **acral lentiginous**. The superficial spreading and nodular types are the most common.

  2. Clinical features

    a. The **superficial spreading** and **nodular** types occur on any part of the body but most often on the legs, shoulders, and upper back. The lesion presents as a gradually enlarging pigmented nodule surrounded by erythema. The nodule may show crusting, bleeding, or ulceration.

    b. Lentigo maligna melanoma occurs in older people or on sun-damaged skin and presents as a pigmented patch.

    c. The uncommon **acral-lentiginous melanoma** presents on the palms, the soles, or the genital or oral mucosa as a pigmented macule that may be deceptively bland and lentigo-like at first, but eventually becomes invasive.

  3. Pathology

    a. Histologically, the tumor originates at the dermoepidermal junction where irregular activity occurs, with streaming of atypical and malignant nevus cells down toward the dermis.

      (1) The tumor cells may vary in size and shape, but most have large nuclei with prominent nucleoli and abundant granular eosinophilic cytoplasm. Multinucleate, bizarre giant cells are present, and mitoses are common. The amount of melanin and inflammatory infiltrate varies greatly from person to person (Figure 24-8).

      (2) In **lentigo maligna melanoma,** an increased number of melanocytes are present in the basal layer of the epidermis, some of which show atypia.

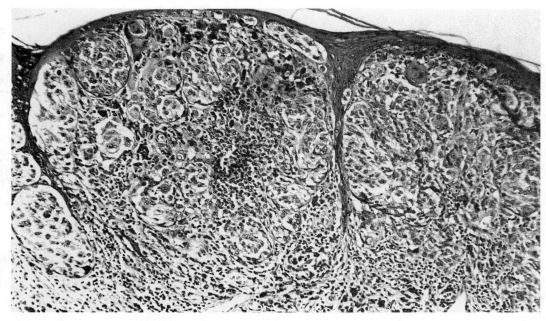

Figure 24-8. Malignant melanoma. The nests of tumor cells infiltrate the upper dermis. A moderate lymphocytic response is also present (high power).

    b. Malignant melanomas have two **growth phases:** the **radial** or **horizontal growth phase** occurs in lentigo maligna and superficial spreading melanoma; the **vertical growth** or **invasive phase** occurs in all four types (see VIII C 1).

    c. Five **levels of invasion** have been established.

        (1) **Level 1:** Tumor cells are limited to the epidermis.

        (2) **Level 2:** Tumor cells extend into the papillary dermis.

        (3) **Level 3:** Tumor cells fill the papillary dermis.

        (4) **Level 4:** Tumor cells invade the reticular dermis.

        (5) **Level 5:** The tumor extends through the skin into the subcutis.

4. Prognosis

    a. Prognosis depends on the type of melanoma, the level of invasion, and the presence or absence of metastases.

        (1) The superficial spreading and lentigo maligna melanomas usually have a better prognosis than the nodular type. Nodular melanoma is the most aggressive variant, in part because diagnosis is rare before deep invasion.

        (2) Of the five levels of invasion, the prognosis is best for the first three.

    b. It is believed that those tumors measuring less than 0.76 mm in thickness (**Breslow's level**) have an excellent prognosis, with low metastatic rates.

5. Metastases. The melanomas that metastasize tend to spread—in early stages—to adjacent skin and regional lymph nodes. In later stages, hematogenous spread occurs, with diffuse visceral involvement.

6. Treatment. Removal of the lesion, with ample uninvolved margins of at least 1 cm, is mandatory.

STUDY QUESTIONS

Directions: Each of the numbered items or incomplete statements in this section is followed by answers or by completions of the statement. Select the **one** lettered answer or completion that is **best** in each case.

1. What is the primary predisposing factor for actinic keratosis?

(A) Autoimmune disease
(B) Chemical exposure
(C) Sunlight exposure
(D) Cigarette smoking
(E) Inheritance

2. Which prognostic factor is the most useful for primary malignant melanoma?

(A) Depth of invasion
(B) Size of malignant cells
(C) Number of multinucleate giant cells
(D) Degree of surrounding inflammation
(E) Amount of melanin produced

3. A middle-aged white man presents with itchy, scaling skin patches on his extensor surfaces. A skin biopsy reveals acanthosis with elongation of the rete ridges into the dermis; rich vascularization of the dermis; and neutrophil infiltration of the epidermis with microabscess formation. The patient's clinical presentation and the histologic findings are most consistent with which diagnosis?

(A) Dermatitis herpetiformis
(B) Tinea versicolor
(C) Pemphigus
(D) Psoriasis
(E) Verruca vulgaris

Directions: The group of items in this section consists of lettered options followed by a set of numbered items. For each item, select the **one** lettered option that is most closely associated with it. Each lettered option may be selected once, more than once, or not at all.

Questions 4–8

The most important superficial fungal infections of the skin are termed dermatophytoses, or tinea. Match the tineal infections with the site of infection.

(A) Scalp
(B) Beard area
(C) Trunk
(D) Scrotum
(E) Toes

4. Tinea barbae

5. Tinea capitis

6. Tinea cruris

7. Tinea pedis

8. Tinea versicolor

1-C	4-B	7-E
2-A	5-A	8-C
3-D	6-D	

ANSWERS AND EXPLANATIONS

1. The answer is C *[III D].*
Actinic keratosis, or solar keratosis, is so named because prolonged exposure to the actinic rays in sunlight is the essential predisposing factor. The lesions usually develop on the face, on the dorsum of the hand, and on other skin surfaces chronically exposed to the sun. Although actinic keratosis is not considered to be malignant per se, the lesions are considered precancerous because of their frequent progression to squamous cell carcinoma (SCC). Treatment is wide-margin surgical excision, although freezing is an alternative approach for smaller lesions.

2. The answer is A *[VIII C].*
In a lesion of primary malignant melanoma, the depth of invasion and the thickness of the lesion are the most important prognostic indicators for the risk of metastatic disease. The size of malignant cells, the number of multinucleate giant cells, the degree of surrounding inflammation, and the amount of melanin produced are features that are found in varying degrees in malignant melanomas but are not useful as prognostic indicators.

3. The answer is D *[II D].*
Acanthosis, elongated rete ridges, and epidermal neutrophil microabscesses are typical features of psoriasis. Verruca vulgaris does not present as scaling patches, and the absence of nuclear and cytoplasmic viral changes plus the presence of the distinctive epidermal microabscesses (Munro's abscesses) distinguish these entities histologically. Dermatitis herpetiformis and pemphigus are bullous diseases, which would not be found clinically or histologically in this patient. Although tinea versicolor may present as scaling patches, widespread involvement of the exterior surface would be unusual, and fungal elements would be found histologically.

4–8. The answers are: 4-B, 5-A, 6-D, 7-E, 8-C *[V B 2].*
The infection of the bearded facial skin in men is termed tinea barbae and is caused by *Trichophyton mentagrophytes*. Tinea capitis is a fungal infection of the scalp caused by *T. tonsurans* or *Microsporum audouinii*. It affects the hair follicles and causes the hair shafts to break off. Tinea cruris, which is caused by the fungus *T. rubrum,* is an erythematous lesion found on the scrotum and inner surfaces of the thigh. *T. rubrum* is also the cause of some cases of tinea pedis, the fungal infection that produces erythema and erosion between the toes. *Pityrosporum orbiculare* produces tinea versicolor, which affects the trunk area where it produces brown discoloration with very fine scales.

25
Soft Tissues
John S. J. Brooks

I. GENERAL CONCEPTS

A. Definition of soft tissues. Soft tissues are those tissues of nonvisceral origin that lie between the dermis and the skeleton. Thus, soft tissues include the muscles, connective tissues, nerves and related paraganglia, blood vessels, and fat.

B. Clinical presentation of soft tissue lesions

1. Most soft tissue lesions produce a noticeable lump, which frequently is painless and often enlarges over a variable period. Importantly, rapid growth of short duration (1 to 2 months) often signifies a benign reactive lesion and should not cause alarm, particularly when the lesion is small (3 cm or less).

2. In some instances, trauma may be related to the development of the lump (as in fasciitis—see II G). True neoplasms probably are not induced by trauma, but trauma may draw a patient's attention to the lesion.

3. A solitary lump may represent anything—an epidermal inclusion cyst (sebaceous cyst), a skin adnexal tumor, a metastasis from a carcinoma elsewhere—but discussion is limited to lesions of **mesenchymal** origin, that is, classic "soft tissue tumors."

C. Biopsy. A biopsy is the only method to ascertain whether a tumorlike mass is reactive, benign, or malignant. Cytologic examination is fraught with difficulty.

II. PSEUDOTUMORS (REACTIVE OR REPARATIVE PROCESSES)

A. General considerations

1. Pseudotumors, although they may resemble tumors, are not true neoplastic growths but reactions to tissue injury. Pseudotumors may be related temporally to a specific traumatic event. They frequently are discovered soon after onset and often are tender or painful.

2. These lesions may vary in size but commonly are under 2 cm. Simple surgical excision is curative; in fact, even if incompletely excised, these lesions are not likely to recur.

3. Variable amounts of inflammatory cells, hemorrhage, and hemosiderin may be found in any individual lesion. Any of these lesions also may include **myofibroblasts,** cells with properties of contraction (**myo-**) and collagen production (**fibroblast**). Such cells participate in normal wound healing as well as in the exaggerated or abnormal processes of repair and regeneration described next.

4. Pseudotumors can be classified into eight types, which are presented in II B to II I in approximate decreasing order of frequency. Any of the first four types can coexist. Note that fasciitis, the two forms of myositis, and occasional vascular reactive tissue may mimic sarcomas histologically.

B. Hematoma

1. This lesion results when extravasation of blood into the soft tissues following vascular disruption (usually posttraumatic) leads to the development of a mass of blood cells, serum, and proteins in a confined space. An inflammatory response proceeds in and around the hematoma, with the presence of granulation tissue and organization of the hematoma, leading to eventual resorption and disappearance of the mass.

2. The reparative process includes the proliferation of many mesenchymal elements. Microscopic examination reveals proliferating capillaries lined by plump endothelial cells, fibroblasts, histiocytes, and red and white blood cells.

3. Sometimes the reparative process shows such marked cellularity as to suggest a sarcoma. Likewise, an organizing thrombus in a greatly dilated small vessel (e.g., on the finger) may contain papillary tufts of endothelial cells mimicking angiosarcoma, but the lesion is encapsulated, unlike that malignancy.

C. Fat necrosis

1. A posttraumatic reaction of adipose tissue, either idiopathic or iatrogenic (e.g., occurring at an injection site), fat necrosis demonstrates a disruption of fat cells, with release of fat and fatty esters and a histiocyte response. A localized liquefaction of fat then occurs, forming a cystic or solid lump that enlarges slowly and may imitate a neoplasm.

2. Ingestion of the liquid fat by phagocytes, the presence of inflammatory cells, and later fibrosis and calcification are notable features. The histiocytes in fat necrosis tend to be mononuclear, with finely granular to bubbly cytoplasm.

D. Foreign-body granuloma

1. This poorly circumscribed mass is composed of an array of inflammatory cells and many histiocytes, predominantly multinucleate forms.

2. The foreign material inciting the reaction may be endogenous (hair shafts, keratin, cholesterol) or exogenous (surgical cotton, suture material, wood or metallic fragments). It usually can be identified readily in the lesion, either in the giant cells or around them. Occasionally, the foreign material may be visible only under polarized light.

E. Xanthogranuloma

1. Some authorities consider xanthogranuloma to be a benign neoplasm rather than a reactive pseudotumor. The lesion is composed of abundant lipid and many histiocytes—thus, the term "xanthogranuloma." It is located most frequently in the retroperitoneum, but may be found in the kidney, lung, mediastinum, or mesentery.
  a. The lesion may grow to a large size; and when it occurs in the retroperitoneum, the lump may be confused clinically with retroperitoneal fibrosis or sarcoma.
  b. **Malacoplakia** (soft plaques that develop on the bladder mucosa or elsewhere) is, in a sense, a type of xanthogranulomatous response to infection with numerous histiocytes. The organisms are ingested by histiocytes or macrophages, but cannot be fully digested due to a cellular defect; they become entombed in calcium salts, forming the so-called **Michaelis-Gutmann bodies**.

2. **Histologically,** xanthogranuloma is distinguished from fat necrosis by the presence of lipid-filled histiocytes (foam cells), which dominate the microscopic field. Xanthogranulomas also contain fibroblasts, giant cells, and capillaries.

F. Myxoma

1. This loose gelatinous mass is a whitish, glistening tumor affecting some parts of the body. It is benign.

2. **Histologically,** this avascular lesion is composed predominantly of a mucinlike, ground substance (proteoglycans) with widely scattered, bland spindle cells. Often a peripheral capsule is present. Although some authorities think of myxoma as a neoplasm, it probably is a peculiar mesenchymal reaction. About 25% of patients have a history of trauma.

3. Common sites of myxomas include the jaw and the intramuscular regions of the thigh and the shoulder. Despite the lack of vascularity, myxomas may reach a considerable size (larger than 10 cm) and clinically can mimic a sarcoma.

G. Pseudosarcomatous (nodular) fasciitis

1. **Pathogenesis.** This form of fasciitis appears as a nodule in the subcutaneous (rarely deeper) tissues. The lesion usually is small, seldom attaining a size of more than 3 cm. It is a nonneoplastic exuberant mesenchymal reaction, which mimics a sarcoma.

    2. Clinical features

      a. The nodule usually is tender, and the patient presents with a history of a rapid growth discovered recently (within 1 week to 2 months). Approximately 30% to 50% of affected patients remember an episode of trauma to the area involved. The favored site is the upper body, particularly the forearm and trunk; the lesion is relatively rare in the lower extremities.

      b. Although it can occur at any age, nodular fasciitis chiefly occurs in young adults. It shows no predilection for either sex.

    3. Pathology. The gross and microscopic infiltrative patterns, mitoses, and dense cellularity can produce diagnostic confusion with malignant mesenchymal tumors (sarcomas).

      a. Histologically, the lesion of nodular fasciitis is composed of highly cellular, well-vascularized tissue, proliferating spindle cells with numerous mitotic figures and foci of myxoid change, and scattered inflammatory cells and erythrocytes. Typically, the lesion is non-encapsulated and interdigitates with surrounding tissue.

      b. Unlike sarcomas, nodular fasciitis (and the myositis types discussed in II I) characteristically display **zonation or a tissue pattern** of organization: A loose central zone lies within a cellular region that is peripherally surrounded by a less cellular zone of fibrous and inflammatory tissue.

      c. To distinguish this lesion from a sarcoma, the recognition of fasciitis must be based on its zonation, inflammatory cell component, and resemblance to exuberant granulation tissue.

    4. Other fasciitis-like pseudosarcomas. Internal organs may be affected by the same reactive repair processes. For example, pseudotumors can develop in the bladder 3 to 6 weeks after a transurethral resection of bladder (TURB). These postsurgical lesions are called postoperative spindle cell nodules, but basically resemble fasciitis with its proliferating myofibroblasts.

H. Proliferative myositis represents a fasciitis-like process in skeletal muscle, which commonly occurs in patients over 50 years of age. The degenerating and regenerating striated muscle cells may assume bizarre configurations that can lead to confusion with rhabdomyosarcoma. As with nodular fasciitis, however, the zonation pattern of growth distinguishes proliferative myositis from a malignancy.

I. Myositis ossificans, probably the result of direct trauma to striated muscle, consists of a mass of bone, cartilage, or both, within a muscle, interdigitating with muscle fibers at the periphery. These lesions probably represent an exaggerated reparative response in the organization of a hematoma involving striated muscle.

    1. Many patients are less than age 30, and the massive calcification occurs fairly rapidly (in 4 to 6 weeks).

    2. Histologically, again, the pattern of growth is one of zonation. The more cellular, nonossified areas tend to be placed centrally, whereas ossified bone in various degrees of maturation is noted near the periphery. Areas of hemorrhage are often seen.

III. NEOPLASMS

A. General concepts

    1. Classification. Soft tissue neoplasms can be divided into benign, locally aggressive, and malignant (Table 25-1; Figure 25-1).

    2. Encapsulation. On physical examination or at surgery, soft tissue lesions may demonstrate **encapsulation,** may be **circumscribed** but without a true capsule, or may show **infiltration** into surrounding tissues. In theory, benign tumors are usually encapsulated, and malignant tumors are not. However, the presence or absence of a capsule cannot be taken as prima facie evidence of benignancy or malignancy.

      a. Grossly, some sarcomas appear encapsulated, but **microscopic examination** usually shows definite invasion outside the gross confines of the lesion; that is, they have a pseudocapsule.

      b. Some soft tissue pseudotumors, which are reactive lesions and not neoplastic, may show both gross and microscopic interdigitation with surrounding tissues (see II).

    3. Necrosis. Necrosis and hemorrhage are features found exclusively in malignant tumors.

Table 25-1. Soft Tissue Tumors

Presumed Origin (or Cells Resembled)	Benign Neoplasms	Locally Aggressive Forms	Malignant Neoplasms
Fibrocytes	Keloid (dermal)	Fibromatosis (desmoid) tumor	Fibrosarcoma
Fibroblasts with histiocyte property	Fibrous histiocytomas (fibrous xanthoma, giant cell tumor of the tendon sheath, sclerosing hemangioma)	Dermatofibrosarcoma protuberans (DFSP)	Malignant fibrous histiocytoma (MFH)
Smooth muscles	Leiomyoma	. . .	Leiomyosarcoma
Striated muscles	Rhabdomyoma	. . .	Rhabdomyosarcoma (embryonal, sarcoma botryoides, alveolar, pleomorphic)
Fat cells	Lipoma Lipoblastoma Hibernoma	Well-differentiated liposarcoma	Liposarcoma
Endothelial cells	Hemangioma	. . .	Angiosarcoma Kaposi's sarcoma
Nerves	Neural sheath tumors [neurofibroma, neurilemmoma (schwannoma), granular cell tumor]	. . .	Malignant peripheral nerve sheath tumors (MPNST, schwannoma)
Neuronal cells	. . .	. . .	Peripheral or primitive neuroectodermal tumors (PNET)
Unknown	. . .	. . .	Synovial sarcoma, epithelioid sarcoma

B. Benign neoplasms. Benign soft tissue tumors frequently are slow-growing masses, which may attain very large sizes. They frequently are encapsulated, they never metastasize, and the prognosis usually is excellent.

1. **Lipoma**
   a. **Clinical features.** The most common soft tissue tumor, a lipoma resembles adipose tissue but is encapsulated and lacks the lobulations of normal fat. Frequently found on the extremities or the back, it may be small or may reach considerable size.
   b. **Transformation** of a lipoma into a liposarcoma has never been convincingly documented.
   c. **Variants**
      (1) A **lipoblastoma** is a rare lobulated, encapsulated, soft tumor that occurs almost exclusively in infants and children. It has a benign clinical course with a low recurrence rate after surgical excision.
      (2) The **hibernoma,** also rare, derives its name from its morphologic resemblance to the brown fat of hibernating animals. It presumably arises from the multivacuolated fat that may occur in the back, hips, or especially the neck in both adults and infants.

2. **Fibrous histiocytoma**
   a. This term encompasses a group of lesions composed of cells that have light microscopic and ultrastructural features of both histiocytes and fibroblasts.
      (1) The **histiocytes** range from mononuclear forms to foam cells, some of which are multinucleate.
      (2) The **fibroblastic component** is arranged in interlacing bundles, or fascicles, which are dispersed among the histiocytes, producing a characteristic whorled appearance called a **storiform pattern**.
   b. These lesions are found most often in the dermis, although they also may occur in deeper tissues. They may recur if not adequately excised.

A

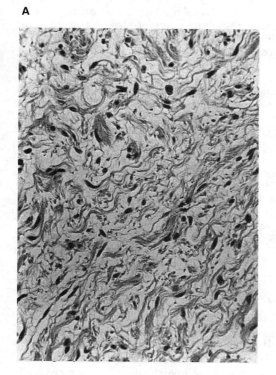

B

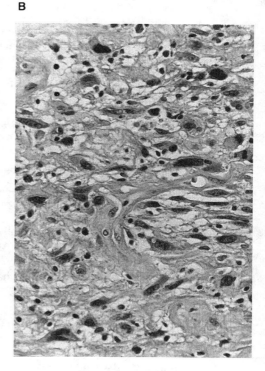

Figure 25-1. (*A*) Benign soft tissue tumor—neurofibroma. At high power, small spindle cells are seen with bland nuclei; there are no mitoses and no necrosis in this relatively hypocellular neoplasm. (*B*) Malignant soft tissue tumor (sarcoma)—malignant fibrous histiocytoma (MFH). In contrast, this tumor at the same high power is more cellular, has very large and atypical nuclei, and scattered mitoses and areas of necrosis (not pictured).

> **c.** Fibrous histiocytomas are subdivided by their most prominent **histologic feature**.
>> **(1) Fibrous xanthoma** is characterized by numerous foam cells within the spindled formation.
>> **(2) Giant cell tumor** of tendon sheaths has many giant cells and is found characteristically on the hands and fingers.
>> **(3) Dermatofibroma** is a term applied to a fibrotic tumor with prominent vascularity. It also may be called a **sclerosing hemangioma**.

3. Hemangioma
> **a.** Composed of newly formed blood channels, hemangiomas are common in infants and are frequently red or blue. They often disappear spontaneously.
> **b. Histologically,** two main types occur, **capillary** and **cavernous,** depending on the size of the channels comprising the lesion. Small channels (capillary) or large channels (cavernous) are lined by bland-appearing endothelial cells.
> **c.** Bleeding is occasionally a clinical problem. Hemangiomas that rapidly reach a large size in newborns may produce thrombocytopenia (**Kasabach-Merritt syndrome**).

4. Keloid is a strictly dermal posttraumatic lesion, a hypertrophic scar with unusually thick collagen bundles. Keloids occur more frequently in blacks and can be associated with pierced ears.

5. Nerve sheath tumors. Usually subcutaneous or dermal tumors (which may be pedunculated), they rarely occur in deeper soft tissues.
> **a.** The following are common **histologic subtypes**.
>> **(1) Neurofibroma** may or may not be circumscribed. It consists of spindle- to comma-shaped cells in a mucus-like (myxoid) background, with the arrangement of cells giving a wavy appearance to the lesion.
>> **(2) Neurilemmoma (schwannoma)** is encapsulated, often has alternating myxoid and cellular areas (**Antoni A** and **Antoni B patterns**), and contains prominent thick-walled blood vessels. Schwannomas can occur as intracranial tumors (see Chapter 21 VIII B 6).

    b. Neurofibromatosis (von Recklinghausen's disease) is an autosomal dominant disorder in which multiple neurofibromas occur in association with multiple café au lait (coffee-colored) spots on the skin. Hamartomatous or neoplastic lesions of other organs may occur as well. The gene for this genetic disorder has been identified as NF1 on chromosome 17.

    c. The **granular cell tumor** is a relatively common lesion believed to be related histogenetically to Schwann cells. (It was formerly called **granular cell myoblastoma,** but a muscle cell origin has been disproved.)

        (1) The lesion, found chiefly in the dermis and submucosal areas (tongue and larynx), is composed of distinctive, large, platelike cells with finely granular cytoplasm.

        (2) Characteristically, the overlying squamous epithelium proliferates at times to such an extent as to simulate a squamous cell carcinoma (SCC)—a condition termed **pseudoepitheliomatous hyperplasia.**

6. Leiomyoma

    a. This benign neoplasm recapitulates smooth muscle and may arise anywhere in soft tissue, often occurring in or near vascular walls. The common uterine leiomyoma is erroneously termed a "fibroid" (see Chapter 18 IV A 1); leiomyomas also are common in the gastrointestinal tract (see Chapter 13 II F 2). In the skin, a leiomyoma must be differentiated from other painful nodules.

    b. Microscopically, the lesion usually is a small, circumscribed nodule that is composed of bundles of elongated, pink cells with fibrillar cytoplasm, resembling smooth muscle. Mitoses are rare, and cellularity usually is even throughout the tumor.

7. Rhabdomyoma is a very rare lesion that resembles mature skeletal muscle. It usually arises in the tongue or vulva.

C. Locally aggressive lesions are a group of nonencapsulated neoplasms that invade surrounding tissues and structures. Frequently, extension of the lesion is greater than can be appreciated grossly, so the tumors are often inadequately excised. The tendency to recur locally is very high. These tumors do not metastasize, but may cause death if local extension involves vital structures.

    1. Fibromatosis (desmoid tumor). This fibrous growth arises from the deep fascia and typically occurs in the shoulder area, the pelvic girdle area, the neck, or the anterior abdominal wall. **Grossly,** it resembles a white, scarlike tumor. **Dupuytren's contracture** (on the palm of the hand) and **Peyronie's disease** (affecting the penis) are special forms of fibromatosis that produce local nodular deformities.

    a. Although composed chiefly of bland collagenous tissue and fibrocytes (like a proliferative scar) with rare mitoses, fibromatosis infiltrates surrounding muscle and soft tissue, often beyond apparent gross limits. Thus, inadequate excisions are often performed, and recurrences are common. Radiation therapy may be given to control recurrences.

    b. Interestingly, **abdominal wall desmoids** occur chiefly in young women. They may contain estrogen receptors and, thus, may respond to hormonal therapy with tamoxifen.

    2. Dermatofibrosarcoma protuberans is a type of fibrohistiocytic lesion that involves the skin and subcutis (see Chapter 24 VII C). Again, multiple local recurrences are common.

    3. Well-differentiated liposarcoma may pursue a locally aggressive course. **Histologically,** it looks like a lipoma but with scattered atypical cells. Excision of a tumor on the extremity may be curative, but complete surgical extirpation of a retroperitoneal tumor often cannot be achieved. It is these latter lesions that gradually grow locally and may result in the patient's death by involvement of vital structures (e.g., the aorta or ureters). Metastases and death do not occur from the more superficial extremity tumors; thus, the name **"atypical lipoma"** is currently used.

D. Malignant neoplasms. Sarcoma is a general term for malignant soft tissue lesions. Sarcomas comprise most pediatric solid tumors but account for 1% to 2% of adult malignancies. These lesions not only infiltrate and invade surrounding tissues but also have the capacity to metastasize. Only sarcomas that arise in extravisceral, extraskeletal, mesenchymal tissues are discussed.

    1. General considerations

        a. Pathogenesis

        (1) Sarcomas are named after the adult tissue that they most closely resemble since most sarcomas partially recapitulate a specific adult tissue, both ultrastructurally and biochemically (determined by immunohistochemical analysis).

        (a) It had been assumed that mature adult cells were directly transformed into a sarcoma, but they probably are not.

(b) Rather, sarcomas probably arise from more primitive precursor cells in damaged or growing tissues. This theory explains why certain tumors occur mainly in the young (e.g., rhabdomyosarcoma in growing muscle tissue) whereas others are found predominantly in elderly persons (e.g., liposarcoma and fibrous tumors in tissues still capable of growth in the adult).

(2) Whether sarcomas arise from committed phenotypic precursors or the uncommitted, pluripotential, mesenchymal cell is under investigation.

b. Classification. Sarcomas may be best considered in three broad categories that highlight differences in occurrence and behavior.

(1) **Round cell sarcomas.** Common in childhood, they have a rapid growth rate, and are lethal unless sensitive to chemotherapy. Examples include rhabdomyosarcoma (chemosensitive), peripheral neuroectodermal tumor (PNET) and extraosseous Ewing's sarcoma.

(2) **Spindle cell sarcomas.** Common in adulthood, they have a slower growth rate and are generally not sensitive to chemotherapy; however, they may be cured if excised completely before metastases have occurred. Examples include leiomyosarcoma, malignant peripheral nerve sheath tumors (MPNSTs), and malignant fibrous histiocytoma (MFH).

(3) **Odd sarcoma types.** A variety of other tumors are idiosyncratic, with unusual biology. Some are indolent but persistent and often deadly (epithelioid sarcoma, alveolar soft part sarcoma), some have an excellent prognosis (myxoid liposarcoma), some are quickly fatal (angiosarcoma), and some are unlike any other sarcoma (Kaposi's sarcoma).

c. Gross appearance

(1) Most sarcomas appear as solitary, deep-seated masses. (Benign tumors and reactive lesions, by contrast, are generally in more superficial tissue; they also tend to be smaller.) The most common sites affected are the extremities and the retroperitoneum.

(2) Sarcomas appear fleshy and often bulge on cut surfaces.

d. Criteria of malignancy

(1) The pathologist utilizes a group of features to diagnose a sarcoma; they include mitotic activity, cellularity and nuclear pleomorphism, and presence of necrosis. These criteria differ according to histologic type and tumor location.

(2) Clinicopathologic correlations and follow-up studies have shown that both site of origin and histology are important predictors when determining the malignancy and, hence, the prognosis of a soft tissue tumor.

(3) Therefore, the criteria for determining malignancy may vary for those tumors that arise in soft tissues as opposed to those lesions that appear identical but arise in viscera. For example, for uterine smooth muscle tumors to be considered sarcomas, average mitotic rates should be 10 per 10 high-power fields; similar smooth muscle tumors in the leg are considered sarcomas with mitotic rates of 1 to 2 per 10 high-power fields.

(4) Clinically benign lesions may partially resemble sarcomas microscopically; for example, they may contain pleomorphic cells and, thus, misdiagnosis can occur. Knowledge of the patient's age, tumor site, and other features such as tumor pattern and mitotic rate are critical for a proper diagnosis. An expert opinion should be sought unless the diagnosis is clinically obvious.

e. Measurement of sarcomas

(1) **Grading.** The grade of a sarcoma is an attempt at prognostication and relates to the degree of differentiation—how closely it resembles adult mesenchymal tissue and its mitotic rate. Low-grade (more differentiated, slow-growing) tumors tend to follow a more indolent course than high-grade (highly mitotic) tumors. Tumors are also given a numeric grade as follows: grade I (low grade), grade II (high grade but intermediate malignancy), grade III (high grade without qualification). Of the sarcomas listed in Table 25-1, rhabdomyosarcoma, synovial sarcoma, and angiosarcoma are always considered grade III because, historically, they have had a uniformly poor prognosis, whatever the degree of differentiation.

(2) **Staging.** Of the four stages established for sarcomas, stages I, II, and III are related to the grade and local involvement of bone or vessels for nonmetastatic tumors; stage IV is for metastatic disease.

(3) **Size** is an important gross feature of prognostic value. As a rule, small tumors (less than 5 cm) have a more favorable outcome.

f. Prognosis

(1) Prognosis depends on the histologic subtype, depth, size, and grade. Tumors that are superficial and small are associated with favorable prognosis. Survival rates, usually poor in the past, have recently shown significant improvement. Although rates vary considerably by type, the overall 5-year survival rate for all types now approaches 70%.

(2) As a group, sarcomas typically **metastasize** hematogenously, most commonly to the lungs and liver. However, they can also extend directly or metastasize to regional lymph nodes. The most common sarcomas to metastasize to lymph nodes are synovial sarcoma and MFH.

g. Treatment. In the treatment of soft tissue sarcomas, the following measures often are used in combination.

(1) Surgical excision is used for localized lesions (i.e., the wide local excision with a 1- to 2-cm margin around the tumor). Often, radical surgery is necessary since these tumors are seen on microscopic examination to be more extensive than is apparent on gross examination.

(2) Radiation therapy is used postoperatively for most tumors in order to sterilize the local tumor bed and to treat inadequately removed tumors (those extending to the margins).

(3) Systemic chemotherapy is given to all patients with advanced (metastatic) disease; complete responses (disappearance of tumor) are the exception, especially in adult tumors. Adjuvant chemotherapy (in the absence of metastases) is given for the chemosensitive childhood round cell sarcomas, but has no proven benefit for the majority of adult spindle cell sarcomas.

2. Round cell sarcomas. Rhabdomyosarcoma is the prototype here and is the most common childhood sarcoma.

a. Rhabdomyosarcoma recapitulates embryonic myogenesis in a disorganized and haphazard pattern. Most cases do not occur on the extremities.

(1) Clinically, the most common complaint is the presence of a mass that is neither painful nor tender despite its rapid growth. Other symptoms relate to the site of the tumor.

(2) Histologic subtypes

(a) Embryonal rhabdomyosarcoma closely resembles the developing muscle of the 7- to 10-week fetus and occurs most commonly in children under age 6.

(i) The tumor usually is located in the head and neck regions, particularly in the orbit, nasopharynx, and middle ear. Another typical location is the paratesticular region.

(ii) Histologically, sheets of small round cells with uniform oval nuclei are noted. Some cells show scanty eosinophilic cytoplasm where cell products, such as the muscle marker desmin, can be demonstrated immunohistochemically. Desmin marks them as rhabdomyoblasts.

(iii) This tumor must be differentiated from other small-cell tumors of childhood, such as malignant lymphoma, leukemia, Ewing's sarcoma, and neuroblastoma.

(b) Sarcoma botryoides is a form of embryonal rhabdomyosarcoma. It tends to occur in the genitourinary, biliary, or upper respiratory tract of very young children.

(i) "Botryoid" refers to the grape-like appearance that the lesion assumes when it grows beneath a mucous membrane. This polypoid, soft tumor looks like jelly or grapes.

(ii) Histologically, the lining epithelium of the mucosa usually is preserved, and a dense zone of undifferentiated rhabdomyoblasts is seen immediately beneath the epithelium (cambium layer). The remainder of the tumor usually appears myxoid with less cellularity. Mitoses are numerous.

(c) Alveolar rhabdomyosarcoma recapitulates cells of a later stage of fetal muscle development than embryonal rhabdomyosarcoma and in an older age-group (10 to 25 years). This type is the least frequent form, but is often deadly.

(i) The tumor commonly occurs in the extremities, particularly the flexor areas of the forearms and hands and the hypothenar eminences.

(ii) Histologically, nests of loosely arranged, small, undifferentiated cells (rhabdomyoblasts) are separated by dense fibrous septa to which only a single layer of tumor cells remains firmly attached, giving an alveolar or pseudoglandular appearance. The rare giant tumor cells aid in the diagnosis.

(d) Rhabdomyosarcoma in older adults. Generally, rhabdomyosarcoma is rare in adults. When it does occur, patients are usually in the fourth to seventh decades of life. About 70% of the tumors arise from the muscles of the lower extremities, particularly the thigh. The tumor is characteristically situated deep within the muscle and can vary from a relatively small to a large and bulky mass. The consistency usually is soft and fleshy, and the color is beefy red-brown.

(3) Prognosis and therapy

 (a) The **prognosis** of rhabdomyosarcoma varies with the site, the histology, and the patient's group level (equivalent to a staging system). Although these tumors are grade III, the prognosis is generally good.

  (i) Site. Prognosis is good for periorbital and paratesticular lesions and poor for lesions located elsewhere in the head, in the extremities, or in the retroperitoneum.

  (ii) Histology. All embryonal types have a favorable histology; the histology for the alveolar type is unfavorable.

  (iii) Group. Patients with completely resected tumors (group I) do extremely well, and 80% to 90% are cured; they are given chemotherapy, which apparently is effective in sterilizing minute metastases. Patients with gross metastatic disease (group IV) uniformly do poorly.

 (b) Significant strides were taken during the 1970s in terms of developing effective **chemotherapy** for rhabdomyosarcoma. It is one of the few sarcomas that are responsive to chemotherapy.

b. Peripheral neuroectodermal tumor (PNET) is also known as neuroepithelioma and is presumably derived from primitive neuronal cells in the peripheral soft tissues.

 (1) Clinically, PNETs arise on the chest wall ("Askin tumor") or extremities of children and young adults between age 5 and 15.

 (2) Histologically, PNET is characterized by small round cells growing in sheets with a high mitotic rate. The formation of so-called **"rosettes"** is virtually diagnostic; a rosette is a ring of cells around an eosinophilic material composed of cell processes. Because not all cases have them, the diagnosis can be difficult. Immunostains for neuronal markers like neurofilament and synaptophysin can be helpful.

 (3) Ultrastructure. Examination with the electron microscope may be necessary for a diagnosis; in PNET, dense core granules may be seen.

 (4) Prognosis and therapy. The prognosis for PNET is uniformly poor because it is currently resistant to known chemotherapy agents. The opposite is true for rhabdomyosarcoma, with which it can be confused. Therefore, it is vital to make a correct diagnosis.

c. Extraosseous Ewing's sarcoma. This prognostically favorable undifferentiated tumor is of unknown origin. Histologically, it resembles PNET but lacks rosettes and neuronal markers. It is a chemosensitive tumor.

d. Molecular biology of round cell sarcomas. Emerging technologies can now assist physicians in making important decisions about clinical management.

 (1) Cytogenetics. Both PNET and Ewing's sarcoma have a similar translocation, t(11,22); rhabdomyosarcoma is different, with abnormalities of chromosomes 2, 3, and 13.

 (2) Specific genes. The MyoD1 gene is important in skeletal muscle differentiation and can be used in the diagnosis of rhabdomyosarcoma. The c-*myc* gene is amplified in PNET whereas the N-*myc* gene is amplified in adrenal neuroblastoma. Other growth-related genes such as p53 and RB1 may or may not have mutations, and the state of these mutations may be of prognostic value in many tumors, including the round cell sarcomas.

3. Spindle cell sarcomas. MFH is the prototype and is the **most common adult sarcoma**.

a. Malignant fibrous histiocytoma

 (1) Clinical features

  (a) In the past, this tumor ranked second to liposarcoma in frequency. It occurs more often in men than in women and may occur at any age.

  (b) The tumor may be found on an extremity, on the head or neck, or in the retroperitoneum. It is the most common tumor of the thigh. MFH may infiltrate widely and may metastasize. The 5-year survival rate is about 60% to 70%.

  (c) The cell of origin of MFH is disputed, and the nomenclature itself has been challenged. No evidence has linked MFH to the monocyte–histiocyte–macrophage lineage of bone marrow origin. Rather, MFH appears derived from a primitive mesenchymal cell with the ability to differentiate along the myofibroblastic phenotype.

(2) Pathology

(a) Grossly, MFH is usually a large (10-cm) tumor with a white to tan-brown cut surface. Occasionally, it may resemble a hematoma. Necrosis and hemorrhage are common.

(b) Histologically, the tumor contains a mixture of "facultative" fibroblasts (sometimes arranged in storiform or pinwheel patterns) and histiocytes. Myofibroblasts often are seen. Cytologic evidence for malignancy includes the pleomorphism, hyperchromatic nuclei, abnormal mitoses, and bizarre tumor giant cells. The tumor is, in fact, the most pleomorphic of sarcomas.

(c) Areas resembling the tumor may occasionally be found in other sarcomas, which are then referred to erroneously as **"dedifferentiated"** (e.g., dedifferentiated chondrosarcoma). For example, a clear-cut chondrosarcoma may show an area no longer like cartilage, but instead like MFH. Thus, the tumor lost its differentiation in the process of tumor progression. This phenomenon may mean that MFH is a type of final common pathway in sarcoma histology.

(3) Atypical fibroxanthoma (atypical fibrous histiocytoma) is a cutaneous lesion of the head or neck seen in elderly patients. It is now considered to be a superficial form of MFH. Although (rarely) it may metastasize, atypical fibroxanthoma generally carries an excellent prognosis because of its resectable superficial location.

b. Leiomyosarcoma, a malignancy of smooth muscle origin, usually arises in the uterus (see Chapter 18 IV A 2) or the gastrointestinal tract (see Chapter 13 II G 3). The tumor also may occur in the retroperitoneum or in an extremity, occasionally originating from large veins.

(1) Pathology

(a) Grossly, leiomyosarcomas range in size from small to very large and have a whorled, fleshy, white appearance.

(b) Histologically, the tumor is composed of elongated smooth muscle cells with pink fibrillary cytoplasm. The pattern of growth is helpful: Alternating bundles and fascicles of cells intersect one another at right angles to the plane of section. Mitoses range in number from as few as 3 per 50 high-power fields to many in a single high-power field. Not infrequently, large bizarre cells are present.

(2) Prognosis of leiomyosarcoma varies by the grade of malignancy and by site; gastrointestinal tumors have a poor prognosis (approximately a 20% 5-year survival rate).

c. Malignant peripheral nerve sheath tumor (MPNST). These tumors have also been called neurofibrosarcomas and malignant schwannomas, but no schwannian differentiation is seen; thus, the noncommittal term.

(1) Site. These malignant tumors usually arise in or near a nerve trunk or in the site of a neurofibroma. Hence, such neurofibrosarcomas may occur anywhere.

(2) Development. Rapid growth of a lesion in a patient who has **neurofibromatosis** usually means that an MPNST has arisen, usually in a central location. Nearly half of all MPNSTs occur in this disease. About 4% to 5% of all neurofibromatosis patients will develop and die from a malignant schwannoma.

(3) Pathology. Generally, these neoplasms are highly malignant tumors composed of cellular spindle cells arranged in a wavy pattern; many mitoses and foci of necrosis are common.

(4) The **prognosis** is quite poor in neurofibromatosis patients. However, other patients typically have smaller and more peripheral tumors, which can be resected earlier, leading to a better prognosis.

d. Prognosis and therapy. All spindle cell sarcomas are treated the same, with wide local excision and radiotherapy. Chemotherapy is given only when metastatic disease is present. Prognosis for this group is generally good, with 5-year survival rates of 50% to 70%. Tumors on the extremities have a more favorable prognosis than those on the trunk or in the retroperitoneum or mesentery.

4. Odd sarcoma types. No prototype exists for this group, as each tumor is different from the others and from the round and spindled sarcomas.

a. Liposarcoma

(1) Clinical features. Liposarcoma is one of the most frequently encountered sarcomas in adults; it is extremely rare in children. Affected patients usually present with a large, bulky mass, most commonly in the thigh or retroperitoneum.

(2) Pathology. Histologically, liposarcoma can be either **myxoid** or **nonmyxoid** (round cell and pleomorphic types). The more common myxoid type is characterized by proliferating lipoblasts in different stages of differentiation, prominent vascularity with a plexiform arrangement of capillaries, and a matrix rich in mucopolysaccharides. The myxoid type is usually hypocellular, and the capillary network resembles a chicken-wire pattern. The round cell type is highly cellular; the pleomorphic type resembles MFH but lipoblasts can be found.

- **(3) Prognosis.** Each type has its own typical course.
  - **(a)** The well-differentiated liposarcoma, also called "atypical lipoma," has an excellent prognosis if on an extremity; retroperitoneal tumors grow slowly and may result in death 5 to 10 years after diagnosis.
  - **(b)** The myxoid tumor has a very good prognosis and most are considered low grade.
  - **(c)** The high-grade round cell and pleomorphic types recur, metastasizing at a high rate; moreover, the prognosis is poor.
- **(4) Treatment** is determined by the histologic type and extent of the tumor.
  - **(a)** Myxoid tumors infiltrate locally, and **wide surgical excision** is the treatment of choice. Many of these tumors are deceiving. They appear to be circumscribed; but if they are simply excised ("shelled out"), the chances of recurrence are high.
  - **(b) Amputation** of an extremity may be advisable when local excision is not feasible or when lesions persist in recurring.
  - **(c) Radiation** is used chiefly as adjuvant therapy: Wound sites are irradiated postoperatively to reduce the risk of local recurrence.

b. Synovial sarcoma
  - **(1) Clinical features**
    - **(a)** Synovial sarcoma may affect patients of all ages, but it is found most frequently in young adults (age 15 to 35). In most series, the tumor has a slight preponderance in men. The name is a misnomer—tumors do not arise from synovial cells, and they rarely are found in joints. However, this familiar name has been retained by convention.
    - **(b)** The tumor commonly occurs in the lower limbs, often in the region of the knee, foot, and ankle. It may develop, however, in any site that has tendons, joints, or bursae. The sarcoma may be small or large, is often well circumscribed, and may be painful. Moreover, it usually has a long clinical duration before diagnosis (6 months to 2 years commonly and perhaps as long as 10 to 20 years). Calcification is commonly seen on x-ray.
  - **(2) Pathology**
    - **(a)** The tumor is typically **biphasic** (i.e., it has a spindle cell fibrosarcoma-like element and a pseudoglandular, or epithelial, element). It has been called the carcinosarcoma of soft tissues. Like true epithelial cells, the glandular spaces have a basement membrane. Calcification often is noted both radiologically and microscopically. Tumor cells express cytokeratin, another feature in common with true epithelial cells.
    - **(b)** Many cases lack glandular formations and are called **monophasic**.
  - **(3)** The long-term **prognosis** generally is poor. Nodal metastases occur in up to 30% of cases, and hematogenous dissemination is common, especially to the lungs. However, recent 5-year survival rates approach 70%.
  - **(4)** The **treatment** of choice is wide excision, which may mean amputation. Because early lesions go unnoticed, surgery usually is performed late in the course of the disease, with involvement of vascular structures. The incidence of local recurrence is, therefore, high. Late metastases (after 5 years) are not uncommon. It seems likely that the prognosis will improve because of recent advances in this chemosensitive tumor.

c. Epithelioid sarcoma may be a related lesion. It arises in distal portions of the extremities, frequently producing multiple nodules along the length of the tendon. This sarcoma may occur on the hand that is otherwise free of sarcomas. It is also a rather superficial tumor and may cause cutaneous nodules with umbilication (ulceration).
  - **(1) Histologically,** this lesion shows granuloma-like features, with large epithelioid cells surrounding zones of necrosis. These findings have led to misdiagnosis of the lesion as a rheumatoid nodule. Like synovial sarcomas and epithelial tumors, the epithelioid sarcoma contains cytokeratin. It has been called the carcinoma of soft tissues.
  - **(2)** The **course** may extend over many years, with multiple recurrences and eventual distant metastasis.

d. Dermatofibrosarcoma (DFSP) protuberans. As the name implies, this cutaneous tumor bulges above the skin surface. It belongs to the fibrohistiocytic family of tumors and occurs on the trunk of middle-aged to elderly patients.
  - **(1) Pathology.** This tumor (DFSP) has a storiform or matlike pattern, and the spindle cells

are bland with few mitoses. Because this pattern is seen in the much smaller dermatofibroma or fibrous histiocytoma, some cases are misdiagnosed. DFSP must be a large lesion (3 cm or greater) clinically.

    (2) Course and prognosis. Local recurrence is common but metastases are rare, as they are for all sarcomas of the skin.

  e. Fibrosarcoma occurs in children and is unusual in adults. It is a highly cellular, uniform, spindle cell tumor without pleomorphism, but with a moderate to high mitotic rate. It is capable of hematogenous metastases. It can be distinguished from MFH by its lack of pleomorphism and from fibromatosis by its cellularity and mitotic rate. Paradoxically, congenital or infantile fibrosarcoma has an excellent prognosis.

  f. Angiosarcoma is an uncommon tumor arising from endothelial cells; it typically occurs in the skin of the elderly (see Chapter 24 VII E) or in the breast, but rarely arises in soft tissues.

    (1) Pathology

      (a) Grossly, the tumor is a hemorrhagic and often necrotic, blue–red lesion. It may rapidly attain a large size and metastasizes readily to the lungs and liver.

      (b) Histologically, the tumor may range from a differentiated tumor (i.e., showing easily recognizable blood vessels) to a solid, anaplastic neoplasm without much noticeable vessel formation.

    (2) The **prognosis** is poor. Death within 2 years is usual, often from exsanguinating hemorrhage. Chemotherapy is not effective.

  g. Kaposi's sarcoma is an unusual form of sarcoma noted for its multicentricity, its symmetry, and its occasional spontaneous regression (although usually only some lesions regress). Because it cannot grow independently and appears to be cytogenetically polyclonal, it may **not** be a fully developed sarcomatous malignancy. For further discussion, see Chapter 24 VII D.

STUDY QUESTIONS

Directions: Each of the numbered items or incomplete statements in this section is followed by answers or by completions of the statement. Select the **one** lettered answer or completion that is **best** in each case.

1. Which of the following is a locally aggressive soft tissue tumor?

(A) Rhabdomyoma
(B) Round cell liposarcoma
(C) Angiosarcoma
(D) Fibromatosis
(E) Nodular fasciitis

2. Which patient is most likely to have nodular fasciitis?

(A) A 52-year-old man who has had a painful 3-cm nodule on his chest for 6 months
(B) A 72-year-old woman who has had a tender 5-cm nodule on her back for 1 year
(C) A 24-year-old woman who has had a tender 2-cm nodule on her right arm for 2 weeks
(D) A 19-year-old man who has had a painless 5-cm nodule on his left leg for 2 months
(E) A 7-year-old boy who has had a painless 1-cm nodule on his left knee as a result of a fall 1 month ago

3. A 15-year-old boy suffered trauma to his leg in late January. By the first week of March, he noted a rapidly growing, extremely firm mass in his thigh. Which conclusion is correct?

(A) A biphasic pattern is likely on biopsy
(B) Trauma called attention to, but did not cause, this lesion
(C) The rapid growth is ominous
(D) An x-ray will be diagnostic
(E) Mitoses alone will determine malignancy

4. A 32-year-old woman notes a 3-cm painless mass, which she attributes to an athletic injury that is lateral to her left popliteal fossa. Three months later, the mass is biopsied, and a diagnosis of synovial sarcoma is made. Which statement accurately describes the prognosis for this patient?

(A) Following radical local excision, the tumor is unlikely to recur
(B) Following radical local excision, the tumor may recur but is unlikely to metastasize
(C) Prophylactic lymph node dissection combined with radical local excision will decrease the chance of tumor recurrence
(D) If the tumor does not recur within 5 years of adequate treatment, it is unlikely ever to recur
(E) The tumor may or may not recur locally but often metastasizes, even after 5–10 years

5. Pseudotumors of soft tissue include all of the following EXCEPT

(A) proliferative myositis
(B) myositis ossificans
(C) nodular fasciitis
(D) fibromatosis
(E) fat necrosis

6. All of the following statements describe therapy for adult spindle cell sarcomas EXCEPT

(A) a wide local excision is critical
(B) postoperative radiation decreases local recurrences
(C) amputation often can be avoided
(D) chemotherapy is effective for many tumors
(E) treatment does not depend on histologic type

7. A soft tissue lesion based in the skin or subcutaneous region can be any of the following EXCEPT

(A) a liposarcoma if on the trunk
(B) an epithelial sarcoma if on the hand
(C) an angiosarcoma if on the head of an elderly patient
(D) an atypical fibroxanthoma if on the neck
(E) an AIDS-associated lesion if a red–purple nodule

1-D	4-E	7-A
2-C	5-D	
3-D	6-D	

8. A 10-cm lump is noted on the thigh of a 50-year-old man. All of the following statements are likely explanations for this lump EXCEPT

(A) the tumor could be a malignant fibrous histiocytoma (MFH)
(B) the tumor could have been there for over 3 months
(C) the tumor could be benign (e.g., a myxoma)
(D) the tumor could be a reactive lesion
(E) the tumor could be calcified

9. A patient with many (> 100) 1-cm polyplike skin lesions is examined by a physician who immediately suspects von Recklinghausen's disease. All of the following statements concerning this disease are true EXCEPT

(A) the skin lesions are neurofibromas
(B) the patient will most likely die of a sarcoma
(C) one of the patient's parents likely has the disease
(D) multiple flat, coffee-colored skin lesions are probably present
(E) the sciatic nerve may be involved

10. A young woman is diagnosed as having sarcoma botryoides of the bladder. All of the following statements about her condition are true EXCEPT

(A) gross examination shows a polypoid growth into the bladder
(B) specific chemotherapy is effective
(C) it is a tumor with a cambium layer
(D) it is a tumor of myofibroblasts
(E) it has a good prognosis

Directions: The group of items in this section consists of lettered options followed by a set of numbered items. For each item, select the **one** lettered option that is most closely associated with it. Each lettered option may be selected once, more than once, or not at all.

Questions 11–18

For each characteristic, select the type of sarcoma.

(A) Round cell sarcoma
(B) Spindle cell sarcoma
(C) Both
(D) Neither

11. Common in adults

12. Chemosensitive

13. Common in childhood

14. Leiomyosarcomatous

15. Peripheral neuroectodermal tumor (PNET)

16. Angiosarcomatous

17. Expert opinion useful

18. Indolent but persistent tumor

8-D	11-B	14-B	17-C
9-B	12-A	15-A	18-D
10-D	13-A	16-D	

ANSWERS AND EXPLANATIONS

1. The answer is D *[II G; III C 1, 3, D 4 f].*
In terms of clinical significance, locally aggressive tumors are considered to be somewhere between benign lesions (e.g., rhabdomyoma) and malignant tumors that are capable of metastasis (e.g., angiosarcoma). Fibromatosis is the most common example of a locally aggressive tumor. Round cell liposarcoma is a fully malignant tumor capable of metastasis. Nodular fasciitis is a woundlike reaction in the deep soft tissues and is a benign lesion without the potential for even local recurrence.

2. The answer is C *[II G 2].*
Nodular (pseudosarcomatous) fasciitis typically affects the upper extremities or trunk of young adults, is noticeable soon after onset, and follows a history of trauma in one-third to one-half of the cases. As with the 24-year-old woman, the nodule produced is characteristically tender and smaller than 3 cm. Larger tumors generally are not fasciitis. However, a nodule on the knee after a fall is more likely to be due to granulation tissue or callus from a fractured bone.

3. The answer is D *[II I].*
The history of the 15-year-old boy described in the question is a classic one for myositis ossificans, a posttraumatic, rapidly enlarging, reactive mass with bone formation. Unlike most soft tissue lesions, an x-ray will indeed be diagnostic, showing massive calcification. Trauma was directly responsible for the development of this reactive lesion. (Trauma is not a cause of sarcoma, although patients often are made aware of sarcoma after trauma.) Rapid growth is a hallmark of reactive lesions, but it is not pathognomonic. Rapid growth also occurs in sarcomas, particularly large lesions with sudden necrosis and hemorrhage; however, rapid growth alone is not ominous and should suggest the possibility of a reaction as well as a neoplasm. Although the biopsy of a myositis could be confusing, it would resemble osteosarcoma with bone formation. A biphasic histology is typical of synovial sarcoma, a tumor that could occur in this age-group, but it would never develop so rapidly.

4. The answer is E *[III D 4 b].*
Synovial sarcomas usually are slow growing and, thus, may have a prolonged natural history, but they metastasize given enough time. Because of a lack of early signs or symptoms, surgical intervention often is performed late in the course of these tumors and often is inadequate. Local recurrences, thus, are frequent. The addition of new therapeutic modalities, such as radiation therapy, to treatment by wide surgical excision (and amputation when possible) has improved the rate of local recurrence. However, late metastases beyond 5 years are common. It may be that some combination chemotherapy will prove to have an effect on prognosis.

5. The answer is D *[II; III C 1].*
Fibromatosis (also called desmoid tumor) is a locally aggressive tumor composed of proliferating fibroblasts. Desmoid tumors of the abdominal wall are particularly common in young women. Fibromatosis never metastasizes but frequently recurs locally; it may even result in death if it invades vital structures. Proliferative myositis, myositis ossificans, nodular fasciitis, and fat necrosis are pseudotumors (i.e., reactive processes), although they present as tumors and are mitotically active like malignancies.

6. The answer is D *[III D 1 g].*
A wide local excision with a 1- to 2-cm margin to decrease local recurrences is the surgical approach of choice. At one time, amputation was performed frequently to achieve local control (lack of local recurrence). However, this procedure is avoided now, where possible, as radiation therapy is capable of sterilizing the area, thereby decreasing local recurrence. Local recurrence, if it occurs, is an unfavorable sign prognostically. Unfortunately, chemotherapy for adult spindle cell sarcomas has not had the major effects seen in treatment of lymphomas; one of the few exceptions is rhabdomyosarcoma (a childhood round cell sarcoma). The therapeutic approach to all adult spindle cell sarcomas is similar regardless of histology.

7. The answer is A *[III D 4 a].*
There are very few superficial sarcomas; most of them are deep to the subcutaneous region, as is particularly true of liposarcoma. The exceptions include the following: Kaposi's sarcoma, the purplish nodules seen in patients with AIDS; epithelioid sarcoma, a tumor that commonly affects the upper extremities, including the hand; angiosarcoma, which occurs on the skin of the head and neck of the elderly; and the atypical fibroxanthoma, a lesion histologically similar to malignant fibrous histiocytoma (MFH), but with a benign course due to its superficial cutaneous location.

8. The answer is D *[I B 1; II F 3; III B 2, D 4 b 1 (b)].*
Size is an important consideration when dealing with a lump of the soft tissues. Reactive lesions certainly mimic sarcomas, both clinically and microscopically, but they rarely grow to be more than 3 cm in size. Anything larger than 3 cm is likely to be a true neoplasm, either benign or malignant. A myxoma may achieve a size greater than 10 cm, and most malignant fibrous histiocytomas (MFHs) are at least that large. Duration of a lesion also is important: If it appeared less than 3 months ago and is small, it could be reactive; most sarcomas have a longer duration. Calcification may be seen in sarcomas secondary to necrosis and calcium precipitation. Calcification is characteristic of synovial sarcoma and extraosseous osteosarcoma, which are rare occurrences.

9. The answer is B *[III B 5 b, D 3 c].*
Von Recklinghausen's disease, or neurofibromatosis, is an autosomal dominant disease. Thus, it is likely that a parent or very close relative of an affected patient also will have the disease. The patient described is classic, but not all patients have as many nodules (which are cutaneous neurofibromas). The peripheral nerves, including large trunk nerves (e.g., the sciatic nerve), may be involved, as may the brain. Café au lait spots are helpful in the diagnosis: These patients usually have at least 5 to 6 such coffee-colored pigmentations. Although malignant transformation (noted as sudden growth in a preexisting neurofibroma) is a well-recognized phenomenon, only 4% to 5% of these patients develop a sarcoma. It is still true that almost half of all malignant potential nerve sheath tumors (MPNSTs, or neurofibrosarcomas) are associated with this disease. Those not associated are said to be "sporadic" neurofibrosarcomas.

10. The answer is D *[III D 2 a (2) (b)].*
A sarcoma botryoides is a special subtype of embryonal rhabdomyosarcoma, a tumor of rhabdomyoblasts. Myofibroblasts are special fibroblasts with contractile properties, seen in wounds and some tumors, such as fibromatosis and malignant fibrous histiocytoma (MFH). The botryoid tumor is a grapelike polypoid tumor that bulges into available spaces. Beneath the bladder epithelium lining the polyp, the dense cluster of tumor cells is the cambium layer. Unlike other sarcomas, rhabdomyosarcoma clearly is responsive to specific chemotherapy, and the botryoid type has an excellent prognosis.

11–18. The answers are: 11-B, 12-A, 13-A, 14-B, 15-A, 16-D, 17-C, 18-D *[III D 1 b].*
Spindle cell sarcomas, like leiomyosarcomas, are common in adults but are not chemosensitive. In contrast, the round cell sarcomas [e.g., peripheral neuroectodermal tumor (PNET)] are more common in childhood and respond to chemotherapy. Angiosarcoma is neither spindled nor round cell in nature and is a highly aggressive but rare sarcoma. Sarcomas are not indolent like the locally aggressive fibromatosis. Due to their rarity, an expert of diagnostic opinion is often sought by both pathologists and clinicians.

Comprehensive
Exam

QUESTIONS

Directions: Each of the numbered items or incomplete statements in this section is followed by answers or by completions of the statement. Select the **one** lettered answer or completion that is **best** in each case.

1. A 58-year-old man is hospitalized for evaluation of recent intermittent upper abdominal pain. History and physical examination reveal a 25-lb weight loss over recent months and upper abdominal tenderness without evidence of a mass, ascites, or jaundice. The best diagnostic approach and most likely preliminary diagnosis would be

(A) abdominal ultrasonography for the diagnosis of chronic cholecystitis with cholelithiasis

(B) serum bilirubin measurement for the diagnosis of chronic cholecystitis with cholelithiasis

(C) endoscopy for the diagnosis of carcinoma of the ampulla of Vater

(D) laparotomy for the diagnosis of carcinoma of the head of the pancreas

(E) computed tomography (CT) for the diagnosis of carcinoma of the body of the pancreas

2. A renal allograft recipient develops bloody diarrhea. A colonic biopsy shows focal necrosis and hemorrhage. Individual endothelial cells are large with prominent nuclear inclusions. The expected copathogen is

(A) Epstein-Barr virus (EBV)

(B) *Candida*

(C) *Pneumocystis*

(D) toxoplasmosis

(E) *Giardia*

3. A 30-year-old woman presents with a gradual onset of hoarseness exacerbated by a recent upper respiratory tract infection. Direct laryngoscopy reveals small papillary excrescences of the true vocal cords. Of the following, the most likely etiology is

(A) autoimmune

(B) bacterial

(C) viral

(D) fungal

4. What is the most common benign mesenchymal tumor of the stomach?

(A) Polypoid adenoma

(B) Leiomyoma (benign stromal tumor)

(C) Glomus tumor

(D) Lipoma

(E) Granular cell tumor

5. A 65-year-old man complains that his hat size is increasing. Physical examination reveals that the patient walks bowlegged because of tibial deformities. Skeletal x-rays are indicative of abnormal bone density confined to the tibias and skull. The most likely etiology is

(A) a pituitary adenoma

(B) a parathyroid adenoma

(C) corticosteroid therapy

(D) a vitamin deficiency

(E) an idiopathic bone disorder

6. A 60-year-old white man with a long history of stable angina complains of a progressive increase in the frequency and severity of his chest pain. About 12 hours after one particularly severe episode of chest pain, he is brought to the emergency room where he is found to be hypotensive and in severe congestive heart failure. An electrocardiogram (ECG) demonstrates significant Q waves as well as ST-segment and T-wave changes. Serum cardiac enzymes demonstrate a markedly elevated MB isoenzyme of creatine kinase (CK). Appropriate medical intervention fails to control the patient's hypotension and cardiac failure. Cardiac arrest ensues, and attempts at resuscitation fail. An autopsy is performed. Which one of the following statements about this patient's condition is true?

(A) A subendocardial myocardial infarct is likely to be found at autopsy

(B) A coronary artery thrombus is unlikely to be found at autopsy

(C) The clinical presentation is classic for constrictive pericarditis

(D) An area of myocardial infarction less than 2 cm in diameter is likely to be found at autopsy

(E) Severe narrowing of at least one coronary artery is an expected finding at autopsy

7. A 10-year-old boy enters the hospital with lethargy, anorexia, and protracted vomiting 1 week after the onset of fever and a presumed viral illness. The patient rapidly develops seizures and metabolic acidosis and lapses into a coma. A liver biopsy demonstrates numerous small cytoplasmic vacuoles (microvesicular steatosis). What is the most likely diagnosis?

(A) Hepatitis A infection
(B) Reye's syndrome
(C) Biliary cirrhosis due to extrahepatic obstruction
(D) Schistosomiasis
(E) Cystic fibrosis

8. Barrett's epithelium is found in what part of the gastrointestinal tract?

(A) Esophagus
(B) Stomach
(C) Small intestine
(D) Large intestine
(E) Rectum

9. A 50-year-old farmer with acute pulmonary edema is examined in the emergency room. The patient is otherwise well and shows no cardiac enlargement on chest x-ray. The most likely diagnosis is

(A) chronic bronchitis from dust inhalation
(B) a pneumoconiosis related to hemp fibers
(C) a hypersensitivity reaction to certain resins
(D) chronic silicosis
(E) silo-filler's disease

10. Which one of the following statements is true regarding glomangiomas?

(A) Glomangiomas arise from specialized structures concerned with temperature
(B) They are typically located adjacent to proximal interphalangeal joints
(C) They are rarely painful
(D) They are malignant
(E) Glomangiomas often surround nerves

11. A 50-year-old white woman complains of fatigue and pruritus of 8 months' duration. Laboratory studies reveal serum transaminase levels that are only minimally elevated, although the serum alkaline phosphatase is measured at 1200 IU/L (normal level is less than 150 IU/L); a serum anti-mitochondrial antibody (AMA) titer is markedly positive. Various imaging modalities demonstrate a normal extrahepatic biliary tree. The characteristic finding on liver biopsy of this patient is

(A) hepatocytes with ground-glass cytoplasm
(B) granulomatous destruction of bile ducts
(C) hepatocytes that demonstrate hepatitis B surface antigen (HBsAg) on immunohistochemical examination
(D) periportal hyaline globules representing α_1-antitrypsin
(E) prominent hepatocyte hemosiderin deposits

12. Which statement describes scleroderma?

(A) Immune complex deposition is extensive
(B) Dense lymphoid infiltrates are the dominant histopathologic change
(C) Vascular sclerosis with myxoid change is a common finding
(D) Fibrosis is found only in the skin
(E) A feature of chronic sclerodermatous renal pathology is fibrinoid necrosis of microvasculature

13. A 1-year-old child develops swelling of the left side of the face following a 1-week episode of diarrhea. Examination of the infant reveals a warm fluctuant mass just lateral and inferior to the ear. What would most likely be revealed by fine-needle aspiration?

(A) Pus
(B) Cells with epithelial lesions
(C) Granulomas
(D) Malignant cells

14. An 80-year-old diabetic patient presents with acute onset of right upper quadrant pain soon after a hypotensive episode. Abdominal ultrasound demonstrates an enlarged gallbladder with a thickened wall. Gallstones are not seen. At the time of cholecystectomy, a perforated gallbladder is found. Which of the following characteristics is most typical of a case of this type?

(A) Large gallstones are frequently missed on an abdominal ultrasound
(B) Gallbladder carcinoma often presents in this manner
(C) Acute acalculous cholecystitis is unlikely in this clinical setting
(D) The gallbladder is likely to show marked acute inflammation, ulceration, and necrosis
(E) The gallbladder is likely to show diffuse cholesterolosis

15. A 50-year-old Cambodian male immigrates to the United States 5 years before presenting to the emergency room with a chronic cough and night sweats. He is admitted and a chest x-ray shows apical infiltrates. Sputum analysis is unrevealing, but a transbronchial biopsy reveals granulomas with giant cells. The diagnosis is

(A) sarcoidosis
(B) berylliosis
(C) tuberculosis
(D) giant cell carcinoma
(E) pneumococcal pneumonia

16. Which feature characterizes acute nonspecific appendicitis?

(A) It primarily affects the elderly but can occur at any age
(B) *Enterobius vermicularis* infestation of the appendix is an important predisposing condition
(C) Luminal obstruction by fecaliths is found in two-thirds of cases
(D) Transmural chronic inflammation is a characteristic consequence
(E) Leukopenia is present

17. The coronary arteries in a failed heart allograft are likely to show

(A) fibrinoid necrosis indicating vascular rejection
(B) granulomatous arteritis indicating vascular rejection
(C) no change, because the coronary arteries are not a target for rejection
(D) transmural hemorrhage indicating vascular rejection
(E) a subintimal and focally transmural infiltrate of macrophages and lymphocytes indicating vascular rejection

18. Which feature is characteristic of acute cholecystitis?

(A) Male predominance
(B) Association with cholelithiasis in 20% to 30% of cases
(C) Gallbladder perforation in most cases
(D) An enlarged and discolored gallbladder
(E) A prominent infiltrate of lymphocytes and plasma cells

19. A 12-year-old boy complains of leg pain and swelling, and an x-ray of the affected limb shows the classic sign of Codman's triangle. What is the most likely diagnosis?

(A) Chondrosarcoma
(B) Osteomyelitis
(C) Osteosarcoma
(D) Multiple myeloma
(E) Aneurysmal bone cyst

Questions 20–21

A 40-year-old woman comes to her physician after noticing a lump in her breast. Physical examination reveals a 3-cm, firm, irregular mass in the lateral aspect of the right breast with dimpling of the overlying skin. A subsequent biopsy of this mass reveals chronic inflammation, necrotic adipose tissue with saponification, and areas of calcification.

20. These histologic findings are consistent with the diagnosis of

(A) comedocarcinoma
(B) fat necrosis
(C) duct ectasia
(D) granulomatous mastitis
(E) adenosis

21. What is the most likely history associated with this lesion?

(A) Nulliparity
(B) Estrogen therapy
(C) Breast-feeding
(D) Previous trauma
(E) Pulmonary tuberculosis

22. Which autoimmune disease is characterized by immune complex deposition in the skin, kidney, and lung?

(A) Systemic lupus erythematosus (SLE)
(B) Sjögren's syndrome
(C) Progressive scleroderma
(D) Graft versus host (GVH) disease
(E) CREST (i.e., calcinosis, Raynaud's phenomenon, esophageal dysfunction, syndactyly, and telangiectasia) syndrome

23. A 50-year-old white woman presents with a pigmented skin lesion of her arm. She states that she has had this "mole" all of her life, but it has been bothering her lately. Examination reveals a 0.5-cm pigmented nodule with an irregular border on one edge, a small area of crusting, and surrounding erythema. The differential diagnosis is traumatized nevocytic nevus versus malignant melanoma. Which histologic feature is the most useful in distinguishing between these two entities?

(A) Nests of melanocytes in the lower one-third of the dermis
(B) Epidermal hyperkeratosis
(C) Numerous mitoses
(D) Multinucleate giant cells
(E) Hair shafts surrounded by nevus cells

24. A 38-year-old man is injured in a head-on automobile collision. When he is brought to the emergency room, he is in shock, unconscious, and requires mechanical respiratory assistance. Despite efforts to save the patient, he dies. Neuropathologic examination on autopsy is most likely to disclose

(A) ruptured basilar artery aneurysm
(B) Duret's hemorrhages
(C) severed medulla oblongata
(D) cerebral infarct
(E) arteriovenous (AV) malformation

25. A 60-year-old man presents with complaints of double vision. Generalized muscle weakness and ptosis are noted on physical examination. A chest radiograph reveals a mass confined to the anterior mediastinum. The histology of the mass will most likely reveal

(A) malignant squamous cells
(B) benign epithelial cells admixed with lymphocytes
(C) Reed-Sternberg cells
(D) mature tissue from all three germ lines
(E) immature malignant cells

26. Which congenital defect of bilirubin metabolism is characterized by increased amounts of conjugated and unconjugated bilirubin in the serum and a black or gray discoloration of the liver due to pigment accumulation in the hepatocytes?

(A) Rotor's syndrome
(B) Crigler-Najjar syndrome, type I
(C) Dubin-Johnson syndrome
(D) Gilbert's syndrome
(E) Reye's syndrome

27. A renal allograft recipient presents with fever and adenopathy 3 months after engraftment. Serum studies show markedly elevated anti–Epstein-Barr virus (EBV) titers. A biopsy of the allograft is most likely to show

(A) fibrinoid necrosis of the small vessels
(B) vascular sclerosis
(C) interstitial fibrosis
(D) a dense lymphoplasmacytic interstitial infiltrate with cytologic atypia
(E) isometric vacuolar change in the tubular epithelial cells

28. A 62-year-old white man presents with a several-year history of heartburn. Upper endoscopy reveals red, velvety, fingerlike projections beginning in the region of the gastroesophageal junction and extending 5 cm into the esophagus. A biopsy reveals intestinal ("specialized")-type columnar epithelium. Which statement about this patient's disorder is true?

(A) This disorder complicates reflux esophagitis in about 10% of patients
(B) Squamous cell carcinoma (SCC) is the most important neoplastic complication of this disorder
(C) The morphologic features are typical of *Candida* esophagitis
(D) Ganglion cells within the myenteric plexus are absent
(E) Tracheoesophageal fistula (TEF) is a common complication

Questions 29–30

A 28-year-old man presents with a single descended testis and a 6-cm solid abdominal mass seen by computed tomography (CT).

29. The most likely diagnosis of the mass is

(A) metastatic prostate cancer
(B) hyperplastic cryptorchid testis
(C) teratoma
(D) adenomatoid tumor
(E) seminoma

30. Which one of the following statements is true regarding the treatment and prognosis of this tumor?

(A) Resection is not indicated
(B) The tumor is radiation sensitive
(C) There is a poor 5-year survival rate
(D) The patient can be followed clinically by measurement of serum levels of prostate-specific antigen
(E) There is no increased risk of malignancy in the descended testis

31. A 42-year-old man presents with acute thrombophlebitis in the leg. After symptomatic therapy and the administration of warfarin for several months, he remains healthy for 1 year. However, another episode of thrombophlebitis occurs—complicated by pulmonary embolism. Appropriate therapy is administered for the acute problems, but the most appropriate diagnostic approach includes

(A) a complete blood count (CBC), bone marrow biopsy, and scan of the liver and spleen
(B) a CBC and measurement of fibrin split products and prothrombin time (PT)
(C) a CBC, clotting factor assay, and abdominal computed tomography (CT) scan
(D) a clotting factor assay, intravenous pyelogram, and bone marrow biopsy
(E) a clotting factor assay, measurement of PT, and a venogram

32. A 16-month-old boy presents with a right-sided abdominal mass, which x-ray reveals to be a partially calcified tumor occupying most of the right abdomen. Microscopic examination of tumor tissue shows cells in rosette patterns. What is the most likely diagnosis?

(A) Wilms' tumor
(B) Hepatoblastoma
(C) Pancreatoblastoma
(D) Neuroblastoma
(E) Pancreatic islet cell tumor

33. A patient complains of nausea, vomiting, and decreased urinary output. Blood pressure is 180/110. Urinalysis shows hematuria and white blood cells (WBCs), but no bacteria. Cultures are negative. Serum creatinine is 3.0 mg/dl. Which pathologic finding can be expected from this patient's kidney?

(A) Nodular glomerulosclerosis
(B) Cellular crescent formation
(C) Basement membrane "spikes"
(D) Positive tissue staining for Congo red
(E) Diffuse podocyte effacement

34. Which condition is most likely to respond to corticosteroid therapy?

(A) Acute vascular rejection
(B) Cyclosporine nephrotoxicity
(C) Acute cellular rejection
(D) "Harvest injury"
(E) Recurrent glomerulosclerosis

35. An adolescent presents with lassitude, jaundice, fever, hypersplenism, and Kayser-Fleischer rings. Which disorder is most likely?

(A) Alpha$_1$-antitrypsin deficiency
(B) Wilson's disease
(C) Hepatitis B infection
(D) Gilbert's syndrome
(E) Genetic hemochromatosis

36. Cytologic examination of a pleural effusion in a 60-year-old man reveals the presence of malignant cells. The most likely primary cancer to be found in this man is

(A) lymphoma
(B) mesothelioma
(C) carcinoma of the colon
(D) carcinoma of the lung
(E) carcinoma of the pancreas

37. A 50-year-old woman complains of pain inside her right cheek and lower lip. Examination reveals multiple white patches of the oral mucosa that can be scraped away, revealing shallow ulcers. Smears of the scrapings from the ulcers fail to reveal viral cellular changes or fungi. These lesions are best described as

(A) ranulas
(B) epulides
(C) leukoplakia
(D) aphthous stomatitis
(E) monilial stomatitis

38. Which statement accurately describes the etiologic agents of viral hepatitis?

(A) Hepatitis B virus (HBV) is the most common cause of post-transfusion hepatitis
(B) Hepatitis D virus (HDV; delta agent) requires help from HBV in order to infect humans
(C) Hepatitis C virus (HCV) is the most common cause of sporadic cases of hepatitis
(D) The genome of HBV is predominantly double-stranded RNA
(E) Chronic hepatitis A develops in 10% to 20% of patients acutely infected with the virus

39. Which statement about Kaposi's sarcoma is true?

(A) The classic form is common in women
(B) Noncutaneous manifestations are common in patients with acquired immune deficiency syndrome (AIDS)
(C) The histology of the different clinical forms varies
(D) Stopping immunosuppressive therapy has no effect on Kaposi's sarcoma in renal transplant cases
(E) The AIDS virus has been shown to cause Kaposi's sarcoma

40. A 32-year-old, previously healthy woman reports a swelling at the angle of her left jaw. Although she has had the condition for 2 months, the mass has not changed in size and is not associated with pain. Physical examination discloses a firm, solitary, 1 × 2-cm mass but no other abnormalities. The most likely diagnosis is

(A) Warthin's tumor
(B) Sjögren's syndrome
(C) malignant mixed tumor (MMT)
(D) parotid sialolithiasis
(E) pleomorphic adenoma

41. A child presents with nephrotic syndrome after a viral illness. Which pathology can be expected?

(A) Diffuse effacement of the visceral epithelial podocytes
(B) About 50% crescent formation
(C) Nodular glomerulosclerosis
(D) Basement membrane spikes
(E) Linear deposition of IgG on the glomerular basement membrane (GBM)

42. A 60-year-old woman with a history of breast carcinoma that had been treated with surgical excision, radiation, and chemotherapy 2 years ago is undergoing routine follow-up. Although she is asymptomatic, her hemoglobin concentration is 8.7 g/dl and hematocrit is 27%. The most likely explanation is

(A) iron deficiency anemia
(B) chemotherapy-induced marrow injury
(C) acute leukemia
(D) metastatic breast cancer
(E) inadequate data are given for a conclusion

43. The most important prognostic factor for human cancer is

(A) tumor grade
(B) tumor stage
(C) lymphocytic infiltration
(D) vascular invasion
(E) mitotic index

44. A gastric carcinoma that metastasizes to the ovary is most likely to be referred to as a

(A) Brenner tumor
(B) Wilms' tumor
(C) Klatskin's tumor
(D) Krukenberg's tumor
(E) Grawitz's tumor

45. A 56-year-old woman has a recurrent myxoid liposarcoma of the upper thigh and inguinal region. The most effective therapy for this patient would be

(A) local excision
(B) local excision and regional lymphadenectomy
(C) hemipelvectomy
(D) localized radiation
(E) chemotherapy with adriamycin

46. A 60-year-old, cachectic, alcoholic patient is found to have bilateral painless enlargement of the parotid glands. The most likely diagnosis is

(A) Sjögren's syndrome
(B) sialadenosis
(C) sialolithiasis
(D) pleomorphic adenoma

47. A 57-year-old man develops swelling and tenderness in his left calf 7 days after undergoing colectomy for colon cancer. He develops acute shortness of breath. A chest x-ray is normal. Which one of the following pathologic descriptions is most likely?

(A) Myocardial hypertrophy and chamber dilatation
(B) Myocardial infarction
(C) Lymphocytic interstitial pneumonitis
(D) Recent pulmonary embolus

48. A 45-year-old woman complains that for 6 months she has experienced increasingly severe headaches associated with right arm weakness and an unsteady gait. Evaluation and subsequent surgery disclose a lesion in the left occipital area, which pathologic examination shows to be a meningioma. The major prognostic determinant in this case is

(A) the histologic subtype of the meningioma
(B) the mitotic index of the tumor
(C) the completeness of surgical removal
(D) tumor vascularity
(E) the patient's amenability to radiation therapy

49. Which one of the following primary hepatic tumors is the most common?

(A) Hepatocellular carcinoma
(B) Angiosarcoma
(C) Cholangiocarcinoma
(D) Cavernous hemangioma
(E) Focal nodular hyperplasia

50. A 6-month-old infant presents with jaundice. The clinical workup includes an abdominal ultrasound followed by endoscopic retrograde cholangiopancreatography (ERCP), which demonstrates diffuse fusiform dilatation of the common bile duct. Which of the following statements best characterizes this patient's condition?

(A) It is more common in males
(B) Patients usually present in adulthood
(C) Cholelithiasis is responsible for this disorder
(D) Adenocarcinoma is not a recognized complication of this disorder
(E) An anomalous pancreaticobiliary union is found in up to 90% of cases

51. A 35-year-old man has been treated for acute bronchopneumonia and appears to be getting better on antibiotics. However, the physician notices a medical student's note in the chart stating that the patient works in a ceramic factory. The next step is to

(A) ask if the factory is old and has asbestos in it
(B) ask if the patient has been taking steroid hormones
(C) reorder a chest x-ray to look for cavitation
(D) perform a skin test for beryllium
(E) ask the patient if he has ever been a coal miner

52. A renal allograft recipient fails to produce urine in the first 48 hours after engraftment. Imaging studies reveal that the allograft is normal size. The graft is well matched. A biopsy is performed and shows needle-shaped crystals within vascular lumens. What is the most likely diagnosis?

(A) Hyperacute rejection
(B) "Harvest injury"
(C) Preexisting atheroembolic disease
(D) Acute cellular rejection
(E) Acute vascular rejection

Questions 53–54

A 35-year-old multiparous woman in the first trimester of a new pregnancy experiences an abnormally rapid increase in uterine size and has an abnormally high serum human chorionic gonadotropin (hCG) level.

53. This clinical history is most compatible with which of the following disorders?

(A) Ectopic pregnancy
(B) Placenta accreta
(C) Leiomyomas
(D) Hydatidiform mole
(E) Chorioangioma

54. Which of the following disorders is a well-known complication of this disease process?

(A) Rupture of the fallopian tube
(B) Leiomyosarcoma
(C) Pseudomyxoma peritonei
(D) Endometrial polyps
(E) Choriocarcinoma

55. The following results are from an adult man's urinalysis—white blood cells, none; red blood cells (RBCs): none; bacteria: none; specific gravity: 1.015; protein: 4 + ; oval fat bodies: present. Which pathological changes can be expected in this patient's kidney?

(A) Cellular crescents
(B) Glomerular necrosis
(C) Basement membrane spikes
(D) Glomerular capillary loop breaks
(E) Vasculitis

56. A 37-year-old white woman comes to a surgeon for a breast biopsy because of a suspicious mammogram. She has had mammograms annually for 5 years. A breast biopsy 3 years ago showed a fibroadenoma and fibrocystic changes, with florid epithelial hyperplasia. When questioned about her relevant family history, she stated that her mother had died of a malignant cystosarcoma phylloides tumor, and that her son had gynecomastia, which was discovered during a physical examination for school sports. Her current breast biopsy reveals lobular carcinoma in situ. Which factor most increases her risk of breast cancer?

(A) Her previous fibroadenoma

(B) Her previous epithelial hyperplasia

(C) Her son's gynecomastia

(D) Her five mammogram exposures

(E) Her age

57. A 32-year-old woman presents with rectal bleeding. Workup includes a barium enema followed by colonoscopy. Both procedures demonstrate numerous polyps carpeting the entire colorectum. Biopsy of one of these reveals a tubular adenoma. A 3-cm mass located in the sigmoid colon is also biopsied, revealing invasive adenocarcinoma. Which statement correctly characterizes this patient's disorder?

(A) It is inherited as an autosomal recessive trait

(B) Adenocarcinoma is usually detected by the second decade

(C) The genetic locus for this disease has been mapped to the short arm of chromosome 14 (14p)

(D) This patient's disorder serves as a model for the adenoma–carcinoma sequence of colorectal carcinoma

(E) Extracolonic adenomas are not found in this disorder

58. A 30-year-old epileptic patient complains that his gums bleed after he brushes his teeth. Gingival hyperplasia is found. The most likely etiology is

(A) epulis

(B) a drug side effect

(C) repeated trauma during seizures

(D) an idiopathic condition associated with epilepsy

59. A 49-year-old man presents with delirium tremens from alcohol withdrawal. Routine blood work reveals that the patient is anemic, with a hemoglobin count of 9 g/dl, a mean corpuscular volume (MCV) of 106 μm^3 (normal = 85–100 μm^3), and a mean corpuscular hemoglobin (MCH) of 34 pg (normal = 28–31 pg). Which one of the following deficiencies is the most likely etiology for this anemia?

(A) Folate

(B) Vitamin D

(C) Vitamin K

(D) Niacin

60. A 16-year-old boy presents with symptoms of nasal obstruction and recurrent epistaxis. Examination reveals a firm, smooth, red–purple polyp in the nasopharynx. An attempted biopsy of the lesion results in uncontrolled bleeding requiring transfusion and emergency surgery. The most likely diagnosis is

(A) verrucous carcinoma

(B) lymphoepithelioma

(C) angiofibroma

(D) nasal polyp

61. A 70-year-old asymptomatic man is found to have bilateral inguinal hernias. At operation for hernia repair, an enlarged lymph node is removed. Pathologic evaluation discloses a metastatic adenocarcinoma. The primary site of such a tumor can best be determined by

(A) barium enema

(B) exploratory laparotomy

(C) immunoperoxidase (IP) localization of specific tumor markers

(D) computed tomography (CT) of the pelvis

(E) electron microscopic (EM) examination of the node

62. Acoustic neuroma is most likely to be found in which of the following patients?

(A) A 16-year-old boy with type III multiple endocrine neoplasia (MEN)

(B) A 49-year-old woman with pigmented macules of the axillary skin

(C) A 28-year-old man with malignant melanoma of the scalp

(D) A 46-year-old woman who received radiation for pituitary adenoma

(E) A 3-month-old boy with ventricular septal defect

63. A child presents with a brief history of upper respiratory infection with rhinorrhea and fever, which has progressed in the last day or two to spiking high fevers and coma. To help in making the diagnosis, the physician should ask the mother whether the child

(A) has been given phenacetin
(B) has ingested Sterno
(C) has been given aspirin during the first part of his illness
(D) is allergic to penicillin
(E) is hyperactive and is taking barbiturates

64. Which immunodeficiency disorder is characterized by a paucity of plasma cells?

(A) DiGeorge syndrome
(B) Bruton's agammaglobulinemia
(C) Chronic mucocutaneous candidiasis
(D) Acquired immunodeficiency syndrome (AIDS)
(E) Immunoglobulin A (IgA) deficiency

65. Synovial sarcoma is most likely to occur in which site?

(A) Head and neck
(B) Knees
(C) Hands
(D) Spine
(E) Shoulders

66. A 14-year-old boy who has difficulty breathing is brought to the emergency room. Examination discloses moderate respiratory distress, a fever of 39°C, and skin pallor. His white blood count (WBC) is 100,000, with 95% lymphoblasts. To evaluate his respiratory distress, a chest x-ray is taken. This film most likely shows

(A) right lower lobe pneumonia
(B) bilateral pleural effusion
(C) cardiomegaly
(D) a mediastinal mass
(E) diffuse pulmonary fibrosis

Questions 67–69

A 19-year-old woman comes to the emergency room with fever and abdominal pain. Examination of the abdomen is limited due to rigidity of the abdominal muscles. Vaginal examination reveals a purulent cervical discharge; bimanual examination of the uterus and adnexa elicits pain.

67. Which of the following diagnostic tests and procedures is most helpful in ruling out an ectopic pregnancy?

(A) Bacterial culture
(B) Serum human chorionic gonadotropin (hCG) measurement
(C) Abdominal ultrasound
(D) Laparoscopy
(E) Endometrial biopsy

68. One month later the same patient again experiences lower abdominal pain. An adnexal mass is discovered during examination. All of the following are likely diagnoses in this clinical setting EXCEPT

(A) tuboovarian abscess
(B) pyosalpinx
(C) hydrosalpinx
(D) ectopic pregnancy
(E) metastatic carcinoma to the ovary

69. Which of the following conditions is a possible long-term consequence of pelvic inflammatory disease (PID)?

(A) Endometriosis
(B) Choriocarcinoma
(C) Eclampsia
(D) Polycystic ovarian syndrome
(E) Infertility

Questions 70–71

A 70-year-old man presents with a history of fevers, night sweats, headache, and facial flushing. Physical examination reveals cyanosis of the face and neck and distended, tortuous, superficial veins over the neck and anterior chest wall. A computed tomography (CT) scan of the thorax reveals an ill-defined solid mass involving the anterior and superior mediastinum.

70. The findings of the physical examination are most likely due to

(A) a paraneoplastic syndrome
(B) heart failure
(C) compression of the superior vena cava
(D) rupture of the esophagus
(E) pulmonary obstruction

71. Possible etiologies of the mass include all of the following EXCEPT

(A) a fungal infection
(B) a granulomatous inflammation
(C) idiopathic fibrosis
(D) an enteric cyst
(E) a malignant tumor

Questions 72–74

A 70-year-old man with a 50-year history of cigarette smoking presents with a productive cough, dyspnea, and cyanosis. An increased chest diameter, decreased respiratory excursion, and end-expiratory wheezes are found during physical examination. No masses are seen on chest radiograph.

72. Cigarette smoke contributes to the pathogenesis of this pulmonary disorder by

(A) reducing α_1-antitrypsin gene transcription
(B) causing pulmonary basement membrane hyalinization
(C) inducing destruction of interalveolar septa
(D) reducing mucus production
(E) causing desquamative interstitial pneumonitis

73. Additional physical findings of hepatomegaly and peripheral edema suggest cor pulmonale. An expected related finding would be

(A) pulmonary veno-occlusive disease
(B) pulmonary arterial hypertension
(C) diffuse alveolar damage
(D) bronchopulmonary dysplasia
(E) pulmonary embolism

74. The expiratory wheezes heard on the chest auscultation may be contributed to by all of the following EXCEPT

(A) interalveolar septal destruction
(B) loss of lung tissue elasticity
(C) chronic bronchiolitis
(D) anthracosis
(E) goblet cell hyperplasia

Questions 75–76

A 60-year-old woman presents with bleeding esophageal varices. Physical examination reveals palmar erythema, caput medusae, and massive ascites. Laboratory data reveals clotting abnormalities and hypoalbuminemia. The patient had a blood transfusion 10 years ago. Serologic studies reveal the following: anti-hepatitis C virus (anti-HCV), positive; anti-hepatitis B surface antigen (anti-HBsAg), negative; HBsAg, negative; anti-hepatitis A virus (anti-HAV) immunoglobulin G (IgG), positive; anti-HAV IgM, negative.

75. Which one of the following statements is NOT true?

(A) Sequelae from blood transfusion-related hepatitis A virus (HAV) infection is most likely responsible for this patient's clinical presentation
(B) Hypoalbuminemia and clotting abnormalities are common findings in patients with cirrhosis
(C) This patient has clinical evidence of portal hypertension
(D) Liver transplantation is a treatment option for this patient

76. All of the following mechanisms would be likely to be causally related to the patient's ascites EXCEPT

(A) sinusoidal vascular blockade related to underlying cirrhosis
(B) posthepatic vascular blockade related to hepatocellular carcinoma
(C) prehepatic vascular blockade related to portal venous thrombosis
(D) postsinusoidal vascular blockade related to underlying cirrhosis
(E) hypoalbuminemia

77. All of the following statements about iron deficiency anemia are true EXCEPT

(A) a hypochromic anemia is present
(B) the cause may be a cecal adenocarcinoma
(C) the serum iron concentration is low
(D) the serum iron-binding capacity is high
(E) the red cells are larger than normal (macrocytic)

78. Hypertension is found in all of the following endocrine disorders EXCEPT

(A) Cushing's syndrome
(B) pheochromocytoma
(C) adrenal medullary hyperplasia
(D) Addison's disease
(E) Conn's syndrome

79. Acute rejection in lung allografts includes all of the following pathologic features EXCEPT

(A) fibrosing obliteration of respiratory bronchioles
(B) perivascular lymphocytic infiltrate
(C) interstitial and alveolar lymphocytic and neutrophilic inflammation
(D) lymphocytic bronchitis
(E) hemorrhagic necrosis and hyaline membrane formation

80. All of the following features are characteristic of atherosclerosis EXCEPT

(A) fatty streaks
(B) cholesterol clefts
(C) hemorrhage
(D) medial granulomas
(E) lymphocytic inflammation

81. Psoriasis is associated with all of the following features EXCEPT

(A) intracytoplasmic inclusions
(B) increased epithelial cell turnover
(C) easy bleeding of skin patches
(D) activation of the complement system
(E) arthritis

82. Complications of acute myocardial infarction include all of the following EXCEPT

(A) fibrinous pericarditis
(B) aortic aneurysms
(C) mural thrombi
(D) cardiac arrhythmia
(E) cardiogenic shock

83. Acquired immune deficiency syndrome (AIDS) patients have an increased susceptibility to all of the following diseases EXCEPT

(A) cytomegalovirus (CMV) infection
(B) Kaposi's sarcoma
(C) lymphoma
(D) pneumococcal pneumonia
(E) mycobacterial infection

84. A 55-year-old man presents with a 1-cm exophytic mass on the prepuce of his penis. The differential diagnosis is condyloma acuminatum versus squamous cell carcinoma. Each of the following clinical features favors the diagnosis of carcinoma EXCEPT

(A) focal ulceration of the lesion
(B) the presence of smegma
(C) elicitation of pain with palpation of the lesion
(D) a firm 2-cm mass in the left inguinal region
(E) multiple lung masses on a chest radiograph

85. True statements concerning tissue repair by granulation tissue formation include all of the following EXCEPT

(A) a wound left open is called secondary healing
(B) granulomas can develop at the site
(C) the body can repair most fistula tracts
(D) granulation tissue formation begins while inflammation is ongoing
(E) a keloid may form

86. All of the following statements about aneurysms are true EXCEPT

(A) syphilitic aneurysms usually occur in the thoracic aorta
(B) berry aneurysms are common in small cerebral arteries
(C) atherosclerotic aneurysms often occur in the abdominal aorta
(D) fusiform aneurysms are balloon-shaped arterial dilatations
(E) cirsoid aneurysms are aneurysmic arteriovenous fistulas

87. A 40-year-old man comes to the physician complaining of a bumpy and nodular irregular masslike lesion of the palm of the hand, which prevents him from fully opening his hand. It would be appropriate for the physician to tell this patient all of the following EXCEPT

(A) it is a classic presentation
(B) surgery will be curative
(C) it is not malignant
(D) it is a type of proliferative scarring process
(E) it is called Dupuytren's contracture

88. Possible autopsy findings in the heart of a patient who died from complications of long-standing hypertension include all of the following EXCEPT

(A) concentric left ventricular hypertrophy
(B) papillary muscle hypertrophy
(C) cardiomegaly
(D) endocardial fibrous thickening
(E) floppy mitral valve

89. All of the following statements about diabetic glomerulosclerosis are true EXCEPT

(A) diabetic glomerulosclerosis is consistently associated with urinary protein loss
(B) diabetic glomerulosclerosis is morphologically characterized by nodular intercapillary sclerosis
(C) diabetic glomerulosclerosis is associated with hematuria
(D) diabetic glomerulosclerosis is usually associated with vasculopathy at other sites such as the retina
(E) early diabetic glomerulosclerosis is morphologically characterized by diffuse glomerular basement membrane (GBM) thickening

90. All of the following findings are associated with varicose veins EXCEPT

(A) cystic medial necrosis
(B) intraluminal thrombosis
(C) portal hypertension induced by liver cirrhosis
(D) hemorrhoids
(E) stasis dermatitis

91. Disorders characterized by granulomatous inflammation include all of the following EXCEPT

(A) cat-scratch disease
(B) tuberculosis
(C) syphilis
(D) sarcoidosis
(E) staphylococcal abscess

92. An 8-year-old girl has a 3-month history of intermittent right lower quadrant pain. Two previous visits to the emergency room have ruled out acute appendicitis. At this visit, a mass is palpated in the lower abdomen. The differential diagnosis includes all of the following conditions EXCEPT

(A) periappendiceal abscess
(B) Burkitt's lymphoma
(C) Crohn's disease (CD)
(D) ovarian germ cell tumor
(E) Hodgkin's disease

93. A 60-year-old man presents with a right facial nerve palsy and a newly noted swelling of his right cheek. A biopsy reveals adenoid cystic carcinoma. All of the following statements are true EXCEPT

(A) recurrence of the tumor following surgical excision is common
(B) facial nerve involvement is a common finding with these tumors
(C) the passage of 5 years with no evidence of recurrent tumor indicates an excellent prognosis
(D) a chest x-ray is indicated

94. All of the following statements concerning the nuclear characteristic of tumors, as determined by DNA flow cytometry, are true EXCEPT

(A) a diploid lesion can be benign or malignant
(B) an aneuploid tumor is a malignant tumor
(C) a malignant tumor can be diploid
(D) reactive lesions should be diploid

95. The prognosis for a patient with sarcoma is related to all of the following EXCEPT

(A) size
(B) stage
(C) grade
(D) depth in the tissues
(E) tumor duration before diagnosis

96. Radiation, in one form or another, is linked to all of the following cancers EXCEPT

(A) squamous cancers of skin
(B) ovarian cancer
(C) thyroid cancer
(D) sarcoma
(E) melanoma

97. All of the following statements regarding acute myocardial infarction are true EXCEPT

(A) most myocardial infarctions are transmural
(B) myocardial infarctions usually involve the left ventricle
(C) subendocardial infarctions usually are circumferential
(D) histologic evidence is seen first at about 24 hours postinfarction
(E) the most sensitive marker within 48 to 72 hours postinfarction is an elevation of the MB isoenzyme of creatine kinase (CK)

98. All of the following statements about lupus nephritis are true EXCEPT

(A) it occurs more frequently in women than in men
(B) variable morphology is the rule
(C) glomerular immune complex deposition is common
(D) autoantibodies to glomerular basement membrane (GBM) are common
(E) clinical evidence for renal involvement often develops

99. Sickle cell disease results in all of the following complications EXCEPT

(A) leg ulcers
(B) spleen infarction
(C) cholelithiasis
(D) pancreatitis
(E) osteomyelitis

100. All of the following statements about malignant fibrous histiocytoma (MFH) are true EXCEPT

(A) it is a deep tumor
(B) it is the most common adult sarcoma
(C) it typically is made up of very bizarre cells
(D) it is also called fibrosarcoma
(E) it is the most common tumor of the thigh

101. All of the following statements concerning radiation are true EXCEPT

(A) the marrow and lymphoid system are the most radiosensitive tissues of the body
(B) a testicular germ cell tumor may be cured by radiotherapy
(C) a dose of 1000 rad of total body radiation would kill all members of an exposed population
(D) postradiation sarcomas may develop after a 20-year interval
(E) cartilage and muscle tissue are relatively radiosensitive

102. Chronic renal allograft rejection involves all of the following EXCEPT

(A) vascular sclerosis
(B) interstitial fibrosis
(C) tubular atrophy
(D) glomerulosclerosis
(E) tubulitis

103. The physician is asked to determine if a young child with chronic respiratory problems has bronchopulmonary dysplasia or congenital adenomatoid malformation. Which of the following is the LEAST helpful in distinguishing between these two entities?

(A) Clinical history
(B) Chest x-ray
(C) Arteriography
(D) Open lung biopsy

104. All of the following statements about oncogenes are thought to be true EXCEPT

(A) quantitative change can be brought about by carcinogenic influence
(B) qualitative change can be brought about by carcinogenic influence
(C) eukaryotic cells contain v-*oncs* and c-*oncs*
(D) oncogenes represent viral DNA
(E) oncogenes appear to code for growth factor receptors

105. All of the following are characteristic of arteriolosclerosis EXCEPT

(A) proliferative thickening of the arteriole wall
(B) association with clinical hypertension
(C) necrosis of the arteriole wall in severe cases
(D) association with diabetes
(E) deposition of amyloid fibrils in the arteriole wall

106. All of the following statements regarding mononuclear phagocytes are true EXCEPT

(A) they generally are fixed cells with little propensity for circulation
(B) they produce growth factors for fibroblasts, myeloid precursors, and endothelial cells
(C) they produce interleukin-1 (IL-1), which acts as an endogenous pyrogen
(D) they normally express major histocompatibility complex (MHC) class II antigens
(E) they are important in antigen presentation

107. A 40-year-old woman presents with bilateral joint pain in her hands. Physical examination reveals symmetric swelling and warmth of the metacarpophalangeal joints. Blood tests reveal a positive rheumatoid factor (RF). The patient is at risk for all of the following conditions EXCEPT

(A) urolithiasis
(B) recurrent fever
(C) amyloidosis
(D) pericarditis
(E) ankylosis

108. Hypopituitarism may be produced by all of the following conditions EXCEPT

(A) pituitary irradiation
(B) chromophobe adenoma
(C) Sheehan's syndrome
(D) basophil adenoma
(E) breast cancer

109. If a bone marrow aspirate or biopsy shows erythroid hyperplasia, suspected causes of an anemia would include all of the following EXCEPT

(A) chronic hemorrhage (e.g., gastric ulcer)
(B) autoimmune hemolytic anemia
(C) hereditary spherocytosis
(D) aplastic anemia
(E) anemia of Hodgkin's disease

Questions 110–111

A 40-year-old black woman comes to the emergency room. She has a 2-year history of congestive heart failure. A murmur characteristic of severe mitral stenosis is heard. Her medical history reveals that at 10 years of age, she developed a severe illness characterized by fever; congestive heart failure; painful, warm joints; and a movement disorder (chorea) 2 weeks after the onset of a severe sore throat.

110. Which one of the following statements about this patient's condition is FALSE?

(A) Her sore throat most likely was caused by infection with group A β-hemolytic streptococci
(B) Her mitral valve is likely to be quite fibrotic and deformed, with fused commissures
(C) Her left atrium is likely to be quite large
(D) The incidence of this patient's disorder has increased dramatically in the United States and Western Europe in the last several decades
(E) The Aschoff body is the classic histologic feature of her childhood illness

Three years later, the patient returns to the emergency room in congestive heart failure. At this time, she is found to have a spiking fever to 40°C and a changing cardiac murmur. Blood cultures grow α-hemolytic (viridans) streptococci. A diagnosis of endocarditis is made. The patient's clinical course includes the development of a right hemiparesis.

111. Which one of the following statements regarding the patient's clinical course is FALSE?

(A) Infective endocarditis is a well recognized complication of chronic rheumatic heart disease
(B) Infection with α-hemolytic (viridans) streptococci is an uncommon cause of endocarditis in patients with damaged heart valves
(C) The patient's right hemiparesis most likely resulted from emboli arising from an infected mitral valve
(D) The valvular vegetations contain fibrin, neutrophils, and gram-positive cocci
(E) The mitral valve is a likely site for the infected vegetations

112. Soft tissue lesions have important features that can be seen grossly or microscopically. All of the following statements about these lesions are true EXCEPT

(A) infiltration of surrounding structures does not necessarily imply sarcoma

(B) encapsulation may be seen in a sarcoma on gross examination

(C) a benign tumor typically shows necrosis

(D) size is an important prognostic feature in a sarcoma

(E) Sarcomas have a very poor prognosis

113. All of the following statements about renal cell carcinoma are true EXCEPT

(A) patients may present with hematuria

(B) lungs and brain are common sites for metastasis

(C) metastatic spread is principally via the bloodstream

(D) peak incidence is in the sixth decade of life

(E) the ratio of men to women with renal cell carcinoma is 1:2

114. True statements about multiple myeloma include all of the following EXCEPT

(A) it may affect several bones simultaneously

(B) it produces abnormal serum protein electrophoresis

(C) it occurs commonly in the young adult

(D) it is not a true bone neoplasm

(E) it produces excessive amounts of immunoglobulins

115. All of the following are features of temporal arteritis EXCEPT

(A) headache pain

(B) intermittent claudication of the jaw muscles

(C) bitter taste sensation

(D) visual disturbances

(E) low-grade fever

116. Usual T-cell functions include all of the following EXCEPT

(A) direct cytolysis

(B) promotion of B-cell activities

(C) suppression of T-cell activities

(D) antigen presentation

(E) lymphokine production

Directions: Each group of items in this section consists of lettered options followed by a set of numbered items. For each item, select the **one** lettered option that is most closely associated with it. Each lettered option may be selected once, more than once, or not at all.

Questions 117–119

Match each clinical history to the most likely diagnosis.

(A) Vitamin A deficiency
(B) Vitamin C deficiency
(C) Vitamin D deficiency
(D) Hyperparathyroidism
(E) Steroid-induced osteopenia

117. A 35-year-old woman with a pathologic fracture of the femur, a tumor of the mandible, and electrocardiographic (ECG) changes

118. A 7-year-old boy with joint pain, bowing of the legs, and swelling of the osteochrondral junctions

119. A 60-year-old woman with a pathologic hip fracture and subsequent biopsy showing abundant uncalcified osteoid cartilage

Questions 120–124

Match each disorder with the associated vitamin lack or excess.

(A) Vitamin A
(B) Vitamin B_{12}
(C) Vitamin C
(D) Vitamin D
(E) Niacin

120. Subacute combined degeneration of the spinal cord

121. Rickets

122. Scurvy

123. Xerophthalmia

124. Megaloblastic anemia

Questions 125–129

Match each symptom complex with the appropriate eponym.

(A) Sheehan's syndrome
(B) Schmidt's syndrome
(C) Sipple's syndrome
(D) Wermer's syndrome
(E) Zollinger-Ellison syndrome

125. Hypothyroidism and hypoadrenalism

126. Hyperparathyroidism and hypoglycemia

127. Gastrointestinal ulcers

128. Postpartum pituitary failure

129. Familial medullary carcinoma of the thyroid

Questions 130–134

For each tumor listed below, select the purported causative agent.

(A) Dietary fat
(B) Vinyl chloride
(C) Asbestos
(D) Cigarette smoking
(E) Cyclamates

130. Angiosarcoma of the liver

131. Transitional cell carcinoma of the bladder

132. Carcinoma of the colon

133. Mesothelioma

134. Carcinoma of the lung

Questions 135–139

Match each immune cell function to the specific type of cell that performs it.

(A) Macrophage
(B) T lympocyte
(C) B lymphocyte
(D) Killer (K) cell
(E) Natural killer (NK) cell

135. Antibody-dependent cytotoxicity

136. Antigen presentation

137. Spontaneous destruction of tumor cells

138. Production of immunoglobulins

139. Production of lymphokines

Questions 140–144

For each type of sarcoma that follows, select the tissue that it recapitulates.

(A) Endothelium
(B) Adipose tissue
(C) Connective tissue
(D) Skeletal muscle
(E) Schwann cell

140. Rhabdomyosarcoma

141. Neurofibrosarcoma

142. Angiosarcoma

143. Liposarcoma

144. Fibrosarcoma

Questions 145–149

Match each ultrastructural finding with the tumor type that is most likely to demonstrate it.

(A) Carcinoid tumor
(B) Rhabdomyosarcoma
(C) Melanoma
(D) Adenocarcinoma
(E) Squamous cell cancer (SCC)

145. Elongated granules

146. Dense core neurosecretory granules

147. Microvilli

148. Tonofilaments

149. Z-bands

Questions 150–153

Match each histologic appearance of the small bowel mucosa with the malabsorptive disorder it characterizes.

(A) Disaccharidase deficiency
(B) Whipple's disease
(C) Celiac disease
(D) Short bowel syndrome
(E) Crohn's disease (CD)

150. Foamy macrophages containing periodic acid–Schiff (PAS)-positive cytoplasmic granules in the lamina propria

151. Normal appearance on small bowel biopsy

152. Mucosal ulceration with cryptitis, crypt abscesses, and granulomas

153. Villous atrophy with crypt hyperplasia

Questions 154–158

For each clinical or pathologic characteristic, select the most closely associated type of leukemia.

(A) Chronic myelogenous leukemia (CML)
(B) Acute myelogenous leukemia (AML)
(C) Acute promyelocytic leukemia
(D) Erythroleukemia
(E) Chronic lymphocytic leukemia (CLL)

154. Bleeding diathesis

155. Philadelphia chromosome

156. Absolute lymphocytosis

157. Thickened gums

158. Mature B-cell origin

Questions 159–163

Match each pathologic feature to the associated pancreatic disorder.

(A) Annular pancreas
(B) Pancreatic pseudocyst
(C) Acute pancreatitis
(D) Chronic pancreatitis
(E) Pancreatic carcinoma

159. Fat and parenchymal necrosis

160. Fibrosis and ductal calcifications

161. Amylase-rich fluid

162. Perineural invasion

163. Duodenal stenosis

Questions 164–168

Match each description of a skin lesion with the name of the lesion.

(A) Macule
(B) Papule
(C) Nodule
(D) Wheal
(E) Vesicle

164. A circumscribed, flat area of skin distinguished by color from the surrounding skin

165. A palpable, solid, round or ellipsoid lesion situated deep in the skin or in the subcutaneous tissue

166. A well-circumscribed solid elevation of the skin

167. A small, circumscribed elevation of the skin containing serum or other fluid

168. A short-lived, circumscribed area of elevated skin produced by focal edema of the upper dermis

Questions 169–172

Match each clinical or pathologic feature with the heart disease it best characterizes.

(A) Coarctation of the aorta
(B) Tetralogy of Fallot
(C) Mitral valve prolapse
(D) Angina pectoris
(E) Atrial myxoma

169. Changing cardiac murmur

170. Normal myocardium or foci of fibrosis

171. Permanent right-to-left shunt

172. Redundant valve

Questions 173–177

For each clinical history, select the central nervous system (CNS) lesion that is most likely to be responsible.

(A) Progressive multifocal leukodystrophy
(B) Malignant lymphoma
(C) Ependymoma
(D) Meningioma
(E) Glioblastoma multiforme

173. A 4-year-old boy with papilledema and headache

174. A 20-year-old man with Hodgkin's disease who develops blindness and aphasia

175. A 52-year-old man with severe headache, double vision, and seizures that have developed over a period of 2 months.

176. A 22-year-old renal transplant patient with a recent onset of visual disturbances and left-sided weakness

177. A 40-year-old woman with gradually increasing headaches and right-sided weakness

Questions 178–182

For each tumor listed below, select the etiologically related agent.

(A) External irradiation
(B) Ultraviolet light
(C) Human papillomavirus (HPV)
(D) Epstein-Barr virus (EBV)
(E) Estrogen

178. Papillary carcinoma of the thyroid

179. Squamous cell carcinoma (SCC) of the cervix

180. Burkitt's lymphoma

181. Clear cell carcinoma of the vagina

182. Malignant melanoma

Questions 183–187

Match each pathologic feature to the associated biliary tract disorder.

(A) Rokitansky-Aschoff sinus
(B) Porcelain gallbladder
(C) Hydrops of the gallbladder
(D) Cholesterol polyp
(E) Primary sclerosing cholangitis

183. Fibrotic, strictured bile duct

184. Foamy, lipid-laden macrophages in the lamina propria

185. Diverticulum-like invaginations of epithelium into and beyond the smooth muscle layer

186. Mural calcification and fibrosis

187. Distended viscus containing cloudy or mucoid fluid

Questions 188–190

For each disease or condition listed, select the bleeding disorder that is most closely associated with it.

(A) Bleeding diathesis
(B) Decreased factor VIII
(C) Both
(D) Neither

188. von Willebrand's disease

189. Hemophilia A

190. Vitamin K deficiency

ANSWERS AND EXPLANATIONS

1. The answer is E *[Chapter 14 III D 3 c].*
This patient's history of abdominal pain and weight loss is suggestive of pancreatic cancer. The least invasive technique that is likely to yield the most diagnostic information is computed tomography (CT), which can detect small mass lesions with great accuracy. The diagnosis of chronic cholecystitis is unlikely in view of the relatively recent onset of symptoms and the marked weight loss. Carcinoma of the ampulla of Vater and the head of the pancreas would most likely produce clinical evidence of jaundice, which is not present in this patient.

2. The answer is B *[Chapter 7 IV A 1 a (2), 3 a].*
The pathologic description of the colonic biopsy is that of cytomegalovirus (CMV) colitis. Hemorrhagic necrosis related to cytomegalic change, with nuclear and cytoplasmic inclusions, is characteristic of CMV colitis. Superinfection with fungus, in particular, *Candida,* is common in CMV infection in immunocompromised patients.

3. The answer is C *[Chapter 22 III B 2].*
The lesions described are consistent with either benign papillomatosis or another neoplastic process. Since neoplasia is not a choice, the best answer is a viral etiology, reflecting the association between papillomatosis and human papillomavirus (HPV) infection. Bacterial and fungal infections do not usually form discrete papillary nodules, and such lesions are not associated with an autoimmune process.

4. The answer is B *[Chapter 13 II F 2].*
Leiomyoma (a benign stromal tumor), is the most common benign mesenchymal tumor of the stomach. These tumors vary in size from 1 to 20 cm; those larger than 3 cm often cause pain or bleeding. Tumors larger than 6 cm need to be extensively evaluated to rule out the possibility of malignancy (leiomyosarcoma, also called malignant stromal tumor). The tumors usually are intramural; some are attached to the muscularis propria by a thin pedicle and, thus, project into the omentum. Microscopically, they consist of spindle and epithelioid mesenchymal cells. The histogenesis of these tumors currently is controversial but most appear to demonstrate some primitive evidence of smooth muscle differentiation. Adenomas are of epithelial, not mesenchymal, origin; glomus tumors, lipomas, and granular cell tumors are distinctly uncommon in the stomach.

5. The answer is E *[Chapter 23 I G 1].*
The clinical history, physical examination, and radiographic findings of a polyostotic disorder characterized by abnormal bone formation are typical of Paget's disease, an idiopathic process. Hyperparathyroidism secondary to parathyroid adenoma, corticosteroid therapy, and vitamin deficiency can all lead to diminished bone density. These processes would be diffuse and would not be related to increased bone remodeling, with changes in skull thickness. Although acromegaly associated with a pituitary adenoma may present with an increase in head size, this disorder does not affect the bone density of long bones.

6. The answer is E *[Chapter 9 III D 2 a (1)–(2), 3 a–d].*
The patient's clinical presentation is typical for a massive transmural myocardial infarct (involving more than 40% of the left ventricular myocardium) that resulted in cardiogenic shock. Transmural infarcts are typically associated with coronary artery thrombosis, which may result from rupture of an atheromatous plaque.

7. The answer is B *[Chapter 15 VII B].*
Reye's syndrome is characterized by acute encephalopathy and hepatic dysfunction. Viral infection, particularly influenza A or B or varicella (chicken pox), appears to be the inciting event. Aspirin ingestion has been noted in more than 90% of cases and may act as a cofactor in the pathogenesis of this disorder. This histologic hallmark of Reye's syndrome is microvesicular steatosis, which can be confirmed by using oil red O on frozen sections to stain for neutral lipid. Necrosis and inflammation are absent. Electron microscopy reveals mitochondrial abnormalities in the brain and in hepatocytes. These mitochondrial defects may lead to impaired fatty acid oxidation and, thus, may be the primary defect in Reye's syndrome.

8. The answer is A *[Chapter 13 I D 2 a (3)].*
In Barrett's epithelium (also called Barrett's esophagus), columnar epithelium replaces the normal squamous epithelium of the distal esophagus as a result of metaplastic change. Chronic peptic ulcers may develop in the setting of Barrett's epithelium. Although the columnar mucosa may resemble either gastric

or intestinal mucosa, it is the intestinal, or "specialized," type that most frequently develops dysplastic changes. From 3% to 10% of patients with Barrett's epithelium have or subsequently develop esophageal adenocarcinoma.

9. The answer is E *[Chapter 4 VI B 1].*
Farmers may be exposed to the noxious fumes of nitrogen oxides when opening and filling a silo; these fumes cause acute pulmonary toxicity, resulting in pulmonary edema. Any chronic process, such as bronchitis, chronic silicosis (as opposed to acute silicosis), or a pneumoconiosis, cannot explain the acute presentation described. Likewise, hypersensitivity reactions may result in gradual dyspnea, but they usually do not produce pulmonary edema.

10. The answer is A *[Chapter 10 IV B].*
Glomangiomas (glomus tumors) are benign tumors composed of vascular channels in a connective tissue stroma surrounded by nests of glomus cells. These tumors arise from the glomus body, which is an arteriovenous shunt richly supplied with nerve fibers; the glomus body is important in temperature regulation. Glomangiomas are often found subungually and can be extremely painful.

11. The answer is B *[Chapter 15 IX A 2–3].*
The woman described presents with signs and symptoms indicative of primary biliary cirrhosis. The histologic features of this disease vary with the duration of the disease and may be variable throughout the liver. The initial insult is to the intermediate-sized bile ducts. A characteristic and nearly pathognomonic lesion is that of granulomatous destruction of these bile ducts (the so-called florid duct lesion). This destruction leads to loss of interlobular bile ducts and a proliferation of small ductules. A portal and periportal infiltrate of chronic inflammatory cells in this disorder can cause diagnostic confusion with the usual causes of chronic active hepatitis. The end stage is a biliary cirrhosis characterized by micronodules of hepatocytes that are surrounded by bands of fibrosis that contain virtually no bile ducts. Changes caused by chronic cholestasis are evident. In chronic hepatitis B, hepatocytes with a ground-glass cytoplasmic appearance often are seen; hepatitis B surface antigen (HBsAg) can be demonstrated in these cells by immunohistochemistry. Hepatitis B core antigen (HBc) also may be demonstrated in the liver of patients with chronic hepatitis B infection. Deposits of α_1-antitrypsin and hemosiderin are not found in this disorder.

12. The answer is C *[Chapter 6 IV D 2].*
Scleroderma is an autoimmune disease characterized by small-vessel destruction and fibrosis of the skin and multiple organs. Vessels often are damaged and sclerotic, with an accumulation of myxoid material in their walls. The microvasculature may also show fibroid necrosis in accelerated cases. The typical pathologic feature of the organs involved in scleroderma is a diffuse accumulation of new collagen. The pathogenesis is not clear; however, immune complex deposition is not a feature. Although edema and perivascular lymphoid infiltrates are seen early in diseased skin, these features are replaced by dense dermal sclerosis.

13. The answer is A *[Chapter 22 V D 1].*
Fine-needle aspiration would likely reveal pus. The physical findings of a warm fluctuant mass in this location are suggestive of a suppurative lesion of the parotid gland. The history of a young child with an illness predisposing to dehydration is a typical setting for acute suppurative parotitis. Viral parotitis, such as that seen in mumps, is usually bilateral, and when it is unilateral, it is not suppurative. Granulomatous parotitis also is not associated with pus formation. A primary malignancy of the parotid gland in an infant is extremely rare and would not typically present as a suppurative process.

14. The answer is D *[Chapter 14 I D 1].*
The clinical picture described is typical for acute acalculous cholecystitis; affected patients are often quite debilitated. The gallbladder demonstrates acute inflammation, ulceration, and necrosis. Diabetes mellitus, hypotension, sepsis, trauma, and arteritis are predisposing conditions. In patients with acquired immunodeficiency syndrome (AIDS), cytomegalovirus (CMV), *Cryptosporidium,* or both may precipitate acute acalculous cholecystitis. Perforation is much more likely to occur in acalculous disease as compared to acute calculous cholecystitis. Abdominal ultrasound is quite sensitive in detecting gallstones greater than 3 mm in diameter.

15. The answer is C *[Chapter 1 V B 2 b].*
Lung infiltrates are found in all the disorders, but only sarcoidosis, berylliosis, and tuberculosis cause granulomas. Apical pulmonary infiltrates and a history of being in a Third-World country are common in tuberculosis, which is recurring with increasing frequency in major cities in the United States.

16. The answer is C *[Chapter 13 VIII B].*
Acute nonspecific appendicitis primarily affects young adults and most commonly is caused by mural ischemia induced by impacted fecaliths. Although *Enterobius vermicularis* (pinworm) may be found in 3% of appendixes, it only rarely causes appendicitis. Histologically, acute appendicitis is characterized by mucosal ulceration and a variable degree of mural necrosis and neutrophilic infiltration. The concept of chronic appendicitis is controversial, with many investigators denying its existence. Leukocytosis often is present.

17. The answer is E *[Chapter 7 III C 6].*
The coronary arteries in cardiac allografts can show subintimal or mural accumulation of foam cells and lymphocytes. This inflammation combined with the accompanying fibrosis has been termed "accelerated atherosclerosis" because of its morphologic similarity to primary coronary atherosclerosis. Since this process may occur within months to years of engraftment, it is thought to be a manifestation of vascular rejection in the coronary arteries. Necrotizing, hemorrhagic, or granulomatous coronary artery disease in allografts is extremely uncommon.

18. The answer is D *[Chapter 14 I D 1 c (1)].*
Macroscopic examination usually shows the enlarged and discolored gallbladder, often with a surface exudate which is characteristic of acute cholecystitis. Fully 90% to 95% of cases of acute cholecystitis are associated with cholelithiasis, with women 1.5 times more likely to be affected than men. Ulceration, edema, and neutrophilic infiltrate are seen microscopically. Perforation occurs in 10% of cases and is more common in acute acalculous cholecystitis. The mortality rate, with free perforation, approaches 30%.

19. The answer is C *[Chapter 23 I H 3 a].*
When an osteogenic sarcoma (osteosarcoma) penetrates the bone cortex, it elevates the periosteum. This periosteal elevation usually produces an acute angle with the underlying remaining cortical bone, which is known as Codman's triangle. As a significant radiographic sign, Codman's triangle aids in the diagnosis of osteogenic sarcoma.

20–21. The answers are: 20-B, 21-D *[Chapter 19 III D].*
Fat necrosis in the breast can form a mass that simulates carcinoma clinically, with retraction of the overlying skin. The lesion is centered in the adipose tissue and does not include ductal dilatation, which occurs in duct ectasia. There is no malignant epithelial proliferation, which occurs in comedocarcinoma. Although macrophages are present in the chronic organizing phase of fat necrosis, granulomatous inflammation is not the primary etiology of fat necrosis. Adenosis refers to the proliferation of lobules and is not a primary feature of fat necrosis.

Fat necrosis of the breast is usually secondary to previous trauma. The injured lipocytes die, and the lipids undergo a degradative process known as saponification. The histologic correlate of this is cell ghosts with a homogeneous eosinophilic appearance to the cytoplasm. Secondary calcification and organization of necrotic tissue, with accumulation of macrophages and mononuclear cells, occur in the chronic phase of the process. Nulliparity, estrogen therapy, breast-feeding, and pulmonary tuberculosis are not directly associated with fat necrosis.

22. The answer is A *[Chapter 6 IV B].*
Systemic lupus erythematosis (SLE) is the prototype disease associated with immune complex deposition in multiple organs. This occurrence reflects polyclonal B-cell activation. Sjögren's syndrome, scleroderma, graft versus host (GVH) disease, and CREST (i.e., calcinosis, Raynaud's phenomenon, esophageal dysfunction, syndactyly, and telangiectasia) syndrome are not particularly associated with immune complex deposition.

23. The answer is C *[Chapter 24 VI C; VIII C].*
Numerous mitoses in a melanocytic lesion of an adult are almost always an indication of malignancy. The presence of multinucleated giant cells, nests of melanocytes deep in the dermis, and epidermal changes can be seen in both benign and malignant melanocytic lesions. The presence of nevus cells surrounding pilar units in an otherwise benign lesion is characteristic of a congenital nevus.

24. The answer is B *[Chapter 21 VI A 5 b; VIII A 3].*
Severe head trauma, as would be expected in this patient, leads to bruising of the brain against the skull. Cerebral edema ensues, with consequent caudal displacement of the midbrain and pons; transtentorial herniation then takes place. The latter results in stretching and tearing of brain stem arteries and veins,

producing parenchymal hemorrhages (Duret's hemorrhages). Although a ruptured aneurysm and an arteriovenous (AV) malformation could result in findings similar to Duret's lesion, these diagnoses would not apply in this instance. Neither a severed medulla oblongata nor a cerebral infarct would be expected findings.

25. The answer is B *[Chapter 12 IV A].*
The most common tumor of the anterior mediastinum is thymoma. The clinical history and physical findings are highly suggestive of myasthenia gravis, a condition that 30% to 45% of patients with thymoma develop. The histologic descriptions correspond to (A) squamous cell carcinoma (SCC), (B) thymoma, (C) Hodgkin's disease, (D) benign teratoma, and (E) malignant germ cell tumor.

26. The answer is C *[Chapter 15 III C 1].*
Dubin-Johnson syndrome is a form of chronic or intermittent jaundice, which is characterized by elevated serum levels of both conjugated and unconjugated bilirubin. Patients generally are asymptomatic. Hepatic excretion of conjugated bilirubin and other organic anions into the bile canaliculus is impaired. The black or gray hepatic discoloration is reflected microscopically by the presence of dark brown, melanin-like pigment in the hepatocyte cytoplasm, predominantly in zone 3. Electron microscopy demonstrates the lysosomal location of the pigment, whose origin and significance are unknown. Rotor's syndrome resembles the Dubin-Johnson syndrome but does not include hepatocyte discoloration. In Crigler-Najjar syndrome, both types I and II, and in Gilbert's syndrome, unconjugated hyperbilirubinemia is associated with a decrease or absence in the activity of the enzyme uridine diphosphate (UDP)-glucuronyl transferase. The liver in these conditions nearly always is histologically normal. Reye's syndrome is a disorder characterized by acute encephalopathy and hepatic dysfunction. Microvesicular steatosis is the characteristic microscopic feature.

27. The answer is D *[Chapter 7 IV B 2 a].*
Transplant recipients are at risk for a variety of opportunistic infections. Epstein-Barr virus (EBV) infection with posttransplant lymphoproliferative disorder (PTLD) is one such complication. In PTLD, the immunosuppressed host suffers from primary or reactivated infection. EBV exerts a proliferative pressure on the B cells. In the absence of regulatory T-cell control, B cells may expand and develop clonal populations (i.e., lymphoma).

28. The answer is A *[Chapter 13 I D 2 a].*
The presence of a red, velvety, distal esophagus that is characterized histologically by a columnar mucosa (particularly the intestinal or "specialized" type) is the hallmark of Barrett's esophagus. This disorder complicates reflux esophagitis in about 10% of patients. Progressive dysplasia of the columnar mucosa may result in the development of adenocarcinoma, which complicates 3% to 10% of cases. Surveillance biopsies are generally performed annually. If high-grade dysplasia or intramucosal carcinoma is found, esophagectomy may be considered for suitable surgical candidates. *Candida* esophagitis is characterized by the presence of yeasts and pseudohyphae, which often invade the esophageal squamous mucosa. Ganglion cells are present in normal numbers in Barrett's esophagus; they are decreased or absent in achalasia. Tracheoesophageal fistula (TEF) is not a complication of Barrett's esophagus, although a fistula could potentially complicate a Barrett's adenocarcinoma.

29–30. The answers are: 29-E *[Chapter 17 I B 2, E 1 d]*, **30-B** *[Chapter 17 I E 1 c].*
The clinical finding of a single testis in the scrotum is consistent with either monorchid (congenital absence of one testis) or cryptorchidism (undescended testis). The additional finding of an abdominal mass in this setting is highly suggestive of a germ cell tumor arising in a cryptorchid testis, since such gonads are normally atrophic and do not undergo hypertrophy. The most common germ cell tumor is seminoma, and the radiographic evidence of a solid mass is most consistent with such a diagnosis since teratomas usually have a cystic component. Prostate cancer is rare in young men, and adenomatoid tumors usually are small tumors of the epididymis.

The treatment of choice for seminoma is resection of the primary lesion followed by radiation therapy. The tumor is exquisitely sensitive to radiation. There is good prognosis for seminoma patients, with a 90%–98% 5-year survival rate. Prostate-specific antigen is a marker of prostate cancer and is not useful in the management of seminoma. Patients with seminoma in one testis have a 2% risk of having a second seminoma in the other testis.

31. The answer is C *[Chapter 8 I B; II A; Chapter 10 II B].*
It is necessary to assess deficiencies or excesses in clotting factors that could lead to increased coagulability; therefore, polycythemia (either primary or secondary) with associated vascular stasis must be

ruled out by a blood count. To rule out an underlying malignant tumor that can produce hypercoagu-lability (especially pancreatic cancer), abdominal computed tomography (CT) is very helpful. By taking a complete blood count (CBC), assessing the clotting factor, and taking an abdominal CT scan, the three most important underlying reasons for the patient's clinical problem are evaluated.

32. The answer is D *[Chapter 20 VI F 2 b].*
The most likely diagnosis is neuroblastoma. Because of the young age of the patient, pancreatic islet cell tumor can be virtually eliminated as a diagnosis. Neuroblastoma, which is the most common extracranial malignant solid tumor of infancy and childhood, frequently is characterized by calcification; Wilms' tu-mor, hepatoblastoma, and pancreatoblastoma do not reveal this feature. Pathologically, the presence of rosettes plus neurofibril formation is pathognomonic for neuroblastoma.

33. The answer is B *[Chapter 16 III A 3 b].*
A patient who presents with nausea and vomiting, oliguria, hematuria, hypertension, and elevated serum creatinine probably suffers from nephritis. Basic pathologic features of nephritis are glomerular prolif-eration and active inflammation. Cellular crescents are extracapillary glomerular proliferation in re-sponse to capillary loop rupture and spillage of plasma proteins into Bowman's space. The other choices are morphologic features associated with nephrotic syndrome [i.e., nodular glomerulosclerosis (diabe-tes), basement membrane spikes (membranous glomerulopathy), tissue congophilia (amyloid), diffuse podocyte effacement (minimal change disease)].

34. The answer is C *[Chapter 7 III A 4].*
Corticosteroids have a lympholytic effect and are good treatment for acute cellular rejection. Acute vas-cular rejection is less responsive to steroid therapy. Steroids have no effect on the renal toxicity of cy-closporine, the tubular damage of "harvest injury," or the fixed structural lesion of the recurrent glo-merulosclerosis.

35. The answer is B *[Chapter 15 IX C 3 b; Table 15-5].*
Wilson's disease represents an inborn error of copper metabolism, which leads to copper accumulation and injury to several organs, most notably the liver, brain, kidney, and eye. The responsible gene, which is located on chromosome 13, is inherited in an autosomal-recessive fashion. The precise excretory defect and the mechanism of copper-induced cellular injury are unknown. The clinical features are dominated by hepatic and neuropsychiatric manifestations as well as hemolytic anemia. Patients can present acutely, with fulminant hepatic failure, or, more commonly, with evidence of chronic hepatitis and cir-rhosis. Kayser-Fleischer rings represent rings of copper deposited in Descemet's membrane of the cornea at the periphery of the iris. They are found in all patients with central nervous system (CNS) involvement but are less frequent in patients without CNS effects. Occasionally, Kayser-Fleischer rings are seen in dis-orders associated with chronic cholestasis, such as primary biliary cirrhosis. Serum free copper, urine copper, and hepatic copper levels are all elevated, whereas the total serum copper and serum cerulo-plasmin levels nearly always are decreased.

36. The answer is D *[Chapter 2 II C 6].*
Numerous studies have shown that most pleural effusions contain adenocarcinoma cells when the ef-fusions are caused by malignant disease in patients without known cancer. Statistically, the usual primary sites for such tumors are the breast in women and the lung in men.

37. The answer is D *[Chapter 22 I C, D].*
Ulceration of the oral mucosa has several etiologies, with similar clinical presentations as shallow ulcers with loosely adherent fibrinopurulent debris. When infectious etiologies such as *Candida albicans* (mo-nilial stomatitis) have been ruled out, the term aphthous stomatitis is used. Leukoplakia will present as white patches on the oral mucosa, but these are not easily scraped away and do not cover ulcers. Both ranulas and epulides form small masses and do not present as ulcers.

38. The answer is B *[Chapter 15 IV B 2–3; Tables 15-1, 15-2].*
The hepatitis D virus (HDV; delta agent) requires the hepatitis B virus (HBV) to act as a helper within the hepatocyte in order to be able to assemble complete viral particles. The complete HDV particle consists of an outer coat of hepatitis B surface antigen (HBsAg) with the RNA core of HDV. HBV is the most com-mon cause of sporadic and fulminant hepatitis. Hepatitis C virus (HCV) is the most common cause of posttransfusion hepatitis. The genome of HBV is predominantly double-stranded DNA, not RNA. In chronic hepatitis B, the HBV genome may be in the episomal state, the integrated state, or both. Patients with acute hepatitis A do not develop chronic liver disease.

39. The answer is B *[Chapter 24 VII D].*
Kaposi's sarcoma, once uncommon, is increasing in incidence because it is one of the problems associated with acquired immune deficiency syndrome (AIDS). However, the AIDS virus does not cause the malignancy; no homology to the viral DNA has been found. In AIDS patients, Kaposi's sarcoma often causes small tumors of the mucous membranes or lymph nodes; these may occur without the more typical cutaneous lesions. Although Kaposi's sarcoma occurs in different clinical forms, the histology is always the same. The classic form of Kaposi's sarcoma is seen in elderly Eastern European Jews; over 90% of patients are men. Rarely, Kaposi's sarcoma develops in renal transplant patients receiving immunosuppressive therapy; stopping this therapy results in regression of the tumor.

40. The answer is E *[Chapter 22 V G 2 a].*
The most likely diagnosis in this young adult with a small, firm lesion but no symptoms is pleomorphic adenoma [also called benign mixed tumor (BMT)]. Warthin's tumor occurs primarily in older men and, therefore, is an unlikely diagnosis in this patient; the lack of associated systemic symptoms eliminates the suspicion of Sjögren's syndrome. The mass does not grow rapidly or become very large, and it is not associated with pain, all of which suggest that the mass is not a malignant mixed tumor (MMT). Similarly, the absence of pain removes the choice of sialolithiasis.

41. The answer is A *[Chapter 16 III A 2 b].*
The most common cause of nephrotic syndrome in children is minimal change disease. In this condition, nephrosis sometimes follows an immunization or infection. The only pathologic finding is diffuse foot process effacement, thus, the name "minimal change" disease.

42. The answer is E *[Chapter 8 I A 3 a–d].*
Iron deficiency anemia, chemotherapy-induced marrow injury, acute leukemia, and metastatic breast cancer are all possible explanations for the low blood values of the 60-year-old woman described. Without detailed peripheral smear morphology and further laboratory data, the diagnosis cannot be determined definitively. Elderly people may have nutritional deficiencies from a poor or inadequate diet; another possibility is gastrointestinal blood loss from an undefined condition (e.g., a cancer). Chemotherapy can depress and injure marrow, producing anemia; and, in some cases, the marrow injury may be prolonged. Cases of postchemotherapy acute leukemia also occur. Finally, metastatic tumors of the bone marrow can produce a marrow-replacement type of anemia.

43. The answer is B *[Chapter 3 V C 3].*
In most human cancers, the stage of the disease is the most important prognostic factor. Stage refers to the extent, or degree of spread, of the disease in the patient (i.e., localized, regional, or distant). Tumor grade (i.e., differentiation), mitotic count, and extent of invasion correlate with the stage of the tumor, in that higher-grade (i.e., less differentiated) tumors and highly invasive tumors tend to be higher-stage lesions.

44. The answer is D *[Chapter 13 II G 1 e].*
The majority of ovarian metastases from gastric adenocarcinoma are composed of signet-ring cells and, thus, conform to the definition of Krukenberg's tumor. Krukenberg's tumors usually are bilateral. By far the most common source for these tumors is the stomach; less commonly, they may disseminate from the colon, breast, appendix, or some other site. A Brenner tumor is a primary epithelial tumor of the ovary, which histologically resembles epithelium found in the urinary tract. A renal cell cancer sometimes is called a Grawitz's tumor. A Klatskin tumor is a bile duct cancer that arises at the junction of the left and right hepatic ducts. Wilms' tumor, also known as nephroblastoma, is a primitive renal tumor generally found in pediatric patients.

45. The answer is C *[Chapter 25 III D 4 a].*
Myxoid liposarcoma infiltrates locally and requires wide surgical excision for a good result. Hemipelvectomy would be the treatment of choice for the patient described, who has a recurring lesion of the upper thigh and inguinal region. Radiation and local excision would be ineffective. Chemotherapy also would not be useful, because myxoid liposarcomas are unlikely to have distant metastases and are not very chemosensitive. Lymphadenectomy would not be necessary since liposarcomas rarely, if ever, spread to nodes.

46. The answer is B *[Chapter 22 V B].*
Sialadenosis is associated with both malnutrition and alcoholism and is the most likely diagnosis. Sjögren's syndrome may present in the same manner, but the clinical setting favors sialadenosis; a biopsy would distinguish the two processes. It would be rare for sialolithiasis or pleomorphic adenoma to present as a simultaneous bilateral process.

47. The answer is D *[Chapter 10 II B].*
Deep venous thrombosis is a complication of surgery and bedrest. Thrombus material in the deep veins may dislodge and travel to the lungs as pulmonary emboli, causing hypoxia and shortness of breath.

48. The answer is C *[Chapter 21 VIII B 4 c].*
Because of their location, meningiomas are not always completely removed surgically and, therefore, may recur. For this reason, the completeness of removal at initial surgery is the most important prognostic feature in the case described. None of the histologic parameters (i.e., histologic subtype, mitotic index, tumor vascularity) are significant if surgery is not complete. The need for radiation therapy implies inadequacy of surgery and, thus, a poorer prognosis.

49. The answer is D *[Chapter 15 XIII A 3 a].*
The cavernous hemangioma is the most common primary hepatic tumor. These lesions usually are incidental findings at autopsy or laparotomy, or they are detected radiographically in the workup for some other unrelated disorder. Cavernous hemangiomas occur at all ages. When symptomatic, they most commonly are found in women who complain of abdominal pain. Rupture is distinctly uncommon; but when it occurs, it usually is in a giant cavernous hemangioma.

50. The answer is E *[Chapter 14 II B 2].*
An anomalous pancreaticobiliary ductal union is found in up to 90% of patients with choledochal cysts. The radiographic features described are typical of a choledochal cyst. The majority of patients present in the first year of life, although some patients do not present until adulthood. Eighty percent of patients are female. The pancreaticobiliary ductal union may allow reflux of pancreatic enzymes into the bile duct, which could weaken the duct wall, leading to the formation of the cyst. Carcinoma (usually adenocarcinoma) may develop within a choledochal cyst; however, usually this complication is not detected until adulthood.

51. The answer is D *[Chapter 4 VI C 6 b].*
In susceptible individuals, exposure to beryllium dust may cause an acute bronchopneumonia. These individuals may show a hypersensitive skin reaction, which is very characteristic of chronic berylliosis. Asbestosis does not present as bronchopneumonia but, rather, as interstitial disease. Steroid hormones rarely cause pulmonary problems unless long-term use has resulted in immunosuppression and pneumocystis pneumonia. However, if that situation had occurred, the patient would not be recovering on ordinary antibiotics, which were used in this case to cover bacterial infection. Cavitation is typical of tuberculosis, which causes small or large nodular granulomas on x-ray. Although coal miners may develop bronchopneumonia, the key factor in this case is the current work in a ceramic factory, where exposure to beryllium is known.

52. The answer is C *[Chapter 7 III A 2 b].*
About 15% of donor kidneys show changes related to preexisting damage prior to harvest. Atheroemboli are pathologically recognized as needlelike spaces within the microvasculature. Atheroembolism is associated with severe atheromatous plaque in the donor vasculature and invasive procedures such as catheterization or vascular surgery. "Primary nonfunction" in a renal allograft may be secondary to a variety of causes, however. Ischemic damage during harvest (i.e., "harvest injury") is most common. Preformed antibody directed against donor tissue can occasionally be missed during pretransplant cross-match testing and cause hyperacute rejection, but this situation is uncommon.

53–54. The answers are: 53-D, 54-E *[Chapter 18 II B 6 a, b].*
Hydatidiform moles are the abnormal villi from a pathologic ovum that can proliferate and enlarge to expand the uterus, and secrete human chorionic gonadotropin (hCG) in levels higher than those associated with a normal pregnancy. The levels of hCG in an ectopic pregnancy are normal, and the uterus is not abnormally enlarged. Placenta accreta is characterized by an abnormally invasive placenta, but it does not abnormally enlarge the uterus or secrete excess hCG. Leiomyomas may enlarge during pregnancy, leading to an unexpectedly large uterus, but do not elevate the hCG level. Chorioangioma is a benign vascular tumor of the placenta that does not appreciably increase its size or alter hCG secretion.
   Choriocarcinoma can follow a normal pregnancy or an abortion but is most commonly associated with previous or concomitant molar pregnancies. Choriocarcinoma can invade through the uterus into the surrounding structures or can metastasize to distant sites. Tubal rupture is associated with ectopic pregnancies and can cause life-threatening hemorrhage; it is not associated with intrauterine molar pregnancies. Pseudomyxoma peritonei is a complication of mucinous epithelial tumors of the ovary, mesothelium, and gastrointestinal tract. Endometrial polyps are usually found in the clinical setting of unopposed estrogen stimulation and are composed of benign endometrial glands and stroma.

55. The answer is C *[Chapter 16 III A 2 d (3)].*
The urinalysis suggests heavy protein loss, a retained ability to concentrate urine, and increased urinary fat (oval fat bodies). These findings are suggestive of nephrosis. Basement membrane spikes are found in membranous glomerulopathy, a leading cause of nephrotic syndrome in adults.

56. The answer is B *[Chapter 19 IV A 4 a; VI 2].*
Florid epithelial hyperplasia is associated with an increased risk of breast cancer; fibroadenomas (unless they contain epithelial hyperplasia) are not. A family history of breast cancer is a risk factor, but a history of gynecomastia is not. The patient's age of 37 years places her in a low-risk age-group. The low dose of radiation received, even after multiple mammographies, does not increase risk.

57. The answer is D *[Chapter 13 IV E 4 c, e].*
This patient's disorder is familial adenomatous polyposis (FAP), which is characterized by innumerable (more than 100) colorectal adenomas. Less frequently, adenomas are found in the small bowel (particularly the duodenum) and stomach. FAP gives strong support to the adenoma–carcinoma sequence of colorectal neoplasia. FAP is inherited as an autosomal dominant trait with genetic linkage to the long arm of chromosome 5 (5q). Adenomas usually occur in the second and third decades, with symptoms appearing one decade later. By the time the symptoms have occurred, roughly two-thirds of patients have developed colorectal carcinoma. Carcinoma only rarely occurs prior to the third decade. If colectomy is not performed prophylactically (usually by age 20), then virtually all patients eventually will develop adenocarcinoma. Adenocarcinoma may also occur at extracolonic sites.

58. The answer is B *[Chapter 22 I D 1].*
Gingival hyperplasia occurs predominantly in patients receiving phenytoin, which is frequently administered to epileptic patients. An epulis would present as a discrete lesion of the gingiva. Gingival hyperplasia is not associated with seizure-related trauma, nor is it idiopathically related to epilepsy.

59. The answer is A *[Chapter 5 IV B 2 f].*
In alcoholic patients, inadequate nutritional intake produces a lack of folate. Folate participates in DNA synthesis therefore, when it is available in insufficient quantities, cellular maturation is impaired. In hematopoietic cells, this deficiency is manifested by macrocytic (large) red cells and by hypersegmented nuclei in leukocytes (white cells).

60. The answer is C *[Chapter 22 II C 2].*
Of the four lesions, only angiofibroma would contain the vascular component that has led to the unfortunate complications of the biopsy. The characteristic color and consistency of the angiofibroma serve as a warning to distinguish it from the more common nasal polyp. A verrucous carcinoma, as its name implies, would not present as a smooth lesion.

61. The answer is C *[Chapter 2 III C 2 b (3) (b)].*
The most likely primary site for a metastatic lesion in an elderly man, as described in the question, is the prostate gland. Immunochemical localization of prostatic acid phosphatase (an enzyme that acts as a tumor marker) or prostate-specific antigen is the least invasive and least expensive technique for determining the site of such a tumor. The other choices—barium enema, laparotomy, computed tomography (CT), and electron microscopic (EM) examination—are less specific, more expensive, and more uncomfortable for the patient.

62. The answer is B *[Chapter 21 VIII B 6; Chapter 25 III B 5 b, D 3].*
Acoustic neuromas occur in middle-aged to elderly people, they affect women more often than men, and they are found commonly in patients with evidence of von Recklinghausen's disease (neurofibromatosis). Neurofibromatosis is characterized by the presence of multiple coffee-colored (café au lait) spots on the skin. Thus, acoustic neuroma is most likely in the 49-year-old woman who presents with pigmented macules of the axillary skin. The patient with type III multiple endocrine neoplasia (MEN) may have colonic ganglioneuromatosis, but he has no apparent increased chance of developing acoustic neuroma. The patient with melanoma (a tumor that is unrelated to neural lesions) would not have an increased propensity for a central nervous system (CNS) tumor. Neither radiation nor congenital abnormalities of other systems are associated with an increased frequency of acoustic neuroma.

63. The answer is C *[Chapter 4 V C 1; Chapter 14 VII].*
The most likely diagnosis of the child's condition is Reye's syndrome following aspirin therapy for a viral cold. For reasons yet unknown, Reye's syndrome has been linked to aspirin use in this situation. Typically, a child suddenly develops protracted vomiting and becomes comatose with signs of liver failure; liver

biopsy usually shows a microvesicular fatty change. Phenacetin in high doses may cause renal papillary necrosis, and Sterno (methyl alcohol) may cause blindness. Although questions relating to allergies and other drugs should always be asked, they are not helpful in this classic presentation.

64. The answer is B *[Chapter 6 V A 1].*
Bruton's (x-linked) agammaglobulinemia is associated with a defect in B-cell immunity that results in a decrease or an absence of circulating immunoglobulins. Of the B-cell immunodeficiency syndromes, only Bruton's agammaglobulinemia and common variable immunodeficiency are characterized by a paucity of plasma cells; in Bruton's agammaglobulinemia, there is a defect in B-cell maturation, so only pre-B cells are present.

65. The answer is B *[Chapter 23 II D 1].*
Approximately 75% of synovial sarcomas develop in the lower extremities. Synovial sarcoma is a malignant neoplasm of the synovial membrane and can occur in the joint synovium, tendons, or bursae. The tumor generally carries a poor prognosis, with fewer than 25% of patients surviving 5 years.

66. The answer is D *[Chapter 8 IV C 3 a, b; VI D 3; Figure 8-8].*
The patient described most likely has T-cell acute lymphocytic leukemia (ALL) or lymphoma with a thymic mass. Although he might have an associated infection, it is not the cause of his respiratory distress. Pleural effusion can occur but is unlikely to be present at the time of the initial diagnosis. Neither cardiomegaly nor diffuse pulmonary fibrosis is relevant to this case.

67–69. The answers are: 67-B *[Chapter 18 I C; II B 4],* **68-E** *[Chapter 18 I C; II B 4],* **69-E** *[Chapter 18 I C 3 c].*
The major differential diagnosis in a young woman with abdominal and pelvic pain includes ectopic pregnancy and pelvic inflammatory disease (PID). These disorders are not mutually exclusive and can occur simultaneously or sequentially. Although the finding of a purulent cervical discharge is most consistent with an infectious process, the presence of an intrauterine or extrauterine pregnancy should be ruled out by measuring serum human chorionic gonadotropin (hCG) levels. Although ultrasound and laparoscopy are useful adjuncts, there are several entities that present as adnexal masses that may not be differentiated by these techniques without knowing the patient's pregnancy status. An endometrial biopsy may not be useful in establishing the diagnosis of an ectopic pregnancy unless a hypersecretory endometrium is found.

Tuboovarian abscess, pyosalpinx, hydrosalpinx, and ectopic pregnancy can present as an enlargement of the fallopian tube, and all are potential sequelae of PID. The contents of a dilated fallopian tube (pus in abscesses and pyosalpinx, serous fluid in hydrosalpinx, and hemorrhage in ectopic pregnancy) suggest the diagnosis at gross examination of the organ, but the diagnosis of an ectopic pregnancy must be confirmed by the identification of chorionic villi, embryonic tissue, or both in histologic section. Malignant tumors are unusual in this age-group and very infrequently will present as primary adnexal masses. The clinical symptoms of fever, pain, and especially purulent vaginal discharge are not often associated with metastases to the ovary.

PID may obliterate the lumens of the fallopian tubes by adhesions and scar tissue, preventing the passage of eggs. Endometriosis, choriocarcinoma, eclampsia, and polycystic ovarian syndrome are not associated with the scarring that occurs in PID.

70–71. The answers are: 70-C *[Chapter 12 III B 2],* **71-D** *[Chapter 12 II B; III B].*
The findings of cyanosis and dilated veins confined to the head, neck, and anterior chest are highly suggestive of superior vena cava syndrome. A helpful clue is the finding of a superior mediastinal mass, which could be responsible for compression of the great vessels, which are also in this compartment. A paraneoplastic syndrome could not explain the vascular findings. The manifestations of heart failure and pulmonary obstruction would not be confined to the head and neck regions. Esophageal rupture, a process of the posterior mediastinum, would not affect the superior vena cava.

Enteric cysts are found in the posterior mediastinum, and, as the name implies, are cystic rather than solid lesions, although conceivably secondary abscess formation in a cyst could mimic a solid mass. Fungal infection granulomatous inflammation, idiopathic fibrosis, and malignant tumors all involve the anterior mediastinum and are more likely causes of this clinical presentation.

72–74. The answers are: 72-C *[Chapter 11 V A, B],* **73-B** *[Chapter 11 III A 2 b; V A 2 c],* **74-D** *[Chapter 11 III A, B].*
The history and clinical findings are consistent with a diagnosis of chronic obstructive pulmonary disease (COPD), with features of both emphysema and chronic bronchiolitis. Cigarette smoking is a chronic irritant that induces inflammation and also reduces antiproteolytic activity, leading to destruction of

pulmonary parenchyma. Cigarette smoke does not affect α_1-antitrypsin gene activity. The pulmonary basement membrane is usually increased in COPD, and desquamative interstitial pneumonitis is not a feature of the disease.

Secondary pulmonary hypertension can occur in COPD, and when it is severe, it can lead to right-sided heart failure (cor pulmonale). Pulmonary veno-occlusive disease and pulmonary thromboembolism can also cause cor pulmonale but are not specifically associated with COPD. Diffuse alveolar damage refers specifically to the hyaline membranes and type II pneumonocyte hyperplasia seen in acute respiratory distress syndromes. Bronchopulmonary dysplasia refers to the chronic sequelae of neonatal respiratory distress syndrome.

Expiratory wheezes heard in COPD patients are produced by narrowing of the airways, which is pronounced by airway collapse. Chronic bronchiolitis causes narrowing of the airways by edema and fibrosis; goblet cell hyperplasia contributes to airway narrowing by mucus secretion. The collapse of the airways by positive intrathoracic pressure during expiration is caused by the loss of lung elasticity found in emphysema due to the destruction of interalveolar septa. Anthracosis refers to the accumulation of carbon pigment within pulmonary macrophages and does not contribute to narrowing of the airways.

75–76. The answers are: 75-A *[Chapter 15 X A 2, B; XI B 1]*, **76-C** *[Chapter 15 XI B 2]*.
This patient most likely has cirrhosis related to infection by the hepatitis C virus (HCV), which she probably contracted through her prior blood transfusion. The patient's hepatitis A virus (HAV) serologies demonstrate prior infection, which is common in the adult population, but HAV does not cause chronic liver disease. Liver transplantation is a treatment option for some patients with end-stage liver disease, although recurrent HCV infection is common. Portal hypertension is a common clinical consequence of cirrhosis.

In most cases, ascites results from portal hypertension related to sinusoidal, postsinusoidal, or posthepatic vascular blockade. These forms of vascular blockade lead to increased hepatic lymph flow and weeping of lymph from the liver surface into the peritoneal cavity. Hypoalbuminemia and secondary hyperaldosteronism may contribute to ascites formation. Patients with hepatitis C virus (HCV)-related cirrhosis are at increased risk for development of hepatocellular carcinoma; this tumor may extensively invade the hepatic vein, leading to posthepatic blockade.

77. The answer is E *[Chapter 8 I A 3 a (1)]*.
Iron deficiency produces red cells that are smaller (microcytic) and paler (hypochromic) than normal, regardless of whether the deficiency is due to dietary inadequacy or other causes. In older patients, a gastrointestinal malignancy, such as a cecal adenocarcinoma, may go unnoticed (e.g., no obstruction) and present only as iron deficiency; it is, therefore, obligatory to assess patients with iron deficiency anemia for this possibility. Laboratory findings confirming iron deficiency are a low serum iron concentration and a high serum iron-binding capacity. (The protein transporting iron, transferrin, has little iron bound and, thus, has a high binding capacity.)

78. The answer is D *[Chapter 20 VI B, C, E 2]*.
Patients with Addison's disease often are hypotensive because of destruction of the adrenal cortex and, thus, mineralocorticoid (aldosterone) deficiency. Cushing's syndrome, which is caused by pituitary or adrenal lesions or by excessive glucocorticoid intake, results in hypertension. Conn's syndrome, which usually is produced by an adrenocortical adenoma, is associated with excessive production of aldosterone; the result is hypertension. Pheochromocytoma and adrenal medullary hyperplasia characteristically produce hypertension by excessive release of catecholamines.

79. The answer is A *[Chapter 7 III D 3 a (1)–(4), 4]*.
Obliterative bronchiolitis (OB) refers to a progressive fibrosing lesion of the membranous and respiratory bronchioles. This chronic change may be seen in rejection, but it can also be seen in infection, ischemia, or graft-versus-host (GVH) disease. The features of acute cellular rejection in the lung depend on the severity of the rejection process. In early rejection, lymphocytic inflammation is confined to the perivascular space. With increasing severity, the inflammation spills into the interstitium and alveolar spaces, and more neutrophils are seen. Severe rejection may have hemorrhage and necrosis accompanied by hyaline membrane formation.

80. The answer is D *[Chapter 10 I B 1]*.
Medial granulomas are not characteristic of atherosclerosis. Fatty streaks and atheromas (intimal plaques) are the classic lesions of artherosclerosis. When atheromas develop ulceration, calcification, thrombosis, intraplaque hemorrhage, or mild lymphocytic inflammation, they are referred to as "complicated plaques." Fatty streaks have been found in children, leading to the speculation that atherosclerosis may begin at a very early age.

81. The answer is A *[Chapter 24 II D].*
Intracytoplasmic inclusions are characteristic of viral infections and are not seen in psoriasis. The rate of epidermal turnover increases sevenfold in psoriasis, and the prominent dermal vascularity is the reason that these lesions bleed easily (Auspitz sign). Activation of the complement system by keratinocytes is the explanation for the epidermal neutrophilic infiltration. Arthritis often accompanies severe psoriatic skin disease.

82. The answer is B *[Chapter 9 III D 3 e].*
Aortic aneurysms are not a complication of acute myocardial infarction but usually are the results of atherosclerosis, various infectious agents, connective tissue abnormalities, or congenital defects. The complications of myocardial infarction are numerous and varied; some may occur within the first hour after the onset of infarction, whereas others may be delayed for months or longer after the acute event. A few (e.g., ventricular arrhythmia, cardiogenic shock, myocardial rupture) are extremely serious and represent common causes of death in patients with myocardial infarction.

83. The answer is D *[Chapter 6 V D 4].*
Acquired immune deficiency syndrome (AIDS) is characterized by a progressive deficiency in cell-mediated immunity. Most severely affected are the helper T cells—cells responsible for "helping" B cells and other T cells to respond appropriately to antigen. Depletion of the helper T-cell population leaves the host susceptible to a variety of infections (especially protozoal, fungal, mycobacterial, and viral) and to secondary malignancies. Resistance to bacterial infections most often is mediated through humoral mechanisms. Therefore, the incidence of pneumococcal pneumonia is not increased in AIDS patients.

84. The answer is B *[Chapter 17 III D 1, 2 b].*
Although chronic irritation by smegma is a postulated predisposing factor to squamous cell carcinoma, its presence during physical examination is not useful in distinguishing clinically between the lesions of condyloma and carcinoma. Ulceration and pain are attributes of carcinoma. The presence of inguinal and lung masses are suggestive of local and distant metastases of carcinoma.

85. The answer is C *[Chapter 1 VI A 1 b, 2 d, B 2].*
Tissues often repair themselves by granulation tissue formation, a process that eventually leads to fibrosis (scar tissue) replacing the defect left by the injury. Granulation tissue begins to form shortly after the onset of inflammation and is well established within 100 hours unless the patient has a malignancy or is malnourished, very old, diabetic, or infected. Granulation tissue does not imply granulomas, although foreign-body granulomas can form in the presence of sutures used to close a surgical wound (in which primary healing is occurring). Sometimes an open wound cannot be closed surgically and, so, undergoes secondary healing, with creation of a large irregular scar. If a person is susceptible, the scar can be excessive, leading to a keloid. Inflammation can lead to fistula formation (i.e., abnormal connection of two structures, often with connection to a lumen, as in an enterocutaneous or a rectovaginal fistula). The body usually cannot heal these structures, which are exposed to continuous insult from inflammation or infection, and surgery is needed to correct the problem.

86. The answer is D *[Chapter 10 I D 1 a–b, 2].*
Berry aneurysms are small saccular (balloon-shaped) aneurysms that most often are congenital and present in the smaller cerebral arteries. Fusiform aneurysms are spindle-shaped dilatations of an artery. Aneurysms secondary to atherosclerosis are the most common type and usually are located in the abdominal aorta below the origin of the renal arteries. Syphilitic aneurysms are relatively infrequent today because of the decrease in the incidence of tertiary syphilis. These aneurysms nearly always are confined to the ascending and transverse portions of the thoracic aorta. Cirsoid aneurysms are dilatations of arteriovenous fistulas.

87. The answer is B *[Chapter 25 III C 1].*
The patient described in the question with an irregular lesion of the palm of his hand has a classic presentation of the proliferative scarring process known as Dupuytren's contracture, a type of fibromatosis. Fibroblasts in collagen are seen with only rare mitoses. It is not a malignancy, although it is locally aggressive. Local recurrence rates are extremely high after surgery, which will be palliative, but probably not curative.

88. The answer is E *[Chapter 9 IV D 1].*
A floppy mitral valve is seen in mitral valve prolapse, but is not a component of hypertensive cardiac disease. Long-standing hypertension leads to serious end-organ effects, particularly involving the heart

and kidneys. The major morphologic changes seen in the heart include cardiomegaly, concentric hypertrophy of the left ventricle, and hypertrophied papillary muscles. Endocardial fibrous thickening may occasionally be present.

89. The answer is C *[Chapter 16 III A 2 e].*
Hematuria is not a prominent feature of diabetic glomerulosclerosis, a form of diabetic nephropathy. Diabetic glomerulosclerosis is characterized in its early stage by diffuse glomerular basement membrane (GBM) thickening. In later stages of diabetic glomerulosclerosis, intercapillary mesangial matrix expansion (diffuse diabetic glomerulosclerosis) eventually becomes nodular (nodular diabetic glomerulosclerosis). This expansion compromises the glomerular capillary lumens. Diabetic glomerulosclerosis is clinically associated with a sequence of microalbuminuria, proteinuria, and eventual renal failure. Diabetic glomerulosclerosis is always found in association with small vessel changes in other sites, such as occur in diabetic retinopathy.

90. The answer is A *[Chapter 10 II C].*
Varicose veins are dilated, tortuous veins often associated with valvular deformities and intraluminal thrombi. Varicose veins frequently are located in the lower extremities, but also may be found at the anorectal junction and in the esophagus in patients with portal hypertension induced by liver cirrhosis. Superficial varicose veins of the lower extremities often are associated with dystrophic tissue changes, stasis dermatitis, and skin ulceration, but not with cystic medial necrosis.

91. The answer is E *[Chapter 1 V B 2 b].*
A bacterial disease typically causes an abscess, which is a collection of neutrophils; a granuloma does not. Several infectious agents cause the distinctive morphologic pattern of inflammation known as granulomatous inflammation. The granulomas consist of nodules that are 1 to 2 mm in diameter and are composed of macrophages (histiocytes) that have been modified to be epithelioid in nature. These epithelioid histiocytes are surrounded by a mononuclear cell infiltrate, which typically is composed mainly of lymphocytes. Although tuberculosis is the classic example of an infectious granulomatous disease, a variety of other infectious disorders are characterized by granuloma formation, including cat-scratch disease, syphilis, certain fungal infections (e.g., histoplasmosis, coccidioidomycosis), and lymphogranuloma venereum. Sarcoidosis, a disease of unknown cause, is another example of a granulomatous inflammatory disorder; in contrast to the other three disorders, noncaseating or nonnecrotizing granulomas are formed in sarcoidosis.

92. The answer is E *[Chapter 8 V A].*
Hodgkin's disease almost never involves the gastrointestinal tract or the reproductive (pelvic) organs. However, Burkitt's lymphoma commonly involves the gastrointestinal tract, especially in children. In the patient described, the possibility of a smoldering periappendiceal abscess must be considered. Crohn's disease (CD) can produce inflammatory fibrous masses. Finally, ovarian germ cell tumors may occur in young girls and must be considered in the diagnosis of this patient.

93. The answer is C *[Chapter 22 V G 3 c].*
Unlike the majority of malignant neoplasms, adenoid cystic carcinoma has a good 5-year survival rate but a poor long-term one. The tumor has a high local recurrence rate and a propensity for nerve involvement. The lung is a common site of metastases.

94. The answer is B *(Chapter 2 IV A 1].*
An aneuploid result does not equate with malignancy. Although most aneuploid lesions are neoplastic, there are exceptions. Flow cytometry can be used to evaluate the nuclear details of a tumor and, in some cases, can provide significant prognostic information. The procedure does have limitations, however, and they are particularly important to know given the relative newness of DNA flow cytometry. A diploid result does not mean that a lesion is benign; diploid lesions may be benign or malignant reactive or neoplastic. A reactive and benign lesion, however, almost always is diploid.

95. The answer is E *[Chapter 25 III D 1 e, f].*
The grade of a sarcoma is a prognostic index based on the tumor's degree of differentiation; low-grade (more-differentiated) tumors tend to have a more indolent course than high-grade (highly mitotic) tumors. Stage also is a prognostic indicator, which is related to the grade of the sarcoma (stages I, II, and III) and to local involvement of bone or vessels and metastatic disease (stage IV). If other factors are equal, the larger a sarcoma, the less favorable the prognosis. Depth is another important factor; superficial tumors in the subcutaneous area carry a far more favorable prognosis than is associated with deep intramuscular tumors. Tumor duration indicates how long a neoplasm could be seen or felt as a lump before diagnosis but has nothing to do with prognosis.

96. The answer is B *[Chapter 4 II D 6; Table 4-1].*
Regular skin cancers [squamous cell carcinoma (SCC)] and melanoma are associated with prolonged exposure to the ultraviolet radiation of the sun. Postradiation therapy tumors may develop in a variety of sites, including the thyroid, soft tissues, or bone; the latter tumors are called sarcomas. However, internal organs, such as the ovary, liver, and kidney, are the least likely to be affected by natural or therapeutic radiation.

97. The answer is D *[Chapter 9 III D 3 b–d].*
Although ultrastructural (electron microscopic) changes can be seen during the first hour after an acute myocardial infarction, the first histologic evidence is seen at about 5 to 12 hours postinfarction (not 24 hours). These changes are characterized by coagulative necrosis, including cytoplasmic hyaline change and eosinophilia, loss of cross-striations, nuclear pyknosis, and karyorrhexis. Neutrophils marginate within capillaries, then exit into the parenchyma at about 24 hours. Another sign of acute myocardial infarction is a serum elevation of the MB isoenzyme of creatine kinase (CK) during the first 48 to 72 hours postinfarction. Most myocardial infarctions are transmural (i.e., they involve virtually the full thickness of the ventricular wall) and involve the left ventricle. Subendocardial (nontransmural) infarctions usually involve one-third to half the thickness of the ventricular wall and are circumferential.

98. The answer is D *[Chapter 16 III A 4 a].*
Lupus nephritis is a term used to describe a range of glomerular nephritides that can occur in systemic lupus erythematosus (SLE). Autoantibodies to a wide variety of antigens can be found in lupus nephritis; however, antibody to glomerular basement membrane (GBM) is distinctly unusual. About 50% to 80% of patients develop some degree of clinical evidence of renal change. The recognition of renal disease usually occurs within 2 years of the onset of systemic illness. The hallmark of lupus nephritis is the extensive glomerular immune complex deposition. A wide variety of histopathologic damage patterns correlate with the severity of the disease. Lupus nephritis is most common in women.

99. The answer is D *[Chapter 8 I A 2 d (1) (b)].*
In sickle cell anemia, leg ulcers and spleen infarction result from small vessel occlusion by sickled red cells. Cholelithiasis results from hemolysis and excessive bilirubin; this problem also occurs in patients with other congenital hemolytic disorders. Sickle cell patients are prone to develop a variety of infections; osteomyelitis, especially that caused by unusual organisms (*Salmonella*), is a very serious infection. Pancreatitis is associated with alcoholism, not sickle cell disease.

100. The answer is D *[Chapter 25 III D 3 a].*
Malignant fibrous histiocytoma (MFH) is a very common adult tumor, which almost always is deep and pleomorphic (with bizarre cells). The thigh is a typical site for this tumor; in fact, MFH is the most common tumor of the thigh in adults. Although the tumor is composed of fibroblasts and myofibroblasts, it is not referred to as a fibrosarcoma because it also has histiocyte-like cells. Fibrosarcoma is seen more often in children and is a nonpleomorphic (uniform) tumor.

101. The answer is E *[Chapter 4 II D].*
Cartilage and muscle tissue are relatively radioresistant. Body cells are affected by ionizing radiation in direct proportion to their rate of turnover and in inverse proportion to their degree of specialization. Thus, the cells of mature cartilage and muscle, which rarely divide, would be relatively less affected by irradiation than the cells of the bone marrow and lymphoid system, which have a high turnover rate. The other statements about radiation are correct.

102. The answer is E *[Chapter 7 III A 6].*
Active lymphocytic inflammation in tubules (so-called "tubulitis") is a feature of acute cellular rejection. Chronic rejection of the kidney is represented by sclerosing pathology. In the vessels, chronic rejection shows vascular sclerosis; in the interstitium, fibrosis and tubular atrophy; and in the glomerular compartment, glomerulosclerosis.

103. The answer is C *[Chapter 11 II C, E].*
Neither bronchopulmonary dysplasia nor congenital adenomatoid malformation is associated with anomalous vasculature, so arteriography is the least useful distinguishing test. Bronchopulmonary dysplasia is an acquired condition. Patients with bronchopulmonary dysplasia typically have a history of respiratory failure and were born prematurely. Although congenital adenomatoid malformation may occasionally present with respiratory distress in the newborn period, the localized cystic nature of the process would differ radiologically from the diffuse nature of bronchopulmonary dysplasia. As reviewed in the text, these two entities exhibit greatly different histologies.

104. The answer is C *[Chapter 3 II C 2].*
Oncogenes are specific DNA nucleotide sequences found in retroviruses (v-*oncs*) and in eukaryote cells (c-*oncs*). The viruses are thought to have acquired v-*oncs* from homologous c-*oncs* during integration into host cells. Oncogenes are thought to play a role in cell growth, since many v-*oncs* code for enzymes that seem to serve as growth factor receptors. Because c-*oncs* have been conserved in eukaryotes throughout evolution, they are presumed to have an important biologic role, perhaps in cell growth, cell differentiation, or both. Viral oncogenes are known to induce malignancies in animals. Although no oncogene is definitely known to produce cancer in humans, certain c-*oncs* are found in association with specific human malignancies, particularly in those also associated with chromosomal abnormalities (e.g., Burkitt's lymphoma).

105. The answer is E *[Chapter 10 I B 3].*
In arteriolosclerosis, no amyloid fibrils are found. Arteriolosclerosis refers to a process of intimal proliferation and sclerosis found in the walls of small arteries and arterioles. Two types of arteriolosclerosis have been described—hyaline arteriolosclerosis and hyperplastic arteriolosclerosis—both of which show a relationship with hypertension. Hyaline arteriolosclerosis also is common in diabetes. In the hyaline type of arteriolosclerosis, the material found is an insudate of plasma constituents into the arteriole wall. In hyperplastic arteriolosclerosis, concentric, laminated thickening of the arteriole wall often is accompanied by fibrin deposits and necrosis.

106. The answer is A *[Chapter 1 II E 2–4; Chapter 6 II B].*
Cells of the mononuclear phagocyte system (also known as the reticuloendothelial system) are widely distributed throughout the body and are named differently depending on location. These cells have a marked propensity for migration toward a site of injury, being stimulated to migrate by chemotatic factors. Cells of the mononuclear phagocyte system perform a variety of functions. They are important phagocytic cells; they process and present foreign antigens to T cells, they express class II major histocompatibility complex (MHC) antigens; and they produce a variety of substances that regulate the inflammatory process [e.g., interleukin-1 (IL-1); growth factors for fibroblasts, myeloid precursors, and endothelial cells; alpha-interferon (IFN-α)].

107. The answer is A *[Chapter 23 II B 2].*
The characteristic symmetric involvement of joints and the presence of rheumatoid factor (RF) are diagnostic of rheumatoid arthritis. Moreover, rheumatoid arthritis may overlap with the symptoms of other collagen-vascular disorders and display systemic symptoms such as fever, malaise, and serositis (including pericarditis). Amyloidosis is also associated with this disorder. The destruction of the joint space may cause fusion (ankylosis) of the affected bones. Urolithiasis is not associated with rheumatoid arthritis.

108. The answer is D *[Chapter 20 II B 1 c (2)].*
Basophil adenomas usually are quite small and do not destroy or replace the pituitary gland; they can, however, lead to pituitary hypersecretion of adrenocorticotropic hormone (ACTH) and, thus, to Cushing's syndrome. Conditions that can produce signs and symptoms of hypopituitarism include pituitary irradiation, pituitary infarction (as is characteristic of Sheehan's syndrome), and tumor replacement of the pituitary gland (by a chromophobe adenoma or breast cancer).

109. The answer is D *[Chapter 8 I A 2 a (2), d (2) (a), e (1), 3 b].*
Erythroid hyperplasia in the marrow signifies a functional marrow capable of reacting to a stimulus (anemia). Thus, erythroid hyperplasia is seen in most common causes of anemia, since these conditions have nonmarrow origins (hemorrhage and hemolysis). In hereditary spherocytosis, the marrow is quite capable of production, and the red cells are destroyed peripherally because of a membrane defect. In Hodgkin's disease, a rare patient may have anemia secondary to an autoantibody. However, in aplastic anemia, the marrow itself is incapable of production; thus, the marrow is nearly empty of cells—aplastic or hypoplastic.

110–111. The answers are: 110-D *[Chapter 9 V A],* **111-B** *[Chapter 9 V B 1].*
The patient's childhood condition was acute rheumatic fever, leading to chronic rheumatic heart disease in adult life. The incidence of rheumatic heart disease has decreased dramatically over the past several decades in the United States and Western Europe, although it continues to be a major cause of cardiac disease in developing countries. Rheumatic fever is a systemic, nonsuppurative inflammatory complication of untreated pharyngeal infection with group A β-hemolytic streptococci. A typical finding in patients with chronic rheumatic heart disease is that of thickened and deformed valve leaflets (as a result of fibrosis) and of fused commissures. Left atrial dilatation, as a result of severe mitral stenosis or insufficiency, may result. The Aschoff body is a classic histologic finding in rheumatic disease.

Streptococci, particularly the α-hemolytic (viridans) variety, account for 65% of cases of infective endocarditis occurring on native heart valves. Typically, the valves have been damaged by prior valve disease. Although rheumatic heart disease was previously the most common cause of the underlying valvular damage found in some cases of infective endocarditis, mitral valve prolapse currently is the most common predisposing valvular abnormality. Because this patient had mitral stenosis, her mitral valve is likely to be affected by the endocarditis. Septic emboli, which originate from the valvular vegetation, may lead to septic infarct in the brain, heart, kidneys, or spleen. The vegetations generally consist of fibrin, inflammatory cells, and the offending organism.

112. The answer is E *[Chapter 25 III A, B, D 1 f].*
Infiltration, although typically seen in sarcomas, is not sufficient evidence for a diagnosis of malignancy; infiltration also is very typical of the locally aggressive tumor fibromatosis. Benign tumors are encapsulated as a rule, both grossly and microscopically. However, the appearance of encapsulation can be seen in a sarcoma on gross examination (i.e., pseudocapsule), and invasion can be seen on microscopic examination. Necrosis in a lesion practically always signifies malignancy, and it is rarely present in a benign soft tissue tumor. Size cannot distinguish between a benign or malignant tumor, but it is very important prognostically once a sarcoma diagnosis is made. Patients with smaller tumors (< 5 cm) do better than patients with larger tumors. Patients with many sarcoma types have good 5-year survival rates and, thus, sarcomas do not necessarily have a very poor prognosis.

113. The answer is E *[Chapter 16 IV B 2].*
Renal cell carcinoma affects men twice as often as it affects women. The carcinoma presents with hematuria, pain, and flank mass. Renal cell carcinoma is one of the most frequently metastasizing tumors, with a major route of metastasis via the bloodstream. Lungs and brain are two of the favorite landing sites. Renal cell carcinoma most frequently affects men near the sixth decade.

114. The answer is C *[Chapter 8 VII A; Chapter 23 I H 3 d].*
Multiple myeloma is most frequently seen in patients between the sixth and eighth decades of life. It is a malignant tumor of the plasma cells growing in the marrow cavity of the bone. Thus, it is not a true primary tumor of bone. The tumor produces excessive amounts of immunoglobulins, which produce the abnormal serum protein electrophoresis.

115. The answer is C *[Chapter 10 I C 2 a].*
As a specific clinical entity, temporal arteritis derives its name from typical involvement of the branches of the carotid artery, in particular, the temporal artery. The symptoms and signs depend on which vessels are affected, but bitter taste sensation has not been reported. Visual disturbances, headache, and intermittent claudication of the jaw muscles often are reported. Low-grade fever is not necessarily a manifestation of involvement of a particular artery but, perhaps, is a reflection of the inflammatory disease process.

116. The answer is D *[Chapter 6 II A 1 a–c].*
T cells perform many important immunologic functions; however, T cells have the ability to recognize foreign antigens only after the antigens have been taken up, processed, and "presented" to them by macrophages. One set of T cells—helper T cells—promotes the activities of both T cells and B cells; another subset—suppressor T cells—suppresses T- and B-cell responses. T cells lyse target cells by direct contact. T cells also participate in the immune response through the production of lymphokines, such as interleukin-2 (IL-2).

117–119. The answers are: 117-D *[Chapter 23 I D],* **118-C** *[Chapter 23 I E 1],* **119-C** *[Chapter 23 I E 1].*
Hyperparathyroidism causes osteoclast activation, which leads to bone resorption and hypercalcemia. Excessive bone resorption may lead to pathologic fractures, and hypercalcemia may affect cardiac contractility. Proliferation of osteoclasts may be so prominent as to form benign tumors, usually found in the jaw (brown tumors).

Vitamin D deficiency in children causes rickets, which is characterized by malformation of bone resulting from decreased calcification. The swelling at sites of new bone formation is best seen at the osteochondral junctions of the rib (rachitic rosary). Deformities can be observed radiographically in every bone; however, rickets is best appreciated clinically as bowing of the tibia in children who are old enough to walk.

In adults, vitamin D deficiency does not present as bone deformities since the epiphyseal plates have closed. However, during normal bone remodeling, a decrease in normal bone calcification causes osteomalacia, with subsequent risk of pathologic bone fractures.

120–124. The answers are: 120-B *[Chapter 5 IV B 2 e (2) (b)]*, **121-D** *[Chapter 5 IV A 3 b (2)]*, **122-C** *[Chapter 5 IV B 3]*, **123-A** *[Chapter 5 IV A 2 a]*, **124-B** *[Chapter 5 IV B 2 e (2) (a)]*.
Subacute combined degeneration of the spinal cord is associated with deficiency of vitamin B_{12}. Both vitamin B_{12} deficiency and folic acid deficiency can result in megaloblastic anemia. The megaloblastic changes are seen in all cell lines of the bone marrow, but they are especially prominent in the red cell series. However, subacute combined degeneration of the spinal cord is seen only in vitamin B_{12} deficiency.
Rickets is the bone disease seen in children with a deficiency of vitamin D. Rickets is characterized by overgrowth of osteoid and the development of bone deformities as the child is growing. The similar bone condition in adults is osteomalacia.
Scurvy is a disease of vitamin C (ascorbic acid) deficiency. The resultant functional and structural abnormalities of connective tissue cause petechial hemorrhages and bleeding gums.
Xerophthalmia, which is associated with vitamin A deficiency, is a condition of extreme conjunctival dryness, leading occasionally to ulceration of the conjunctiva.

125–129. The answers are: 125-B *[Chapter 20 VI E 1 a (1) (a)]*, **126-D** *[Chapter 20 IV C]*, **127-E** *[Chapter 20 V C 2 c; Table 20-4]*, **128-A** *[Chapter 20 B 1 c]*, **129-C** *[Chapter 20 III B 8 c]*.
Autoimmune destruction of multiple endocrine glands can occur in a variety of combinations. Thyroiditis is common; Addison's disease (i.e., hypoadrenalism) is unusual. Sometimes, both of these disorders coexist in one patient (a condition referred to as Schmidt's syndrome), with pathologic and clinical evidence indicating an autoimmune etiology.
Polyendocrine neoplasia characterizes Wermer's syndrome, or multiple endocrine neoplasia (MEN) type I. Parathyroid abnormalities are prominent in MEN type I; pancreatic islet cell tumors (e.g., insulinoma) also are characteristic components of this syndrome.
Gastrointestinal ulcers are common in the duodenum and stomach and usually are solitary. If ulcers exist in several sites and in uncommon locations, a gastrin-producing tumor (usually of pancreatic islet cell origin) is likely; this condition is referred to as Zollinger-Ellison syndrome.
The presence of hypopituitarism in a woman shortly after pregnancy is termed Sheehan's syndrome. It is believed that pituitary gland infarction occurs because of shock resulting from excessive blood loss at delivery or because of thrombosis of the arteries that supply the pituitary, possibly as a result of coagulation abnormalities at term.
The association of medullary carcinoma of the thyroid gland with adrenal pheochromocytoma and parathyroid hyperplasia has been named Sipple's syndrome. This is a familial form of MEN syndrome.

130–134. The answers are: 130-B *[Chapter 15 XIII B 5 a]* **131-D** *[Chapter 16 V C 1 b]*, **132-A** *[Chapter 13 IV F 1 a (2)]*, **133-C** *[Chapter 4 VI C 5 b (2) (a)]*, **134-D** *[Chapter 11 VIII B 1 b]*.
An association between a very rare liver tumor (angiosarcoma) and occupational exposure to vinyl chloride has been established. The epidemiology is indicated by the unusual histology of the tumor.
Although furor raged over governmental studies showing the development of bladder cancer in animals fed large amounts of cyclamates, this association in man is far from clear. Factors that have been linked to urinary bladder cancers in humans include exposure to carcinogens contained in aniline dyes and cigarette smoke.
Epidemiologic studies from many areas of the world have indicated an association between diet and colonic neoplasia. One dietary agent implicated is fat; the incidence of colon cancer is high in countries in which the diet is rich in fat.
Asbestos exposure has been implicated in a variety of cancers, especially cancer of the lung. Mesothelioma, however, develops in a disproportionate number of individuals who have been exposed to asbestos. The rarity of mesothelioma in the general population supports a theory of "causative" association with asbestos.
The link between cigarette smoking and lung cancer (usually squamous and small cell types) is well established and is of major significance because the number of cigarette smokers is large.

135–139. The answers are: 135-D *[Chapter 1 II F 4 b]*, **136-A** *[Chapter 1 II E 3 a (1)]*, **137-E** *[Chapter 1 II F 4 a (2)]*, **138-C** *[Chapter 1 II F 3 a (2)]*, **139-B** *[Chapter 1 II F 2 b (1)]*.
The cells of the immune system represent an elaborate and highly specialized defense mechanism. When an antigen is encountered by these cells, a well-coordinated immune response follows, which may be humoral, cell-mediated, or both. The primary cells involved in the immune response are lymphocytes, of which there are two major types: T lymphocytes (T cells) and B lymphocytes (B cells). A third group of lymphocytes, termed null cells, divide into natural killer (NK) cells, killer (K) cells, and lymphocyte-activated killer (LAK) cells. Macrophages—in addition to their functions in the acute inflammatory response—also play an important role in the immune response.

Lysis of target cells that are antibody-dependent is the main function of K cells. In antibody-dependent cytotoxic reactions, the antibody (usually immunoglobulin G) binds to the Fc receptor on the K cell and to the antibody combining site on the target cell.

In the cell-mediated immune response to certain microorganisms (e.g., *Mycobacterium tuberculosis*), activated macrophages are the first cells to come in contact with the antigen. The macrophage ingests the organism and "processes" the antigen into a form recognizable to T cells. It then presents the antigen to T cells in conjunction with major histocompatibility complex (MHC) molecules on the macrophage surface. This activity is called antigen presentation.

NK cells, in contrast to K cells, kill target cells without an antibody signal. NK cells are capable of killing several tumor cell lines in vitro, and they do so without prior sensitization. NK cells attach to target cells via a receptor, in a process that does not require divalent calcium.

B cells—with stimulation by antigen, T cells, and other cells—differentiate into plasma cells. Plasma cells are responsible for the production of the five types of immunoglobulins; each plasma cell produces only one type of immunoglobulin.

Sensitized T cells produce and release a variety of soluble substances (called lymphokines) during immune reactions, particularly cell-mediated immune reactions and antibody responses. Lymphokines function in many ways to regulate and intensify the immune response. Interleukin-2 (IL-2) and interferon are examples of lymphokines.

140–144. The answers are: 140-D, 141-E, 142-A, 143-B, 144-C *[Chapter 25 III D 1 a; Table 25-1].*
The histologic pattern of most sarcomas recapitulates a particular type of mesenchymal tissue, and the tumors originally were named for such tissues. Thus, rhabdomyosarcoma is a sarcoma that recapitulates striated (skeletal) muscle; neurofibrosarcoma, nerve (Schwann) cells; angiosarcoma, blood vessels (endothelium); liposarcoma, fat cells (adipose tissue); and fibrosarcoma, fibrocytes (connective tissue). Although some authorities believe that most sarcomas arise from a totipotential mesenchymal stem cell, phenotypic fidelity (i.e., leiomyosarcoma remaining recognizable as such throughout a patient's course) would not be explained by that theory. Suffice it to say that the cell of origin or histogenesis of sarcomas is unclear and a subject of debate.

145–149. The answers are: 145-C, 146-A, 147-D, 148-E, 149-B *[Chapter 2 V C, D; Table 2-2].*
Ultrastructural analysis can help in the diagnosis of neoplastic diseases by disclosing information about the nature of a neoplasm and the cells of its origin. Electron microscopy (EM) can reveal a variety of changes at the cellular level, including changes in nuclei, junctional complexes, surface villi, granules, and interdigitating processes.

The diagnosis of melanomas can be aided by EM, which reveals characteristic elongated granules (premelanosomes). If the melanoma is undifferentiated (i.e., has inconspicuous pigment), diagnosis can be difficult.

Carcinoid tumors are low-grade neuroendocrine carcinomas that, like melanomas, have ultrastructural granules. In carcinoids, the granules are present in a dense core that can be recognized by EM.

Adenocarcinomas display microvilli, whereas the villi seen in mesotheliomas are quite long. The diagnostic ultrastructural finding in squamous cell cancers (SCCs) is the presence of abundant tonofilaments, which probably represent sheaves of cytokeratin filaments.

The skeletal muscle tumor rhabdomyosarcoma recapitulates the normal cell by exhibiting Z-bands on EM.

150–153. The answers are: 150-B *[Chapter 13 III C 3 d],* **151-A** *[Chapter 13 III C 3 c],* **152-E** *[Chapter 13 V B 3],* **153-C** *[Chapter 13 III C 3 a].*
Malabsorption of dietary nutrients can result from a defect at any step in digestion or in any of the organs involved in the digestive process. Several small bowel diseases can cause malabsorption.

Whipple's disease is a systemic disorder that causes mucosal damage and lymphatic obstruction. In this disorder, the lamina propria of the small bowel becomes glutted with foamy macrophages, and a periodic acid–Schiff (PAS) stain demonstrates numerous positively staining cytoplasmic granules. Electron microscopic examination reveals bacillary bodies in the cytoplasm (often within lysosomes) and in the extracellular space.

Recent molecular biologic studies suggest that the causative organism is an unusual actinomycete, provisionally named *Tropheryma whippelii*. AIDS patients infected with *Mycobacterium avium-intracellulare* may demonstrate similar foamy macrophages with PAS positivity in the small bowel, but the organisms also are acid-fast ("pseudo-Whipple's disease").

Disaccharidase deficiency is a collective term used for several malabsorptive states in which a disaccharide cannot be digested because of the absence of one or more enzymes that are localized to the brush border of the small bowel epithelium. Lactase deficiency is the most common of these disorders. Although the histologic appearance of the small bowel is normal, specific enzyme assays can identify the defect.

Crohn's disease (CD) is a chronic inflammatory and ulcerative disease that can cause malabsorption by mucosal damage or by multiple strictures with bowel overgrowth. Transmural chronic inflammation is the histologic hallmark of CD and often is accompanied by granulomas. Characteristic mucosal changes include ulcerations, cryptitis, and crypt abscesses.

Celiac disease results from an abnormal immune response to gliadin (a glycoprotein in gluten), with resultant damage to the epithelial cells lining the villi of the small bowel. The villi become atrophic (which produces the characteristic "flat biopsy"), and the crypts, in an attempt to produce more lining cells, become hyperplastic. Chronic inflammatory cell infiltration is seen in the lamina propria, with an increased number of intraepithelial lymphocytes.

154–158. The answers are: 154-C *[Chapter 8 IV B 2 b (1)]*, **155-A** *[Chapter 8 IV B 1]*, **156-E** *[Chapter 8 IV C 2]*, **157-B** *[Chapter 8 IV B 2 a (1)]*, **158-E** *[Chapter 8 IV C 2]*.
Acute promyelocytic leukemia is characterized by prominent primary cytoplasmic granules, as seen in normal promyelocytes. Due to granule release of a procoagulant factor with thromboplastin activity, 75% of patients either present with a significant bleeding diathesis or develop this condition during therapy.

Chronic myelogenous leukemia (CML) is a marrow-derived neoplasm composed principally of granulocytic cells in various stages of maturation. White blood cell counts (WBCs) usually are greater than 50,000/μl. The Philadelphia chromosome is present in the bone marrow in 90% of patients.

Chronic lymphocytic leukemia (CLL) is a lesion of the mature small lymphocyte and has a low proliferative rate. Fully 98% of cases are of B-cell origin. This common form of leukemia affects the elderly, who present with splenomegaly and symptoms related to anemia. Most patients present with a marked lymphocytosis (above 20,000/μl).

Acute myelogenous leukemia (AML) primarily affects adults and is preceded by a few days to weeks of weakness, bleeding, and fever. Physical examination shows petechiae, sternal tenderness, thickened gums, adenopathy, splenomegaly, and hepatomegaly. Untreated, this form of leukemia causes death in 1 to 3 months.

Erythroleukemia is a special subtype of AML in which the marrow shows vastly increased numbers of erythroid precursors in addition to the myeloblastic proliferation.

159–163. The answers are: 159-C *[Chapter 14 III C 1 d]*, **160-D** *[Chapter 14 III C 2 c (1)]*, **161-B** *[Chapter 14 III C 2 d (1)]*, **162-E** *[Chapter 14 III D 3 d (2)]*, **163-A** *[Chapter 14 III B 1 b]*.
Acute pancreatitis is characterized by edema, fat and parenchymal necrosis, and a neutrophilic infiltrate. Most cases are associated with alcoholism or impaction of a gallstone in a region of the ampulla of Vater. Proteases, elastases, and lipases cause enzymatic digestion of the pancreas.

Chronic pancreatitis is characterized by fibrosis and chronic inflammation. Ductal calcifications are a prominent finding in cases associated with chronic ethanol abuse (a form referred to as chronic calcifying pancreatitis).

Pancreatic pseudocyst may result from either acute or chronic pancreatitis. The pseudocyst is an encapsulated collection of amylase-rich fluid; the wall of the pseudocyst consists of fibroinflammatory tissue.

Nearly all pancreatic exocrine carcinomas are ductal in origin and are adenocarcinomas. Perineural invasion by the tumor often is quite conspicuous.

Annular pancreas is a congenital anomaly characterized by a ring of tissue from the head of the pancreas that encircles the descending portion of the duodenum. The resulting duodenal stenosis causes vomiting and failure to thrive.

164–168. The answers are: 164-A, 165-C, 166-B, 167-E, 168-D *[Chapter 24 I C]*.
Macule, papule, nodule, wheal, and vesicle are all terms that describe the lesions that are produced by various diseases of the skin. For example, tender red nodules, which are found in the pretibial skin surfaces, are the classic findings in erythema nodosum, an inflammatory disease of the skin and subcutaneous tissue. Molluscum contagiosum is a poxvirus infection characterized by flesh-colored, smooth papules of the skin. Macules varying from white to brown are seen in tinea versicolor—a yeast infection caused by *Pityrosporum orbiculare*. Wheals and vesicles characterize the various eruptions that may follow oral or parenteral administration of a drug.

169–172. The answers are: 169-E *[Chapter 9 VII C 1 a]*, **170-D** *[Chapter 9 III D 2 b]*, **171-B** *[Chapter 9 VI B]*, **172-C** *[Chapter 9 VII A]*.
Primary cardiac tumors are quite rare and are much less frequent than metastatic tumors to the heart. Atrial myxoma is the most frequent primary cardiac tumor in adults, whereas rhabdomyoma is most common in the pediatric age-group. Both are benign. Atrial myxoma, which is most commonly found in the left atrium, often causes a changing cardiac murmur and systemic emboli.

Angina pectoris is characterized by severe precordial or substernal chest pain of limited duration. Alone, stable angina may be associated with no discernible histologic changes in the myocardium. More commonly, angina patients examined at autopsy demonstrate foci of interstitial fibrosis or evidence of old myocardial infarction.

Tetralogy of Fallot is associated with a permanent right-to-left shunt due to the pulmonic outflow obstruction (usually subpulmonic) and associated ventricular septal defect. This disorder is fatal early in life unless surgical correction is performed. Coarctation of the aorta is not associated with a shunt.

Mitral valve prolapse is characterized by prolapse of one or both cusps of the mitral valve into the left atrium. The affected leaflets are redundant and often slightly thickened, causing mitral insufficiency.

173–177. The answers are: 173-C *[Chapter 21 VIII B 2]*, **174-A** *[Chapter 21 III B 6]*, **175-E** *[Chapter 21 VIII B 1 d]*, **176-B** *[Chapter 21 VIII B 10]*, **177-D** *[Chapter 21 VIII B 4]*.
Ependymoma is the most common central nervous system (CNS) tumor in young children, with the highest incidence at about age 3 to 4 years. Affected children characteristically present with papilledema and headache.

Progressive multifocal leukodystrophy is a rare progressive disorder that primarily occurs in adults with a debilitating illness, such as Hodgkin's disease. Multiple unusual neurologic abnormalities (e.g., hemiparesis, blindness, aphasia) reflect the predominant cerebral involvement.

Glioblastoma multiforme is a rapidly growing CNS lesion most commonly seen in men. The relatively rapid course (2 months) and severe neurologic symptoms described in the 52-year-old man are strongly indicative of this malignant lesion.

Lymphoma of the brain is an uncommon malignancy that may occur in immunocompromised patients. The history of renal transplantation in the 22-year-old patient with recent visual disturbances and left-sided weakness is suggestive of lymphoma.

Meningioma is a slow-growing tumor. The slowly progressive neurologic problems in the middle-aged woman are indicative of this tumor.

178–182. The answers are: 178-A *[Chapter 20 III B 8 a (1)]*, **179-C** *[Chapter 18 IV B 6 c (3)]*, **180-D** *[Chapter 8 VI C 5]*, **181-E** *[Chapter 18 VIII B 2]*, **182-B** *[Chapter 4 II D 1 a; Chapter 24 VIII C]*.
External irradiation to the neck (usually low dose) has been implicated in papillary thyroid cancer, although doses of radiation high enough to destroy the thyroid gland do not have this neoplastic effect. Most series have reported that the association of thyroid cancer and radiation is strongest when the radiation exposure occurred in childhood.

There are strong indications for a viral etiology of neoplasia. Epidemiologic, serologic, and biochemical evidence closely link cervical cancer and human papillomavirus (HPV). Another neoplastic–viral association is Burkitt's lymphoma and Epstein-Barr virus (EBV); although the evidence for the association is less strong than that for cervical cancer and papillomavirus, it is nonetheless intriguing.

Clear cell carcinoma of the vagina is a very rare tumor, and until recently it was virtually unheard of in young women. When a series of these tumors was diagnosed, epidemiologic evidence showed that the patients had been exposed in utero to diethylstilbestrol (DES), a synthetic estrogen.

Melanoma may be related to ultraviolet light, since epidemiologic studies indicate that the tumor is more common in areas of strong sunlight; it is almost epidemic in Australia.

183–187. The answers are: 183-E *[Chapter 14 II D 4 a]*, **184-D** *[Chapter 14 I F 1 a (1) (b)]*, **185-A** *[Chapter 14 I D 2 b (2) (b)]*, **186-B** *[Chapter 14 I D 2 b (2) (c)]*, **187-C** *[Chapter 14 I E]*.
Primary sclerosing cholangitis is a rare disorder associated with fibrotic strictures of the biliary tree. It most commonly involves both the extrahepatic and intrahepatic bile ducts. Patients usually are young males who also have ulcerative colitis. Some patients have other fibrosing disorders, such as retroperitoneal fibrosis and orbital inflammatory pseudotumors.

Cholesterol polyps are relatively common, small, innocuous lesions of the gallbladder. They are characterized histologically by polypoid elevation of the epithelium by an infiltrate of foamy, lipid-laden (cholesterol-rich) macrophages. When the foamy macrophages are diffusely distributed throughout the gallbladder mucosa, the term strawberry gallbladder often is used.

Chronic cholecystitis is characterized by mural thickening. Fibrosis and chronic inflammation are the histologic hallmarks of this disorder. Rokitansky-Aschoff sinuses are found in 90% of patients; these sinuses represent diverticulum-like herniations of the gallbladder epithelium into and beyond the muscular layer.

Porcelain gallbladder is the term used to describe mural calcification seen in patients with chronic cholecystitis. The radiopaque calcium can be seen in abnormal radiographs. Porcelain gallbladder is associated with an increased frequency of gallbladder carcinoma.

Hydrops (mucocele) of the gallbladder may result when a stone becomes impacted in the cystic duct. The gallbladder becomes distended by cloudy or mucoid fluid. Much less commonly, obstruction of the cystic duct by tumor can cause hydrops.

188–190. The answers are: 188-C *[Chapter 8 II C 3 b]*, **189-C** *[Chapter 8 II B 1]*, **190-A** *[Chapter 8 II B 2 a, c]*.

Hemophilia A, von Willebrand's disease, and vitamin K deficiency all are coagulation disorders that may result in bleeding; however, individuals with these coagulation defects must receive an injury before they bleed. Vitamin K deficiency can be identified by decreased serum levels of prothrombin and factors VII, IX, and X in combination with normal levels of factors V, VIII, and fibrinogen. Hemophilia is caused by defective or deficient factor VIII. Diagnosis of this x-linked disorder is made by the clinical picture, family pedigree, and factor VIII level in serum. von Willebrand's disease is characterized by defects of factor VIII and von Willebrand's factor, a glycoprotein synthesized by endothelial cells and megakaryocytes and released into the circulation. This latter factor aids in platelet adhesion to endothelium.

Index